# The
# Menopause
## Endocrinologic Basis and
## Management Options

# Dedication

This fifth edition is dedicated to the late Georgeanna Seegar Jones MD, who was a professor emerita of obstetrics and gynecology at Eastern Virginia Medical School, which houses the Jones Institute for Reproductive Medicine. She was a gynecological endocrinologist, who devoted years to improving infertility for women. In 1980, Dr Jones and her husband Howard W Jones Jr, MD, together created the first in vitro fertilization program in the United States.

She had been director of Johns Hopkins' Laboratory of Reproductive Physiology and initiated the hospital's gynecological endocrine clinics. Her interests included research on the hormonal changes in the perimenopause, which she described and defined in the first three editions of this textbook.

I am proud to have known her as my teacher, my colleague, and my friend.

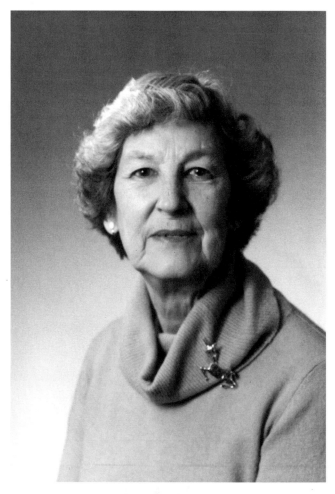

The photograph of Dr Georgeanna S Jones was kindly supplied by Dr Howard W Jones Jr, The Jones Institute for Reproductive Medicine, Norfolk, Virginia, USA.

# The
# Menopause
## Endocrinologic Basis and Management Options

### Fifth Edition

Bernard A Eskin MS MD

*Professor of Obstetrics and Gynecology;*
*Director of Menopause and Geripause Center;*
*Gynecology and Endocrinology*
*Drexel University College of Medicine*
*Philadelphia, PA, USA*

informa
healthcare

© 2007 Informa UK Ltd

Fourth edition published in the United Kingdom in 2000 by Parthenon Publishing Group
Fifth edition published in the United Kingdom in 2007 by Informa Healthcare, 4 Park Square, Milton Park, Abingdon, Oxon OX14 4RN. Informa Healthcare is a trading division of Informa UK Ltd. Registered Office: 37/41 Mortimer Street, London W1T 3JH. Registered in England and Wales number 1072954.

Tel: +44 (0)20 7017 6000
Fax: +44 (0)20 7017 6699
E-mail: info.medicine@tandf.co.uk
Website: www.informahealthcare.com

A CIP record for this book is available from the British Library.

Library of Congress Cataloging-in-Publication Data

Data available on application

ISBN-10: 1 84214 327 1
ISBN-13: 978 1 84214 327 8

Distributed in North and South America by
Taylor & Francis
6000 Broken Sound Parkway, NW, (Suite 300)
Boca Raton, FL 33487, USA

*Within Continental USA*
Tel: 1 (800) 272 7737; Fax: 1 (800) 374 3401

**Outside Continental USA**
Tel: (561) 994 0555; Fax: (561) 361 6018
Email: orders@crcpress.com

Distributed in the rest of the world by
Thomson Publishing Services
Cheriton House
North Way
Andover, Hampshire SP10 5BE, UK
Tel: +44 (0)1264 332424
Email: tps.tandfsalesorder@thomson.com

Composition by J&L Composition, Filey, North Yorkshire
Printed and bound in India by Replika Press Pvt Ltd

# Contents

# Contributors

**Mason C Andrews MD**
Professor of Obstetrics and Gynecology
Eastern Virginia Medical School
Department of Obstetrics and Gynecology
The Jones Institute for Reproductive Medicine
Norfolk, VA
USA

**Hugh RK Barber MD**
Lenox Hill Hospital
New York, NY;
Cornell College of Medicine
New York, NY
USA

**Rosemary Basson MD FRCP (UK)**
UBC Departments of Psychiatry and Obstetrics
and Gynecology;
Director, UBC Sexual Medicine Program
Vancouver General Hospital
Vancouver, BC
Canada

**Brian M Berger MD**
Division of Reproductive Endocrinology
Department of Obstetrics and Gynecology
Harvard Medical School;
Medical Director of Donor Egg and Gestational
Carrier Program
Boston IVF
Quincy, MA
USA

**Bhagu R Bhavnani MD**
Professor, Faculty of Medicine
Department of Obstetrics and Gynecology
University of Toronto;
Institute of Medical Sciences
St Michael's Hospital
Toronto, Ontario
Canada

**Ari D Brooks MD**
Associate Professor
Department of Surgery
Drexel University School of Medicine
Philadelphia, PA
USA

**William P Castelli MD**
Framingham Cardiovascular Institute;
Boston University School of Medicine
Boston, MA
USA

**Jane Cleary-Goldman MD**
Division of Maternal-Fetal Medicine
Department of Obstetrics and Gynecology
Columbia University
New York, NY
USA

**Karen L Dahlman PhD**
Department of Psychiatry
Mount Sinai School of Medicine
New York, NY
USA

**Mary D'Alton MD**
Chair, Department of Obstetrics and Gynecology
Columbia University
New York, NY
USA

**Nina S Davis MD FACS**
Associate Professor Urology/Urogynecology
Oregon Health and Science University;
Portland VA Medical Center
Portland, OR
USA

**Alan H DeCherney MD**
Chief, Reproductive Biology and Medicine
National Institutes of Health
Washington, DC
USA

**Edzard Ernst MD PhD FRCP FRCPEd**
Department of Complementary Medicine
Peninsula Medical School
Universities of Exeter and Plymouth
Exeter
UK

**Bernard A Eskin MS MD**
Professor of Obstetrics and Gynecology;
Director of Menopause and Geripause Center;
Gynecology and Endocrinology
Drexel University College of Medicine
Philadelphia, PA
USA

**Jesse J Hade**
Department of Obstetrics and Gynecology
UCLA School of Medicine
Los Angeles, CA
USA

**Lothar AJ Heinemann MD PhD DSc MSc**
Director
Center for Epidemiology and Health Research
Berlin
Germany

**Debra S Heller MD**
Professor of Pathology and Laboratory Medicine
and of Obstetrics, Gynecology and Women's
Health
UMDNJ-New Jersey Medical School
Newark, NJ
USA

**Lenora R Johnson MA CCC-A Audiology**
Associated Audiologic Consultants, Inc
Philadelphia, PA
USA

**Edward W Keels MA CCC-A Audiology**
Associated Audiologic Consultants, Inc
Philadelphia, PA
USA

**Kim Kelly PhD**
Department of Psychiatry
Mount Sinai School of Medicine
New York, NY
USA

**Laura E Post Kornegay MD**
Lexington Internists PC
Lexington, VA
USA

**Frank I Marlowe MD FACS**
Professor, Otolaryngology and Head & Neck
Surgery
Drexel University College of Medicine
Philadelphia, PA
Philadelphia College of Osteopathic Medicine
Philadelphia, PA
USA

**Martin A Martino MD**
Division of Gynecologic Oncology
Department of Obstetrics and Gynecology
Penn State College of Medicine;
Penn State Cancer Institute;
Minimally Invasive Surgery Center for
Gynecologic Oncology
Lehigh Valley Hospital
Allentown, PA
USA

**Donna Mueller PhD RD FADA LDN**
Department of Bioscience and Biotechnology
Drexel University
Philadelphia, PA
USA

**Parveen K Nagra MD**
Department of Ophthalmology
Drexel University School of Medicine
Philadelphia, PA
USA

**Miguel Paniagua MD**
Geriatric Research Education and Clinical Center
Research Service
Miami Veterans Affairs Medical Center
Geriatrics Institute and Division of Gerontology
and Geriatrics
Miller School of Medicine
University of Miami, Miami, FL
USA


**Honesto Poblete MD**
Department of Surgery
Drexel University School of Medicine
Philadelphia, PA
USA


**Hermann PG Schneider MD PhD**
Professor Emeritus
Department of Obstetrics and Gynecology
University of Münster
Münster
Germany


**Lee P Shulman MD**
Northwestern Memorial Hospital
Division of Reproductive Genetics
Department of Obstetrics and Gynecology;
Northwestern Ovarian Cancer Early Detection
Program
Feinberg School of Medicine
Northwestern University
Chicago, IL
USA


**Mona R Sutnick EdD RD**
2135 St. James Place
Philadelphia, PA
USA


**Bruce R Troen MD**
Geriatric Research Education and Clinical Center
Research Service
Miami Veterans Affairs Medical Center
Geriatrics Institute and Division of Gerontology
and Geriatrics
Miller School of Medicine
University of Miami
Miami, FL
USA


**Shira Varon MD**
Department of Obstetrics and Gynecology
George Washington University
Washington, DC
USA


**Ronald J Wapner MD**
Maternal-Fetal Medicine
Department of Obstetrics and Gynecology
Columbia University
New York, NY
USA

# Acknowledgements

As editor and author of this fifth edition of *The Menopause: Endocrinologic Basis and Management Options* textbook I would like to thank the many contributors to this update. We have all traveled the complex road of differentiating between aging and reproductive loss and have tried to share our observations with our readers.

On the physical and technical side my thanks go to our publisher and trouble-shooter Nick Dunton for his persistence and words of encouragement.

The copy editors, and especially Abigail Griffin, our senior editor, deserve much credit for their help publishing the book.

I particularly give a generous thank you to my wife, Lynn Eskin, for her help in collating, researching and computing, but especially coping with my absences to complete this update of all the new information since the last edition.

My best wishes to all who helped me.

# Foreword

The timing of the fifth edition of *The Menopause: Endocrinologic Basis and Management Options* couldn't be better. There are multiple factors contributing to its importance: the growth of our older population, scientific and pharmacologic advances in knowledge, new attitudes regarding the menopause, and confusion sowed by conflicting data and media reports. The role of the clinician has never been more essential in helping women deal with all of these issues.

Clinicians who interact with women at the time of the menopause have a wonderful opportunity and, at the same time, an important obligation. Medical involvement at this point in life offers women years of benefit from preventive health care. This is the opportunity that should be seized. Although it is logical to argue that health programs should be directed to the young because it makes sense to create good lifelong health behavior, the impact of teaching preventive care is even more observable and more tangible at middle age. The prospects of limited mortality and the morbidity of chronic diseases are now viewed with belief, understanding, and even fear during these older years. The chance of illness is higher, but the impact of preventive health care is greater.

In the 21st century, our focus will be on the prevention of disease and maintenance of function in old age. Our success will be measured by how well we perform not only as an individual patient's advocate, but how responsive we are to society and to the population of the world. Physicians will learn to be less of a rugged individualist and more responsive to new social obligations, more active as members of teams in our health care systems, hospitals, and organizations.

How are we going to do this? I believe there will be at least three important changes.

1. There will be a tremendous application of the technology of information. Of course, this new technology will be applied to medical education, but patient education and participation in decision-making will reach new high levels. Global health will be influenced by pervasive communication. All public health agencies in the world will be connected with each other.
2. Specialists and generalists will learn to work together as the health care system recognizes the clinician's role as patient's advocate and the need to provide and measure quality care.
3. We will increasingly use new measures of medical decision-making. Decisions today are being based on the results of clinical studies, not anecdotal experience. When I was a resident and a young faculty member, I didn't know what a confidence interval was and couldn't tell a case-control study from a cohort study. We are now teaching epidemiology, biostatistics, ethics, cost awareness, and outcome analysis.

Sometimes, young clinicians fear that medicine will be reduced to molecular biology. Very often, a patient comes to us because of symptoms generated by distress secondary to life's circumstances. Only the clinician who is sensitive to an individual's interactions with people and environment can help a patient identify the sources of distress and to deal with them. We will continue to practice people medicine, and therein lies the secret. The patient–clinician interaction is the feature of our lives that makes medicine special, interesting, and fun. If this were not so, the same disease would present in the same way in every patient, and it would be simple, non-challenging, and boring.

The menopause is a prime example of clinical decision making that is broadly based, including knowledge gained from books and journals and a clinician's personal experience, all uniquely modified by an understanding of each individual patient. Changes in menstrual function are not symbols of some ominous 'change'. There are good physiologic reasons for changing menstrual function, and understanding the physiology will do much to reinforce a healthy, normal attitude. Attitudes and expectations about the menopause are very important. It is important, therefore, that clinicians not only are familiar with the facts relative to the menopause but also have an appropriate attitude and philosophy regarding this period of life.

The menopause serves a useful purpose. The menopause should remind women and clinicians that this is a time for education. This physiologic event brings clinicians and patients together, providing the opportunity to enroll patients in a preventive health care program. Contrary to popular opinion, the menopause is not a signal of impending decline, but rather a wonderful phenomenon that can signal the start of something positive, a good health program. Rather than being a lightning rod for social and personal problems, the menopause can be a signal for the future.

This book, edited by Bernard Eskin, is unique in its broad spectrum, covering the physiology and pathology commonly encountered in older women. Mastering its content will enhance the ability of clinicians in the 21st century to meet the current challenges in helping women to be educated regarding this time in their lives and to maximize the quality and length of each individual lifespan.

*Leon Speroff MD*
*Department of Obstetrics and Gynecology, Oregon*
*Health Sciences University, Portland, OR, USA*

# Preface

This fifth edition of *The Menopause: Endocrinologic Basis and Management Options* provides a new and upbeat approach for the overall care of the late reproductive woman. Women have advanced impressively during the last fifty years in politics, professions and business. This change in status brings with it the desire to overcome those obstacles that midlife reproductive and hormonal changes may present. It is then a responsible demand that research should be expanded to allow women to continue to succeed in their respective roles by overcoming barriers caused by menopausal problems. The textbook is divided into four major sections: Aging and the Menopause, Endocrinology of the Menopause, Clinical Problems in the Menopause, and Treatment of the Menopausal Woman. Each section is subdivided into a number of chapters that elaborate on the major entities involved.

Women begin to feel older – well before they should – because of the onset of menstrual-affiliated symptoms that occur because of reproductive dysfunctions. The menopause transitions may begin prematurely as early as her mid-thirties. Hormonal modifications occur due to declining ovum maturation and reduced sex steroid metabolism in the ovaries. As a result, there is reduced estrogen available for target tissues. Estrogen receptor inhibition further lessens the hormonal functions in the pudenda, skin, hair, breasts, and probably, bone. In this time frame decreasing sexual desire, unexplained mood changes, and irregular hot flashes may occur. These clinical events intensify the anxieties of aging in these young women already worried by persistent media and commercial advice.

Factually, women are encumbered with the actual menopause at a time when the effects of anatomic aging begin to be more apparent. This textbook endeavors to separate the acute symptomatology of hormonal transition at menopause from the chronic problems of aging. This is a difficult task since sex hormone secretions and target cellular responses require normal functioning tissues, and these may have become depleted or distorted with aging. Reproduction is gradually lost in the menopause because of gonadal atrophy, while other highly fundamental processes seem only minimally reduced. In the male, generally with gonadal survival, reproductive loss is gradual and may not be totally withdrawn throughout life. However, the other aging processes seem to diminish similarly in both men and women.

In the menopause, estrogen deficiency appears as the responsible cause of the many undesirable conditions that have been described, thus, estrogen replacement seems reasonable. Many other endocrine tissues also suffer secretory loss, which is adequately, but carefully replaced with desirable results. Unrestricted estrogen replacement, given in high and variable doses, modified by added progesterone (for uterine protection) were used commonly. Presumably, these therapies provided reduced menopausal symptomatology; however, in recent large trials and studies they produced side-effects, contraindications, and complications as well. These undesirable findings were considered to be in greater numbers than could be justified for a medication for non-critical symptomatic improvement. Thus, estrogen therapy needs to be contained and limited to be successful. The individualization of the use of these medications to patients with serious difficulties has been suggested. Newer treatment methods that are being discovered and used in recent trials are described in the text. The increase in available lower doses of approved medication provides the observant therapist with an acceptable dose-response fine-tuning result. Added to the therapeutics is the rigorous use of early prophylactic tactics and increased personal self-help maintenance.

Along with these changes, currently there is increased longevity, particularly in women, due to the availability of effective general medical prophylaxis and treatment. The most rapidly increasing age segment is those women over 85 years of age. With this prolongation of the life span, the 'pursuit of happiness' or quality of life (QOL) becomes the eminent factor. While these remain vague entities and are remarkably individual, the physician can help in many ways to make the desired improvements partially attainable.

This textbook describes the changes in a woman's survivance from the early premeno-pausal transitions through the late geripause. As with the first four editions, it is meant to serve as an accurate reference and a current resource. This includes the medical, physiologic, biochemical, pharmacologic, sexual, endocrine, and now, sensory results of aging and sex hormonal loss.

We have endeavored to redefine aging and hormonal loss further and introduced the care and outcomes that may currently satisfy the expectations of the healthy, maturing women of today.

*Bernard A Eskin*

# Section I

# Aging and the menopause

# Chapter 1

# The menopause and aging

Bernard A Eskin

## INTRODUCTION

The menopause has been reconceived in the 21st century. Particularly, recognition of genetic and genomic conditioning as a major influence has evolved to explain the potential timing and severity of the transitions. These basic stimulators work on both the endocrine system and the aging process. The direct action and influence of these characteristics are discussed in Chapter 4. Section I will deal with the aging phenomenon and how it influences the many transitions and final domain of the menopause.

Essentially, aging in women occurs in both reproductive (germ) and somatic cells. Reproductive aging is an aggregate of many factors. The effectiveness of the entire endocrine system, including the gonads, deteriorates as a result of systemic aging. In the chapters that follow, the anatomical and endocrine decline that occurs during the years of transition, pre- and postmenopause, and geripause (late postmenopause) are presented. These modifications are the results of the progressive aging within tissues, the reduced ability of cells to respond to stimulus, and modifications of the intrinsic factors that activate cells.

The philosophical debate continues concerning the etiology of reproductive aging. Is aging the result of target organ degeneration with tissue loss or regression of neurotransmission from the central nervous system? From the most recent data it becomes apparent that these conditions coexist. In women, the obvious losses of first, reproduction, and later, menses are results of many biological and chemical temporal changes brought about by aging.

Why aging occurs remains unknown and its course still unalterable. Most research had been directed towards describing the anatomical and physiological changes; however, manipulations of the genetic code provides a vestige of penetration into this mystery. The recent gene insertion for the protein component of telomerases in senescent human cells re-extends their telomerases to lengths typical of young cells.[1] Intracellular and molecular biological techniques have brought new insight by describing the biochemical alterations of growth and metabolism seen in the elderly. From these observations, many new hypotheses have evolved, mostly generated by animal research. The accelerated interest shown since the turn of the century is the result of an increased visibility of the aged segment of our population, and their spiraling social and economic impact.

The need for improving the quality of life for postmenopausal women has become a serious matter in medical care (Chapter 7).[2] Longevity has naturally improved, and with it, quality of life has become considerably more important. Of note has been the entrance of many human 'old age' illnesses requiring intense clinical research and care. The 'baby boomer' generation is now over 60 years of age, with new demands. The scientific promise of a 100 plus age carries with it the demands for parallel quality years.

Regardless of the fact that much has been written concerning the aging processes related to biological reproduction, the relevant questions in correlating aging and menopause remain the same. These are:

1. does menopause affect life expectancy?
2. does aging cause reproductive failure and menopause?
3. is the rate of cellular senescence increased with reproductive senescence?

Practically, clinical problems that must be considered are:

4. is cellular deterioration due to lack of estrogen?
5. do the available replacement therapies prevent any sequelae of aging?

These questions are considered and discussed throughout this book. In this chapter, the direct questions relating to the aging phenomenon are addressed in light of both knowledge and hypotheses that continue to accrue. After a general review of the basic theories of aging, specific information concerning aging and reproduction is presented. The readers are then asked to judge our conclusions and form their own.

## GENERAL THEORIES OF AGING

Molecular chemical research and genetic expression experience of intracellular changes caused by aging have led to several theories (Table 1).[3-5] These theories recognize a series of events within the cell which prevent the orderly processes of growth and metabolism, and remain formidable despite recent knowledge. No single theory for human aging satisfies totally all the biological phenomena that occur. This categorization of theories continues.

### Genetic

The 'genetically determined' theories consider biological life to have a predetermined longevity and perhaps quality of living owing to persistence of the individual genetic code. Genetic expression, therefore, is a result of preformed biological conditioning provided by a preconceived template.[6] This hypothesis has remained extant over many decades because of results obtained from epidemiological statistics by life insurance actuaries,

intraspecies records and longevity data for identical versus non-identical twins.[7] Computer-tabulated research indicates that the primary basis for longevity of an individual strain, or a species, appears to be the sum of the genetic material incorporated in the fertilized egg at the climactic moment when the spermatozoon meets the unfertilized egg.

### Stem cell depletion

The regenerative power of stem cells has raised issues about their relation to aging.[8] There appears to be an implicit two-fold question: (1) does functional depletion of stem cells affect the accumulation of aging-related deficits, and (2) can activation of stem cells alleviate deficits? These authors provide two types of systems: (1) the remarkably depleted pool of ovarian follicles, and (2) the reserve hematopoietic stem cells.[8] It is essential to this text that loss of follicles leads to menopause. This certainly provides an additional potential for intervention into the aging agenda (Chapter 4).

### Programming

Within the cell there are biochemical factors that occur genetically, which have been chemically pre-programmed. Evidence of the DNA code biochemically visualizes this theory. This concept provides a mechanism by which the genetic theory can function. Stepwise changes occur within these cells, leading to degeneration within the cytosol or nuclear materials on a pretimed basis. Although not universally true, this thesis is more widely applicable than most others. Concurrently, this theory provides opportunities for treatment with optimism for the reversal of some aging conditions. Early results show that mechanisms may evolve which inhibit or modify the genetic signals that cause health hazards.

### Somatic mutations

The mutation theory refers to environmental insults, i.e. extrinsic effects on the cells in the body. Practicably, examples might be the results of laser, radiation, medication or normal biological reactions. This theory seems compatible with other approaches to aging, as most species are vulnerable to fairly random molecular events. The nature of the mutation is influenced by the factors that

| Table 1.1 | Theories of cellular aging |
|---|---|
| 1. | Genetic |
| 2. | Stem cell depletion |
| 3. | Programmed aging |
| 4. | Mutation theory |
| 5. | Autoimmune |
| 6. | Cross-linkages |
| 7. | Extracellular factors |
| 8. | Combination |

affect cell function. This theory is applicable particularly to reproductive tissues, such as in the ovary, where serious alterations could result in the transmission of mutations to succeeding generations. Cloning provides evidence, to date in animals, that all cells are transmissible and, thus, liable to extreme manipulation. A concept that appears viable is that cloned anlage that has aged maintains the level of cellular disintegration garnered from these older tissues. Since the female gamete is present from birth, arrested in the first meiotic division, irreparable modifications may occur by environmental damage.

## Autoimmune

Autoimmune protection is reduced or lost with aging. The immune factors circulating throughout the body can then overwhelm the individual cells, causing cellular destruction. In addition to the autoimmune loss, there is a marked decline with aging in both availability and activity of the total immune systems. Thus, there is a decrease in defense against infections, immune complex diseases and carcinogenesis, all of which contributes further to an acceleration of the intracellular aging processes. The potential effect of the loss of cellular resistance to the immune system has become an important condition. In the geripause age, a new series of heretofore casual diseases may become more threatening. Upon losing immunological safeguards, the affected cells are destroyed or modified by infiltration by the lymphatics and circulating lymphatic cells.

## Cross-links

The cross-linkage theory deals with a complex series of biochemical events that can inhibit the function of the cells throughout the aging process. There is evidence that some molecules present in the cytoplasm of old tissue cells comprise atypical or transformed components of DNA, RNA and peptides, covalently bound together. This reflects age-dependent deterioration of molecules with possible loss of continuity or bonding weakened by age. Tissues could lose differentiation by that mechanism, with possible reduction in function.

One concept postulates that aging is a specific biological function which promotes the progressive evolution of sexually reproducing species. Like any other important function, aging is mediated by several molecular mechanisms working simultaneously. Three such mechanisms have been postulated to date:

1. Telomere shortening due to suppression of telomerase at early stages of embryogenesis
2. Age-related mechanisms that induce the synthesis of heat shock proteins in response to denaturing stimuli
3. Incomplete suppression of the generation and scavenging of reactive oxygen species (ROS).

None of these phenomena can kill the organism, but only weaken it, which becomes crucial under extreme conditions.[9]

## Extracellular factors

The impact of extracellular factors upon cellular performance is impressive. Extrinsic as well as intrinsic factors contribute to organizational decline during aging. Most apparent is a condition which disturbs the cells by changing the proper sequence of biochemical events, such as incorrect neurogenic or trophic stimulation. Transport mechanisms as well as membrane energy and chemistry reactions could be restricted. When aging affects enzyme systems, for example, an inappropriate reaction occurs which disturbs the entire cell.

## Combination theories

These hypotheses can be combined to satisfy the individual conditions. Within the cell molecular physiology, aging could affect a series of disruptions which radically prevent outside stimuli from reacting in an expected manner. The cell response may not only be diminished, but if it is effectual, it may result in developmental 'errors'. Therefore, this leads to intracellular disease states, such as seen in histological dysplasias and neoplasias, and tissue and organ degradation.

Medawar,[10] as quoted by Strehler,[3] described aging as the result of genetic and stochastic processes. The latter represents the accumulated sum of the effects of recent stress, injury or infection. These are environmental in origin and thus, in a paradoxically technical sense, the effects of 'nature'. While we have added many scientific data to these general theories in the subsequent century, the basis of aging remains 'genetic versus environmental'!

## ALTERATIONS IN AGING IN ALL ENDOCRINE TISSUES

The theories of aging described pertain to intracellular changes seen in all elements of the body, although many investigators consider them to be appropriate only to those tissues we associate with clinical aging, i.e. skin, neurological and vascular tissues, muscle, and bone. Anatomical and physiological modifications caused by the aging process have been established in these specific areas.

The endocrine system is unique in that, besides obvious losses of tissue growth and metabolism, secretory activity may be inhibited, modified or even completely reversed by the aging process. Secretions generally required for normal physiological function of other parts of the body may be lost.[11] Particularly applicable is a reduction in muscle strength, which leads to frailty.[12]

A series of histological modifications that are not unique occurs in the endocrine glands as a result of aging.[11] Connective tissue increases in the gland capsule, and connective tissue elements replace secretory cells. In the endocrine cell, mitotic rate decreases and fragmentation of mitochondria and nuclear damage often appear.

Thus, alterations in the endocrine tissues with aging relate to both secretory and target organ functions.[13] The changes are:

1. primary loss of functional tissue by hypoplastic or atrophic changes in secreting cells
2. decrease in secretory rate as a result of these cellular changes
3. decrease of metabolic clearance of hormones produced
4. decrease in end-organ response to hormone stimulation.

## MENOPAUSE AND LONGEVITY

There have been several research programs which compare longevity after menopause in the woman with that in other mammalian females.[14–17]

Women live the longest after menopause relative to their total life span, when compared with all other mammals. During the 20th century, longevity for women has increased two-fold. Maximum reproductive age has been unaffected by this increased life expectancy.[18] More than 33% of a woman's life remains after the cessation of menses; conversely, in the monkey, the mouse, the

rat and other mammals, unless genetically altered this period is short, usually 10–15% (Figure 1.1) of life span.[17] The reproductive span in one strain of mice (CBA) has been genetically reduced, compared with other mouse strains.[19] In these mice the total life span was unchanged; only the percentage of time in the postcyclic period was increased (47%). These data provide evidence that the life span is unassociated with postreproductive percentiles (Figure 1.1). Interestingly, a review from medieval times until early this century showed that the effects of senescence rarely became a consideration, because of the short life span seen in women in those eras.[16,20] Considerably more astounding is the promulgation of research seen in *Drosophila melanogaster* which promoted the 'disposable SOMA' theory: that longevity requires investments in somatic maintenance which reduce the resources available for reproduction. A recent series of statistical historical studies has indicated that a trade-off existed.[21]

The four representative periods of the life span in all females were defined as prepuberty, regular reproductive cyclic activity, irregular cyclic activity and postmenopausal or senile anestrous phase (geripause).[17,22] Clinically, these have been defined more elaborately as prepuberty, puberty, active reproductive, decelerating reproductive, perimenopause (premenopause) and postmenopause.[23] A statistical analysis of these phases has been compiled to ascertain the relative proportions of the life span of each, using actuarial longevity projections.

Conclusions reached by Jones show several characteristic features:[17]

1. the proportion of the life span spent in sexually immature condition is by far the greatest in women
2. under the sheltered conditions afforded by industrial civilization or laboratory existence, all females become infertile well before the end of the total life span
3. the end of the reproductive life span in women occurs shortly after reproductive cycles stop
4. the proportion of the life span in primates characterized by total absence of reproductive cycles is the longest in humans (Figure 1.1).

Recently scientists at the Julius Center in Utrecht, the Netherlands stated that age-adjusted mortality is reduced 2% with each increasing year of age at menopause; in particular, ischemic heart disease

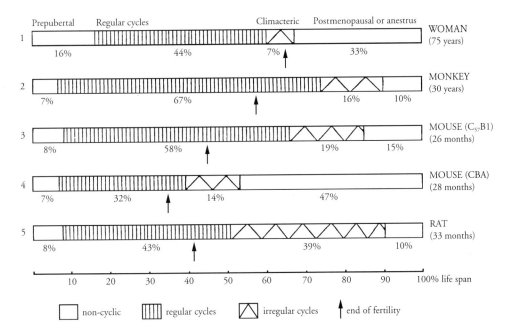

**Figure 1.1** Reproductive cyclic activity expressed as a percentage of total life span. Reproduced from Jones. Front Horm Res 1975; 3: 1,[17] with permission from the publisher.

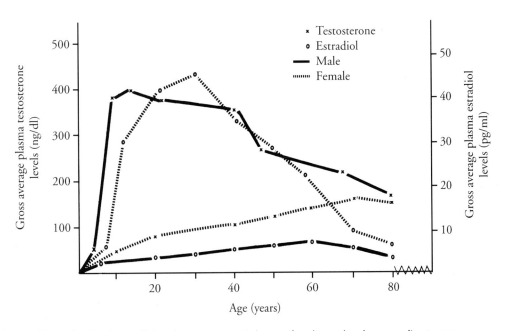

**Figure 1.2** Plasma levels of estradiol and testosterone in human females and males according to age.

mortality is 2% lower. They also indicated that the risk of death from uterine or ovarian cancer is increased by 5%; the net effect of later menopause is an increased life span.[24] At the same center, another group has provided evidence that candi-date genes affect pathogenesis, and linkage genes provide the aging responses.[25]

For practical follow-up reasons, much of the basic biological research in gerontology has been limited to small mammals. Specifically, for many years the relationship of aging to the reproductive cycle has been studied in mice,[19] and rats.[26] However, human ovaries differ from those of most other mammals because they continue to secrete hormones that are capable of maintaining subclinical cycles for a comparatively long time after overt reproduction ceases. The reproductive cycles may be re-established in old rats by the use of L-dopa; however, no evidence of a statistically valid extension of the life span has resulted from this treatment. Changes in the neuroendocrine system due to the loss of ovarian activity at menopause have been cited to have important biological roles in the control of reproductive and extra-reproductive functions. In review this may regulate mood, memory, cognition, behavior, immune function, locomotor system, and some cardiovascular conditions. These are essentially deficits also due to aging.[27]

The distinguishing histological and endocrine characteristics of the human ovary are discussed in Chapter 3 on pathology. The number of oocytes remaining in the ovary may account for cyclicity as well as fertility at an unexpectedly older age. Since the number of viable oocytes in women at a given range of years (such as 40–44) may vary as much as 100-fold, the age of menopause is an individual response.[28,29] Women who become menopausal by 45 years of age have experienced an accelerated decline of their fertility before the age of 32 years. This estimate is suitable for recommending screening.[30] Additionally, since the time of natural menopause has been shown to be heritable, natural menopause in the normal age range has not been recognized in the spectrum of phenotypes determined by the mutations of the follicle-stimulating hormone (FSH)-receptor genes.

Surgical menopause by bilateral ovariectomy with or without hysterectomy does not appear to change the longevity of the woman, when the surgery is performed for benign disease. Using the evidence available, there appears to be no reduction in the duration of life with premature ovarian failure. Since both of these conditions have usually been treated with estrogen replacement because of potential medical problems, we must rely on prior interpretation of these results. Although there has been no extension of reproductive life, the longevity of the female is currently 80+ years, and may increase to 85 years during the coming decade.[31]

Longevity seems to be a combination of conditions. It would appear from the statistics available that, in the woman, it is not related to the time of menopause. From these data, the length of the postmenopausal period relates to the mean life span in the human female, and can be documented in lower mammals.[32] Conversely, extension of cyclic reproduction by ovulatory techniques would not seem to be a potential mechanism for lengthening the life span. Both basic and clinical research into cyclic extension, fertility notwithstanding, shows no improvement in tissues that would lengthen life span. The commentary of Weismann continues to be as valid as it was 100 years ago:[14,31]

'Death itself, and the longer or short duration of life, both depend entirely on adaptation. Death is not an essential attribute of living matter; it is neither associated with reproduction, nor a necessary consequence of it . . .'.

## AGING AS A CAUSE OF REPRODUCTIVE FAILURE

In the human, reproduction may serve as a biological model for aging.[30] This is particularly true in the female, where decreasing sex hormone production eventually results in the demise of a dynamic physiological system (Figure 1.2).[33] The gradual reduction in estrogen secretion due to fading follicular growth and development in the ovary has been shown. An age-related decline in the process of folliculogenesis results in reduced oocyte quality. The well-characterized age-related increase in meiotic non-dysfunction is one symptom of compromised oocyte growth.[34]

Appropriate levels of estrogen cause both negative and positive feedback stimuli to the hypothalamic-pituitary axis, which maintains cyclicity in the reproductive process.[35] Secondary to this major goal, estrogen maintains sexual end-organ tissue structures.[36] In the aging woman, when ovarian estrogen secretions are reduced, available extra-ovarian levels continue to prevent many degenerative changes for a limited time. When body estrogen is severely depleted, senescence of the secondary sexual organs occurs.[36] Neurochemical changes appear to be the combined result of increase mitotic signaling by gonadotropins and gonadotrophin-releasing hormone (GnRH), decreased differentiative and neuroprotective signaling via sex steroids, and increased differentiative signaling via activins.[36]

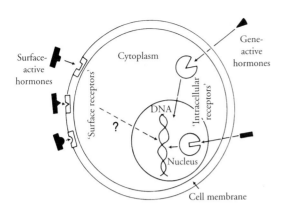

**Figure 1.3** Subcellular location of receptors for different hormone classes. Cells consist of an outer surface membrane, enclosing the soluble cytoplasm and the DNA-containing nucleus. Hormones whose receptors are located on the membrane include pituitary hormones, insulin, epinephrine (adrenaline), and glucagon. Receptors for steroids and thyroid hormones are found inside the cell, in the cytoplasm, and in the nucleus. Hormones of this latter category act more or less directly on the genome. Surface-active hormones may in some cases act indirectly on the genome, although their initial actions are on the cell membrane. Reproduced from Behnke et al. The Biology of Aging. New York: Plenum Press 1978: 291,[33] with permission from the publisher.

In a man, testosterone appears to maintain a threshold level well into the seventh decade, while his estradiol levels are slightly increased. The woman has a mild increase in androgen blood titers with the elevation of serum testosterone. These are usually the result of persistent activity of the extragonadal steroid pathways (Figure 1.2) and reduced aromatization.

## Alterations in reproductive tissues with aging

Ovaries differ from other endocrine organs in women because they function for only a limited period during the life span.[30] Other endocrine glands continue to secrete throughout life, and require therapeutic replacement when they become deficient. The aging cellular events and apoptosis (programmed cell death) described for all the endocrine glands pertain similarly to the reproductive system. The reproductive aging process seems to occur over a short period of time as a result of a predetermined series of events. Most likely, this is precipitated by both ovarian

and pertinent neuroendocrine failure, then further enhanced by the obsolescence of the tissues throughout the reproductive axis. The ability to maintain the regulation of the various reproductive functions is complicated, and results in the onset of premenopause.

This biological aging occurs in the female reproductive organs. Hormonal secretion diminishes almost linearly, and hormonal effectiveness is depressed further by reduced end-organ responses. The ovarian effluent decreases invariably from a peak in the reproductive years, through the perimenopausal era, and into the geripause, the postmenopausal reproductive senescence (Figure 1.2). Geripause is a new descriptive term, introduced here to represent the late postmenopause (after age 65 years). This phase is becoming longer and more significant in the 21st century (Chapter 2). The once-functional reproductive system shows well-documented evidence of decreasing efficiency and activity at each level.

Most of the research done by biologists and endocrinologists has been with regard to singular biological events in the reproductive axis. Thus, it is difficult to determine where the reduction in activity begins, or whether it has a multiple-level origin. Receptor systems exist at target cells for both pituitary hormones (FSH; luteinizing hormone, LH) in the ovary, and steroid hormones (estrogen, progesterone, androgens) in the target cells. These differ, as pituitary hormones are proteinaceous and act on surface receptors, and steroid hormones respond with intracellular (cytosol or nuclear) receptors (Figure 1.3).[37] The functional efficiency of the systems is an elemental factor in cellular aging.[36,38]

## Hypothalamic and pituitary senescence

The central nervous system initiates the cyclic reproductive response when a 'mature' hypothalamic-pituitary axis reacts to estrogen feedback.[36] At puberty, this lessening of the resistance by the hypothalamus provides the first cyclicity. In monitoring the roles of the various levels as they may be implicated, the hypothalamic-pituitary axis appears to be most vulnerable.

Aging of the hypothalamic-pituitary-ovarian axis parallels that of other organ systems. Longitudinal analyses have not been done, and are necessary to ascertain whether these measures will predict reproductive reserve before irreversible dysfunction occurs.[12] The hypothalamus and pituitary glands must remain efficient to

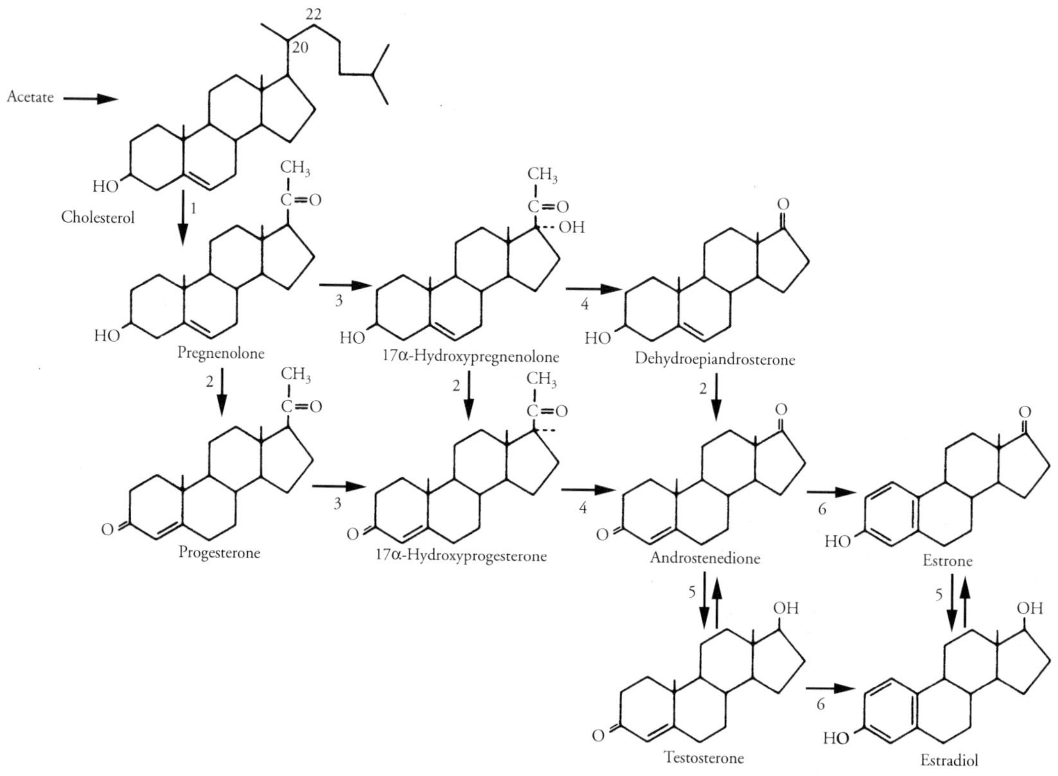

**Figure 1.4** Steroid biosynthetic pathways. The following enzymes are required where indicated: (1) 20-hydroxylase, 22-hydroxylase and 20,22-desmolase; (2) 3β-ol-dehydrogenase and o4–o5 isomerase; (3) 17α-hydroxylase; (4) 17,20-desmolase; (5) 17β-ol-dehydrogenase; (6) aromatizing enzyme system. Reproduced from Mishell and Davajan. Reproductive Endocrinology, Infertility and Contraception. Philadelphia: FA Davis, 1979: 42–54,[37] with permission from the publisher.

provide reproductive cyclicity, as programming for ovulation is provided by this axis. Cytological studies in postreproductive animals, and post-mortem studies on postmenopausal humans have yet to reveal any modifications that could be associated with aging. Additionally, the initial rise in gonadotropins in the menopause would seem to make the consideration of pituitary senescence difficult to accept.[35] The later postmenopausal decreases in gonadotropins are more consistent with the atrophism of the secreting cells.[36,39]

A theoretical possibility, which has research support, shows that aging of the neuroendocrine reproductive system causes a reversal of its pubertal onset.[30,40,41] In order to provide ovulation, the anterior pituitary must have the qualitative capability to respond to a moderate estrogen increase with a negative feedback of gonadotropin release. Additionally, a severely positive gonadotropin feedback (surge) must occur at a high level of

estrogen. The feedback mechanism in women appears to become less efficient in the later reproductive phases. This may be responsible for the increased infertility seen in women who have waited until their late 30s to begin child-bearing.[42,43] Thus, it becomes apparent that aging reverses an important feedback function rather than causing a direct pituitary disruption. This subtle differentiation in pituitary activity seems less intrusive on the general endocrine health of menopausal women.

The neuroendocrinology of aging has been well reviewed.[27,44–47] Clinical experiments with epinephrine (adrenaline) or progesterone, or by stimulation of the preoptic area of the hypothalamus, showed that ovulation could be restimulated in the senescent rat.[48,49] There have been several recent studies on the effect of agonal therapy with L-dopa and bromergocryptine, in recycling rodents in the postestrus (senescent) period. These therapies, considered to have a releasing hormone action similar to a dopamine surge, cause secretion of a pulse of gonadotropin from the pituitary, which stimulates ovarian tissue more readily than the existing intrinsic hormones. The significance of this effect remains difficult to define.[44,49] At present, these results have not been completely confirmed by controlled studies with humans, although elderly women treated with L-dopa or bromergocriptine for parkinsonism have been noted on occasions to cycle after the menopause. The further evidence of the benefits of psychoactive medications for menopausal problems, and the success of monamine regulators as well, causes much reflection on the possible etiologies for the symptomatology.[50]

## Absence of primordial or sensitive follicles

Convincing histological evidence has shown that the aging cells lose the ability to regrow and develop into active follicles, even with adequate stimulation (Chapter 10).[51,52] The remaining follicles tend to have a reduced sensitivity to the intrinsic gonadotropin, which may be due to the biological character of the older follicles, or a reduction in gonadotropin receptor in the cells.[35,53]

The hormonal pathway involved in steroid synthesis has been hypothetically shown to be dependent upon a two-cell response. The two cells involved are the granulosa and theca cells, which surround the follicles that are developing during each cycle. Several studies have shown that the steroid pathway requires both of these cells for the formation of estrogen. Observations from clinically assisted reproductive support have shown that the time interval between the onset of accelerated decline of the ovarian reserve and menopause is eventually fixed.[30] Androgens result from the cholesterol to pregnenolone responses (Figure 1.4),[54] and intermediate androgens such as dehydroepiandrosterone and androstenedione are formed within the theca cells. Androgens are transported from the theca cells to the granulosa cells, where aromatizing enzymes produce estrogens. The primary non-pregnant estrogens – estradiol and estrone – are then secreted into the vascular system.

Estrogens and gonadotropins are required for the formation of receptors for gonadotropins. Estrogen has the capacity to form both FSH and LH receptors on either the theca or granulosa cells; LH has the ability to form FSH receptors, particularly on the granulosa cells; and FSH has the

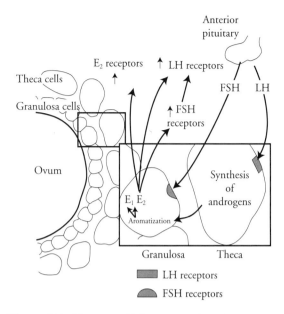

**Figure 1.5** The two-cell theory: granulosa-theca steroid pathway; follicle-stimulating hormone (FSH), and luteinizing hormone (LH) activity on cell receptors. Reproduced from Eskin. Issues in Reproductive Endocrinology. New York: Medical Arts Press 1984: 99,[54] with permission from the publisher.

capability of forming both FSH and LH receptors on either cell (Figure 1.5). In addition, it appears that estrogen forms its own estrogen nuclear receptors on any of these cells involved. At the present time two distinct estradiol receptors exist – alpha (α) and beta (β). The α-receptor is fundamentally found in reproductive cells, while β-cells are seen in somatic tissues. The beta estrogen receptor has been divided for clarity into $ER\beta_1$ and $ER\beta_2$, each being defined by specific entities with which they may respond.[55] Other estrogen receptors have been mentioned, but are not yet fully recognized. During the aging phenomena, many of these responses are not adequate or effective, with a resulting reduction in follicular growth and development.[52,56]

Evidently, many of the enzymes are reduced in numbers and effectiveness during the aging process. This causes the hormone pathway to malfunction and, in fact, may bring about an increase in intermediate hormonal release. When aromatization does not occur, intermediate androgens continue to be formed and secreted directly into the blood. The increase in the amount of androgens present may cause serious clinical symptoms in women.[57]

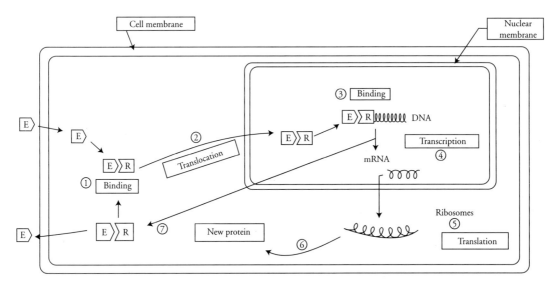

**Figure 1.6** The mechanism of action of estradiol. Estradiol enters through the membrane by diffusion and is (1) bound to the receptor. The complex is (2) translocated to the nucleus where it is (3) bound to the chromatin material. The DNA (4) transcription to mRNA results in (5) ribosomal translation in the cytoplasm. New protein (6) is formed and utilized in cell metabolic processes. The estradiol–receptor complex leaves the nucleus (7), where it is dissociated to estradiol (which presumably leaves the cell) and receptor protein, which is reused in the binding process.

Functional loss of stroma occurs in biological aging intracellularly, with increased fibrosis.[48,58] Because of this, there is diminished active cellular milieu needed to produce the steroid fractions required for appropriate hormonal secretions.[59,60] This may also be a reason for the enzyme letdown that has been described (Figure 1.5).

### Alterations in sensitivity to gonadotropins

As stated above, these changes may be due to reduction in gonadotropin receptors by modification or loss.[61] These proteinaceous receptors act on the surface of the cells, and may respond by providing the specific enzyme systems required for intracellular biochemical pathways (Chapter 20). The expected steroidogenesis in the ovary leading to the secretion of estrogens may be interrupted by receptor alterations.[62] The changes that occur could be precipitated by factors such as toxicity, mutations, or immunological damage. The results of the loss of gonadotropin activity would be a sex steroid shift in the secretion of intermediary metabolites (Figure 1.4). Some of these androgenic steroids are clinically active, and may be responsible for postmenopausal symptomatology.

Sensitivity of the follicle to gonadotropins has been considered to be a requirement for the function of the secretory cells. In the ovary, the loss of receptor at the molecular level reduces the activity of the gonad and its vitality for further responsiveness. It has become evident that gonadotropins may be qualitatively altered and, thus, less effective at the specific target cell.[63,64] Some studies have indicated environmental effects that cause central nervous system changes capable of influencing the hypothalamic discharge and, by that means, of modifying gonadotropin release.[65]

### Steroid receptor loss

One important theory depends on reduced receptor response with biochemical modifications of the cytosol protein necessary for estrogen action. Research from many laboratories, including our own,[16,66,67] shows modifications in the aging cell that may limit capability for the specific steroid action expected. While the appropriate estrogen is present, a decrease in target cell sensitivity depresses the reproductive organs and requires an increased estrogen level for restoration of activity.[63] Studies have shown also that a single gene (*ESR1*) has variations in gene response, which may be a determining factor for postmenopausal estradiol levels.[68] These estrogen receptor α gene polymorphisms may be an essential cause of the variability of activity among same-age postmenopausal women. Since estrogens act also on the ovary, the reduction in end-organ response causes the ovary to decrease steroid output, resulting in an impasse.

This short summation of the arguments for reproductive failure and aging serves to introduce the many controversies. Cessation of reproductive activity is secondary to the loss of many physiological and biochemical events, and occurs either genetically or environmentally. Any level of the reproductive system may be causative, although ovarian senescence appears to be the most common. The effect of estrogen and estrogen receptors on the aging organs is discussed in the following section.

## CELLULAR SENESCENCE AS A RESULT OF MENOPAUSE

Gonadal secretion of estrogen and progesterone wanes, and the ovulatory ability of the ovary decreases. The loss of these hormones, which are responsible for secondary sexual characteristics in women, causes changes that are initially subtle, but which cannot be easily separated from those resulting from aging. The clinical symptomatology seen is remarkably variegated (Table 1.2). The signs and symptoms of the disorders that appear to be the result of estrogen deficiency are not limited to the reproductive system. Estrogen affects tissues throughout the body, and receptors for this steroid have been isolated in non-sexual tissues.

These clinical conditions show a different hormone threshold level for each individual. The variation appears to be due to end-organ response

rather than steroid level. Radioimmunoassay studies in aging women show that metabolic clearance rates are modified, and almost always decrease when estrogen production wanes. This might be responsible for a progressively higher level of circulating steroid, which could lead to tissue pathology, especially if exogenous hormone is also being given. However, most gerontologists feel that intracellular control occurs, which modifies the response to the estrogen stimulus.[27,57,63]

Estrogen has been described as decreasing initially between the ages of 26 and 29 years; however, most evident effects are seen in the decelerating reproductive (36–43), perimenopausal (42–51), and postmenopausal (51–65) years (Chapter 8).[23] As estrogen decreases, menstrual problems evolve such as amenorrhea (cessation of menses), oligomenorrhea (prolongation of cycles), hypomenorrhea (reduction in amount of bleeding), and menorrhagia (heavy menstrual bleeding).

Ovarian hormones are quantitatively and qualitatively transformed in aging (Figure 1.4). Intermediate steroids increase, and may act peripherally to bring about the clinical changes with advancing age.[23] The effect of progesterone, which is only minimally measurable in the postmenopausal serum, has been under considerable investigation for therapeutic use, an area that is reviewed in the therapy section of this book.

### Tissue effects of sex hormones

Data on intracellular receptors for estrogen and progesterone in hormone-specific target tissues (i.e. breast, uterus, pituitary, etc) have accumulated since the initial hypotheses were presented.[69–71] These reproductive hormone-target cell responses depend on unidentified intracellular binding proteins having attributes which include high specificity and affinity for each steroid (Figure 1.6).[33] When estrogen or progestin passes through the membrane into the cell cytosol, a complex consisting of steroid and receptor protein is formed, which can then be translocated as a unit from the cytoplasm through the nuclear membrane into the nuclear compartment.[72] Receptor transformations occur within the nucleus and, under specific conditions, nuclear mRNA synthesis results. Following this, mRNA translation in the ribosomes can lead to protein synthesis. Thus, the initial steroid has caused a series of intracellular events to occur which stimulate the affected tissues to growth and

**Table 1.2** Disorders related to hypoestrinism

*Directly*
Atrophic vulvovaginitis
Urethral syndrome
Skin, hair, and breast changes

*Indirectly*
Hot flushes
Osteoporosis
Psychosexual problems
Functional cardiac diseases

*Probably*
Psychological conditions
Atherosclerotic heart disease
Lipid metabolism

Control by hormones and/or other biochemical agents

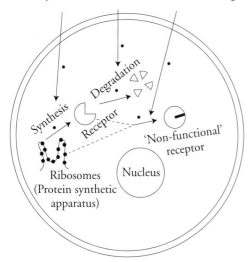

**Figure 1.7**   Theoretical positions where hormones or other biochemical agents could control receptor changes during aging. Reproduced from Behnke et al. The Biology of Aging. New York: Plenum Press 1978: 291,[33] with permission from the publisher.

development, according to the set pattern generated by the chromosomal genes (genome) of the nucleus.[68,72] Receptor research has shown that the steroid receptor system may be more simplistic, and may be present on the cell nuclear membrane, thus reducing the complexity involved with a cytosol protein receptor (Figures 1.3 and 1.6).[73,74]

Some steroids related to estradiol cause incomplete responses because the duration of residence in the nucleus is altered.[57,59,68,71] It has been hypothesized that the endogenous estrogens – estrone, estradiol and estriol – have a different response according to the target organ. The metabolic action may depend on the time that the steroid–receptor complexes of these estrogens remain in the nucleus. When the complex remains within the nucleus for a longer time, a greater effect on the cell results. Metabolism and growth may follow, even when the cell has evident resistance to the stimulating complex, if prolonged binding to the nuclear substance can occur.[75]

The quantity of receptor available in the cytosol of the target cells is an important condition which can regulate the response by a cell to a specific steroid hormone. The levels of the receptors are specific to target tissue, and appear to be unalterable. However, estrogen therapy increases the number of receptors available for estrogen

action.[76] Another possible source of receptor supply is from those reclaimable after the receptor complex has affected the nuclear response. After such exposure to estrogens, the estrogen receptor moves to the cell nucleus and gradually dissociates, returning to the cytoplasm in a free condition, and, thus, can be recycled (Figure 1.6). The number of free estrogen receptors available is an important control for further activity of the cell by this steroid.[69]

On the other hand, certain non-steroidal anti-estrogens act as antagonists to the cell metabolism by competing for the available receptors.[77] Some of these anti-estrogens act initially in a manner similar to estrogens by stimulating the same metabolic and regulatory pathways that cause uterine and endometrial growth. The responses may be lessened because of the reduced efficiency of the estrogen employed.

Another means of endogenous control over steroid receptor levels is the influence that one steroid exerts on the receptor levels of others. For example, estrogens can induce progesterone receptors in human breast cells, while progesterone can impair the replenishment of the estrogen receptor in the rat uterus. This type of effect reduces the sensitivity of the uterus to subsequent estrogen exposure after a single estrogen bolus. This cross-reaction may be due to an inhibition of receptor synthesis, or to increased inactivation. If progesterone is an antagonist to estrogen reception, obviously it can cause the estrogen to be even less effective although the quantities available are extremely low.

Mechanisms available at present to change receptor responses are essentially limited to seven alternatives and their combinations (Table 1.3). One of the important factors in the study of aging concerns the innate loss of receptors in the cells of the aging reproductive tract.[62]

| Table 1.3   Determinants of estrogen response |
| --- |
| 1.   Levels and availability of estrogen receptors in target tissue |
| 2.   Hormone quality and quantity |
| 3.   Level of ligand affinity |
| 4.   Interference by other steroids |
| 5.   Temporal effect of the complex in the nucleus |
| 6.   Level of protein response |
| 7.   Measurement of how readily the receptor complex separates from the hormone and whether it can provide reusable receptors |

There has been rapid progress in the field of receptors for reproductive hormones. Estrogen α-receptor (ERα) analysis to determine estrogen-responsive tumors has been utilized in breast cancer therapeutics for many years.[78] Progestin usage in uterine dysplasia has been included as an antagonist in several treatment programs. Anti-estrogen therapy for estrogen-dependent cancer has been effectively used. Research into receptors and neoplasia in aging has shown some interaction, but still requires further data.[67] Laboratory studies in capillary endothelial cells in human prostate, cerebellum, and capillary endothelial tissues of the heart have identified the presence of β-estrogen receptors. These antipolyclonal estrogen $\beta_1$- and $\beta_2$-receptors still require a simpler technique before a positive elaboration of their other qualities can be made.[79] Several studies have recently characterized other possible estrogen receptors by immunohistochemical techniques.

Current investigations show that receptor loss with aging results in decreased intracellular metabolism. Thus, when estrogen receptors decrease, there may be a loss of function at specific reproductive target cells and other less obvious tissues in the body. With cellular aging, peripheral endocrine changes occur, which in themselves can be responsible for the deterioration of many bodily systems besides reproduction.

## Changes in receptor systems in aging

The conditions for secretion from the follicular cells in the ovary have been described. In the two-cell theory (Figure 1.5), the theca and granulosa cells receive signals, presumably through gonadotropin membrane receptors for LH and FSH. The two cells respond in tandem by secreting steroids into the circulating system. Thus, the active ovary has appropriate secretory cells which are stimulated by gonadotropins secreted from the pituitary. These hormones signal the ovarian cells through receptor systems on the membranes. This results in the secretion of estrogens, primarily as estradiol, and other intermediate steroids including progesterone (Figure 1.4). Estrogens and progesterone, thus secreted, act at the appropriate target organs and require their own intracellular or nuclear receptors for response. Additionally, estrogens provide specific ovulatory functions in the scheme of follicular growth through the presence of estrogen receptors in the ovary.[46]

Specific research into estrogen receptor systems is ongoing, and has shown that they are not lim-ited to the ovary and secondary sexual tissues, but are also found to a lesser degree in other tissues as indicated by ERα and ERβ. Advances in the measurement of estrogen α-receptors provide several new medical applications.[80] Successful production of non-specific antisera to purified estrogen receptor has led to the development of sensitive radioimmunoassays for this receptor. Rapid and accurate estrogen α-receptor determination has become available for the diagnosis of reproductive disease states, and for evaluating cancer treatment. Recent studies have also implicated ERβ in menopausal symptomatology. It has become apparent that cytosine-adenine polymorphism of the *ERβ* gene has been associated with menopausal and premenopausal symptoms.[57] Additional findings of ERβ as well as ERα in the brain has caused an increase in evaluation of estradiol as an effector of neuroendocrine menopausal problems.[55,57]

Eukaryotic gene structure has shown that mutations involving the intermediate sequences of steroid-hormone regulation may be phenotypically silent. These may not influence the expression of the signal under usual circumstances. However, in aging and cancer or other genetically effected illnesses, gene structure could be altered, and the mutations effected by these previously silent responses would become evident.[80]

The mechanisms for intracellular systems for the estradiol α-receptor have been generally outlined (Figure 1.6). More detailed evaluation is shown in Chapter 20. These receptor systems appear to control steroid hormone action. However, a recent question has arisen whether these receptors are present directly on the nuclear membrane,[73] rather than only effected through a specific cytoplasmic receptor, or both. Another receptor system, the eosinophil binding system, which may be responsible for some of the early estrogen responses – for example water inhibition, increased vascular permeability and histamine release – has also been described.[81]

Until the advent of receptor biochemistry, therapy could not be conceivably thought effective on target cells affected by histological aging. Molecular biological research, actively done in many laboratories, shows the changes that occur within the aging cells by receptor systems. These data have been fully summarized,[62] and indicate that steroids appear to have intracellular or nuclear receptors, while other hormones such as gonadotropins have surface receptors (Figures 1.5 and 1.6). Hormones require a receptor system in order to transmit the specific biochemical purpose. While the specific mechanisms of translation in the nucleus are not yet fully understood, several steps appear to be necessary for activation of the chromatin material. These biochemical events may be changed by aging, and may be responsible for reduced or modified hormonal behavior.[33,82] The ability of many of the hormones to stimulate DNA synthesis and cell division has been observed to decrease with aging.[46]

Changes in cell responsiveness during aging have been ascribed to a wide variety of hormones and neurotransmitters, and a great number of target cells and tissues. This has been shown in various animal species as well as in man, and for a wide variety of physiological and biochemical processes.[75] In this research, the time and rate of change with age varies, depending upon the variables noted. In this book, the basic mechanisms by which hormones and neurotransmitters act at the cellular and molecular levels under normal conditions, independent of the aging process, are presented.[62,63] Any of the changes that occur within the cell can mediate hormone and neurotransmitter action and modify it according to the age of the individual.[83] This could result in altered hormonal and neurotransmitter responsiveness, with a completely different end result. The major emphasis at present is on the differentiation between changes in receptor and post-receptor events causing altered functional responses during the aging process.[63] In addition, the ability of a number of hormones to stimulate DNA synthesis and cell division has been observed to decrease with aging.

In an early review, 200 different receptor systems were studied as a function of age during the adult portion of the life span.[84] The various types of receptor alterations were catalogued and reported as they occurred during the aging process. In general, 50% of the studies reported showed reduced receptor concentration with increased age, 35% reported no changes whatsoever, 10% found increased receptor concentrations with increased age, and 5% reported changes in affinity which generally decreased with increased age. Discrepancies were noted in independent work from many other laboratories over many years. The need for resolution of these controversies by standardization of experimental models and methodology was recognized. Reasonably close, if not causal, relationships between receptor and response loss exist in about 35 cases. Since it is apparent that correlations alone do not establish causality, receptor loss may not necessarily be totally responsible for reduced responsiveness in

some of these systems;[62] however, the importance of receptor dysfunction remains unquestionable.

The mechanisms of hormone receptor loss from target cells during aging have been investigated.[33,62,63] Molecular processes that are altered during aging result in decreased cellular concentrations of functional hormone receptors. These include abnormal synthesis (assembly), degradation (disassembly), and possible presence of receptors in a non-functional state, and the negative state, and the negative effect of other hormones and biochemical agents on the processes (Figure 1.7). These destructive events could account for the reduction in activity shown in cells affected by toxic substances as well as aging.

Using radioactive labeling, the concentrations and affinity of receptors were determined in aging tissues in rats. Steroid hormone concentrations appear to be reduced during aging in a number of tissues, including brain, fat, liver, muscle, and prostate gland. The binding affinity is not changed, but seems to depend on the ability of the tissues to maintain normal receptor concentrations, and not on the ability of the receptors to respond. This finding is not universal to all of the hormones studied, but may be a response that is undetectable by present research techniques.[84] In rodents, glucocorticoids have shown a reduction of 60% in the ability to control nutrient transport and metabolism between maturity and senescence.[85] This is paralleled by a 60% reduction in glucocorticoid receptor concentrates. Estrogens have been shown to have a reduced ability to provide certain enzymes required for the proper transmission of nerve impulses in the brain. Estrogen receptor concentrations in the brain were also noted to have decreased with aging, an important preliminary finding.

Starting with the perimenopausal period, estrogen concentrations decrease in both production and serum levels. Estrogen appears to have ubiquitous activity in cells throughout the body, and the primary method of expression is through intracellular estrogen receptors (Figure 1.7). If receptors decrease with aging, a further reduction in cellular activity would result. Not all the cells of the body appear to age equally, and a differential in the receptor systems may be responsible for the uneven results which have been seen.

In our laboratory, we have isolated iodinated proteins in breast tissues, which act within the cytosol and appear to be required for normal estrogen receptor action.[86] Estradiol receptor protein changes occur qualitatively and quantitatively in the cytosol in breast tissue from rats made iodine deficient.[87] Progesterone receptor is also affected by a lack of iodine, and varies indirectly with the estradiol receptor levels;[88] thus, iodine appears to be a determinant of receptor availability and action in rat breast tissues.[89] When older rat models were used, dietary deficiency or blockade of iodine caused histological atypism in the mammary tissues, which was sharply increased compared with that seen in younger animals.[67] These abnormal mammary glands were also seen to show differences in receptor levels according to advancing age. Microarray studies on human breast carcinoma cultures show the effective concentrations of estrogen receptors activated by iodine. The pathways indicate the increase in enzyme activity and response necessary for nuclear action.[90]

Studies of the effects of aging on estrogen metabolism in the rat uterus have revealed several variables in receptor responses. The probability of non-functional receptors in aged uteri has been described, although it is particularly difficult to separate active from non-active receptors. The likely explanation for apparent steroid receptor loss during aging in the rat uterus is an altered control of the biosynthetic pathway, rather than a change in the molecular structure of the receptor itself. Further research being carried out in several laboratories is studying post-receptor responses.[63] Measuring RNA polymerase II activity following estrogen administration, the absolute magnitude of response was not shown to diminish with age. Impaired responsiveness of senescent nuclei was seen in the presence of mature receptor preparations. This would show that aging may affect cellular components and/or processes in the scheme of estrogen action distal to cytoplasmic receptor activation, and the number of molecular sites in which this could occur has been described, but not separated. Age-associated defects for estrogen stimulation occur at various levels in the transduction apparatus of the cells found in the rat uterus. These may range from quantitative and possibly qualitative deficits in the receptors themselves, to nuclear changes involved in the activation of RNA polymerase II.[75]

While these receptor aging studies were mostly in rodents, the data seem remarkably similar to the information known in the human. Difficulties in quantitation and evaluation of the research have led to conflicting evidence. There has been indirect evidence of reduced estrogen receptor protein in the breasts of menopausal women; whether this is due to aging or estrogen loss is controversial.[78] Uterine endometrial cell loss has been previously reported.[91,92] Resistant arteries from postmenopausal women show functional and morphological abnormalities. ERα contributes to vascular protection by estrogen in the peripheral resistance circulation.[93] The evidence that the loss of estrogen and progesterone may reduce cell metabolism in various tissues of the body is likely to be correct. Research is active in this field, as both neurotransmitters, receptors, and receptor modulators are fundamental to end-organ expression of hormones.

Aging has been considered by gerontologists for many years to be a response to decline of both the neurogenic and endocrine systems.[4] The question is whether reproductive loss due to aging stems from depletion of stimulation in the central nervous system, or from failure of target tissue action, or perhaps anywhere along the intermediate axis. This remains unanswered, and a matter for continuing research. These problems in aging and reproduction require competent solution if treatment and/or quality and longevity in the postmenopausal period of life is expected to improve.

## CELLULAR DETERIORATION AND ESTROGEN

Non-reproductive somatic cells go through a series of events that promote growth and development. Such cells range from cell populations that are consistently proliferating (skin, gastrointestinal lining, blood-forming elements) to those that are non-growing (nervous tissue, muscle).[5] As discussed above, the endocrine system lies between these extremes as it requires stimulation for preparation and secretion of the specific hormones involved.

When estrogen diminishes, intracellular activity decreases in estrogen-dependent tissues. These tissues appear to be limited to primary and secondary sexual organs as well as specific areas of the central nervous system. Atrophism is most apparent in the vulvar, vaginal and urethral regions, also as a result of cellular aging. Cellular changes are detailed in Chapter 3 and the clinical problems in later chapters.

When estrogen replacement is given, the affected tissues are still not fully restored, indicating that end-organ failure continues regardless of available hormone. Secretions from the higher endocrine centers (pituitary and hypothalamus) increase initially, responding to the changes and feedback from the cellular milieu at the target organ. These modifications in molecular structure in the estrogen-dependent cells cannot be defined clearly by present research techniques. However, new enzyme models with rat uteri have shown anion differences.[75] These models and other similar responses in women remain an important step to further basic and clinical research to assist therapeutic improvement.

It is apparent that non-reproductive tissues are affected on an individual basis, according to functional receptors that are present. Whether specific estrogen receptors are the required cell stimulators in these sites is unknown. Several clinical problems which focus on symptoms in the skeletal and central nervous systems have been studied. Osteoporosis, neurovascular phenomena (such as hot flushes), and cardiovascular diseases are the serious postmenopausal conditions encountered. Cardiac protection by estrogen seems clinically tenuous, and some basic research is needed to enlighten this area.[94,95] The combination of both a neuroendocrine and a neurocardiac basis for protection by estrogen in the presynaptic ganglia of the heart has been suggested.[96,97]

However, no estrogen receptors have been measured in bone, and the effects of estrogen on nervous tissue has remained difficult to define. The possibility that there may be nuclear receptors that are not measurable in specific estrogen β-receptor form has been considered.[55,73] These systems may be the reason for a lack of correlation in these tissues when effects are compared with laboratory receptor measurements.

## ESTROGEN REPLACEMENT AND AGING

If estrogen is responsible for cellular senescence of reproductive tissues, replacement therapy should be fully effective as a restorative measure. However, the legendary 'fountain of youth' remains elusive. Treatments of many kinds have been used in an attempt to turn back the clock. At present, gerontologists strive to improve the quality of life as longevity increases. The use of hormones, from the mystical transplants of Brown-Sequard in the 19th century, to the 'estrogen forever' phase at the beginning of the 20th century remains obscure.

Estrogen increases estrogen receptors and, therefore, enhances bodily cellular responses under their control.[76] Nevertheless, aging itself reduces endocrine activity by the deterioration of the secretory mechanisms, and decreases the metabolism within the responding cells by modifying receptors and other unknown factors (Figure 1.7). Estrogen appears to have specific effects on the central nervous system, hypothalamus and pituitary gland. Further modifications of these higher centers by aging may be restrictive or even non-responsive to the needs of the reproductive system.

Estrogen has been described as providing variable clinical improvement, and several chapters discuss the advantages and disadvantages of its use. Experimental work continues with estrogen, estrogen analogs and intermediate sex steroids in an effort to change intracellular pathways and receptor action. Estrogen replacement therapy has been considered as a potent method for improving the quality of life for the menopausal woman if properly indicated.[98] Pharmaceutical research is dedicated to producing therapeutic hormones that are safer and more effective.

Progesterone as a therapy for the menopause may serve as a substitute for estrogen in certain target organs. The clinical use of progesterone to protect some estrogen-dependent tissues from neoplastic changes during estrogen therapy in the postmenopause has been suggested. Changes in central nervous system stimuli, as seen by secondary hypothalamic pulses, appear to be the basis for hot flushes. The resulting elevations of gonadotropin (LH) are considered by some to be responsible for a limited response. This hypothalamic thermal action is being treated by anti-GnRH substances as an alternative to estrogen.[99] The use of anti-estrogenic compounds (SERMS) are in trial.

Throughout the research and clinical history of estrogen replacement, there has been no evidence that estrogen or other hormonal therapies are effective in deterring aging. On the other hand, aging can block the effect of estrogen in reproductive tissues and other hormone-affected tissues. Estrogen, while initially useful in the perimenopause, can change only modestly the atrophism of aging in the postmenopausal period. Thus, aging is intrusive on reproduction, and our present knowledge does not provide complete replacement therapies that can revitalize the system.

## CONCLUSIONS

1. Menopause does not appear to affect longevity nor is postmenopause or geripause affected by increased life expectancy.
2. Cellular aging is a direct cause of reproductive failure, which leads to the menopause.
3. Estrogen-dependent tissues have an increased rate of senescence in the perimenopause and menopause.
4. Intracellular deterioration is more dependent on aging than menopause, or the lack of sex steroids.
5. Aging of the reproductive stimulatory centers is responsible for reduction in target cellular activity and leads to eventual intracellular demise.
6. Hormonal replacement has limitations in reparation of hypoestrinism and aging cells.

The success of sex hormone therapies in aging is dependent on the response of the altered cells of the woman. The changes in intracellular metabolism may be focally distributed throughout the body. Thus the use of estrogen replacement therapy must be considered on the basis of individual effectiveness versus risk.

## REFERENCES

1. Miller PB, Soules MR. Correlation of reproductive aging with function in selected organ systems. Fertil Steril 1997; 68: 443–8.
2. Zoellner YF, Oliver P, Brazier JE et al. Reliability and validity of a newly developed menopause-specific quality-of-life questionnaire, the QualiPause Inventory (QPI). Qual Life Res 2001; 10: 260.
3. Strehler BL. Time, Cells, and Aging, 2nd edn. New York: Academic Press, 1974.
4. Rockstein M. Theoretical Aspects of Aging. New York: Academic Press, 1974.
5. Shock NW. Physiologic theories of aging. In: Rockstein M, ed. Theoretical Aspects of Aging. New York: Academic Press, 1984: 119–28.
6. Fossel M. Telomerase and the aging cell. J Am Med Assoc 1998; 279: 1732–5.
7. van Asselt KM, Kok HS, Pearson PL, Dubas JS, van Noord PA. Heredibility of menopausal age in mothers and daughters. Fertil Steril 2004; 82: 1348–51.
8. Schlessinger D, Van Zant G. Does functional depletion of stem cells drive aging? Mech Ageing Dev 2001; 122: 1537–53.
9. Skulachev VP. Aging is a specific biological function rather than the result of a disorder in complex living systems: biochemical evidence in support of Weismann's hypothesis. Biochemistry 1977; 62: 1191–5.
10. Medawar PB. An Unsolved Problem of Biology. London: Lewis, 1951.
11. Leathem JH. Endocrine changes with age. In: Ostfeld AM, ed. Epidemiology of Aging. DHEW Publication 75–711. Washington DC: DHEW, 1972: 224–32.
12. Fiatarone MA, O'Neill EF, Ryan ND et al. Exercise training and nutritional supplementation for physical frailty in very elderly people. N Engl J Med 1994; 330: 1769–75.
13. Gusseck DJ. Endocrine mechanisms and aging. Adv Gerontol Res 1972; 4: 105.
14. Weismann A. Essays Upon Hereditary and Kindred Biologic Problems. London: Oxford University Press, 1981.
15. Tietze C. Reproductive span and rate reproduction among Hutterite women. Fertil Steril 1957; 8: 89.
16. Young JZ. An Introduction into the Study of Man. Oxford: Clarendon Press, 1971.
17. Jones EC. The post-reproductive phase in mammals. Front Horm Res 1975; 3: 1.
18. Brody JA, Grand MD, Frateschi LJ et al. Epidemiology and aging: maximum reproductive age unaffected by increased life expectancy in the twentieth century. Aging 1998; 10: 170–1.
19. Thung PJ, Boot LM, Muhlbock D. Senile changes in the oestrous cycle and in ovarian structure in some inbred strains of mice. Acta Endocrinol 1956; 23: 8.
20. Amundsen DW, Diers CJ. Age of menopause in medieval Europe. Hum Biol 1973; 45: 605.
21. Westendorp RG, Kirkwood TB. Human longevity at the cost of reproductive success. Nature 1998; 396: 743–6.
22. Eskin BA, Troen BR. The Geripause: The Postmenopausal Woman. New York and London: CRC Parthenon Publishing, 2003.
23. Eskin BA. Menopause hormones and drug therapy during reproductive senescence. In: Cooper RK, Walker RF, eds. Experimental and Clinical Interventions in Aging. New York: Marcel Dekker, 1983: 85–117.
24. Ossewaarde ME, Bots ML, Verbeek AL, Peeters PH, vander Graaf Y. Age at menopause, cause-specific mortality and total life expectancy. Epidemiology 2005; 16: 556–62.
25. Kok HS, van Asselt KM, Van der Schouw YT, Peeters PH. Genetic studies to identify genes underlying menopausal age. Hum Reprod Update 2005; 11: 483–93.
26. Bloch S. Studies on climacterium and menopause in albino rats. III. Histological observations on the aging genital tract. Gynecologica 1961; 152: 414.
27. Rehman HU, Masson EA. Neuroendocrinology of female aging. Gend Med 2005; 2: 41–56.
28. Block E. Quantitative morphologic investigations of the follicular system in women. Variations at different ages. Acta Anat 1952; 14: 108.
29. Maszmann L. Epidemiology of climacteric and post-climacteric complaints. Front Horm Res 1973; 2: 22.
30. Nikolaou D, Templeton A. Early ovarian ageing. Eur J Obstet Gynecol Reprod Biol 2004; 113: 126–33.
31. Fries JF. Aging, natural death, and the compression of morbidity. N Engl J Med 1980; 303: 130–5.
32. Keefe DL. Reproductive aging is an evolutionarily programmed strategy that no longer provides adaptive value. Fertil Steril 1998; 70: 204–6.
33. Roth GS. Altered biochemical responsiveness and hormone receptor changes during aging. In: Bejnke J, Finch G, Momeut G, eds. The Biology of Aging. New York: Plenum Press, 1978: 291.
34. Volarcik K, Sheean L, Goldfarb J et al. The meiotic competence of in vitro matured human oocytes is influenced

by donor age: evidence that folliculogenesis is compromised in the reproductively aged ovary. Hum Reprod 1998; 13: 154–60.

35. Kok HS, Peeters PH, Grobbee DE, Pearson PL, Wijmenga C. Age at natural menopause is not linked with FSH receptor region: a sib-pair study. Fertil Steril 2004; 81: 611–16.

36. Atwood CS, Meethal SV, Liu T, Wilson AC, Gallego M, Smith MA, Bowen BL. Dysregulation of the hypothalamic-pituitary-gonadal axis with menopause and andropause promotes neurodegenerative senescence. J Neuropathol Exp Neurol 2005; 64: 93–103.

37. Goebelsmann U. Steroidogenesis. In: Mishell DR Jr, Davajan V, eds. Reproductive Endocrinology, Infertility and Contraception. Philadelphia: FA Davis, 1979: 42–54.

38. Lamberts SWJ, van den Beld AW, van der Lely A-J. The endocrinology of aging. Science 1997; 278: 419–23.

39. Metcalf MG, Donald RA, Livesey JH. Pituitary-ovarian function in normal women during the menopausal transition. J Endocrinol 1980; 87: 191.

40. Eskin BA. Clinical consideration of age-related changes in serotonin and norepinephrine metabolism of reproductive function. Neurobiol Aging 1984; 5: 151.

41. Atit R, Eskin BA, Walker RF. Comparison of gonadotropin secretion in women and female rats during aging. Age 1986; 9: 10.

42. Simon JA, Bustillo M, Thorneycroft IH. Variability of midcycle estradiol positive feedback: evidence for unique pituitary response in individual women. J Clin Endocrinol Metab 1987; 64: 789.

43. Eskin BA, Trivedi RA, Weideman CA, Walker RF. Positive feedback disturbances and infertility in women over thirty. Am J Gynecol Health 1988; 2: 110.

44. Finch CE. Neuroendocrinology of aging: a view of an emerging area. Biol Sci 1975; 25: 645.

45. Finch CG, Tanzi RE. Genetics of aging. Science 1997; 278: 407–11.

46. Wilkes MM, Lu KH, Hopper BR, Yen SSC. Altered neuroendocrine status of middle-aged rats prior to the onset of senescent anovulation. Neuroendocrinology 1979; 29: 255.

47. Morrison JH, Hof PR. Life and death of neurons in the aging brain. Science 1972; 278: 412–19.

48. Clemens JA, Ameromoni Y, Jenkins T, Meites J. Effects of hypothalamic stimulation, hormones, and drugs on ovarian function in old female rats. Proc Soc Exp Biol Med 1969; 132: 561.

49. Miller AE, Riegle GD. Serum LH levels following multiple LHRH injections in aging rats. Proc Soc Exp Biol Med 1978; 157: 494–9.

50. Joffe H, Soares CN, Cohen LS. Assessment and treatment of hot flushes and menopausal mood disturbance. Psychiatr Clin North Am 2003; 26: 563–80.

51. Greenblatt RB, Colle ML, Mahesh VB. Ovarian and adrenal steroid production in postmenopausal woman. Obstet Gynecol 1976; 47: 383.

52. Meredith S, Butcher RL. Role of decreased numbers of follicles in reproductive performance in young and aged rats. Biol Reprod 1985; 32: 788–94.

53. Butcher RL. Effect of reduced ovarian tissue on cyclicity, basal hormone levels and follicular development in old rats. Biol Reprod 1985; 32: 315–21.

54. Eskin BA. Physiology of gonadotropins LH/FSH. In: Eskin BA, Issues in Reproductive Endocrinology. New York: Medical Arts Press 1984: 99.

55. Eskin BA, Aloyo VJ. Cellular senescence and estrogen. In: Schneider HPG, ed. Nenopause: The State of the Art – in Research and Management. New York and London: The Parthenon Publishing Group 2003: 211–17.

56. Page RD, Butler RL. Follicular and plasma patterns of steroids in young and old rats during normal and prolonged estrous cycles. Biol Reprod 1982; 27: 383.

57. Takeo C, Negishi E, Nakajima A, Ueno K. Association of cytosine-adenine repeat polymorphism of the ERα gene with menopausal symptoms. Gend Med 2005; 2: 96–105.

58. Thung PJ. Ageing changes in the ovary. In: Bourne J, ed. Structural Aspects of Aging. New York: Hafner 1961: 109.

59. Mattingly RF, Huang WY. Steroidogenesis of the menopausal and postmenopausal ovary. Am J Obstet Gynecol 1969; 103: 679.

60. Vermeulen A. The hormonal activity of the postmenopausal ovary. J Clin Endocrinol Metab 1976; 42: 247.

61. Channing CP, Tsafriri A. Mechanism of action of luteinizing hormone and follicle stimulating hormone on the ovary in vitro. Metabolism 1977; 26: 413.

62. Hess GD, Roth GS. Receptors and aging. In Johnson JE, ed. Aging and Cell Functions. New York: Plenum Press 1985: 149–85.

63. Roth GS, Hess GD. Changes in the mechanisms of hormone and neurotransmitter action during aging: current status of the role of receptor and postreceptor alternatives. Mech Aging Dev 1982; 20: 175.

64. Cooper RL, Roberts B, Rogers DC, Seay SG, Conn PM. Endocrine status versus chronological age as predictors of altered LH secretion in the aging rat. Endocrinology 1984; 114: 391–6.

65. Cooper RL. Pharmacological and dietary manipulations of reproductive aging in the rat: significance to central nervous system aging. In: Cooper RL, Walker RF, eds. Experimental and Clinical Interventions in Aging. New York: Marcel Dekker 1983: 27–44.

66. Moudgil VK, Kanugro MS. Effect of age of rat on the induction of acetylcholinesterase of the brain by 17-beta estradiol. Biochim Biophys Acta 1973; 329: 211.

67. Krouse TB, Eskin BA, Mobini J. Age-related changes resembling fibrocystic disease in iodine-blocked rat breasts. Arch Pathol Lab Med 1979; 103: 631.

68. Schuit SC, de Jong FH, Stolk L, Koek WN. Estrogen receptor (ERα) gene polymorphisims are associated with estradiol levels in postmenopausal women. Eur J Endocrinol 2005; 153: 327–33.

69. Jensen EV, Suzuki T, Kawashina T. A two-step mechanism for the interaction of estradiol with rat uterus. Proc Natl Acad Sci USA 1968; 59: 632.

70. Shyamala G, Gorski J. Interrelationships of estrogen receptors in the nucleus and cytosol. J Cell Biol 1967; 35: 125A.

71. Mylonas I, Jeschke U, Shabani N et al. Immunohistochemical analysis of ERα, ERβ and progesterone receptor in normal human endometrium. Acta Histochemica 2004; 106: 245–52.

72. Jensen EV, Mohle S, Brecher PI, DeSombre ER. Estrogen receptor transformation and nuclear RNA synthesis. In: O'Malley BW, Means AR, eds. Receptors for Reproductive Hormones. New York: Plenum Press 1973. 122–36.

73. Gorski J. Evolution of a model of estrogen action. Rec Prog Horm Res 1986; 42: 297–9.

74. Anderson JN, Peck EJ, Clark JH. Estrogen-induced uterine responses and growth. Endocrinology 1975; 96: 160.

75. Roth GS. Effects of aging in the mechanisms of estrogen action in rat uterus. Adv Exp Med Biol 1986; 196: 347–60.

76. Little M, Szendro P, Teran C, Hughes A, Jungblut PW. Biosynthesis and transformation of microsomal and cytosol estradiol receptors. J Steroid Biochem 1975; 6: 493.

77. Clark JH, Peck EJ, Anderson JN. Nafoxidine, mode or action on estrogen receptor systems. Nature 1974; 251: 446.

78. McGuire WL, Carbone PP, Vollmer EP. Estrogen Receptors in Human Breast Cancer. New York: Raven Press 1975.

79. Lindner V, Kim SK, Karas RH. Increased expression of estrogen receptor beta in RNA in male blood vessels after vascular injury. Clin Res 1998; 83: 224–9.

80. Chan L, O'Malley BW. Mechanism of action of the sex steroid hormones. N Engl J Med 1976; 294: 1322.

81. Tchermitchin A, Tchermitchin X, Galand P. Correlation of estrogen-induced uterine eosinophilia with other parameters of estrogen stimulation produced with estradiol and estriol. Experimentia 1975; 31: 993.

82. Roth GS, Adelman RV. Age related changes in hormone binding by target cells and tissues: possible role in altered adaptive responsiveness. Exp Gerontol 1975; 10: 1.

83. Snyder DL, Johnson DM, Eskin BA et al. Effect of age on cardiac norepinephrine release in female rats. Aging Clin Exp Res 1995; 7: 210–17.

84. Roth GS. Hormone receptor changes during adulthood and senescence: significance for aging research. Fed Proc 1979; 38: 910.

85. Roth GS, Livingston JN. Reductions in glucocorticoid inhibition of glucose oxidation and presumptive glucocorticoid receptor content in rat adiposities during aging. Endocrinology 1976; 99: 831.

86. Eskin BA, Sparks CE, LaMont BI. The intracellular metabolism of iodine in carcinogenesis. Biol Trace Elem Res 1979; 1: 101.

87. Eskin BA, Jacobson HI, Bolmarich V, Murray JA. Breast atypia in altered thyroid states: intracellular changes. Senologia 1977; 4: 114.

88. Eskin BA, Mitchell MA, Modhera PR. Mammary gland hormone receptors in iodine deficiency. Proc Endocrinol Soc 1985; 67: 24.

89. Eskin BA. Iodine and breast cancer: an update 1982. Biol Trace Elem Res 1983; 5: 399.

90. Eskin BA, Stoddard II F, Brooks AD. Microarray characterization of iodine metabolic pathways in breast cancer. Proceedings of the International Thyroid Conference. Thyroid 2005; 15 (Suppl 1): S179–S180.

91. Gosden RG. Uptakes and metabolism in vivo of tritiated estradiol-17 beta in tissue of aging female mice. J Endocrinol 1976; 68: 153.

92. Nelson JF, Holinka CF, Finch CE. Loss of cytoplasmic estradiol binding capacity during aging in uteri of 57/6 mice. Proc Endocrinol Soc 1976; 58: 349.

93. Kublickiene K, Svedas E, Landgren BM et al. Small artery endothelial dysfunction in postmenopausal women. J Clin Endocrinol Metab 2005; 90: 6113–22.

94. Grodstein F, Stampfer M. The epidemiology of coronary heart disease and estrogen replacement in postmenopausal women. Prog Cardiovasc Dis 1995; 38: 199–210.

95. Hulley S, Grady D. Bush T et al. Randomized trial of estrogen plus progesterone for secondary prevention of coronary heart disease in postmenopausal women. J Am Med Assoc 1992; 280: 605–13.

96. Eskin BA, Snyder DL, Gayheart P, Roberts J. The protective effect of estrogen on the cardiac adrenergic nervous system. In: Roberts J, Cardiovascular Disease in Women. Dallas: American Heart Association, 1997: 23–30.

97. Martino M, Eskin BA. Estrogen and the postmenopausal heart: advances in protection. Female Patient 1999; 24: 19–28.

98. Eskin BA. Sex hormones and aging. In: Roberts J, Adelman RC, Cristofalo VJ, eds. Pharmacologic Interventions in the Aging Process. New York: Plenum Press 1978: 207–24.

99. Yen SSC, Tsai CC, Naftolin F, Vandenburg G, Ajabor L. Pulsatile patterns in gonadotropin release in subjects with or without ovarian function. J Clin Endocrinol Metab 1972; 34: 671.

# Chapter 2

# The demographics of aging women

Miguel Paniagua and Bruce R Troen

## INTRODUCTION

A demographic revolution is occurring that will change the landscape of healthcare. The growth in numbers of people aged 65 years and older is greater than that of the general population, and the most rapid increase is occurring in the group aged 85 years and above, the so-called 'oldest old'. This pattern will be maintained and even accelerate in the next 35 years. Today, one out of every ten persons in the US is 60 years or older; by 2050, one out of five will be 60 years or older. Those 85 years and over currently make up 11% of the 60 and over age group and will grow to 19% by 2050. The ramifications of such a population shift are profound, and will force us to reassess our notions of 'old age' and the approach to delivering medical care to these individuals. This will be especially important for women, who comprise a significant majority of those aged 65 years and older. Until recently, the phases of maturity for a woman comprised childbearing age (premenopausal), followed by the menopause (or a perimenopausal period), and ending in a postmenopausal state. It is now clear that the term 'postmenopausal' insufficiently describes the years following menopause. Instead, the postmenopausal period is more the penultimate stage of life, and is increasingly often the prelude to a prolonged epoch for many women – the geripause. In order to provide the best possible care, we must approach the geripausal patient in a manner that recognizes that the patient's physiology and response to stress and illness are markedly different than at earlier times in life.

## DEMOGRAPHY

The average/median life span (also known as life expectancy) is represented by the age at which 50% of a given population survives, and maximum life span potential (MLSP) represents the longest-lived member(s) of the population or species. The average life span of humans has increased dramatically over time, yet the MLSP has remained approximately constant, and is usually stated to be 90 to 100 years.[1] For 99% of our existence as a species, the average life expectancy for humans was very short compared to the present. During the Bronze Age (circa 3000 BC), the average life expectancy was 18 years due to disease and accidents. Average life expectancy in 275 BC was still only 26 years. By 1900 improved sanitation helped to improve the average life expectancy at birth for humans to 47 years, but infectious disease was still a major killer. As of 2002, better diet, health care, and reduced infant mortality had resulted in an average life expectancy of 77.3 years.[2] These trends are reflected in dramatic difference in the survival curves for women in the US from 1901 and 1998 (Figure 2.1).[3] The increase in the average life expectancy has resulted in a compression of morbidity and mortality (a rectangularization of the survival curve) towards the end of the lifespan (Figure 2.1). Evidence for the continuation of this trend is the increase in life expectancy at the age of 65 by 3.3 years since 1960.[4] Life expectancy at birth in Japan and Singapore has reached 80 years, the highest level of all the world's major countries, and has reached 79 years in several other developed nations (e.g. Australia, Canada, Italy, Iceland, Sweden, and Switzerland). Levels for the US and most other developed countries fall into the 76–78

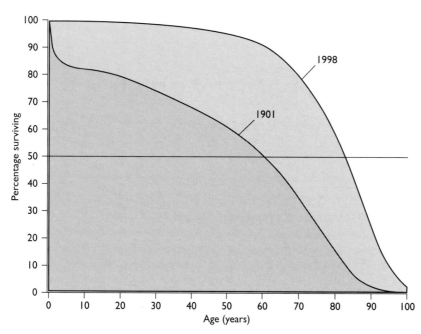

**Figure 2.1** Percentage survival curve for females in the US in 1901 and 1998. The 50% survival values have improved, but maximum life span potential has remained the same. The data from 1901 refer to white females. (Reproduced from Kinsella and Velkoff. In: US Bureau of the Census. Series P95/01-1. Washington DC: US Government Printing Office, 2001.[3])

year range (Figure 2.2). Of note, the longest-lived human for whom documentation exists was Jeanne Calment, who died at the age of 122 in August 1997. The longest-lived male was Christian Mortensen, who died in 1998 at the age of 115. As causes of early mortality have been eliminated through public health measures and improved medical care, more individuals have approached the maximum life span. Between 1960 and 1994, the population of those aged 85 years and over grew by 274%, whereas the elderly population in general rose 100% and the entire US population grew only 45%.[5] Of note, life expectancy at birth in the US varies depending upon gender and race; in 2002 it was 80.3 years for white females, 75.6 years for black females, 75.1 years for white males, and 68.8 years for black males (Figure 2.3). The widening of the sex differential in life expectancy has been a central feature of mortality trends in developed countries in the 20th century. In 1900, in Europe and North America, women typically outlived men by two or three years. Today, the average gap between the sexes is roughly 7 years, but exceeds 12 years in parts of the former Soviet Union, as a result of the unusually high levels of male mortality (Figure 2.4). Of note, the difference in life expectancy between males and females in the US has gradually declined during the past three decades (Figure 2.5), and the difference between white and black individuals has resumed its decline since a widening in

the gap between 1982 and 1989 (Figure 2.5). Continued increases in life expectancy in the next century, the greater life expectancy for women, and the tendency for women to marry men older than they are lead to the projection that 70% of 'baby boom' women will outlive their husbands and can expect to be widows for 15 or more years.

In 2000, there were an estimated 35 million people age 65 years or older in the US, accounting for almost 13% of the total population. The number of older Americans has increased more than ten-fold since 1900, when there were 3 million people age 65 years or older (4% of the total population). Despite the growth of the older population, the US is a relatively young country when compared with other developed nations. In many industrialized countries, older persons account for 15% or more of the total population.[3] As in most countries of the world, there are more older women than older men in the US, and the proportion of the population that is female increases with age. In 2000, women were estimated to account for 58% of the population aged 65 and older, and 70% of the population aged 85 and older.[6] Similarly, the number of centenarians will increase 15-fold, from approximately 145 000 in 1999 to 2.2 million by 2050. The disparity between sexes is also evident in sex ratios as we age. There are approximately 83 males per 100 females in the age group 65 to 74 years. This ratio decreases to 46 per 100 in the age group

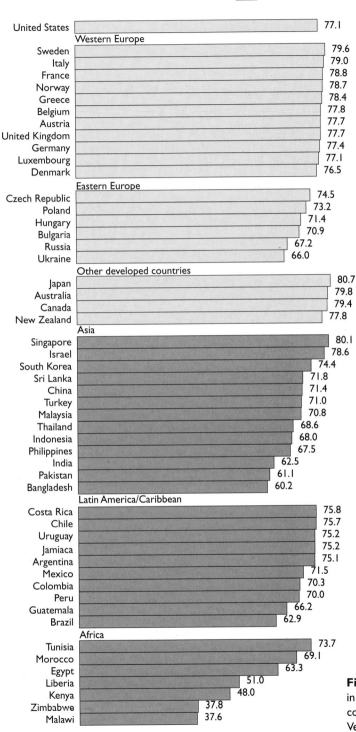

**Figure 2.2** Life expectancy at birth (2000), in years, in developed and developing countries. (Reproduced from Kinsella and Velkoff. In: US Bureau of the Census. Series P95/01-1. Washington DC: US Government Printing Office, 2001.[3])

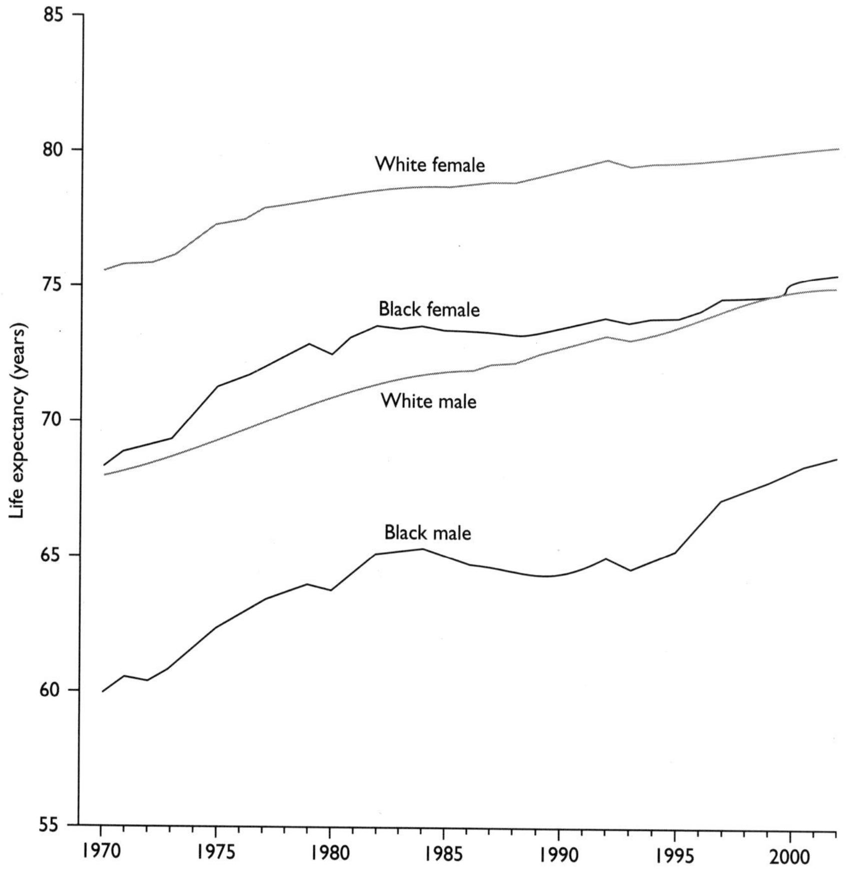

**Figure 2.3** Life expectancy at birth in the US as a function of sex and race. (Reproduced from Kochanek KD et al. National Vital Statistics Report 2004; 53(5): 1–115.[2])

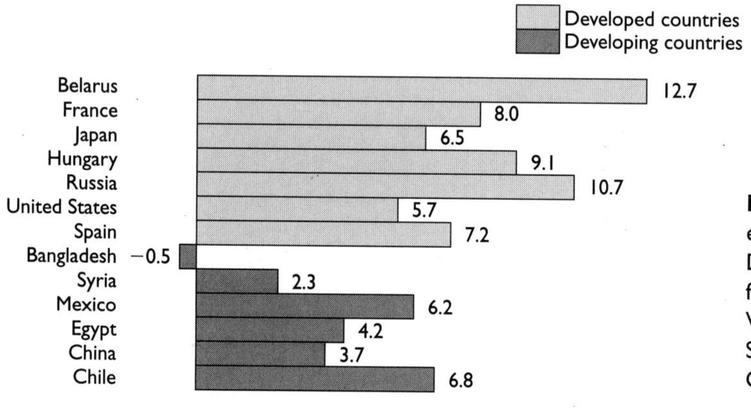

**Figure 2.4** Female advantage in life expectancy at birth in the year 2000. Differences in years between males and females. (Reproduced from Kinsella and Velkoff. In: US Bureau of the Census. Series P95/01-1. Washington DC: US Government Printing Office, 2001.[3])

over 85 years. It stands to reason that women aged 65 years and older are four times as likely to be widowed as their male counterparts. The older population will continue to grow significantly in the upcoming decades (Figure 2.6). Growth slowed during the 1990s because of the relatively small number born during the Great Depression of the 1930s. By 2010, the first group of 'baby boomers' will reach the age of 65 years. Consequently, between 2010 and 2030, the older population will mushroom.[7] Between now and 2030, the number of people aged 65 and older will double and account for 20% of the population. By 2050 almost 25% of the elderly will be 85 years and

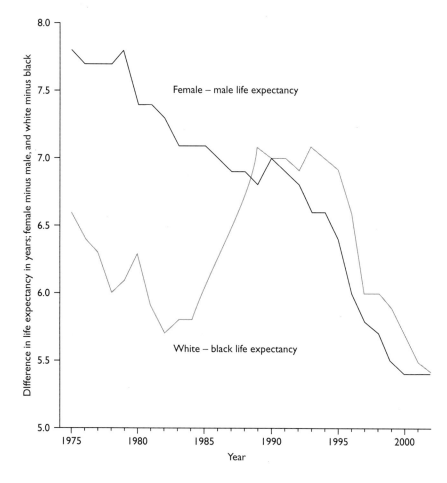

**Figure 2.5** Differences in life expectancy between females and males and between white and black individuals in the US, 1975–2002. (Reproduced from Sahyoun NR et al. Aging Trends 2001(1): 1–10.[30])

older. One can appreciate further the increasing longevity of those who reach the age of 65 by considering the following: 14% of 65 year olds in 1960 were expected to reach the age of 90, 26% of 65 year olds in 2000 will be expected to reach the age of 90, and 42% of 65 year olds in 2050 will probably live to the age of 90.[4]

This is not a phenomenon unique to the US, as the entire world's elderly population is projected to grow considerably in both absolute and relative terms. By 2050, the world's elderly will comprise nearly 17% of the global population, as compared to only 7% in 2002. The effect in underdeveloped nations could be profound, in that they may have less time to adapt to the consequences of continued rapid population aging than developed nations.

## NORMAL AGING

There is evidence supporting at least five common characteristics of aging:

1. *increased mortality with age after maturation.* In the early 19th century, Gompertz first described the exponential increase in mortality with aging due to various causes, a phenomenon that still pertains today.[8] In 1995, the death rate for all causes between the ages of 25 and 44 years was 189.5/100 000, and for the ages of 65 years and over was 5069.0/100 000: a more than 25-fold increase[9]

2. *changes in biochemical composition in tissues with age.* There are notable age-related decreases in lean body mass and total bone mass in humans.[10,11] Although subcutaneous fat is unchanged or declining, total fat remains the

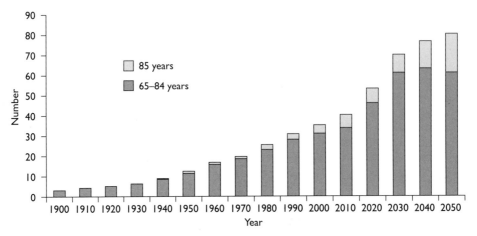

**Figure 2.6**   Number of persons aged 65 years or over, 1900 to 2050 (numbers in millions). (Data taken from Hobbs and Damon. In: US Bureau of the Census, Current Population Report. Washington DC: US Government Printing Office, 1996; P23–190.[4])

same.[10] Consequently, the percentage of adipose tissue increases with age. At the cellular level, many markers of aging have been described in various tissues from different organisms.[12] Two of the first to be described were increases in lipofuscin (age pigment),[13] and increased cross-linking in extracellular matrix molecules such as collagen.[14,15] Additional examples include age-related changes in both the rates of transcription of specific genes and the rate of protein synthesis and numerous age-related alterations in post-translational protein modifications, such as glycation and oxidation.[16,17]

3. *progressive decrease in physiological capacity with age.* Many physiological changes have been documented in both cross-sectional and longitudinal studies.[18–20] Declines in various organ systems include: cardiac output and heart rate in response to stress, peripheral blood vessel compliance, bone mineral density, cartilaginous resiliency, creatinine clearance, renal blood flow, maximum urine osmolality, forced vital capacity and expiratory volume, maximal oxygen uptake, intestinal motility, visual accommodation and acuity, color sensitivity, depth perception, high-frequency perception, speech discrimination, T-cell immune response, total sleep time and time in REM sleep, and psychomotor performance. These decreases occur linearly from about the age of 30 years, however the rate of physiological decline is quite heterogeneous from organ to organ and individual to individual.[21,22] As

described in detail elsewhere in this book, women experience a dramatic decline in estrogen at the time of the menopause. Growing evidence suggests that testosterone, dehydroepiandrosterone, and growth hormone levels also decline with age.[23]

4. *reduced ability to respond adaptively to environmental stimuli with age.* A fundamental feature of senescence is the diminished ability to maintain homeostasis.[24] This is manifest, not primarily by changes in resting or basal parameters, but in the altered response to an external stimulus such as exercise or fasting. The loss of 'reserve' can result in blunted maximum responses, as well as in delays in reaching peak levels and in returning to basal levels. For example, the responses of heart rate and cardiac output to exercise and sympathetic nervous system stimulation are significantly reduced in the elderly.[25]

5. *increased susceptibility and vulnerability to disease.* The incidence and mortality rates for many diseases increase with age and parallel the exponential increase in mortality with age.[26] For the five leading causes of death for people over 65 years, the relative increase in death rates compared to people aged 25–44 years is: heart disease – 92-fold, cancer – 43-fold, stroke – >100-fold, chronic lung disease – >100-fold, and pneumonia and influenza – 89-fold.[9] The basis for these dramatic rises in mortality is incompletely understood, but presumably involves changes in the function of many types of

cells that lead to tissue/organ dysfunction and systemic illness.

## HEALTH STATUS

Increasing age is accompanied by poorer health, as manifested by higher disease rates and increasing levels of frailty and disability. More than a quarter of those over 65 years categorize their own health as fair or poor.[27] The leading causes of death in the elderly are listed in Table 2.1. Cardiovascular disease caused the most deaths in this age group in 1996. Cancer was responsible for the second highest number of deaths. Given the growth of the elderly population, the number of incident cancers is projected to more than double in the first part of this century.[28] The leading causes of death among the elderly as reported in 2002 continued to be heart disease, followed by cancer, stroke, chronic lower respiratory diseases, influenza and pneumonia, and diabetes.[29] Alzheimer's disease is a more prominent cause of death in women, particularly those aged 85 years and over (Table 2.2). Among elderly women, chronic bronchitis, emphysema, and other chronic respiratory conditions especially increased.[30] Interestingly, age-adjusted death rates for all causes of death in people aged 65 years and over declined by 12% between 1981 and 2001.[2] Notably, death rates for diseases of vascular origin, such as heart disease and stroke, declined by one-third,

whereas death rates due to diabetes and chronic lower respiratory diseases increased by 43% and 62% respectively.[2] When considering that multiple causes may contribute to death, diabetes, chronic obstructive pulmonary disease, and atherosclerosis are much more likely to to be identified as a comorbid condition at the time of death.[30]

Most people over 65 years report at least one chronic ailment, including (in descending prevalence) arthritis, hypertension, heart disease, diminished hearing, cataracts, orthopedic impairment, sinusitis, and diabetes (Table 2.3). Cerebrovascular disease rates quadruple, heart disease rates triple, and arthritis and hypertension rates double between the perimenopausal era (45–64 years) and the geripause ≥65 years). Women suffer from higher rates of arthritis and hypertension, whereas men have higher rates of heart disease and hearing impairment. These trends and gender differences persist in self-reported conditions by those aged 65 and older (Figure 2.7). Several conditions that do not explicitly appear in Table 2.3 merit mention. There are more than 1.3 million osteoporotic fractures a year in the US, including 500 000 in the spine, 250 000 in the hip, and 240 000 in the wrist.[31] This results in significant morbidity (manifest often in decreased mobility) and economic cost. Up to 50% of women above the age of 50 years are osteopenic, and 18% are frankly osteoporotic.[32] One-third of all women and one-sixth of all men who reach the age of 90 years suffer a hip fracture;

| Cause | All people % | All people Rate[a] | Men % | Men Rate[a] | Women % | Women Rate[a] |
|---|---|---|---|---|---|---|
| Cardiovascular | 35.7 | 1808 | 35.2 | 1983 | 36.2 | 1686 |
| Cancer | 22.3 | 1131 | 25.6 | 1442 | 19.6 | 915 |
| Cerebrovascular | 8.2 | 415 | 6.6 | 374 | 9.5 | 443 |
| COPD[b] and allied conditions | 5.3 | 270 | 6.0 | 338 | 4.8 | 223 |
| Pneumonia and influenza | 4.4 | 221 | 4.2 | 236 | 4.5 | 212 |
| Diabetes | 2.7 | 137 | 2.5 | 139 | 2.9 | 136 |
| Accidents and adverse effects | 1.8 | 91 | 1.9 | 110 | 1.7 | 78 |
| Alzheimer's disease | 1.3 | 62 | 0.9 | 49 | 1.5 | 71 |
| Renal | 1.2 | 62 | 1.2 | 70 | 1.2 | 56 |
| Septicemia | 1.0 | 51 | 0.9 | 50 | 1.1 | 52 |

**Table 2.1**  Leading causes of death in people 65 years and over in the US in 1996

[a]Rate per 100 000 population. Adapted from Peters KD et al. National Vital Statistics Report 1998; 47.[49]
[b]COPD: chronic obstructive pulmonary disease.

**Table 2.2**   Leading causes of death among people in the US in 2001

| People aged 65 years and over | | People aged 85 years and over | |
| --- | --- | --- | --- |
| **Men** | **Women** | **Men** | **Women** |
| Heart disease | Heart disease | Heart disease | Heart disease |
| Malignant neoplasms | Malignant neoplasms | Malignant neoplasms | Cerebrovascular disease |
| Cerebrovascular disease | Cerebrovascular disease | Cerebrovascular disease | Malignant neoplasms |
| Chronic lower respiratory diseases | Chronic lower respiratory diseases | Chronic lower respiratory diseases | Alzheimer's disease |
| Influenza and pneumonia | Alzheimer's disease | Influenza and pneumonia | Influenza and pneumonia |
| Diabetes mellitus | Influenza and pneumonia | Alzheimer's disease | Chronic lower respiratory diseases |
| Accidents | Diabetes mellitus | Renal disease | Diabetes |
| Alzheimer's disease | Renal disease | Accidents | Renal disease |
| Renal disease | Accidents | Diabetes | Accidents |
| Septicemia | Septicemia | Pneumonitis due to solids and liquids | Septicemia |

Data taken from Statistics FIFoA-R. Washington DC: US Government Printing Office, 2004.[29]

**Table 2.3**   Chronic conditions by age in the United States in 1996[a]

| Condition | All 45–64 years | All ≥65 years | Male ≥65 years | Female ≥65 years |
| --- | --- | --- | --- | --- |
| Arthritis | 233 | 490 | 405 | 550 |
| Hypertension | 223 | 403 | 349 | 442 |
| Heart disease | 121 | 308 | 367 | 224 |
| Hearing impairment | 145 | 284 | 362 | 268 |
| Deformity/orthopedic impairment | 176 | 178 | 166 | 187 |
| Chronic sinusitis | 179 | 153 | 135 | 167 |
| Diabetes mellitus | 64 | 126 | 124 | 128 |
| Cerebrovascular disease | 15 | 71 | 80 | 65 |

[a]Rates given are conditions/1000 persons.
Data from Benson and Marano. National Center for Health Statistics, Vital Health and Statistics 1998; 10(199).[27]

26% of hospital discharges for hip fracture in 1994 were for men.[32] Urinary incontinence affects 15–30% of community-dwelling elderly, and up to 50% of those in long-term care facilities.[33] Perimenopausal-aged women experience more stress incontinence, whereas urge and mixed incontinence predominate in the elderly.[34] Incontinence is associated with isolation, depression, and the risk of institutionalization. Dementia is one of the most common causes of disability in the elderly. More than 25% those aged 85 years, and more than 50% of those aged 95 years and over suffer dementia.[35] Alzheimer's disease accounts for two-thirds or more of dementia, with a prevalence in community dwellers of 10% of those over 65 years and 47% of those older than 85.[36] Because women have a longer life expectancy, they experience a higher rate of dementia. It is interesting to note that outpatient screening for breast and cervical cancer is decreased in women with a higher number of chronic conditions.[37]

Frailty in the elderly has a distinct phenotype that includes unexplained weight loss, exhaustion, weak grip, slow walking speed, and low energy.[38] Of those aged 65 years and older living alone, 7% had at least three criteria for frailty,

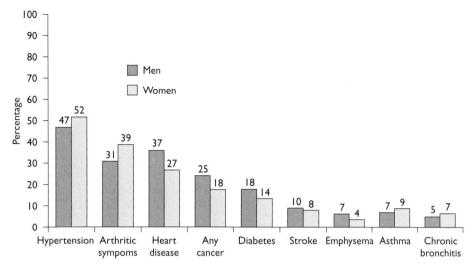

**Figure 2.7**  Percentage of people aged 65 years and over who reported selected chronic conditions, 2001–2002. (Adapted from Statistics FIFoA-R. Washington DC: US Government Printing Office, 2004.[29])

while 46% had none. Women, African-Americans, people aged 75 years and older, the less educated, and the poor are more likely to be frail. The most common coexisting illnesses in the frail include arthritis, hypertension, and diabetes. Over a period of three years, frail elderly suffered more falls, worsening mobility and disability, hospitalization, and, most importantly, death. After seven years, 43% of those who were frail died, compared to 12% of those who had no initial indicators of frailty. Increasing numbers of studies now show that frail elders are more likely to suffer prolonged or repeated hospitalizations, and undergo protracted or limited recovery.[39] Triggers for such events often include multiple co-morbid conditions, and possibly a fall and/or fracture. In one cohort study of 558 community-dwelling older women with at least moderate disability, physical decline was associated with increasing age, nonwhite race, former smoking, abnormal baseline walking speed, and instrumental activities of daily living (IADL) impairment. Cognitive decline was associated with age and baseline mini-mental status examination score. Combined cognitive and physical decline was associated with age, baseline walking speed, mini-mental status examination score, IADL impairment, as well as current smoking (odds ratio (OR) = 5.66) and hemoglobin level (OR = 0.68). This may represent potentially modifiable risk factors in those women at risk for cognitive and functional decline.[40] The loss of homeostatic reserve (including increased reaction

time, decreased strength, decreased vision) and the presence of osteoporosis and/or polypharmacy probably play important roles in worsening the outcomes of acute illness in the frail elderly. Fortunately, knowledge of the phenotype of frailty will hopefully permit the development of better assessment tools and interventions to enhance the health of frail elders.

Many of the elderly suffer from multiple conditions, and these restrict the activities of older people. Over 50% of those aged 65 years and older reported at least one disability, with one-third experiencing severe disabilities. According to the 2003 National Health Interview Survey (NHIS), about 34 million persons (12%) were limited in their usual activities due to one or more chronic health conditions, and about 4 million persons (2%) required the help of another person with activities of daily living (ADL).[41] Women spend approximately twice as many years disabled prior to death as their male counterparts.[42] With increasing age, disabilities and difficulties performing ADLs and instrumental activities of daily living (IADL) become more prevalent (Figure 2.8). ADL include bathing, dressing, eating, and ambulation.[43] IADL include meal preparation, shopping, managing money, using the telephone, doing housework and laundry, ability to travel, and taking medication.[44] It is important to note, however, that over 70% of people aged 65 years and over-report their health status as good, very good, or excellent, despite the prevalence of chronic conditions in this group.[27] In a study of 5395 Canadians aged 65 years and older, 4.6% reported using a wheelchair, and older adults who reported greater dependence in basic self-care and IADL were more likely to use a wheelchair. However, the effects of self-care dependence on wheelchair use varied by gender, with men being more likely than women to use wheelchairs with increasing self-care dependence. The number of chronic health conditions and being unmarried also increased the odds of wheelchair use.[45] Despite the prevalence of chronic conditions and increasing disability, more than 90% of the elderly live in the community, and 75% of those aged 85 years and older still live at home.

## CONCLUSION

As described above, the number of people aged 65 years and older will continue to dramatically increase well into the next century. The physiology of the elderly and their response to pathology markedly differ from younger individuals, espe-

cially women who are premenopausal and perimenopausal. Furthermore, the most explosive growth will occur in the group of people aged 85 years and older. We are beginning to learn that these 'old' old may represent a distinct subgroup in the elderly population. Indeed, in the not too distant future, we may use the term 'elderly' to refer to those aged 85 years and over. Despite the prevalence of chronic illness and the rapid age-related increase in mortality in those aged 65 years and over, there is some evidence to suggest that future cohorts may be healthier. Manton et al. report that age-related disability declined between 1982 and 1994.[46] In addition, since 1953, Americans have engaged in healthier behaviors: per capita tobacco consumption has declined by 40%, butter consumption is down by one-third, use of whole milk and cream is down 25% and the use of saturated animal fats in cooking is down 40%.[47] It is possible that such behaviors, often associated with the 'baby boomers' as they have matured, may reduce future rates of chronic diseases. These changes, along with advances in health care, may continue to fuel the increase in life expectancies that has been driving the rectangularization of the survivorship curve. It is unknown what impact there will be on health care utilization. It also stands to reason that despite the higher life expectancy in women versus men, the unfortunate trade-off may be more years at the end of life spent in disability, and perhaps in institutional care. At the very least, it has become increasingly clear that the demographic shift towards a progressively aged and aging population will necessitate that providers pay more and more attention to maintaining and enhancing the health and quality of life of the elderly.

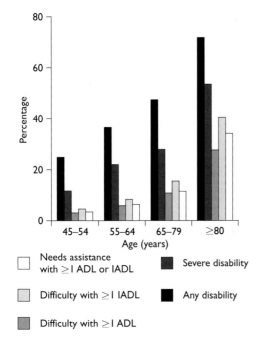

**Figure 2.8** Disability prevalence with age. (Data from McNeil J. Population Reports 1997; P70–61.[48])

## REFERENCES

1. Cutler RG. Evolutionary perspective of human longevity. In: Hazzard WR, Andres R, Bierman EL et al., eds. Principles of Geriatric Medicine and Gerontology, 2nd edn. New York: McGraw-Hill, 1985; 16.
2. Kochanek KD, Murphy SL, Anderson RN, Scott C. Deaths: Final Data for 2002. National Vital Statistics Report 2004; 53(5): 1–115.
3. Kinsella K, Velkoff VA. An Aging World: 2001. In: US Bureau of the Census. Series P95/01-1. Washington DC: US Government Printing Office, 2001.
4. Hobbs FB, Damon BL. 65+ in the United States. In: US Bureau of the Census, Current Population Report.

Washington DC: US Government Printing Office, 1996; P23–190.

5. Sixty-Five Plus in the United States. US Bureau of the Census, Statistical Brief. Washington DC: US Government Printing Office, 1995; 95(8).

6. Projections of the Total Resident Population by 5-Year Age Groups, and Sex with Special Age Categories: Middle Series, 1999 to 2000. In: US Bureau of the Census, Population Projections Program PD. Washington DC: US Government Printing Office, 2000; 202–33.

7. Day JC. Population Projections of the United States by Age, Sex, Race, and Hispanic Origin: 1995 to 2050. US Bureau of the Census, Current Population Reports. Washington DC: US Government Printing Office, 1996; P25–1130.

8. Gompertz B. On the nature of the function expressive of the law of human mortality and on a new mode of determining life contingencies. Philos Trans R Soc Lond B Biol Sci 1825; 115: 513.

9. Rosenberg HM, Ventura SJ, Maurer JD et al. Births and deaths: United States, 1995. Monthly Vital Statistics Report 1996; 45 (3(S2): 31–3.

10. Shock NW, Greulich RC, Andres R et al. Normal Human Aging: The Baltimore Longitudinal Study of Aging. Washington, DC: US Department of Health and Human Services, 1984.

11. Riggs BL, Melton LD. Involutional osteoporosis. N Engl J Med 1986; 314: 1676–86.

12. Florini JR, ed. Composition and function of cells and tissues. Handbook of Biolochemistry in Aging. Boca Raton: CRC Press, 1981.

13. Strehler BL. Time, Cells, and Aging, 2ne edn. New York: Academic Press, 1977.

14. Bjorksten J. Cross linkage and the aging process. In: Rothstein M, ed. Theoretical Aspects of Aging. New York: Academic Press, 1974; 43.

15. Kohn RR. Aging of animals: possible mechanisms. In: Principles of Mammalian Aging, 2nd edn, Kohn RR, ed. Englewood Cliffs, NJ: Prentice-Hall, 1978.

16. Finch CE. Introduction: Definitions and concepts. In: Longevity, Senescence, and the Genome, Finch CE, ed. Chicago: University of Chicago Press, 1990, 3–42.

17. Levine RL, Stadtman ER. Protein Modifications with Aging. In: Schneider EL, Rowe JW, eds. Handbook of the Biology of Aging, 4th edn. San Diego: Academic Press, 1996; 184–97.

18. Shock NW. Longitudinal studies of aging in humans. In: Finch CE, Schneider EL, eds. Handbook of the Biology of Aging, 2nd edn. New York: Van Nostrand Reinhold, 1985; 721.

19. Kane RL, Ouslander JG, Abrass IB. Clinical Implications of the Aging Process. Essentials of Clinical Geriatrics, 4th edn. New York: McGraw-Hill Health Professions Division, 1999; 3–18.

20. Taffet GE. Age-Related Physiologic Changes. In: Cobbs EL, Duthie EH, Murphy JB, eds. Geriatric Review Syllabus, 4th edn. Dubuque, Iowa: Kendall/Hunt Publishing Company, 1999; 10–23.

21. Lakatta EG. Changes in cardiovascular function with aging. Eur Heart J 1990; 11 (Suppl C): 22–9.

22. Lindeman RD, Tobin J, Shock NW. Longitudinal studies on the rate of decline in renal function with age. J Am Geriatr Soc 1985; 33: 278–85.

23. Roshan S, Nader S, Orlander P. Review: ageing and hormones. Eur J Clin Invest 1999; 29: 210–3.

24. Adelman RC, Britton GW, Rotenberg S et al. Endocrine regulation of gene activity in aging animals of different genotypes. In: Bergsma D, Harrison DE, eds. Genetic Effects on Aging. New York: Alan R Liss, 1978; 355.

25. Lakatta EG. Cardiovascular aging research: the next horizons. J Am Geriatr Soc 1999; 47: 613–25.

26. Brody JA, Brock DB: Epidemiological and statistical characteristics of the United States elderly population. In: Finch CE, Schneider EL, eds. Handbook of the Biology of Aging, 2nd edn. New York: Van Nostrand Reinhold, 1985; 3.

27. Benson V, Marano MA. Current Estimates from the National Health Interview Survey, 1995. Hyattsville, MD: National Center for Health Statistics, Vital Health and Statistics 1998; 10(199).

28. Polednak AP. Projected numbers of cancers diagnosed in the US elderly population, 1990 through 2030. Am J Public Health 1994; 84: 1313–16.

29. Older Americans 2004: Key Indicators of Well-Being, November 2004. Appendix A. In: Statistics FIFoA-R. Washington DC: US Government Printing Office, 2004.

30. Sahyoun NR, Lentzner H, Hoyert D, Robinson KN. Trends in causes of death among the elderly. Aging Trends 2001(1): 1–10.

31. Christiansen C. Consensus development conference: diagnosis, prophylaxis, and treatment of osteoporosis. Am J Med 1993; 94: 646–50.

32. Looker AC, Orwoll ES, Johnston CC Jr et al. Prevalence of low femoral bone density in older US adults from NHANES III [see comments]. J Bone Miner Res 1997; 12: 1761–8.

33. Resnick NM. Urinary incontinence. Lancet 1995; 346: 94–9.

34. Thom D. Variation in estimates of urinary incontinence prevalence in the community: effects of differences in definition, population characteristics, and study type. J Am Geriatr Soc 1998; 46: 473–80.

35. Ebly EM, Parhad IM, Hogan DB, Fung TS. Prevalence and types of dementia in the very old: results from the Canadian Study of Health and Aging [see comments]. Neurology 1994; 44: 1593–600.

36. Evans DA, Funkenstein HH, Albert MS et al. Prevalence of Alzheimer's disease in a community population of older persons. Higher than previously reported [see comments]. JAMA 1989; 262(18): 2551–6.

37. Kiefe CI, Funkhouser E, Fouad MN, May DS. Chronic disease as a barrier to breast and cervical cancer screening [see comments]. J Gen Intern Med 1998; 13: 357–65.

38. Fried LP, Tangen CM, Walston J et al. Frailty in older adults: evidence for a phenotype. J Gerontol A Biol Sci Med Sci 2001; 56: M146–56.

39. Perry HM 3rd. The endocrinology of aging. Clin Chem 1999; 45(8 Pt 2): 1369–76.
40. Atkinson HH, Cesari M, Kritchevsky SB et al. Predictors of combined cognitive and physical decline. J Am Geriatr Soc 2005; 53(7): 1197–202.
41. Schiller JS, Adams PF, Nelson ZC. Summary health statistics for the US population: National Health Interview Survey, 2003. Vital Health Stat 2005; 10(224): 1–104.
42. La Croix AZ, Newton KM, Leveille SG, Wallace J. Healthy aging. A women's issue. West J Med 1997; 167: 220–32.
43. Katz S, Downs TD, Cash HR, Grotz RC. Progress in development of the index of ADL. Gerontologist 1970; 10: 20–30.
44. Lawton MP, Brody EM. Assessment of older people: self-maintaining and instrumental activities of daily living. Gerontologist 1969; 9: 179–86.
45. Clarke P, Colantonio A. Wheelchair use among community-dwelling older adults: prevalence and risk factors in a national sample. Can J Aging 2005; 24: 191–8.
46. Manton KG, Stallard E, Corder LS. The dynamics of dimensions of age-related disability 1982 to 1994 in the U.S. elderly population. J Gerontol A Biol Sci Med Sci 1998; 53: B59–70.
47. Longino CF. Myths of An Aging America. American Demographics, August 1994, 36–42.
48. McNeil J. Americans with Disabilities: 1994–1995. Current Population Reports 1997. Washington DC: US Department of Commerce, Bureau of the Census, 1997, 70–61.
49. Peters KD, Kochanek KD, Murphy SL. Deaths: Final Data for 1996, National Vital Statistics Report 1998; 47.

# Chapter 3

# Pathology of the menopause

Debra S Heller

## INTRODUCTION

Menopause is defined as the permanent cessation of menses due to loss of ovarian follicular activity. A woman is considered menopausal when she has not had a menstrual period for a year. The perimenopausal period, when ovarian function declines, generally extends for 2–8 years prior to, and one year after, the last menstrual period. The median age of menopause in the US is 51 years.[1] At the turn of the 19th century, female life expectancy coincided with the menopause. In the 21st century, many women live more than one-third of their lives after the menopause.[2] It is predicted that over 50 million women in the US will be postmenopausal after the year 2000.[3] Apart from natural menopause, many women experience surgical menopause. During this period, many changes occur in a woman's body. This chapter reviews pathology associated with menopause.

## THE FEMALE REPRODUCTIVE TRACT

Some of the most profound physical changes at menopause occur in the reproductive tract. Estrogen deficiency, aging, previous birth trauma and genetics play roles in the physiological changes and potential disease states of the menopause. In one two-year study of gynecological admissions, 10.04% of the women were postmenopausal.[4] The most common diagnoses were postmenopausal bleeding (32.72%) due either to atrophy or hyperplasia in almost equal proportion, vaginoperineal lacerations with cystorectocele, with or without incontinence (10.9%), cancer (11.21%; of these 25.45% were endometrial or ovarian), benign ovarian cysts (11.21%), uterine

prolapse (9.3%), endometrial polyps (9.09%), leiomyomata (3.93%), and cervical cancer (3.93%). The most common category was uterine pathology (68.78%), followed by ovarian pathology (15.15%), prolapse-related (10.9%), vulvar (2.72%) and vaginal (1.51%).

### The vulva

Changes in the vulva are related to age and estrogen deficiency. There is a decrease in the number and coarsening of the texture of the pubic hair, as the hair follicles age. The labia majora decrease in size, with loss of elastic and fatty subcutaneous tissue. Histologically, there is thinning of the epidermis and dermis.[5] Vulvar conditions seen with increasing frequency in this age group include the non-neoplastic epithelial disorders lichen sclerosus, and squamous cell hyperplasia. Paget's disease of the vulva and squamous cell carcinoma are also more common in postmenopausal women. Any suspicious lesion of the vulva must be biopsied.

The non-neoplastic epithelial disorders of the vulva, according to the International Society for the Study of Vulvovaginal Diseases (ISSVD), comprise lichen sclerosus, squamous cell hyperplasia, and others. These conditions often present with pruritus. Lichen sclerosus leads to gross thinning and whitening of the vulva, with narrowing of the introitus. Histologically, there is loss of rete pegs, thinning of the epithelium, and a zone of dermal homogenization with variable chronic inflammation (Figure 3.1). Squamous hyperplasia may be secondary to an uninterrupted itch–scratch cycle. Histologically, there is hyperkeratosis, acanthosis and chronic inflammation. Both conditions are often treated with topical steroids.

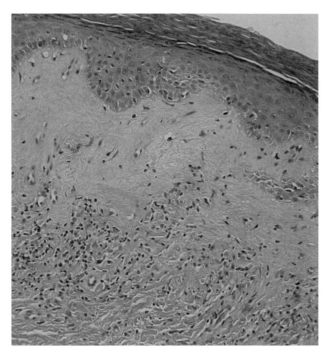

**Figure 3.1** Lichen sclerosus: there is thinning of the epithelium, with flattening of the rete pegs, dermal homogenization, and hyperkeratosis. Dermal inflammation is variable.

Paget's disease of the vulva is most often an in situ lesion. It may be associated with underlying adenocarcinoma in the vulva, as well as extragenital carcinomas, and these should be searched for. Grossly, the vulva appears red and velvety, with white patches. Histologically, the large Paget cells can be seen at the dermal–epidermal junction, percolating up (Figure 3.2). Excision is the treatment of choice; however, the lesion tends to recur, possibly because of the microscopic margins often extending beyond the grossly visible ones.

The most common malignancy of the vulva is squamous cell carcinoma (Figure 3.3). While the incidence is increasing in the premenopausal age group in association with human papillomavirus, the majority of cases are still seen in elderly women. Recent advances in surgical therapy, with separate vulvar and groin incisions, has led to decreased postoperative morbidity in these women.

### The vagina

With estrogen deficiency the vagina shortens, with loss of rugae, and becomes pale and friable. There is loss of elasticity. Atrophy of the Bartholin's glands contributes to decreased lubrication. Dyspareunia may be a problem.

Histologically, loss of glycogen and flattening of the epithelium can be noted. The loss of glycogen leads to decreased Döderlein bacilli with their production of lactic acid. This leads to an alkaline pH, which predisposes to atrophic vaginitis.[5] Overgrowth of enteric bacteria at this pH also predisposes to urinary tract infections.[6] Although no longer much utilized in clinical practice, with sensitive blood tests available, some indication of estrogen deficiency in the region can be obtained by determining a maturation index. Vaginal symptoms do not necessarily correlate with the index. A swab taken from the lateral vaginal wall is examined in the cytology laboratory, and the number and maturation of the cells is evaluated. There are three types of squamous cells potentially present in the vagina: superficial cells, intermediate cells, and parabasal cells. In cycling women, the superficial and intermediate cells predominate. With estrogen deficiency, there is a shift towards intermediate and parabasal cells. The index is reported as the proportions of 100 cells counted in terms of parabasal-intermediate-superficial. A cycling woman will have superficial and intermediate cells in varying proportions, while postmenopausal smears are more likely to contain intermediate and parabasal cells (Figure 3.4). It should be noted that the ratios are variable for all age groups, and cannot be relied upon in the face of inflammation.

Loss of pelvic fascial support is multifactorial, and relates to estrogen, genetics, parity, birth

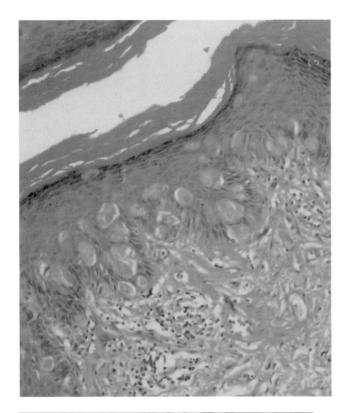

**Figure 3.2**  Paget's disease of the vulva: the large pale Paget cells are seen at the dermal–epidermal junction, and percolating up the epithelium.

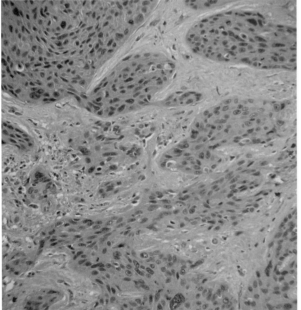

**Figure 3.3**  Squamous cell carcinoma of the vulva: this keratinizing tumor infiltrates in characteristic nests.

trauma and conditions of excess intra-abdominal pressure such as obesity, chronic obstructive pulmonary disease (COPD) and constipation. In addition, skeletal muscle is replaced by fat and connective tissue with aging, contributing to the loss of pelvic support.[5] Women may experience cystoceles, rectoceles, enteroceles and uterine prolapse. Stress incontinence may accompany these changes. Estrogen therapy may be utilized to prepare the vaginal mucosa for reparative surgery.

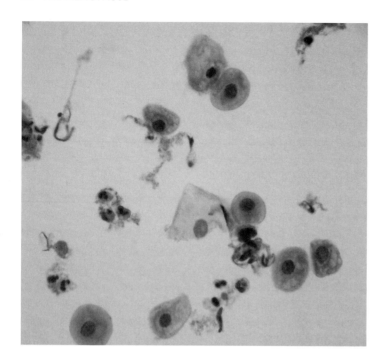

**Figure 3.4** A menopausal Pap smear containing abundant parabasal cells.

Sufficient estrogen may be absorbed to stimulate the previously atrophic endometrium.

Primary vaginal squamous cell carcinoma does occur in postmenopausal women; however, a primary vulvar or cervical carcinoma with vaginal spread must be considered first.

## The cervix

With menopause, the cervix decreases in size, with decreased stroma and epithelial atrophy, and may become flush with the vaginal vault.[5] The squamocolumnar junction tends to move upwards, making colposcopic evaluation for neoplastic and preneoplastic disease more difficult. Cervical stenosis may occur, and may lead to pyometra or hematometra. The cervix may show erosion: the loss of superficial epithelial layers, or true ulceration with loss of epithelium and formation of granulation tissue. Cervical ectropion, the presence of endocervix on the portio, may be seen secondary to bilateral lacerations at childbirth.[5]

Many squamous cell carcinomas that occur in the cervix are seen in postmenopausal women. Many women with cervical cancer have not received a Pap smear for several years prior to diagnosis. It is critical for postmenopausal women to continue to receive gynecological care. Grossly, squamous cell carcinoma of the cervix may be exophytic or endophytic. Histological appearance is similar to squamous cell carcinomas arising elsewhere. Adenocarcinomas of the endocervix may also be seen in perimenopausal women.

## The endometrium

In one study of 801 perimenopausal and postmenopausal women screened prior to estrogen replacement therapy, there was one carcinoma (0.13%), four atypias (0.63%), 373 cases of atrophic endometrium (46.9%), 133 proliferative endometria (16.7%), 54 secretory endometria (6.8%), 41 hyperplasias (5.2%), and 195 specimens of tissue insufficient for diagnosis (24.5%).[7] The sampling instrument was not described. These authors concluded that screening biopsy of asymptomatic women was not justifiable. In another study, 68% of endometrial samples prior to hormone replacement therapy (HRT) were atrophic, 23.5% proliferative, 0.5% secretory, 0.6% hyperplastic, 0.07% carcinoma, and 6.6% insufficient tissue.[8] Biopsies were performed with a Vabra aspirator. Forty-six cases (1.6%) had polyps, which may be missed by in-office sampling. The authors felt that the low cancer yield reflected the younger patients in this group: most were 45–55 years. They also concluded that a biopsy was not necessary in asymptomatic women prior to instituting HRT.

In the untreated menopausal woman, the endometrium is often thin and inactive. It is easily inflamed, and this may lead to bleeding. All post-menopausal bleeding must be investigated to rule out carcinoma; however, in many cases the bleeding is due to atrophy. In a literature review, the most common pathological diagnoses on endometrial sampling performed for postmenopausal bleeding were carcinoma, polyp, pyometra, atrophy, proliferative endometrium, secretory endometrium, hyperplasia, and insufficient tissue.[4]

A large number of postmenopausal women will be treated with tamoxifen for breast cancer. Tamoxifen, while utilized for its antiestrogenic activity in the breast, exerts a weak estrogenic effect on the postmenopausal uterus. Endometrial polyps, hyperplasias, carcinomas and other conditions associated with estrogen may be seen in the uterus. Malignant mixed mesodermal tumors and sarcomas are also increased.[9] The literature has been somewhat controversial as to whether tamoxifen-associated uterine malignancies are of low- or high-risk types. Screening for uterine disease in women taking tamoxifen has included transvaginal ultrasound and biopsy. Many women are currently followed with ultrasound, with biopsy reserved for bleeding.[10]

Endometrial sampling performed in-office often produces a scant specimen in postmenopausal women. The clinician may be under the impression that a sample is abundant when most of the aspirated material is actually blood. While the majority of these cases are due to atrophy, it is up to the clinician to determine whether scant tissue in the sample signifies scant tissue in the uterus, or insufficient sampling. A normal variant of atrophy, cystic atrophy, can be distinguished from simple hyperplasia by the flattened epithelium of the glands in the former.

Endometrial polyps often occur in the perimenopausal and postmenopausal woman. Endometrial polyps have a surface lining, are polypoid in shape, and contain irregular glands in a fibrotic stroma. The stalk contains thick blood vessels. Polyps may be fragmented during removal, and difficult to diagnose histologically with certainty. The polyps seen in association with tamoxifen tend to be large, multiple, and with a very fibrotic stroma, although this is not pathognomonic.

Owing to the unopposed estrogen associated with anovulation in the perimenopausal period, endometrial hyperstimulation can occur. Some postmenopausal women also have excess endogenous estrogen, particularly if obese, or in the case of an estrogen-secreting ovarian neoplasm. The endometrium may initially show disordered proliferation, with occasional cystic glands in a proliferative background, insufficient for a diagnosis of hyperplasia. Endometrial hyperplasia is classified by architecture and the presence or absence of cytological atypia. Simple hyperplasia consists of a mild increase in the gland/stroma ratio, while complex hyperplasia shows greater crowding, still with intervening stroma. Either may occur with or without cytological atypia. Simple hyperplasia with atypia is unusual, so many pathologists shorten the diagnoses to simple, complex or atypical (complex with atypia) hyperplasia. It has been shown that only complex hyperplasia with atypia poses a significant risk of development of endometrial carcinoma.[11] A concurrent unsampled carcinoma may also be present when an endometrial biopsy shows atypical hyperplasia.[12] There is interpathologist variability in the diagnosis of endometrial hyperplasia, and recent studies have suggested an alternate way to histologically detect precancerous endometrial lesions. Studies have shown that the loss of *PTEN* tumor suppressor gene function, which can be demonstrated by loss of immunohistochemical staining, is characteristic of most endometrial cancers and precancers, although PTEN-negative glands may be seen admixed with positive ones in normal endometrium as well.[13] When a monoclonal proliferation of these PTEN-negative glands occurs, Mutter terms these lesions endometrial intraepithelial neoplasia (EIN), and describes the morphology of these precancerous lesions as having a volume percentage stroma of <55%.[14]

Endometrial carcinoma may actually arise by two pathogenic disease mechanisms. Estrogen-related neoplasms tend to be well differentiated, less aggressive endometrioid carcinomas (Figure 3.5), occurring in younger, heavier women, as opposed to the more aggressive non-estrogen-related neoplasms, uterine papillary serous (Figure 3.6), and clear-cell carcinoma, which are more likely to occur in the older, thinner patient. Malignant mixed mesodermal tumors also tend to occur in the older postmenopausal patient. For the usual endometrioid endometrial carcinoma confined to the uterus, prognosis relates to tumor grade and depth of invasion, and the pathologist may be called upon to perform an intraoperative consultation to assess depth of invasion.

Endometrial biopsies from women experiencing abnormal bleeding while on HRT are often

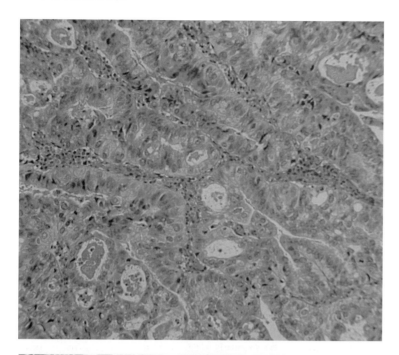

**Figure 3.5**  Well-differentiated (International Federation of Gynecology and Obstetrics (FIGO) grade 1) endometrial adenocarcinoma, showing back-to-back glands with no intervening stroma.

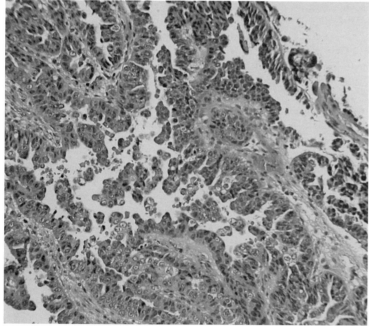

**Figure 3.6**  Uterine (papillary) serous carcinoma: note the papillary configuration and marked cytological atypia.

received by the pathology laboratory. Many times, a history of hormonal therapy is not given, and is important for accurate evaluation. Patterns seen reflect the therapy effect as well as the underlying hormonal milieu of the woman. Atrophic, and normal proliferative and secretory patterns are sometimes seen, as are the occasional hyperplasia or carcinoma. Sometimes an irregular pattern of mixed proliferative and secretory changes is seen. If the history is known to the pathologist, the diagnosis can state that the irregular pattern is consistent with HRT. On occasion, these mixed patterns do show worrisome glandular crowding, suggestive of an excess estrogen effect.

## The myometrium

The myometrium is also an estrogen target tissue. The size of the uterus decreases with the menopause, bringing the corpus/cervix ratio from 2:1 to 1:1. Uterine weight decreases from an average of 100 g down to 50–60 g, and may be as low as 25–30 g. Uterine fibroids decrease in size, and may show hyalinization and calcification.[5] Uterine vessels often show atherosclerotic changes.

## The Fallopian tube

The Fallopian tubes are estrogen target tissues. At menopause, there is atrophy of epithelium and muscle, with a decrease in tubal length and diameter.[5] It has been shown that Fallopian tube epithelial atrophy mimics endometrial changes in the postmenopausal woman not on HRT.[15]

## The ovary

During the fifth month of fetal life, there are approximately 6–7 million oogonia present, with 1–2 million germ cells at birth, and 300 000 at puberty. By three years after the menopause, there is virtual depletion of germ cells.[16] The menopausal ovary decreases in size. The stroma becomes fibrotic, the surface cerebriform. There is depletion of primordial follicles, and the ovary is peppered with corpora albicans. Stromal hyperthecosis, a hyperplastic change consisting of nests of luteinized stromal cells, may occasionally occur in the postmenopausal woman. These ovaries appear enlarged and yellow on cut section, and masculinization of the patient due to hyperandrogenism as a result of the production of androstenedione may lead the clinician to suspect a masculinizing neoplasm. Aromatization of the androstenedione in the patient's adipose tissue may lead to increased production of estrone and hyperestrogenic effects as well.

The risk of ovarian cancer increases with age. Unfortunately, the majority of ovarian carcinomas are diagnosed at an advanced stage, owing to lack of early symptomatology. No efficient mass screening method yet exists. In one study, screening was performed initially by transvaginal ultrasound, followed by CA-125, pelvic examination and exploratory laparotomy after two abnormal transvaginal ultrasonic studies.[17] A few early cancers were detected. However, widespread screening for ovarian carcinoma has not been shown to be cost-effective.

Ovarian neoplasms are divided into those of surface epithelial origin, those of stromal origin, and those of germ cell origin. Germ cell tumors are usually seen in younger patients, and are not further considered here. Among epithelial neoplasms, the most common are benign serous cystadenomas and cystadenofibromas. The most common type of ovarian carcinoma seen is the papillary serous cystadenocarcinoma, which is histologically similar to uterine papillary serous carcinoma. Endometrioid carcinoma of the ovary, which resembles endometrial carcinoma histologically, is almost as common. Stromal tumors of the ovary occurring commonly in the postmenopausal woman include the benign fibrothecoma and the granulosa cell tumor, which is a slow-growing but malignant neoplasm. Both may produce estrogen, which can lead to endometrial hyperstimulation and subsequent pathology.

## THE GENITOURINARY SYSTEM (BLADDER/URETHRA)

Urogenital mucosal atrophic changes are due to a combination of age and estrogen deficiency. The proximal urethra, lined by squamous epithelium, undergoes atrophy with estrogen deficiency. Urethral caruncles, ectropion of the mucosa, may occur. The trigone also has estrogen receptors. The risk of urinary outflow obstruction increases with age, because of possible narrowing of the distal urethra. Thus, menopausal women are at increased risk of atrophic trigonitis and the urethral syndrome, with urgency, burning, hesitancy, frequency and nocturia. Stress and urge incontinence can occur. Urinary symptoms may relate to a combination of atrophy, prolapse, susceptibility to infection, decreased bladder capacity, increased intra-abdominal pressure, genetics, and superimposed conditions such as congestive heart failure, diabetes and neurological impairment.[5,6]

## BONE

Approximately 1.5 million fractures per year are attributable to osteoporosis (Figure 3.7) in the US. With osteoporosis comes increased risk of vertebral, wrist and hip fractures. Two-thirds of these patients are women.[18] Bone loss starts at around age 30 years, and accelerates after the menopause.[19] There is a ten-fold increase in bone loss for about 10 years after loss of ovarian function. The rate of

Colles' fractures increases ten-fold from age 35 to 60 years. Hip fractures are the 12th leading cause of female death,[20] with up to 20% of hip fracture patients dying within a year of the injury.[18] Biochemical markers of bone turnover are increased with menopause.[1] The risk of osteoporosis increases owing to a variety of factors at the menopause, some related to estrogen deficiency, some to aging. These include low calcium intake, early menopause, family history, increasing age, lack of exercise, nulliparity, cigarettes and alcohol, thinness and small bones, and White or Asian race.[21]

## THE CARDIOVASCULAR SYSTEM

Cardiovascular risk after the menopause is associated with less favorable lipid and coagulation profiles, changes in vascular reactivity and other tissue effects.[22] Although many women fear death by cancer the most, the fact is that cardiovascular disease is the leading cause of death in women (Figure 3.8). Heart disease deaths in women are 10 times as frequent as breast cancer deaths.[20] Heart disease accounts for over 50% of postmenopausal deaths, and morbidity and mortality are greater in women.[3] Some evidence suggests that the risk of heart disease is even greater with surgical than

with natural menopause.[16] This may be due to the longer hypoestrogenic state.

## THE CENTRAL NERVOUS SYSTEM

Alzheimer's disease, a condition strongly affected by genetics, may also be influenced by the hormonal state of menopause.[23] It has been suggested that estrogen may work by improving blood flow and stimulating neurons, and may interact with genetic factors.[24] Alzheimer's disease is characterized histologically by neuritic plaques with deposition of β-amyloid in the plaques and cerebral blood vessels, and the development of neurofibrillary tangles. There are pronounced neurochemical deficits.[24]

## THE SKIN

Collagen synthesis and maturation are stimulated by estrogen.[1] In one study, postmenopausal women taking HRT were shown to have increased skin thickness and sebum production, compared to a group not taking HRT.[25] Pierard and colleagues have also suggested that HRT has beneficial effects on some mechanical properties of skin, and may slow intrinsic cutaneous aging.[26]

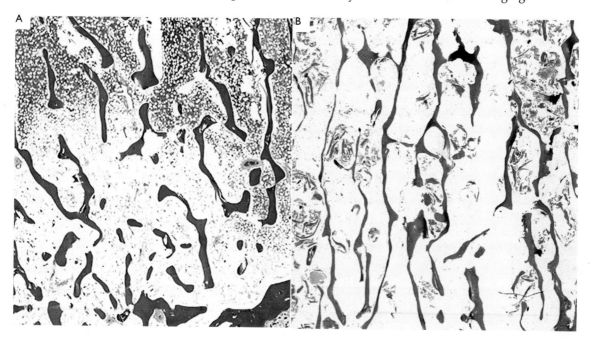

**Figure 3.7** Osteoporosis: note the normal bone on the left (A), and the decreased bone density of the osteoporotic bone on the right (B).

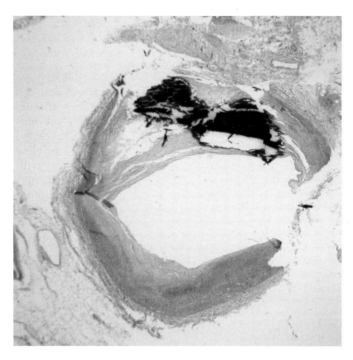

**Figure 3.8**  Atherosclerosis: a coronary artery branch shows luminal narrowing.

## THE BREAST

There is a decrease in the size of the glands and subcutaneous fat of the breast, as well as a loss of elasticity of Cooper's ligament, leading to a change of shape, with flattening.[5,27] Nipples become smaller and flatter, and lose their erectile properties. The risk of breast cancer increases, with most cases occurring after the menopause.[28] There is an approximately 8% overall lifetime risk of breast cancer, which increases with age (Figure 3.9).

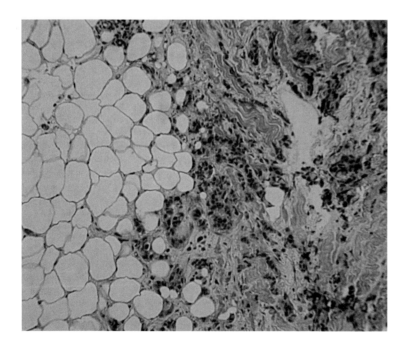

**Figure 3.9**  Infiltrating duct carcinoma of the breast.

# REFERENCES

1. Greendale GA, Sowers M. The menopause transition. Endocrinol Metab Clin North Am 1997; 26: 261–77.
2. Wich BK, Carnes M. Menopause and the aging female reproductive system [Review]. Endocrinol Metab Clin North Am 1995; 24: 273–95.
3. Villablanca A. Coronary heart disease in women. Gender differences and effects of menopause [Review]. Postgrad Med 1996; 100: 191–6.
4. Pepe F, Panella M, Pepe G et al. Current aspects of gynecological pathology in postmenopause. Clin Exp Obstet Gynecol 1988; 15: 80–3.
5. Brown KH, Hammond CB. Urogenital atrophy. Obstet Gynecol Clin North Am 1987; 14: 13–32.
6. Schaffe J, Fantl JA. Urogenital effects of the menopause. Baillière's Clin Obstet Gynaecol 1996; 10: 401–17.
7. Archer DF, McIntyre-Seltman K, Wilborn WW Jr et al. Endometrial morphology in asymptomatic postmenopausal women. Am J Obstet Gynecol 1991; 165: 317–20.
8. Korhonen MO, Symons JP, Hyde BM et al. Histologic classification and pathologic findings for endometrial biopsy specimens obtained from 2964 perimenopausal and postmenopausal women undergoing screening for continuous hormones as replacement therapy. Am J Obstet Gynecol 1997; 176: 377–80.
9. Cohen I. Endometrial pathologies associated with postmenopausal tamoxifen treatment. Gynecol Oncol 2004; 94: 356–66.
10. Barakat RR. Tamoxifen and the endometrium. Cancer Treat Res 1998; 94: 195–207.
11. Kurman RJ, Kaminski PF, Norris HJ. The behavior of endometrial hyperplasia. A long-term study of 'untreated' hyperplasia in 170 patients. Cancer 1985; 56: 403–12.
12. Bilgin T, Ozuysal S, Ozan H, Atakan T. Coexisting endometrial cancer in patients with a preoperative diagnosis of atypical endometrial hyperplasia. J Obstet Gynaecol Res 2004; 30: 205–9.
13. Zheng W, Baker HE, Mutter GL. Involution of PTEN-null glands with progestin therapy. Gynecol Oncol 2004; 92: 1008–13.
14. Mutter GL. Histopathology of genetically defined endometrial precancers. Int J Gynecol Pathol 2000; 19: 301–9.
15. Amso NN, Crow J, Lewin J et al. A comparative morphological and ultrastructural study of endometrial gland and fallopian tube epithelia at different stages of the menstrual cycle and menopause. Hum Reprod 1994; 9: 2234–41.
16. Richardson SJ. The biological history of menopause. Baillière's Clin Endocrinol Metab 1993; 7: 1–16.
17. DePriest PD, van Nagell JR Jr, Gallion HH et al. Ovarian cancer screening in asymptomatic postmenopausal women. Gynecol Oncol 1993; 51: 205–9.
18. Agarwal SK, Judd HL. Menopause. Curr Ther Endocrinol Metab 1997; 6: 624–31.
19. Heersche JN, Bellows CG, Ishida Y. The decrease in bone mass associated with aging and menopause [Review]. J Prosth Dent 1998; 79: 14–16.
20. Smith RP. Modern menopause management. Curr Opin Obstet Gynecol 1994; 6: 495–8.
21. Kain CD, Reilly N, Schultz ED. The older adult. A comparative assessment. Nurs Clin North Am 1990; 25: 833–48.
22. Prelevic GM, Jacobs HS. Menopause and postmenopause. Baillière's Clin Endocrinol Metab 1997; 11: 311–40.
23. Massart F, Reginster JY, Brandi ML. Genetics of menopause-associated diseases. Maturitas 2001; 40: 103–11.
24. van Duijn CM. Menopause and the brain. J Psychosom Obstet Gynecol 1997; 18: 121–5.
25. Callens A, Vaillant L, LeCompte P et al. Does hormonal skin aging exist? A study of the influence of different hormone therapy regimens on the skin of postmenopausal women using non-invasive measurement techniques. Dermatology 1996; 193: 289–94.
26. Pierard GE, Letawe C, Dowlati A et al. Effects of hormonal replacement therapy for menopause on the mechanical properties of skin. J Am Geriatr Soc 1995; 43: 662–5.
27. Utian WH. The fate of the untreated menopause. Obstet Gynecol Clin North Am 1987; 14: 1–11.
28. Wren BG. The breast and the menopause. Baillière's Clin Obstet Gynaecol 1996; 10: 433–47.

# Chapter 4

# Genetic and genomic factors in the menopause

Lee P Shulman

## INTRODUCTION

The onset of menopause, along with all its associated symptoms and conditions, appears to be directly related to the diminution in circulating estradiol. However, the timing, extent and impact of menopause are not solely related to this eventual loss of ability to produce physiologic levels of sex steroids. The cause of the loss of endogenous estradiol in women who undergo ovarian extirpative procedures is clear; however, the gradual decrease and eventual loss of physiological levels of estradiol that characterizes the reproductive years appears to be the result of the gradual loss and eventual exhaustion of the ovarian follicle pool.[1] This process begins in utero as maximum follicular complement (millions) occurs during fetal life with reduction continuing until natural menopause when only a few (several hundred) follicles remain. As so few follicles are able to maintain normal menstrual activity, the age of the onset of natural menopause appears to be related to both the initial number of follicles and the rate of follicular decline.

Genetic and environmental factors are clearly integral to this process. Indeed, nuclear,[2] as well as mitochondrial genes,[3] appear to have important roles in the timing and extent of this ongoing follicle loss process. In addition, environmental factors including drugs may adversely impact genetic mechanisms associated with a variety of organic functions,[4,5] some of which are associated with menopause and menopause-related outcomes.

In order to better understand menopause and its impact on women, it is necessary to understand all the processes that lead to its onset and presentation. The delineation of exact mechanisms, genes and environmental factors associated with the onset of non-premature natural menopause is not yet available. What is known is that the genetic and genomic processes are major determinants of the onset and presentation of menopause,[2,6] and that the recognition and delineation of these genetic and genomic contributions to menopause are vital to better understanding the pathophysiology of menopause and thus to develop effective preventive and therapeutic modalities.[7]

It is also clear that genetic and genomic factors impact many of the disease states that characterize the menopausal years, including cancer, cardiovascular disease and depression among other menopause-related health and lifestyle conditions. This chapter will not attempt to undertake an examination of such an enormous wealth of information and ongoing study. Rather, it will present a review of the genetic and genomic impact on the onset and presentation of menopause, including premature ovarian failure. Although the role of genetics and genomics is critical to the pathophysiology of menopause-related morbidities and mortalities, and menopause-specific genes probably affect some of these disease processes, our current understanding of such complex gene interactions is 'embryonic' in nature, and thus not amenable to a review. This chapter will thus present our current understanding of the genetic role in premature ovarian failure and menopause, and review the role of counseling for affected women and their families.

## PREMATURE OVARIAN FAILURE

Premature ovarian failure (POF) is defined as a lack of ovulation, with reduced serum sex steroid levels, and elevated gonadotropin levels occurring before the age of 40 years.[8] Ovarian failure leads to a constellation of health and lifestyle issues including menopause, reduced libido, osteoporosis, urogenital atrophy, and infertility. Autosomal genes and sex chromosome aberrations are known to cause POF, as well as environmental factors that lead to ovarian dysfunction and adversely affect the production of ovarian sex steroids.

Whether a woman is believed to have POF as result of inability to conceive, or changes in menstrual activities or the presentation of menopause-like symptoms attributable to ovarian failure and the subsequent reduction in serum sex steroid levels, counseling and genetic testing are warranted, and an important part of the evaluation of such women. POF can result from the following genetic etiologies:

- X chromosome abnormalities and translocations;
- Autosomal chromosome translocations;
- Autosomal recessive disorders;
- Autosomal dominant disorders.

Because of the wide variety of etiologies of POF, a thorough personal and family history along with a detailed physical examination should be the first step in the diagnostic process. The presence of similarly affected relatives as well as other somatic abnormalities can provide critical information concerning the etiology of POF. For example, the finding of several females within a family with POF can indicate a potential autosomal recessive form of POF, whereas mild stigmata associated with Turner's syndrome can be suggestive of a mosaic or non-mosaic X chromosome etiology for the POF.

## X chromosome abnormalities and translocations

Many X chromosome deletions result in a Turner syndrome-like presentation with primary amenorrhea and incomplete or absent secondary sexual development. Spontaneous menstruation occurs in approximately 50% of women with a 46,X,del(X)(p11) and in most women with 46,X,del(X)p21 or distal deletions. However, among those with spontaneous menstruation, most will develop secondary amenorrhea and POF.[9,10] Most deletions involving the long arm of the X chromosome also lead to infertility and ovarian failure, with more proximal deletions tending to lead to more severe clinical presentations than the more distal deletions.[11] Indeed, translocations and deletions from Xq21 to Xq26 are more likely to be associated with POF than complete ovarian failure.[12] X:autosome translocations can lead to a wide spectrum of abnormality ranging from complete ovarian failure to POF. Severity of symptoms is related to the X chromosome breakpoints as well as the non-translocated X chromosome that is more likely to be inactivated, as inactivating the translocated X chromosome would also inacitivate the autosome involved in the translocation, leading to a de facto unbalanced autosomal complement and a marked increased risk for considerable developmental and anatomical abnormality or lethality.[13,14]

In addition, fragile X (FMR1) premutation carriers are at increased risk of developing POF, with 2–4% of women with POF being premutation carriers. In families of women with POF, the risk of a woman with POF being in the premutation range can be as high as 15%.[15]

## Autosomal chromosome translocations

Balanced autosomal translocations can also be associated with POF.[16] According to, the probable etiology for the POF is meiotic breakdown secondary to failure of synapsis resulting from the translocated chromosomes.[12] Once counseling has been provided, chromosome analysis should be the initial genetic test offered to individuals with signs and symptoms of POF. A normal outcome should be followed by a FMR1 gene assay to determine whether the woman is a premutation carrier.

## Autosomal recessive disorders

Autosomal XX gonadal dygenesis genes are probably responsible for some familial presentations of POF. In such cases, siblings demonstrate a spectrum of ovarian abnormalities from complete failure to POF, all with normal cytogenetic outcomes. Aittomaki and colleagues showed that an FSH receptor (FSHR) mutation could result in complete ovarian failure in one sibling and POF in another.[17] In women with POF who have affected first-degree relatives with premature reduction or absence of ovarian function, with normal chromosomes and no evidence of environmental disruption of ovarian function (e.g. chemotherapy), consideration of an autosomal recessive condition as an etiology for the POF is warranted.

## Autosomal dominant disorders

Autosomal dominant heritability in women with POF who have a normal chromosome complement and a family history of multigenerational affected women has been considered a likely etiology for POF, and thus could explain a new onset of POF as a new mutation dominant condition. A recent study by Vegetti and colleagues (1998) details an analysis of 71 women with POF, normal chromosome analyses and no other known cause for POF.[18] This study found that 22, or 31%, of the probands had other affected relatives. Another study by Vegetti and colleagues (2000) of an expanded sample of similarly affected women found that 29% had affected relatives.[19] Assessment of these familial aggregates showed inheritance patterns consistent with autosomal dominant and X-linked dominant heritability. Such epidemiological evidence may correlate well with molecular studies seeking to identify genes associated with POF.

In contradistinction to the current role of genetic counseling and testing in the clinical management of many gynecological conditions, genetic counseling and testing has a central role in the evaluation of women with POF. A considerable percentage of affected women will be found to have a genetic cause for POF, with chromosome aberrations being the most likely finding in such women. Even among women who are not found to have a detectable genetic cause, the delineation of a heritability pattern and the counseling process itself may provide valuable information for the patient and her family members.

## MENOPAUSE

There is great variability in the age of onset of natural menopause, ranging from the early 40s through the early 60s, with the mean age of onset of natural menopause among women in the US being in the early 50s.[2,20–22] Early onset of menopause is associated with a variety of postmenopausal health problems and a higher risk of mortality resulting from the premature exposure to low levels of estrogens and other ovarian sex steroids. Indeed, it is estimated that deaths from cardiovascular disease fall by 2% for each year that menopause is delayed.[23] Lifestyle factors play an important role in the onset and impact of menopause, with smoking, alcohol, and breastfeeding associated with an earlier onset of menopause,[21–23] and body mass index and oral contraceptive use inversely related to early menopause.

Although the role of heritable factors in the age of onset of menopause has long been discussed, it was Cramer and colleagues in 1995 who suggested that familial or heritable factors were a component of the determination of the age of onset of menopause.[24] Murabito and colleagues report that at least 50% of inter-individual variability in the onset of menopause is attributable to genetic factors, with hertiability accounting for 74% of the variation in menopause onset in the original cohort, and 45% among offspring of the original cohort.[25] Other studies have found similar outcomes. van Asselt and colleagues found that heritability accounted for approximately 44% of the age of menopause,[26] and Kok and colleagues similarly estimated that genetic factors were the main source of variation in the age of onset of menopause.[2]

As with other phenotypic or disease-specific analyses, twin studies are valuable in determining the role, if any, of genetics in the expression of the particular feature or condition. Sneider and colleagues found that the age of onset of menopause was approximately 63% due to heritable factors rather than environmental factors or chance,[27] whereas Treloar and colleagues found heritability to be responsible for 31% to 53% of the age of onset of menopause.[28] de Bruin and colleagues found the highest heritability estimates, with a value of 0.85–0.87 for singleton sisters, and 0.71–0.72 for twins.[1]

As opposed to the occasionally distinctive heritability patterns observed with POF, the lack of a specific heritability pattern associated with the age of menopause is strongly suggestive of an independent contribution of multiple genes to the varying ages of menopausal onset. Indeed, in the analysis of traits in which the variation is predominantly genetically determined, it is assumed that numerous genes make independent and additive contributions to the variation.[1] In addition, as progression through the reproductive years and into menopause is also associated with reducing fertility and increasing risks for a variety of conditions including cancer and cardiovascular disease, it is quite possible that some of the genes that are eventually found to be associated with the onset of menopause may also be associated with reproductive failure, or with the development of a variety of age-related morbidities. With the almost universal acceptance of the important role of genetics and genomics in the determination of the onset and extent of menopause, the identification of those genes and proteins that impact menopause should now proceed. To this end, Murabito and colleagues have recently reported the initial identification of novel loci suggestive for linkage to the age of menopause.[29] Further research will be needed to identify unique and specific genes associated with the onset of menopause and its impact on morbidity and mortality.

Whether the genes that are ultimately found to be associated with the onset of menopause are nuclear or mitochondrial, are unique to the menopausal process, or associated with fertility or other health-related concerns, it is clear that these genes play an important role in determining the age of menopause and thus its impact on the health, quality of life, and longevity of each woman. Whereas health care providers must remain diligent in encouraging women to change those lifestyle issues such as smoking and excessive alcohol consumption that are associated with early menopause, the recognition of genetic and genomic influences and the eventual detection of specific genes and proteins will probably provide considerably more information that will allow for more accurate and effective diagnostic and therapeutic modalities for menopausal women, and probably also for many more women with varied medical and health care problems.

## CONCLUSIONS

Although it is clear that genetics and genomics will probably provide more accurate information concerning the onset and health and lifestyle impact of menopause, advances in molecular technologies will surely provide new, novel and more effective therapeutic interventions to a wide variety of menopausal-related conditions. From advances in pharmacogenomics allowing for the production of more effective and safe pharmacological interventions,[30] to ongoing work in stem cell research that promises to change our entire approach to therapeutic intervention for a variety of conditions from cancer to cardiovascular disease,[31,32] our ability to prevent, detect and treat a wide variety of menopausal-related conditions is changing and will continue to do so, with the continuing incorporation of genetic and genomic information into clinical practice.

## REFERENCES

1. de Bruin JP, Bovenhuis H, van Noord PAH et al. The role of genetic factors in age at natural menopause. Hum Reprod 2001; 16: 2014–18.
2. Kok HS, van Asselt KM, van der Schouw YT et al. Genetic studies to identify genes underlying menopausal age. Hum Reprod Update 2005; 11: 483–93.
3. Jansen RP. Germline passage of mitochondria: quantitative considerations and possible embryological sequelae. Hum Reprod 2000; 15 (Suppl 2): 112–28.
4. Bosse R, Rivest R, Di Paolo T. Ovariectomy and estradiol treatment affect the dopamine transporter and its gene expression in the rat brain. Brain Res Mol Brain Res 1997; 46: 343–6.
5. Stopper H, Schmitt E, Kobras K. Genotoxicity of phytoestrogens. Mutat Res 2005; 574: 139–55.
6. Murabito JM, Yang Q, Fox C et al. Heritability of age at natural menopause in the Framingham Heart Study. J Clin Endocrinol Metab 2005; 90: 3427–30.
7. Shostak S. Locating gene-environment interaction: at the intersection of genetics and public health. Soc Sci Med 2003; 56: 2327–42.
8. Goswami D, Conway GS. Premature ovarian failure. Hum Reprod Update 2005; 11: 391–410.
9. Simpson JL, Rajkovic A. Ovarian differentiation and gonadal failure. Am J Med Genet 1999; 89: 186–200.
10. Panasiuk B, Usinskiene R, Kostyk E et al. Genetic counselling in carriers of reciprocal chromosomal translocations involving the short arm of chromosome X. Ann Genet 2004; 47: 11–28.
11. Layman LC. Genetic causes of infertility. Endocrinol Metab Clin North Am 2003; 32: 549–72.
12. Simpson JL, Elias S. Common gynecologic disorders. In: Genetics in Obstetrics and Gynecology, 3rd edn. Philadelphia: Saunders, 2003: 171–210.
13. Mumm S, Herrera L, Waeltz PW et al. X/autosomal translocations in the Xq critical region associated with premature ovarian failure fall within and outside genes. Genomics 2001; 76: 30–6.
14. Prueitt RL, Chen H, Barnes RI et al. Most X;autosome translocations associated with premature ovarian failure do not interrupt X-linked genes. Cytogenet Genome Res 2002; 97: 32–8.
15. Uzielli ML, Guarducci S, Lapi E et al. Premature ovarian failure (POF) and fragile X premutation females: from POF to fragile X carrier identification, from fragile X carrier diagnosis to POF association data. Am J Med Genet 1999; 84: 300–3.
16. Burton KA, Van Ee CC, Purcell K et al. Autosomal translocation associated with premature ovarian failure. J Med Genet 2000; 37: E2.
17. Aittomaki K, Herva R, Stenman UH et al. Clinical features of primary ovarian failure caused by a point mutation in the follicle-stimulating hormone receptor gene. J Clin Endocrinol Metab 1996; 81: 3722–6.
18. Vegetti W, Grazia Tibiletti M, Testa G et al. Inheritance in idiopathic premature ovarian failure: analysis of 71 cases. Hum Reprod 1998; 13: 1796–800.
19. Vegetti W, Marozzi A, Manfredini E et al. Premature ovarian failure. Mol Cell Endocrinol 2000; 161: 53–7.
20. Schildkraut JM, Cooper GS, Halabi S et al. Age at natural menopause and the risk of epithelial ovarian cancer. Obstet Gynecol 2001; 98: 85–90.

21. van Noord PAH, Dubas JS, Dorland M et al. Age at natural menopause in a population-based screening cohort: the role of menarche, fecundity, and lifestyle factors. Fertil Steril 1998; 68: 95–102.

22. Palmer JR, Rosenberg L, Wise LA et al. Onset of natural menopause in African American women. Am J Public Health 2003; 93: 299–306.

23. Dvornyk V, Long JR, Liu PY et al. Predictive factors for age at menopause in Caucasian females. Maturitas 2006; 54: 19–26.

24. Cramer DW, Xu H, Harlow BL. Family history as a predictor of early menopause. Fertil Steril 1995; 64: 740–5.

25. Murabito JM, Yang Q, Fox C et al. Heritability of age at natural menopause in the Framingham Heart Study. Obstet Gynecol Surv 2005; 60: 656–7.

26. van Asselt KM, Kok HS, Pearson PL et al. Heritability of menopausal age in mothers and daughters. Fertil Steril 2004; 82: 1348–51.

27. Snieder H, MacGregor AJ, Spector TD. Genes control the cessation of a woman's reproductive life: a twin study of hysterectomy and age at menopause. J Clin Endocrinol Metab 1998; 83: 1875–80.

28. Treloar SA, Do K-A, Martin NG. Genetic influences on the age of menopause. Lancet 1998; 352: 1084–5.

29. Murabito JM, Yang Q, Fox C et al. Genome-wide linkage analysis to age at natural menopause in a community-aged sample: the Framingham Heart Study. Fertil Steril 2005; 84: 1674–9.

30. Piccioni P, Scirpa P, D'Emilio I et al. Hormonal replacement therapy after stem cell transplantation. Maturitas 2004; 49: 327–33.

31. Pathak S, Multani AS. Aneuploidy, stem cells and cancer. EXS 2006; 96: 49–64.

32. Perin EC. The use of stem cell therapy for cardiovascular disease. Tex Heart Inst J 2005; 32: 390–2.

# Chapter 5

# Pregnancy in the perimenopause

Jane Cleary-Goldman, Mary D'Alton and Ronald J Wapner

## INTRODUCTION

Due to advances in assisted reproductive technology (ART), it is now possible for women aged 50 years and older to become pregnant and to have successful pregnancies. Nonetheless, pregnancy in this age group is rare and has been associated with perinatal complications such as pre-eclampsia, gestational diabetes, and Cesarean delivery.[1–7] Due to small numbers of patients, recommendations for pregnancy management are based on retrospective studies, cases series, and expert opinion. This chapter will review the current literature on pregnancy outcomes in the perimenopause and up-to-date recommendations for management of these patients.

## EPIDEMIOLOGY

Pregnancy during the perimenopause is rare. In the most recent Center for Disease Control Vital Statistics for 2003, 323 births to women aged 50 to 54 years were recorded which was a 23% increase over the 263 births reported in 2002. Since 1997, the number of births for women aged 50 to 54 years has increased with an average annual gain of 14%.[8]

## SUMMARY OF PREGNANCY OUTCOMES

Due to the fact that few women become pregnant during the perimenopause, there are few studies regarding the perinatal outcomes of these women. Most recently, Salihu et al performed a retrospective review of all births in the US from 1997 to 1999, using the National Center for Health Statistics public access vital records files.[7] Women were broken down into four groups to assess risk gradients for adverse perinatal outcomes:

1. 20–29 years
2. 30–39 years
3. 40–49 years
4. greater than 50 years.

There were 539 patients in the fourth group ranging in age from 50 to 54 years (54 years of age is the oldest age included in the database). Thirty-seven per cent of cases were multiples. Covariates considered included race, marital status, education, prenatal care utilization, smoking, and alcohol consumption. Use of ART and multifetal pregnancy reduction were not commented on. Main birth outcomes included intrauterine fetal demise (IUFD), low and very low birth weight, preterm and very preterm delivery, and small for gestational age. Maternal complications evaluated included anemia, cardiac disease, diabetes, chronic hypertension, pre-eclampsia, eclampsia, abruption, and placenta previa.

For women aged over 50 years, rates of cardiac disease, chronic hypertension, diabetes, pre-eclampsia, abruption, and placenta previa were elevated. The risks for low birth weight and very low birth weight (adjusted odds ratio (AOR) 3.00 and AOR 1.85), preterm and very preterm births (AOR 3.00 and AOR 3.35), small gestational age (SGA) (AOR 1.67), and fetal mortality (AOR 2.20) were significantly elevated with increasing maternal age, even after adjusting for confounding factors such as parity, marital status, education, and alcohol consumption. It was interesting to note that older mothers were at higher risk for fetal morbidity and mortality when carrying multiples.

The magnitude of these differences was less marked than for those observed among singletons.

Paulson et al performed a retrospective analysis of all in vitro fertilization (IVF) cycles conducted at one US ART program from 1991 to 2001 in patients aged over 50 years.[6] Seventy-seven patients between the ages of 50 and 63 years underwent IVF, resulting in 55 pregnancies and 45 live births (data were ascertained from 40 deliveries). There were 31 singleton, 12 twin, and 2 triplet pregnancies. The mean gestational age at delivery was 38.4 weeks, 35.8 weeks, and 32.2 weeks, respectively. The mean birth weights were 3039 g, 2254 g, and 1913 g, respectively. Sixty-eight per cent of the singletons and 100% of the multiples were delivered by Cesarean. Twenty-five per cent of patients were diagnosed with mild preeclampsia and 10% were diagnosed with severe pre-eclampsia. Approximately 18% of patients were diagnosed with non-insulin-requiring gestational diabetes, while less than 3% were diagnosed with insulin-requiring gestational diabetes.

It was interesting to note that adverse outcomes increased with increasing age. Among women younger than 55 years of age, pre-eclampsia was noted in 26% of patients, while it was noted in 60% of patients greater than 55 years of age. Gestational diabetes was more common in women greater than 55 years of age (40%) compared to women younger than 55 years of age (13%).

In addition, one patient carrying a singleton experienced premature rupture of membranes at 29 weeks, and delivered 10 days later. One patient delivered twins at 30 weeks for acute onset of severe pre-eclampsia. One patient underwent hysterectomy for placenta accreta, and one patient received a blood transfusion after Cesarean delivery for placenta previa. There were no neonatal or maternal deaths.

## MANAGEMENT STRATEGIES

Prior to commencing fertility treatment, these patients should be counseled about the complications associated with pregnancy in this age group. Risks include multiple gestation and its inherent complications, gestational hypertension, pre-eclampsia, gestational diabetes, abnormal placentation, stillbirth, Cesarean delivery, and possibly cardiac complications. Patients should also undergo a thorough work-up (cardiac, renal, and metabolic) prior to undergoing fertility treat-

ments, to confirm that they are healthy. Once pregnant, patients should be seen frequently to monitor their blood pressure. Most often, these pregnancies are conceived with egg donation. As a result, the risk for fetal aneuploidy is that of the egg donor. First trimester screening, chorionic villus sampling, second trimester screening, and amniocenteses are all options for these women. An anatomical survey should be scheduled in the middle trimetser. Glucose tolerance testing in the early third trimester is also suggested. Fetal surveillance in the third trimester should be considered, due to the possible increased risk for intrauterine fetal demise. Long-term outcomes regarding parenting and the impact of childbearing over 50 years of age on pediatric and maternal outcomes are unknown.

## CONCLUSION

In summary, pregnancy in the perimenopause is feasible due to advances in assisted conception techniques. While many patients who become pregnant in the sixth decade of life have successful outcomes, these patients are at risk for obstetric complications. A thorough medical work-up prior to undergoing fertility treatment is suggested. Counseling regarding the perinatal risks associated with pregnancy at this age is also suggested. Once pregnant, it is recommended that these patients undergo surveillance for signs and symptoms of hypertensive and cardiac issues throughout the antepartum and postpartum periods. Fetal surveillance is also reasonable for this age group.

## REFERENCES

1. Sauer MV, Paulson RJ, Lobo RA. Pregnancy after age 50: application of oocyte donation to women after natural menopause. Lancet 1993; 341: 321–3.
2. Narayan H, Buckett W, McDougall W, Cullimore J. Pregnancy after fifty: profile and pregnancy outcome in a series of elderly multigravidae. Eur J Obstet Gynecol Reprod Biol 1992; 47: 47–51.
3. Antinori S, Versaci C, Panci C, Caffa B, Gholami GH. Fetal and maternal morbidity and mortality in menopausal women aged 45–63 years. Hum Reprod 1995; 10: 464–9.
4. Paulson JR, Thornton MH, Francis MM, Salvador HS. Successful pregnancy in a 63-year-old woman. Fert Steril 1997; 67: 949–51.
5. Sauer MV. Motherhood at any age? Egg donation was not intended for everyone. Fert Steril 1998; 69: 187–8.

6. Paulson JR, Boostanfar R, Saadat P et al. Pregnancy in the sixth decade of life: obstetric outcomes in women of advanced reproductive age. JAMA 2002; 288: 2320–3.

7. Salihu HM, Shumpert MN, Slay M, Kirby RS, Alexander GR. Childbearing beyond maternal age 50 and fetal out-comes in the United States. Obstet Gynecol 2003; 102: 1006–14.

8. National Vital Statistics Report, September 8 2005; 54(2). Center for Disease Control and Prevention.

# Chapter 6

# Sexuality during and after the menopause

Rosemary Basson

## INTRODUCTION

Psychological, interpersonal, cultural, and biological factors modulate women's sexual experiences and sexual function. Aging and menopause are associated with an inevitable reduction of sex hormones. The supply of dehydroepiandrosterone (DHEA), its sulfate DHEAS, androstene-5-ene-3β,17β-diol and androstenedione to peripheral cells for intracellular production of testosterone and estrogen declines with age; ovarian production of estrogen ceases with menopause, while ovarian production of testosterone is variable in later life. These hormonal changes may or may not negatively influence sexual function. Rather than inevitable sexual decline from lower hormone levels, the evidence is that certain factors, e.g. strongly positive feelings for the partner,[1,2] and emotional and mental wellbeing,[1,3] and prior rewarding sexual experiences,[2] protect from potential dysfunction. Given that a woman's sexuality is so highly contextual, the presence of her needed emotional intimacy, erotic stimulation, privacy, safety, freedom from distractions (e.g. from poverty or family illness), and absence of partner sexual dysfunction strongly modulate women's sexual response cycles (Figure 6.1).[4]

Even in female rodents, there exist complex brain networks whereby environmental cues and past experience modulate sexual behavior.[5–7] Female rodents prefer to regulate the frequency of being mounted, and will choose the cage associated with memories with this preferred style of copulation. Moreover, the same increase in sexual behaviour, afforded by giving progesterone to an oophorectomized but estrogen-replete rodent (which also can be obtained by administration of dopamine rather than the sex steroid), can be entirely replicated by placing a male animal in the cage next door. There is some evidence that supplementing testosterone to older women can increase their sexual responsiveness,[8] and early data suggesting a dopaminergic drug can do the same,[9] but these changes are more clearly evident in response to a new partner.[2,3,10]

Thus hormonal change is one contributing rather than overriding factor modulating the sexual experience of midlife and older women. Nevertheless, as clinicians, we do see women whose careful detailed assessment does not identify contextual, interpersonal, or personal psychological issues accounting for midlife changes in sexual response. The complexities of hormone activity, particularly androgen activity, will be discussed, and an attempt will be made to identify basic data that are still needed for a scientific approach to hormone therapy for sexual dysfunction. Given the evidence of the importance of psychosexual factors, even as the role of hormonal reduction becomes clearer, it will remain necessary to assess and manage sexual problems in midlife and older women, with a holistic biopsychosexual approach.

## WOMEN'S SEXUAL RESPONSE: CHARACTERISTICS AND PHYSIOLOGY

In order to assess the endocrine, psychological and interpersonal factors affecting midlife and older women's sexuality, it is helpful to recall basic characteristics of female sexual function and physiology.

## Women have many reasons for engaging in sex

Reasons women engage in sexual activity with partners are varied, and constitute an ongoing subject of research.[11] Enhancement of emotional closeness is a strong motivating factor. Other reasons or incentives include to increase the woman's own sense of wellbeing, to feel more 'normal', more attractive, more committed and loved and to please the partner. Available data indicate sexual desire is an infrequent reason for women's sexual engagement in a majority of established relationships.[11–13] Most studies focus on heterosexual couples, but clinical experience suggests similarity in lesbian couples. It is clear that this type of sexual motivation is dependent on the expectation and realization of emotionally and physically rewarding experiences and outcomes.

## Phases of sexual response overlap and their order varies

Beginning then for reasons that may not be strictly sexual, the first phase of responding is that of arousal, consisting of subjective sexual arousal/sexual excitement, plus alterations in physiology. Breast, genital, and facial blood flow increases, along with changes in respiration, blood pressure, heart rate, muscle tension and renal

function. If the subjective arousal is enjoyed, the woman remains focused, and if the stimuli are continued for sufficient time, she may then become very aware of sexual desire. Desire and arousal then co-occur and compound. Sexual satisfaction may include one or many (or no) discrete orgasms. More intense arousal can follow the first orgasm. So, sexual response is circular rather than linear, phases are not discrete and the order is variable (Figure 6.1).

Any initial 'spontaneous' desire augments the cycle as shown in the figure.

## Subjective sexual excitement correlates poorly with measured increases in genital congestion

When increases in genital congestion in response to sexual visual erotic stimuli are recorded by means of a tampon-like device known as a vaginal photoplethysmograph, there is highly variable correlation with subjective arousal. This is true for sexually healthy women, as well as those complaining of lack of sexual desire, lack of sexual arousal, and sexual pain.[14,15] Typically, women with chronic lack of sexual arousal show prompt (within seconds) increases in vaginal congestion comparable to control women, but report no subjective sexual excitement in response to the erotic

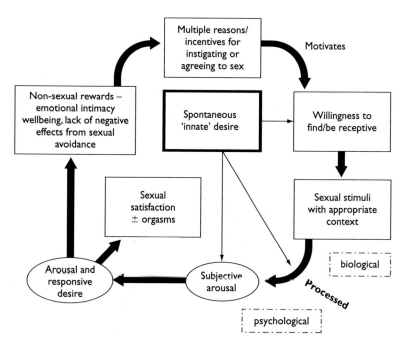

**Figure 6.1**  Circular sex response cycle showing multiple reasons over and beyond sexual desire motivate women to sexually engage. Arousal often precedes desire and the two coexist and reinforce. (Adapted from Figure 1 in Basson R. Female sexual response: the role of drugs in the management of sexual dysfunction. ACOG 2001; 98: 350–3, with permission from Lipincott, Williams & Wilkins.)

stimuli. Such women may even report negative emotions, e.g. anxiety, embarrassment, sadness. Functional magnetic resonance imaging (MRI) studies show areas of the brain that are activated during the watching of erotic videos. Unlike the situation in men, activation of the areas organizing the genital vasocongestive response does not correlate with the woman's subjective sexual arousal as she views the erotic video while in the MRI tube.[16]

## Physiology of genital engorgement

A number of physical changes occur in response to erotic sexual stimulation, including genital swelling, increased vaginal lubrication, as well as engorgement of the breasts, nipple erection, increases in skin sensitivity to sexual stimulation, changes in heart rate, blood pressure, muscle tone, breathing, body temperature, and skin circulation, with mottling of the skin and a 'sex flush' of vasodilation over the chest, breasts and face. Research has focused on the genital changes in congestion arising from active neurogenic dilation of blood spaces and blood vessels within the vulvar tissues and the submucosal vaginal vascular plexus. With sexual stimulation, brain activity in the hypothalamus, and other areas subserving the genital response, are activated such that the autonomic nervous system directs increased blood flow to the vagina. This causes an increase in the transudation of interstitial fluid from the submucosal capillaries, moving between the epithelial intracellular spaces and on to the vaginal lumen. Simultaneously, the autonomic nervous system allows relaxation of the smooth muscle cells surrounding the blood spaces (sinusoids) in clitoral tissue, causing swelling. There is also vasodilatation of labial blood vessels causing swelling of the labia. Depicted by recent immunohistological studies of the genital skin covering the clitoris and labia, are nerves containing nitric oxide (NO) – the major neurotransmitter underlying vulvar vascular smooth muscle relaxation.[17]

Although the underlying neurobiology is incompletely understood, this genital vasocongestive response appears to be highly automated, occurring within seconds of an erotic stimulus.[14] Parasympathetic nerves release NO and vasointestinal polypeptide (VIP) mediating vasodilatation. Also released is acetylcholine (ACh) which blocks noradrenergic vasoconstricting mechanisms and promotes NO release from the endothelium. Parasympathetic and sympathetic pathways and somatic pathways are far less separate than was previously believed. For instance, communication between the NO-containing cavernous nerve to the clitoris and the distal portion of the somatic dorsal nerve of the clitoris from the pudendal nerve, has been identified.[17] The pelvic sympathetic nerves primarily release vasoconstrictive norepinephrine (noradrenaline), epinephrine (adrenaline) and adenosine triphosphate, but some release ACh, NO and VIP. Of note, it has been repeatedly demonstrated in sexually healthy women that anxiety can *increase* the vasocongestive response of the genitalia to erotic stimulation.[18] Although NO is thought to be the major neurotransmitter mediating vulval engorgement, in the vagina, VIP, NO and another unidentified neurotransmitter are involved.[19]

Coincident with the relaxation of vascular smooth muscle, there is lengthening, distension, and dilatation of the vagina, and the uterus moves up out of the pelvis. There may be a 'cervical motor reflex' whereby touch to the cervix leads to reduction in pressure of the upper portion of the vagina and an increase in pressure of the middle and lower portions, accompanied by an increase in electromyographic activity in the levator ani and puborectalis muscles. Thus it is hypothesized that during intercourse, penile thrusting on the cervix might cause contraction of the pelvic muscles facilitating upwards 'ballooning' of the vagina, while the same muscle contraction constricts the lower vagina.[20] A further reflex demonstrated recently shows reduced uterine tone in response to mechanical or electrical stimulation of the clitoral glans. The background tonic contraction of the uterus was abolished by clitoral stimulation. Simultaneously, uterine pressure declined. It is hypothesized that this reflex might contribute to the known increase in size and elevation of the uterus with sexual arousal.[21]

For the majority of women, the clitoris is the most sexually sensitive area of their anatomy. However, for many women, clitoral stimulation is only enjoyable if non-physical and non-genital physical stimulation have occurred first. Without preceding arousal, direct clitoral stimulation can be unpleasant, 'too intense', and even painful. Recent immunohistological studies have identified neurotransmitters thought to be associated with sensation (substance P and calcitonin gene-related peptide – CGRP), concentrated immediately under the epithelium of the glans clitoris.[17] Clitoral tissue extends far beyond the portion visible when the clitoral hood is retracted. It includes the clitoral glans, corpora, crura, running along the pubic rami, peri-urethral tissue in front of the anterior vaginal wall, and the 'bulbs' under the superficial perineal muscles surrounding the anterior distal vagina contiguous with the periurethral tissue and the corpora (Figure 6.2).

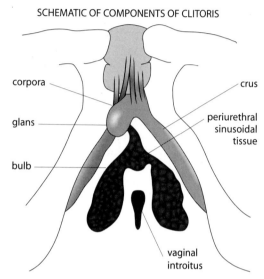

SCHEMATIC OF COMPONENTS OF CLITORIS

corpora

glans

bulb

crus

periurethral sinusoidal tissue

vaginal introitus

**Figure 6.2**   Clitoral tissue in the vulva is extensive. The palpable portion under the clitoral head being less than 10% of the total. (Adapted from Figure 3 in Basson R. The female sexual response revisited. J SOGC 2000; 22: 383–7, with permission from the Society of Obstetricians and Gynecologists of Canada.)

## Causes of distress with sexual experiences

In a recent national probability sample of North American women aged 20–65 years, the major determinants of whether or not a woman experiences distress about her sexual life were found to be her emotional relationship with her partner during sexual activity, and her general emotional wellbeing.[1] Physical aspects of sexual response, including awareness of arousal, vaginal lubrication and orgasm, were poor predictors.

## Subjective arousal is modulated by psychological and biological factors

The reflexive highly automated physical genital response of vasocongestion has been mentioned. The processing of the erotic stimuli, their context and the feelings generated by sexual arousal is a slower entity. Different areas of the brain are involved, as shown in Figure 6.3.

Psychological factors that influence the processing of erotic stimuli, i.e. the woman's arousability, include non-sexual distractions, her sexual self-confidence, expectations of reward, feelings for her partner at that time and generally, as well as safety issues including adequate birth control, safety from sexually transmitted diseases, unplanned pregnancies, plus privacy issues. Themes from childhood and adolescence that negatively affect her arousability may assume greater importance in midlife. This may be due to the increased vulnerability as formerly robust levels of sex hormones decline. Alternatively, unresolved anger, and resentment towards parental figures may be

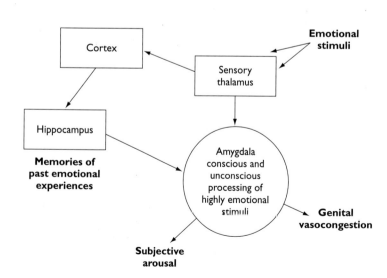

Cortex

Sensory thalamus

Emotional stimuli

Hippocampus

**Memories of past emotional experiences**

Amygdala conscious and unconscious processing of highly emotional stimuli

**Subjective arousal**

**Genital vasocongestion**

**Figure 6.3**   The rapid genital congestive response is thought to be the result of unconscious automatic processing that is possibly innately programmed. Subjective sexual arousal may or may not be experienced. (Adapted from Figure 1 in Basson R. A model of women's sexual arousal. J Sex Marital Ther 2002; 28: 1–10, with permission from Taylor & Francis Group.)

revived by current circumstances – for instance, now having to provide care for a previously abusive parent, or watching the effects of divorce on grandchildren, thereby reviving memories of similar unhappiness/anger experienced in the woman's childhood. As women attempt to suppress these negative emotions, they often succeed – but inevitably other emotions are suppressed in the process, including sexual arousal and sexual desire.

Biological factors include fatigue (e.g. from shift work, menopause-related insomnia, partner's snoring, her own possible undiagnosed sleep apnea), medication effects, chronic illness, markedly low levels of androgen activity (see later), and, far less commonly, undiagnosed or untreated hypo- or hyperthyroid states, or hyperprolactinemia.

## CHARACTERISTICS OF SEXUAL FUNCTION TYPICAL OF MID-AGED AND OLDER WOMEN

### Changes in desire and arousal

A lessening of desire and responsivity with age and with menopause is identified in some studies of postmenopausal women but not in others.[2,22–24] In 13 500 recently studied men from 29 countries, older age, net of other factors, consistently increased the likelihood that sexual problems will occur. In 13 500 women studied in the same countries, only lubrication difficulties were positively associated with age.[24] Sexual feelings for the partner, mental and emotional wellbeing, absence of partner's sexual dysfunction, and expectation of sexual satisfaction due to rewarding past sexual experiences have all been shown to mitigate sexual problems and protect from distress about sex.[1–3,23,24]

### Changes in genital blood flow in response to sexual stimulation

Research into increases in genital congestion in response to erotic stimuli in pre- and postmenopausal women who are and are not subjectively aroused by those stimuli are of particular interest. Whether or not the woman is aroused subjectively, the percentage increase in genital congestion appears similar in pre- and postmenopausal women.[14] The technique of vaginal

photoplethysmography (VPP) does not record actual blood flow but if operators, settings, and techniques are standardized, baseline values can be compared for the most frequently recorded measure of the vaginal pulse amplitude (VPA), (that is to say, the increase in pulse amplitude with each heart beat).[14] The baseline measure is lower in postmenopausal women. Therefore, even though the percentage increase is similar in pre- and postmenopausal women, actual blood flow, and therefore lubrication production, may sometimes be insufficient to allow comfortable intercourse postmenopausally unless estrogen is given. Other estrogen-deficient women may lubricate sufficiently for coital comfort, assuming the stimulus is sufficiently erotic. Clearly, not all postmenopausal women need to use estrogen or a topical lubricant. It has been hypothesized that estrogen protects the woman from pain and discomfort, even if the context and the stimuli are insufficiently erotic, whereas the estrogen-deficient woman with lower baseline congestion is very dependent upon useful sexual stimulation.[14]

### Increased importance of low-key sexual pleasuring, non-penetrative sex

Available data indicate the importance of affectionate sensual touching and caressing, non-genital sexual touching and stimulation that is genital but not focused on the act of intercourse.[25] These normal requirements of more leisurely, playful, non-goal-oriented interaction may not be met when a male partner has erectile dysfunction and moves quickly onto intercourse in case his erection fades and cannot be regained.

## FACTORS AFFECTING SEXUAL FUNCTION IN MIDLIFE AND OLDER WOMEN

### Sexual self-view

Known to markedly affect sexual desire and responsivity, a woman's sexual self-view may change in mid- and later life. In societies where youth and beauty are equated with sexual attractiveness, sexual self-view may suffer. Lack of menses and permanent infertility may represent loss of sexual attractiveness. For other women, the changes have positive effects. The end of possible menorrhagia, polymenorrhea and unpredictable cycles, as well as birth control concerns, allows a new sexual freedom.

## Distractions

A common cause of lack of subjective arousal, the number and intensity of distractions may reduce or increase with menopause depending on life's circumstances. Children may have left home but yet be ongoing causes of concern. Renewed interest in career or change of career may increase sexual interest and response in association with increased self-confidence generally, or may constitute new, possibly potent distractions when attempting to be sexual.

## Emotional intimacy

Emotional closeness to the partner may well increase now the couple can focus more on themselves. However, for troubled relationships, a previous endeavor to keep the peace, coexist amicably 'for the sake of the children' is now questioned, and may or may not lead to effort to improve the relationship. Negative consequences of refusing the partner's requests for sexual activity may appear less threatening since the option of ending the relationship may now be seriously considered.

## Culture

Recent baseline data from a longitudinal study of 3300 multi-ethnic premenopausal North American women, aged 42–52 years, confirmed that women of different ethnicities endorsed the various reasons given in the study for engaging in sexual activity with a partner (to express love, for pleasure, because the partner wanted to, to relieve tension). However, Hispanic women were the least likely to indicate that they engage in sex for pleasure. Also the proportion of women responding that they engage in sex because their partner wanted them to was lowest for African-American and highest for Hispanic and Japanese women. African-American, Chinese and Japanese women reported less desire than Caucasian women.[26] Hispanic women reported low physical pleasure and arousal. Chinese women reported more pain and less arousal than the Caucasian women, as did the Japanese women, although the only significant difference was for arousal.[26]

## Menopausal symptoms

Mood instability, vasomotor symptoms and vaginal dryness reduce sexual motivation, arousability and enjoyment. Studying 354 Australian women transitioning menopause, bothersome menopausal symptoms negatively affected the woman's well-being which influenced her sexual responsivity, which in turn, influenced sexual desire.[27]

## Androgen production

Testosterone production within cells in the brain and elsewhere from adrenal precursors including DHEA, DHEAS, androst-5-ene-3β,17β-diol and androstenedione, accounts for the majority of testosterone activity in older naturally menopausal women, and close to 100% in surgically menopausal women. Such a local biosynthesis and action of androgens in target tissues eliminates the exposure of other tissues to androgens, and thus minimizes the risk of undesirable masculinizing or other androgen-related side-effects.[28] However, from the third decade onwards, androgen precursor production progressively declines, such that in the 50–60-year-old age group, serum DHEA has already decreased by 70% compared with the 20–30-year-old peak values.[28] This cellular deprivation is difficult to measure in individual women. Less than 10% of the testosterone produced in cells outside of the gonads and adrenal glands, spills back into the bloodstream.[29] Thus serum levels of testosterone reflect mainly gonadal production. Moreover, the assays for serum testosterone (free, bioavailable, total) are not designed for the female range, and are very unreliable.[30] Mass spectrometry methods or equilibrium dialysis for the measurement of free testosterone are recommended, but are rarely available to clinicians and often are not chosen by researchers. Metabolites resulting from the breakdown of testosterone – wherever it has been produced – can be measured. The recommended assays are for serum concentrations of androsterone glucuronide (ADT-G), androstane 3α, 17β-diol glucuronide (3α-diol-G), and androstane 3β, 17β-diol glucuronide, (3β-diol-G).[29] However, these are currently only available on a research basis. Moreover, age-related values in women with and without sexual dysfunction have yet to be established.

Sudden loss of androgen can result in a syndrome whereby formerly useful sexual stimuli – mental, visual, non-genital touch, genital touch, intercourse – all fail to arouse. Any former awareness of genital swelling, throbbing and lubrication is lost. Similarly, former innate or spontaneous desire is now absent. Chemotherapy-induced or surgical menopause, especially in younger women, may be associated with this syndrome.[31,32] However, other women with induced menopause report no sexual changes. Middle-aged and older women may be less likely to report such symptoms: a recent prospective non-randomized study showed that 106 perimenopausal women requiring hysterectomy for benign pathology, choosing hysterectomy and bilateral salpingo-oophorectomy (BSO) over hysterectomy alone, showed no deterioration in sexual function at one year postsurgery compared to pre-operative assessment.[33] A majority of women choosing BSO received estrogen supplementation as did those with hysterectomy alone, if they had menopausal symptoms. There were decreased scores in 3 of 24 sexual variables in the women receiving hysterectomy alone. There is minimal evidence correlating sexual function with serum androgen levels in postmenopausal women with and without sexual dysfunction. Studying 2900 pre- and perimenopausal multi-ethnic North American women, aged 42–52 years in the SWAN (Study of Women's Health Across the Nation) study, total testosterone and free androgen index (FAI) showed minimal correlation with sexual function.[34] Similarly, measures of free and total testosterone failed to correlate with sexual function in a study of 1021 Australian women, aged 18–75 years. A low score for sexual response for those over 45 years of age was associated with higher odds of having a serum DHEAS level below the tenth percentile for this age group. However, the majority of women with low DHEAS did not have reduced sexual function.[35] Clearly, questions related to variable amounts of remaining adrenal precursors of testosterone, reductions in steroidogenic enzymes, changes in number and sensitivity of androgen receptors, levels of specific coactivator and corepressor proteins that modify transcription and interplay between estrogen and androgen, need much more research.

## Estrogen production

Ovarian estrogen production ceases after menopause. Intracellular production of estrogen from testosterone, DHEA, DHEAS and androstenedione depends on adrenal and ovarian production of these precursors, numbers of fat cells (an important site of aromatization of testosterone to estradiol), and the presence of the appropriate steroidogenic enzymes to synthesize estrogen or testosterone and dihydrotestosterone (DHT) from the precursors in the tissue concerned. Elucidation of the structure of most of the tissue-specific genes that encode for steroidogenic enzymes responsible for transforming precursors into androgens and/or estrogens, is ongoing. Particular focus is on 3β-HSD (hydroxysteroid dehydrogenase), 17β-HSD, 5α-reductase and aromatase – enzymes involved in the synthesis from DHEA of the most potent natural androgen, namely DHT, and the most potent natural estrogen, namely estradiol.[29] Thus in the older woman, the importance of local biosynthesis of sex hormones applies to estrogens as well as to androgens (although a reliable parameter of total estrogen secretion comparable to the glucuronides identified for androgens has yet to be determined).

The role of low estrogen in loss of sexual desire and arousability remains unanswered. Sexual responsivity was improved in a recent study of Australian women receiving estrogen therapy, provided the estrogen levels reached between 650 and 758 pmol/l – approximately twice the level required to improve local symptoms of vaginal dryness.[36] Whether the documented effect of supplemental testosterone in increasing desire and arousability is via the androgen receptor or via the estrogen receptor after aromatization, is unclear. One recent study suggests benefit is via the androgen receptor, as the addition of aromatase inhibitor did not negate the benefit of supplemental testosterone given to postmenopausal women using transdermal estrogen therapy.[37] Whether testosterone allows benefit simply by reducing sex hormone-binding globulin (SHBG), and therefore frees estrogen to be more bioavailable, is also unclear.

The role of estrogen in tissue health also requires further research. The pallor of vulvar vaginal atrophy may be obvious. Estrogen levels directly correlate with the ratios between para-basal, intermediate and superficial vaginal cells, as in the Maturation Index.[38] However, symptoms of vaginal dryness, pain, and difficulty with intercourse correlate poorly with visual changes, with estrogen levels, and with duration of estrogen lack. Symptoms sometimes occur perimenopausally, and sometimes only decades postmenopause. The role of permeability of vaginal epithelial cells is unclear. Nerve endings containing calcitonin gene-related peptide (CGRP) are present in the vaginal epithelial cells, possibly modulating their permeability.[39]

Low estrogen levels lead to increase in pH of the vaginal lumen, predisposing to vaginal infections which undermine women's sexual self-confidence, and contribute to dyspareunia. The mechanism of estrogenic acidification of the vagina has been recently reviewed.[40] Traditionally, this was attributed to hydrogen peroxide and protons secreted by Doderlein lactobacilli in the estrogen-replete tissues. There is now some evidence that vaginal-ectocervical cells acidify the lumen by the secretion of protons across the apical plasma membrane. It is thought that this active proton secretion occurs throughout life but that it is upregulated by estrogen.[40]

### Altered sexual sensitivity of non-genital skin, the breasts, clitoris, and other genital tissues

Reduced sexual sensitivity of non-genital skin and of the breast has received little scientific study. A small number of studies using pressure thresholds have demonstrated reduced vulval sensitivity with postmenopausal states, and increased sensitivity with the use of topical estrogen.[41] Recently, both age and postmenopausal state have been associated with reduced vibratory sensation of the genital tract. Age by itself, affects peripheral non-genital sensation.[42]

The 'genital deadness' underlying the diagnosis of genital arousal disorder is not well understood.[43] Early research indicates that despite useful erotic stimulation, reduced genital vasocongestion is identified only in a subgroup of women diagnosed with genital arousal disorder.[44] The suspected role of reduced androgen activity in this lost sexual genital sensitivity despite apparent engorgement, awaits scientific study.

## DEFINITIONS OF WOMEN'S SEXUAL DYSFUNCTION

Just as phases of sexual response overlap, so do women's sexual dysfunctions.[23] Revision and expansion to the definitions of women's sexual disorders found in the American Psychiatric Association's Diagnostic and Statistical Manual of Mental Disorders (DSM-IVTR) were developed by an international committee organized by the American Urological Association Foundation.[43] The Second International Consensus on Sexual Dysfunctions in Men and Women under the aus-

pices of the International Consultation on Urological Disease and the International Societies of Urology and Sexual and Impotence Research, has recently provided evidence-based recommendations on assessment and management of men and women's sexual dysfunction. Their recommendations included acceptance of these revised definitions of women's sexual disorders.[45] Table 6.1 lists these revised definitions.

Each disorder is then further clarified with the following descriptors:

1. lifelong or acquired
2. generalized or situational
3. the degree of distress – mild, moderate or marked
4. the presence of contextual factors:
   - past factors from developmental history affecting psychosexual development
   - present factors – interpersonal, environmental, societal, cultural
   - medical factors.

## ASSESSMENT AND MANAGEMENT OF SEXUAL DYSFUNCTIONS IN MIDLIFE AND OLDER WOMEN

### Sexual desire/interest disorder and subjective and combined arousal disorders

Using the framework of women's circular sex response cycle (Figure 6.1), it is necessary to assess the various sexual motivations/incentives and the degree of intimacy, trust, respect, and attraction within the relationship. The sexual context and suitability of the stimuli when sexual activity is attempted, as well as the outcome in terms of both physical and emotional satisfaction, must be clarified. Frequently this assessment is itself highly therapeutic. The woman and her partner see the logic to their situation, and they can choose whether they wish to address the problematic areas.

It is also recommended that each partner is seen alone to carefully identify personal and interpersonal psychological factors, as well as contextual factors. Careful exclusion of depression or other mood disorder is necessary. Table 6.2 outlines sexual assessment.

Behavioral, cognitive and sexual therapies have been the mainstay of therapy once etiological factors have been clarified. Cognitive behavioral therapy (CBT) addresses the problematic areas in

**Table 6.1**    Definitions of women's sexual dysfunction[43]

| Diagnosis | Definition | Comments |
|---|---|---|
| Sexual desire/interest disorder | Absent or diminished feelings of sexual interest or desire, absent sexual thoughts or fantasies *and* a lack of responsive desire. Motivations (here defined as reasons/incentives), for attempting to become sexually aroused are scarce or absent. The lack of interest is beyond a normative lessening with life cycle and relationship duration. | Minimal spontaneous sexual thinking or desiring of sex ahead of sexual experiences does not necessarily constitute disorder. Additional lack of responsive desire is integral to the diagnosis. |
| Combined sexual arousal disorder | Absent or markedly reduced feelings of sexual arousal (sexual excitement and sexual pleasure) from any type of stimulation, and absent or impaired genital sexual arousal (vulval swelling and lubrication). | There is minimal sexual excitement (subjective arousal) from any type of stimulation – erotic material, stimulating the partner, genital and non-genital stimulation. There is no *awareness* of the reflexive genital vasocongestion (swelling/lubrication). |
| Subjective sexual arousal disorder | Absent or markedly reduced feelings of sexual arousal (sexual excitement and sexual pleasure) from any type of stimulation. Vaginal lubrication and other signs of physical response still occur. | Despite lack of sexual excitement/subjective arousal, lubrication is noted by the woman or partner. Intercourse is comfortable without use of external lubricant. |
| Genital arousal disorder | Absent or impaired genital sexual arousal – minimal vulval swelling or vaginal lubrication from any type of sexual stimulation, and reduced sexual sensations from caressing genitalia. *Subjective sexual excitement still occurs from non-genital sexual stimuli.* | The presence of subjective arousal (sexual excitement) from non-genital stimuli (erotica, stimulating the partner, receiving breast stimulation, kissing) is key to this diagnosis. |
| Orgasmic disorder | Despite the self-report of high sexual arousal/excitement, there is either lack of orgasm, markedly diminished intensity of orgasmic sensations, or marked delay of orgasm from any kind of stimulation. | Of course, women with arousal disorders will rarely or never experience orgasm. |
| Vaginismus | Persistent or recurrent difficulties of the women to allow vaginal entry of a penis, finger or any object despite the woman's expressed wish to do so. There is often (phobic) avoidance and anticipation/fear/experience of pain, along with variable and involuntary pelvic muscle contraction. Structural or other physical abnormalities must be ruled out/addressed. | Confirmation of this diagnosis is not possible until there has been therapy sufficient to allow a careful introital and vaginal examination. It is a presumptive diagnosis initially. |
| Dyspareunia | Persistent or recurrent pain with attempted or complete vaginal entry and/or penile vaginal intercourse. | There are many causes, including vulvovaginal atrophy from estrogen deficiency and vulvar vestibulitis syndrome. |

**Table 6.2** Assessment of sexual dysfunction

The following questions can be directed at the sexual couple:

1. *sexual problem in patient's own words*: clarify further with direct questions, giving options rather than leading questions, giving support and encouragement, acknowledgement of embarrassment and reassurance that sexual problems are common
2. *duration, consistency, priority*: are problems present in all situations, and which problem is most severe?
3. *context of sexual problems*: emotional intimacy with partner, activity/behavior just prior to sexual activity, privacy, birth control, risk of sexually transmitted disease, usefulness of sexual stimulation, sexual skills of partner, sexual communication, time of day/fatigue level
4. *the rest of each partner's sexual response*: check this currently and prior to the onset of the sexual problems
5. *the reaction of each partner*: how each has reacted emotionally, sexually and behaviorally
6. *previous help*: compliance with recommendations and effectiveness
7. *reason for presenting now*: what has precipitated this request for help?

The following questions are asked from each partner when seen alone:

1. *partner's own assessment of the situation*: sometimes it is easier to talk about symptom severity, e.g. total lack of desire, in the partner's absence
2. *sex response with self-stimulation*: also enquire about sexual thoughts and fantasies
3. *past sexual experiences*: positive, negative aspects
4. *developmental history*: relationships to others in the home while growing up; losses, traumas, to whom (if anyone) were they close, were they shown physical affection, love, respect?
5. *enquire about sexual, emotional and physical abuse*: explain that abuse questions are routine and do not necessarily imply causation of the problems.

The following areas must also be assessed:

1. *physical health including medications*: specifically ask about medications with known sexual side-effects, including SSRIs, β-blockers, anti-androgens, gonadotrophin-releasing hormone agonists, hormonal contraceptives
2. *evaluation of mood*: a significant correlation of sexual function and mood warrants routine screening for mood disorder.

Items 3–5 of the single patient interview may sometimes be omitted (e.g. for a recent problem after decades of healthy sexual function).
Adapted from Table 3 in Basson R. Assessment and management of women's sexual dysfunctions: desire and arousal disorders. New Engl J Med 2006; 354: 1497–506. ©2006 Massachusetts Medical Society. All rights reserved.

the woman's sex response cycle, including inappropriate sexual context, behaviors in either partner which reduce attractiveness/trust, as well as distractions. More distant factors, for instance, when sexual symptoms are thought to result from past (non-sexual) themes from childhood and from low sexual self-image, may require short-term psychotherapy. Sex therapy focuses on the interpersonal issues as well as the sexual details. 'Sensate focus techniques' consist of exchanging physical touch, moving from non-sexual to sexual areas of the body, similar to systematic desensitization in other behavioral therapies that reduce anxiety. Unfortunately, outcome data for all the above types of interventions are limited. Also, control groups are rarely included, but one study of CBT showed improvement in 74% receiving CBT that was maintained in 64% at one year.

There was minimal improvement in the control group.[46] One study of sex therapy of 365 married couples showed that 65% were improved by clinical judgment at the end of therapy.[47]

## Investigational therapy

For some couples, the emotional closeness, sexual context, and previously rewarding sexual stimuli, all appear to be in place and without any interference by psychological or psychiatric issues – yet the woman's sexual response has faded. Some physicians are gaining experience in the investigational use of systemic testosterone, along with systemic estrogen, after careful exclusion of the above non-hormonal factors. However, this presents a major clinical dilemma arising from the factors shown in Table 6.3.

**Table 6.3**    Major difficulties regarding testosterone supplementation

- The need for (time-consuming) comprehensive biopsychosocial assessment
- Unavailability of measures of total androgen activity
- Presence of expected long-term dysfunction from presumed hormonal lack but absence of long-term data of hormone administration
- The need for concomitant systemic estrogen therapy. There is documented risk if estrogen therapy is started some years postmenopause, and unknown risk/benefit when started for sexual symptoms at the time of menopause
- Current lack of formulations of systemic androgen for women
- Lack of availability of sensitive accurate assays of testosterone levels to monitor testosterone supplementation (assays designed for higher male range)

The studies supporting the role of androgen therapy in older women, have focused mainly on surgically menopausal women. There are now five published studies where an attempt was made to replete the testosterone levels to the upper limit for normal premenopausal women.[8,48–51] Benefit was seen with 350 but not 150 or 450 μg transdermal testosterone daily. The oldest study[8] showed benefit in terms of arousal and response and pleasure and orgasm but not in parameters of desire.[48–50] By contrast, the more recent studies also show increases in the desire domain in the questionnaires used as part of the clinical trials. Data from a similar randomized controlled trial involving *naturally* menopausal women showed similar improvement in response and desire.[52] Earlier studies employed supraphysiological doses of testosterone or involved the use of methyl testosterone. The latter leads to reduced high-density lipoprotein (HDL) cholesterol and cannot be ensured to be supplying androgen within a physiological (for premenopausal women) range. This is because the methyl testosterone, as well as the testosterone freed by a methyl testosterone-induced reduction of SHBG, both act on the androgen receptor. However, only testosterone is measured in the available assays.

Safety data are needed for long-term estrogen therapy commenced at around the time of the menopause in non-obese healthy women. Similarly, long-term safety data are needed for any concomitant testosterone administration. Of particular cause for concern is a possible increased incidence of metabolic syndrome. Baseline data from the SWAN study show strong correlation between low SHBG (with corresponding high endogenous androgen levels) and the incidence of metabolic syndrome.[34] Also, despite in vitro studies suggesting testosterone may protect from breast cancer, the question of a possible increased risk with supplemental testosterone remains.

Physicians prescribing testosterone (along with estrogen and progestin if the uterus is in place), must explain the investigational nature of this therapy and arrange follow-up which should include:

- clinical tracking of sexual function
- examination re weight, blood pressure, upper abdominal obesity, hirsutism, acne, scalp hair loss, clitoromegaly, breast changes
- measurement of lipids, hematocrit, fasting blood glucose
- mammography, uterine ultrasound.

The possibility of increasing androgen availability by changing from oral to transdermal estrogen, thereby lowering SHBG, should always be first explored.[53]

Table 6.4 lists the potential risks of androgen administration.

Currently, accurate guidelines regarding androgen therapy are not possible because the science is imprecise. However, recommendations that invite caution about the investigational nature of such therapy are in place.[54,55]

**Table 6.4**    Risks of androgen administration

- Risks from concomitant long-term estrogen
- Potential increase in insulin resistance and increase in upper abdominal obesity[34]
- Hirsutism, acne, loss of scalp hair
- Clitoromegaly and voice deepening
- Fluid retention
- Endometrial and breast hyperplasia/neoplasia
- Reduced HDL cholesterol if methyl testosterone (available in US) is used
- Sleep apnea
- Emotional lability
- Unknown (due to lack of long-term data)

## Management of genital arousal disorder

The management of the 'genital deadness' that typifies genital arousal disorder is unclear. Early research suggests that some, but only some of these women have demonstrably reduced genital vasocongestion in response to erotic stimuli found to create subjective arousal.[44] Thus those with reduced vasocongestion may benefit from investigational use of a phosphodiesterase inhibitor.[44] Unfortunately, the place of psychophysiological study to monitor increases in pelvic vasocongestion in response to erotic stimuli in clinical practice, is still quite unclear. These tests are not generally available. The provisional recommendation is that when local estrogen does not relieve this lack of genital sensitivity, then the investigational use of phosphodiesterase inhibitors may be suggested with due precaution against concomitant use of nitrates or alpha-blockers. Similarly, a role for the investigational use of topical testosterone, e.g. 0.2 ml of 2% testosterone to the clitoral area is hypothesized due to the large number of androgen receptors in the vulva,[56] this loss of genital sensitivity may be in part due to lack of androgen effect. Scientific study is awaited.

Diagnosis of genital arousal disorder may be made subsequent to a denervating radical hysterectomy. However, techniques for avoiding the portions of the inferior hypogastric plexus in the cardinal and broad ligaments have been developed.[57] Sexual outcome studies of women who have received radical hysterectomies using these nerve-sparing techniques are now awaited. In one small study, 12 women with simple hysterectomy, and 12 with radical hysterectomy (Piver Rutledge Class III) were compared to 17 sexual healthy controls. Of note, these women were not postmenopausal nor did they have major complaints of sexual dysfunction. The results are of some interest, given the maximum increase in vaginal congestion was certainly highest in the controls and lowest in those women receiving non-sparing radical hysterectomies. Counterintuitively, it was found that subjective arousal was lowest in the women who had received simple hysterectomy. Furthermore, there was no difference in subjective arousal/excitement between control women and the women receiving radical hysterectomies.[58]

A recent Croatian study has shown the importance of fear of dyspareunia due to dryness after radical hysterectomy. Of 210 women treated with combinations of surgery, radiation and chemotherapy for cancer of the cervix, some 50% endorsed a marked fear of pain, whereas only six women apparently identified actual dyspareunia, and a further three identified impossible penetration.[59] In keeping with the biopsychosocial conceptualization of sexual function and dysfunction, a marked synergy between untoward sexual outcome of nerve damage from treatment of cancer of the cervix and history of sexual abuse, has been noted.[60] An absence of sexual satisfaction was reported by 20% of women with neither abuse nor cancer of the cervix, by 31% who had been sexually abused but had no history of cancer of the cervix, and by 28% of women with cancer but without abuse, but by 45% of women with both abuse and cancer of the cervix. This lack of sexual satisfaction caused far more distress in the women with both abuse and cancer histories than in any of the other groups. Dyspareunia as a component of sexual dysfunction was extremely rare in women without cancer of the cervix, and was reported by 12% of those with cancer of the cervix, but by 30% of those with cancer of the cervix and past abuse.

## Assessment and management of dyspareunia

Dyspareunia requires careful assessment (Tables 6.5 and 6.6). Loss of vaginal elasticity with thinning of the vaginal epithelium, reduced lubrication, and lost vulval sexual sensitivity, all associated with vulvovaginal atrophy, may be improved with local estrogen.[61]

| Table 6.5   Assessment of chronic dyspareunia: history |
| --- |
| • Ask if vaginal entry is possible at all (i.e. with finger, penis, speculum, tampon) |
| • Ask if subjective sexual arousal (excitement) is experienced when intercourse is attempted and as it progresses |
| • Enquire exactly when the pain is experienced: <br> – with attempted entry of penile head or dildo <br> – with partial entry of penis or dildo <br> – with deep thrusting <br> – with penile movement <br> – with the man's ejaculation <br> – with the woman's subsequent urination <br> – for hours or minutes after attempted or completed intercourse or other vaginal stimulation attempts |
| • Enquire whether on some occasions there is less/no pain and if so, what is different? |

**Table 6.6**    Assessment of chronic dyspareunia: physical examination

- *External genitalia*: sparsity of pubic hair suggesting low adrenal androgens, vulval skin disorders e.g. lichen sclerosis causing soreness with sexual stimulation. Cracks/fissures in the interlabial folds suggestive of chronic candidiasis. Dermatological conditions and vulvar dystrophies requiring biopsy and definitive diagnosis even if sexually asymptomatic.
- *Introitus*: vulval disease involving introitus, e.g. vulval atrophy, lichen sclerosis, signs of recurrent splitting of the posterior fourchette, abnormalities of the hymen, adhesions of the labia minora, swellings in the area of the major vestibular glands, allodynia (pain sensation from touch stimulus) of Skene's duct openings and of the crease between the outer hymenal edge and inner edge of labia minora – typical of of vulvar vestibulitis syndrome (VVS) as causes of introital dyspareunia. Presence of cystocele, rectocele, prolapse interfering with the woman's sexual self-image. Abnormal vaginal discharge associated with burning dyspareunia.
- *Internal examination*: hypertonicity of the pelvic muscles associated with mid-vaginal dyspareunia. Tenderness – trigger points on palpating the deep levator ani due to underlying hypertonicity, vaginal atrophy, all as causes of deeper dyspareunia.
- *Full bimanual examination*: presence of nodules and/or tenderness in the cul-de-sac, fornices, along the uterosacral ligaments, retroverted fixed uterus, tenderness palpating the anterior or posterior vaginal wall suggestive of uterine, bladder or rectal pathology, all as causes of deeper dyspareunia.

Adapted from Table 4 in Basson R. Assessment and management of women's sexual dysfunctions: desire and arousal disorders. New Engl J Med 2006; 354: 1497–506. ©2006 Massachusetts Medical Society. All rights reserved.

Vulvar vestibulitis is seen in midlife women as well as in younger women.[62] At present, there are a number of therapies addressing central and peripheral sensitization associated with neurogenic inflammation, which, in turn, leads to the familiar discrete areas of allodynia around the introital rim.[63] These therapies include chronic pain medications such as anticonvulsants and tricyclic antidepressants, topical local anesthetics, topical anti-inflammatory drugs such as cromoglycate, and vestibulectomy as well as sexual therapy, and psychotherapy. There are no evidence-based recommendations. Because hypertonicity of pelvic muscles is thought to contribute to the pain in many women, pelvic muscle physiotherapy may be recommended.[64]

Pain relief may be partial and/or delayed, so it is important to assist the couple to create rewarding erotic sexual interactions that do not involve anything entering the vagina. Acceptance of non-penetrative sex by both partners will be necessary. Chronic dyspareunia leads to lost arousability and lack of desire at any stage of the sexual experience if the painful component, namely intercourse, persists.

### Assessment and management of orgasmic disorder defined as lack of orgasm despite high arousal

More often a lifelong concern, orgasmic disorder acquired in mid or later life may be associated with the use of serotonergic antidepressants, changes in the sexual relationship from trust/control/vulnerability issues, neurological disease, or nerve damage. It should be clarified whether the woman can experience orgasms with self-stimulation. If so, this would direct therapy towards interpersonal issues, e.g. of trust, and/or the need for the woman to guide her partner on the specific type of stimulation she requires. More prolonged, direct vulval and clitoral stimulation may now be needed.

Amelioration of selective serotonin reuptake inhibitor (SSRI)-induced orgasmic disorder is difficult. A recent Cochrane review made no recommendation of medication to reverse medication-induced orgasmic disorder in women.[65] However, benefit of bupropion shown in one of two randomized controlled trials was noted to be of interest.[66,67] The addition or substitution of bupropion is often tried, but the focus of therapy should be to assist the couple in making the stimulus and the context more exciting. This may include vibrostimulation to the mons or clitoral area. Sometimes, adaptation to high arousal without orgasmic release, focusing on the pleasure of the arousal rather than orgasm, again allows for satisfying experiences.

The majority of middle-aged women presenting with loss of orgasm have an underlying arousal disorder. Loss of genital sexual sensitivity and response may predominate, or, more commonly, there is a global lack of mental excitement as well as lack of the body's former response. Either way, the diagnosis is arousal disorder rather than orgasmic disorder.

## CONCLUSION

Many midlife and older women have sexual difficulties. When these difficulties amount to a sexual disorder is an ongoing subject of research and debate. Current revisions to the definition of disorder no longer focus on 'spontaneous desire/fantasies' as the hallmark of healthy sexual desire. The evidence is that this aspect of sexuality has a broad spectrum of frequency across women, and is not the reason why they engage in sex. It is now more appropriate to focus the assessment and management on the woman's subjective arousal/excitement/pleasure. The interplay of psychosocial factors and sex hormone activity is currently under scrutiny. An accurate measurement of androgen activity that reflects the intracellular production of testosterone is awaited. Longer-term safety data for supplemental estrogen and testosterone for sexual dysfunction are urgently required.

*Acknowledgement*
My sincere thanks to Dr Peter Rees for his helpful review of the manuscript, and to Mrs Maureen Piper for her excellent secretarial skills.

## REFERENCES

1. Bancroft J, Loftus J, Long JS. Distress about sex: a national survey of women in heterosexual relationships. Arch Sex Behav 2003; 32: 193–211.
2. Dennerstein L, Lehert P. Modeling mid-aged women's sexual functioning: a prospective, population-based study. J Sex Marital Ther 2004; 30: 173–83.
3. Avis NE, Stellato R, Crawford S et al. Is there an association between menopause status and sexual functioning? Menopause 2000; 7: 297–309.
4. Basson R. Rethinking low sexual desire in women. BJOG 2002; 109: 357–63.
5. Pfaus JG, Kippin TE, Centeno S. Conditioning and sexual behaviour: a review. Horm Behav 2001; 40: 291–321.
6. Blaustein JD. Progestin receptors: Neuronal integrators of hormonal and environmental stimulation. Ann NY Acad Sci 2003; 1007: 1–13.
7. Mani SK, Allen JMC, Clark JH et al. Convergent pathways of steroid hormone and neurotransmitter-induced rat sexual behaviour. Science 1994; 265: 1246–9.
8. Shifren JL, Braunstein GD, Simon JA et al. Transdermal testosterone treatment in women with impaired sexual function after oophorectomy. N Engl J Med 2000; 343: 682–8.
9. Segraves RT. Bupropion sustained release for the treatment of hypoactive sexual desire disorder in premenopausal women. J Clin Psychopharmacol 2004; 25: 339–42.
10. Klusmann D. Sexual motivation and the duration of partnership. Arch Sex Behav 2002; 31: 275–87.
11. Cain VS, Johannes CB, Avis NE. Sexual functioning and practices in a multi-ethnic study of mid-life women: Baseline results from SWAN. J Sex Res 2003; 40: 266–76.
12. Regan P, Berscheid E. Belief about the state, goals and objects of sexual desire. J Sex Marital Ther 1996; 2: 10–120.
13. Galyer KT, Conaglen HM, Hare A et al. JV. The effect of gynecological surgery on sexual desire. J Sex Marital Ther 1999; 25: 81–8.
14. van Lunsen RHW, Laan E. Genital vascular responsive and sexual feelings in midlife women: Psychophysiologic, brain and genital imaging studies. Menopause 2004; 11: 741–8.
15. Meston CM, Gozalka BB. Differential effects of sympathetic activation on sexual arousal and sexually dysfunctional and functional women. J Abnorm Psychol 1996; 105: 582–91.
16. Karama S, Lecours AR, Leroux JM et al. Areas of brain activation in males and females during viewing of erotic film excerpts. Hum Brain Mapp 2002; 16: 1–13.
17. Yucel S, de Souza A, Baskin LS. Neuroanatomy of the human female lower urogenital tract. J Urol 2004; 172: 191–5.
18. Palace EM, Gozalka BB. The enhancing effects of anxiety on arousal in sexually dysfunctional and functional women. J Abnorm Psychol 1990; 99: 403–11.
19. Creighton SM, Crouch NS, Foxwell NA et al. Functional evidence for nitrergic neurotransmission in human clitoral corpus cavernosum: a case study. Int J Impot Res 2004; 16: 319–24.
20. Schäfer A. Cervico motor reflex: Description of the reflex and role in sexual acts. J Sex Res 1996; 33: 153–7.
21. Shafik A, El-Sibai O, Mostafa R et al. Response of the internal reproductive organs to clitoral stimulation: The clitoro-uterine reflex. Int J Impot Res 2005; 17: 121–6.
22. Laumann EL, Paik A, Rosen RC. Sexual dysfunction in United States: prevalence and predictors. JAMA 1999; 10: 537–45.
23. Fugl-Myer AR, Sröjens Fugl-Myer K. Sexual disabilities, problems and satisfaction in 18–74-year-old Swedes. Scand J Sexology 1999; 2: 79–105.
24. Laumann, EO, Nicolosi A, Glasser DB et al. Sexual problems among women and men, aged 40–80 years: Prevalence and correlates identified in the global study of sexual attitudes and behaviours. Int J Impot Res 2005; 17: 39–57.
25. Hajjar RR, Kamel HK. Sex in the nursing home. Clin Geriatric Med 2003; 19: 575–86.
26. Avis NE, Zhao X, Johannes CB et al. Correlates of sexual function among multi-ethnic middle-aged women: results from the Study of Women's Health Across the Nation (SWAN). Menopause 2005; 12: 385–98.
27. Dennerstein L. Lehert P, Burger H et al. Factors affecting sexual functioning of women in the midlife years. Climacteric 1999; 2: 254–62.
28. Labrie F, Bélanger A, Tusan L et al. Marked decline in serum concentrations of adrenal C19 sex steroid precursors and conjugated androgen metabolites during aging. J Clin Endocrinol Metab 1997; 82: 2396–402.
29. Labrie F, Bélanger A, Bélanger P, et al. Androgen glucuronides, instead of testosterone, as the new markers of androgenic activity in women. J Steroid Biochem Mol Biol 2006; Apr 16; [E-pub ahead of print].

30. Davis SR, Guay AT, Shifren JL et al. Endocrine aspects of female sexual dysfunction. J Sex Marital Ther 2004; 1: 82–6.

31. Padero MCM, Bhasin S, Friedman TC. Androgen supplementation in older women: too much hype, not enough data. J Am Geriatr Soc 2002; 50: 1131–40.

32. Ganz PA, Desmond KA, Belin TR et al. Predictors of sexual health in women after a breast cancer diagnosis. J Clin Oncol 1999; 17: 2371–80.

33. Aziz A, Brännström M, Bergquist C et al. Perimenopausal androgen decline after oophorectomy does not influence sexuality or psychological wellbeing. Fertil Steril 2005; 83: 1021–8.

34. Santoro N, Torrens J, Crawford S et al. Correlates of circulating androgens in mid-life women: The Study of Women's Health Across the Nation (SWAN). J Clin Endocrinol Metabol 2005; 90: 4836–45.

35. Davis SR, Davison SL, Donath S et al. Circulating androgen levels in self-reported sexual function in women. JAMA 2005; 294: 91–6.

36. Dennerstein L, Lehert P, Burger H. The relative effects of hormone and relationship factors on sexual function of women through the natural menopausal transition. Fertil Steril 2005; 84: 174–80.

37. Davis SR, Goldstat R, Papalia MA et al. Effects of aromatase inhibition on sexual function and wellbeing in postmenopausal women treated with testosterone: a randomized placebo controlled trail. Menopause 2006; 13: 37–45.

38. Utian WH. Definitive symptoms of postmenopause. Incorporating use of vaginal parabasal cell index. Estrogens in the postmenopause. Front Hormone Res 1975; 3: 74–93.

39. Hoyle CHV, Stones RW, Robson T et al. Innervation of vasculature and microvasculature of the human vagina by NOS and neuropeptide-containing nerves. J Anat 1996; 188: 633–44.

40. Gorodeski GI, Hopfer U, Liu CC et al. Estrogen acidifies vaginal pH by up-regulation of proton secretion via the apical membrane of vaginal-ectocervical epithelial cells. Endocrinol 2005; 146: 816–24.

41. Foster DC, Palmer M, Marks J. Effect of vulvovaginal estrogen on sensorimotor response of the lower genital tract: a randomized control trial. Obstet Gynecol 1999; 94: 232–7.

42. Connell K, Guess MK, Bleustein CB et al. Effects of age, menopause, and comorbidities on neurological function of the female genitalia. Int J Impot Res 2005; 17: 63–70.

43. Basson R, Leiblum S, Brotto L et al. Definitions of women's sexual dysfunctions reconsidered: advocating expansion and revision. J Psychosom Obstet Gynecol 2003; 24: 221–9.

44. Basson R, Brotto L. Sexual psychophysiology and effects of sildenafil citrate in estrogenized women with acquired genital arousal disorder and impaired orgasm. Br J Obstet Gynecol 2003; 110: 1–11.

45. Basson R, Althof S, David S et al. Summary of the recommendations on sexual dysfunctions in women. J Sex Med 2004; 1: 24–34.

46. Trudel G, Marchand A, Ravart M et al. The effect of a cognitive behavioral group treatment program on hypoactive sexual desire in women. Sex Rel Ther 2001; 16: 145–64.

47. Sarwer DB, Durlak, JA. A field trial of the effectiveness of behavioral treatment for sexual dysfunctions. J Sex Marital Ther 1997; 23: 87–97.

48. Buster J E, Kingsberg S A, Aguirre O et al. Testosterone patch for low sexual desire in surgically menopausal women: a randomised trial. Obstet Gynecol 2005; 105: 944–52.

49. Davis SR, van der Mooren MJ, van Lunsen RHW et al. The efficacy and safety of a testosterone patch for the treatment of hypoactive sexual desire disorder in surgically menopausal women: a randomized, placebo-controlled trial. J Menopause 2006.

50. Braunstein GD, Sundwall DA, Katz M et al. Safety and efficacy of a testosterone patch for the treatment of hypoactive sexual desire disorder in surgically menopausal women: A randomized, placebo-controlled trial. Arch Intern Med 2005; 165: 1582–9.

51. Simon J, Braunstein G, Nachtigall L et al. Testosterone patch increases sexual activity and desire in surgically menopausal women with hypoactive sexual disorder. J Clin Endocrinol Metab 2005; 90: 5226–33.

52. Kroll R, Davis S, Moreau M, Waldbaum A, Shifren J. Wekselman K. Testosterone transdermal patch (TTP) significantly improved sexual function in naturally menopausal women in a large phase III study. Fertil Steril 2004; 82 (Suppl 2): S77.

53. Kraemer GR, Kraemer RR, Ogden BW et al. Variability of serum estrogens among postmenopausal women treated with the same transdermal estrogen therapy and the effects on androgens and sex hormone binding globulin. Fertil Steril 2003; 79: 534–42.

54. Wierman ME, Basson R, Davis SR et al. The Therapeutic Use of Androgens in Women: An Endocrine Society Clinical Practice Guideline. J Clin Endocrinol Metab (in press).

55. Belisle S, Blake J, Basson R, et al. SOGC Clinical Practice Guideline: Canadian Consensus on menopause and osteoporosis. 2006 Update. J Obstet Gynecol Can 2006; 28: 1–112.

56. Hodgins MB, Spike RC, Mackie RM et al. An immunohistochemical study of androgen, estrogen and progesterone receptors in the vulva and vagina. Br J Obstet Gynecol 1988; 105: 216–22.

57. Yabuki Y, Asamoto A, Hoshiba T et al. A new proposal for radical hysterectomy. Gynecol Oncol 1996; 62: 370–8.

58. Maas CP, ter Kuile MM, Laan E et al. Objective assessment of sexual arousal in women with a history of hysterectomy. Br J Obstet Gynecol 2004; 111: 456–62.

59. Buković D, Strinić T, Habek M et al. Sexual life after cervical carcinoma. Coll Antropol 2003; 27: 173–80.

60. Bergmark K, Åvall-Lundqvist E, Dickman PW et al. Synergy between sexual abuse and cervical cancer in causing sexual dysfunction. J Sex Marital Ther 2005; 31: 361–83.

61. Cardozo L, Bachmann G, McClish D et al. Meta analysis of estrogen therapy in the management of urogenital atrophy in postmenopausal women: Second report of the Hormones and Urogenital Therapy Committee. Obstet Gynecol 1998; 92(4) Part II: 722–7.

62. Harlow B, Gunther Stewart G. A population-based assessment of chronic unexplained vulvar pain: Have

we underestimated the prevalence of vulvodynia? J Am Med Wom Assoc 2003; 58: 82–8.

63. Reed BD, Haefner HK, Cantor L. Vulvar dysesthesia (vulvodynia), a follow-up study. J Reprod Med 2003; 48: 409–16.

64. Glazer HI, Rodke G, Swencionis C. Treatment of vulvar vestibulitis syndrome with electromyographic biofeedback of pelvic floor musculature. J Reprod Med 1995; 40: 283–290.

65. Rudkin L, Taylor MJ, Hawton K. Strategies for managing sexual dysfunction induced by antidepression med-

ication (Cochrane Review). The Cochrane Library Issue. Oxford: Update Software, 2004.

66. Clayton AH, Warnock JK, Kornstein SG et al. Placebo-controlled trial of bupropion SR as an antidote for selective serotonin reuptake inhibitor-induced sexual dysfunction. J Clin Psychol 2004; 65: 62–7.

67. Masand PS, Ashton AK, Gupta S et al. Sustained-release bupropion for selective serotonin reuptake inhibitor-induced sexual dysfunction: a randomized double-blind, placebo-controlled, parallel-group study. Am J Psychiatry 2001; 158: 805–7.

# Chapter 7

# Quality of life assessment in the menopause

Lothar AJ Heinemann and Hermann PG Schneider

## INTRODUCTION

Symptoms such as impaired memory, lack of concentration, nervousness, depression, insomnia, periodic sweating or hot flushes, bone and joint complaints, and reduction of muscle mass occur during menopausal transition.

The first widely accepted attempt to document the severity of menopausal complaints in women was the Kupperman Index,[1,2] a listing of the relevant symptomatology in this age-span. This questionnaire, developed in the 1950s, focused primarily on symptomatic relief, assessed on the basis of the physician's summary of the severity of the climacteric complaints, and assisted by a weighting index, rather than letting women assess their perceived symptoms. This is an example of a simple symptoms inventory without attempts to standardize it or to apply psychometric methodology. Only two decades later, the time had come for the development of more specific symptom lists or other questionnaires as instruments to measure changes, and to validate them in a scientific manner. Psychometric methods were more frequently applied in the 1950s and 1960s, but this knowledge was greatly restricted to psychology and social science and not yet common in medicine. Test theory and test construction developed rapidly in the 1960s also, spreading to the medical field.

It was the period of time when social scientists became more and more aware of only gradual differences between the so-called 'objective hard data' and 'subjective soft data', as different degrees of proof (hardness) had to be acknowledged. All measurements underlie similar rules, and could be of the same 'quality' if an adequate and rigorous quality assessment is applied to reduce the existing measurement error to the lowest possible level and to secure the highest possible validity. Principally, even symptom lists could be transformed into measurement tools applying appropriate methods. This theoretical approach was put into practice with the development of many (health-related) quality of life scales (HRQoL) during the last three decades.

Finally, increased awareness emanated of subjectively perceived QoL to best serve the description of treatment benefits; and this with much the same scrutiny as high-tech lab standards. This article briefly reviews some QoL-related instruments to measure the level of menopausal complaints and possible changes after treatment. We focus our attention on instruments with applied psychometrics to develop the scale and evaluate their basic properties – such as dimensions (domain) of a scale to measure complex human characteristics. This would require analysis of the structure of constructs such as menopausal complaints and assessment of the different aspects of this 'syndrome'. The way it is achieved is by analyzing the possible intercorrelations of all possible symptom combinations. As a result, symptoms will cluster into 'factors', which allow assessment of variation. This is the principle of factor analysis. The factors represent the 'domains or subscales' of a complex construct (like menopause). Our review will only consider scales that have undergone factor analysis and developed subscales, in order to better understand the multifaceted menopausal symptomatology (Chapter 6).

Another important trend to be considered is the increasing recognition in recent years among clinicians and researchers of the role of patient-reported data as outcome measures for clinical and drug research. Health authorities are in support of this growing interest. As a reflection, we can observe multiple attempts for a state-of-the-art development of health-related QoL scales applicable to women in their menopausal transition.

## SCALES AVAILABLE FOR ASSESSMENT OF MENOPAUSAL SYMPTOMS AND QUALITY OF LIFE

As this report is not intended for global reviewing, a selection of the most widely practiced questionnaires and measuring instruments is presented.

Half a century ago, the *Kupperman Index* was introduced to assist in the documentation of menopause-related symptoms, without having ever been subjected to psychometric analysis.[1,2] The first properly analyzed climacteric symptom scale was the *Greene Climacteric Scale*. This 22-item questionnaire with a rating of symptom severity (four rating points) specifies the three domains – vasomotoric, somatic, and psychological.[3] Its practical application and further validation finally resulted in the current scale of 21 items; this analytical process required the omission of five items and introduction of four new ones. The factor analysis of the final 21-item scale discovered four domains (vasomotor, somatic, anxiety, and depression).[4] Its relation to generic quality of life assessment apparently is not clarified.

Factor analysis also played a central role in the development of the *Menopausal Symptom Checklist*.[5] It consists of 25 items with a six-point scale for each item. Three subscales were generated: general somatic, vasomotoric, and psychological. This list allows a separate evaluation of both frequency and severity.

Another widely used inventory is the *Women's Health Questionnaire*, also based on an initial factor analysis. It consists of a rather complex scale with 32 items but only two rating points (present or absent). Thus, frequency but not severity is evaluated. Eight domains are described (vasomotor, somatic, anxiety, depression, cognitive difficulties, sleep problems, sexual behavior, and menstrual symptoms).[6] Its established general quality of life perspective is seen as an advantage. Norm values have been established for middle-aged women's perception of their emotional and physical health.[7]

The *Utian Quality-of-Life Score* is focused on general QoL rather than QoL in menopausal women. This instrument was also developed with a two-stage application of factor analysis: The 23-item instrument with a five-point rating scale for each item has four subscales (occupational, health, emotional, and sexual). This scale can measure severity of QoL burden. Only limited data on reliability and validity are as yet available. A relatively low number of menopausal symptom-specific items may require a parallel application of another more menopausal symptom-related scale for the most widely practiced application of such scales, which is during the menopausal transition.

The *QualiFemme Questionnaire* is a health-related QoL questionnaire based on factor analysis of 32 selected items. It consists of five relevant dimensions (principal components), which are defined as the general, psychological, vasomotoric, and urogenital domain plus one additional domain related to skin and hair problems. A 15-item version is readily available.[8]

The *QualiPause Inventory* (QPI) is a recently developed scale with 20 specific and some general items to evaluate symptoms and undesirable treatment effects with special regard to menopausal complaints.[9,10] Following factor analysis, six dimensions of the instrument were identified: psychosocial, vasomotor, physical, sexual, menstrual, and androgenic. This scale serves as a basis for a more advanced instrument applicable to pharmaco-economy, currently under investigation with testing and validation (personal communication: YF Zoellner).[11] The QPI has favorable psychometric characteristics concerning reliability and validity.[10]

All the above-mentioned questionnaires and inventories more or less consider sexual behavior a separate domain or item. More specific treatment options as well as considerable variation across populations urged clinical scientists to develop broader profiles of female sexual function and appropriate ways of assessment. Hypoactive sexual desire disorder (HSDD) is defined as a persistent deficiency or absence of sexual fantasies and desire for sexual activity that causes marked distress or interpersonal difficulty (American Psychiatric Association, 1994).[12] Women who have undergone menopause, whether natural or surgical, may experience a significant reduction in sexual desire. The *Profile of Female Sexual Function* (PFSF) is a new, self-report, multinational instrument designed to measure sexual desire and associated symptoms in women with HSDD following menopause. Specifically, this instrument, which contains 37 items in seven separate domains and an overall sexual satisfaction question, has been developed to reflect the clinical phenomenology of this disorder and its effects on the patients' thoughts, feelings, behaviors, and emotions. The initial development of the PFSF was performed in North America, Europe, and Australia. The PFSF is reliable and valid for use in women with HSDD and was demonstrated to have robust psychometric properties across numerous geographies.[13]

Sexuality certainly has great bearing on quality of life. Recent European questionnaires in four to six different countries agree that reduced sex drive concerns a good third of women aged 50 to 60 years. Of these, only small proportions of up to 10% ever seek treatment. In a scale of 1 (extremely unhappy) to 10 (extremely happy), sexual satisfaction of the average European woman was rated around 6, vaginal pain being the leading symptom. These women also admit 'increased sex life would make me feel more feminine and helps confidence and self-esteem'.[14]

Standard hormone replacement therapy (HRT) will significantly reduce both the frequency and severity of classical menopausal symptoms. Hogervorst et al (2002) systematically reviewed the effect of HRT on the cognitive function. Their study included 15 publications with a total of 566 postmenopausal women. This meta-analysis did not report any favorable effect of HRT on cognitive functions (verbal measures, spatial measures, speed of reading, or memory).[15]

In the Women's Health Initiative (WHI) Study, no favorable effect on cognitive function associated with the use of HRT was found.[16] Overall, randomized data systematically report that HRT improves a QoL that is hampered by the presence of climacteric symptoms. When symptoms are not present, HRT does not improve QoL, and would not do so in elderly women. Therefore, clinical practice would foster the application of menopause-specific questionnaires and their validated association with QoL in women of transient menopausal age. A validated and short symptom scale would optimally serve such practical purposes. One such example is the *Menopause Rating Scale*.[17]

## THE MENOPAUSE RATING SCALE

In addition to menopause-specific scales,[17,18] the first version of the Menopause Rating Scale (MRS) has been used since 1992.[19,20] It was initially developed to provide the physician with a tool to document specific climacteric symptoms and their

changes during treatment and was seen as an improvement over the commonly applied Kupperman Index.

A critical assessment of this new scale, however, disclosed methodological deficiencies, which, both in theory and practice, limited its use. This resulted in proposals to improve the physician-based scale:

- application of the scale in a representative sample of women after questionnaire revision
- revision of the questionnaire such that women will complete it themselves; first of all because self-assessment is more sensitive, and second, a self-administered questionnaire would not limit future application
- modification of the wording of items to a simple, laymen-appropriate form
- proper psychometric evaluation of the revised scale based on a representative sample and development of simple-to-use standardized items with clear dimensions
- classification of the severity of complaints based on a normal population sample
- provision of normative data, representative for the climacteric age in the female population.

In early 1996, the MRS questionnaire was standardized using a representative random sample of 689 German women aged 40 to 60 years, in order to obtain a new and standardized MRS.[21] The first revision of the questionnaire mainly concerned the layout, and some adjustments regarding the number, structure, and wording of items; these were made to support the applicability as a self-administered questionnaire. The MRS was formally standardized following up-to-date psychometric rules. The revised scale consists of a list of 11 items to be answered: the respondent has a choice among five categories – no symptom, mild, moderate, marked, or severe complaints/symptoms (Appendix 7.1).

*The factor analysis was performed as the first step of standardization of this instrument*

Three dimensions were identified explaining 58.8% of the total variance: psychological, somato-vegetative, and urogenital dimension. A five-point rating of severity was applied to each of the eleven items of the MRS: 0 (no symptom) or up to four scoring points (severe symptom), i.e. depending on the severity of the complaints perceived by the women completing the MRS (ticking the appropriate box in Appendix 7.1).

## Evaluation of the MRS

The scoring scheme is simple, i.e. the score increases point by point with increasing severity of subjectively perceived complaints in each of the 11 items (from 0 to 4 points). By checking one of five possible boxes of 'severity' for each of the items, the respondent provides her subjective status. This can be read from the questionnaire (Appendix 7.1).

The *total score* of the MRS ranges from 0 (asymptomatic) to 44 (highest degree of complaints). The minimal/maximal scores vary between the three dimensions, depending on the number of complaints allocated to the respective dimension of symptoms (see also the evaluation form in Appendix 7.2):

- psychological symptoms: 0 to 16 scoring points (four symptoms: depressed, irritable, anxious, exhausted)
- somato-vegetative symptoms: 0 to 16 points (four symptoms: sweating/flush, cardiac complaints, sleeping disorders, joint and muscle complaints)
- urogenital symptoms: 0 to 12 points (three symptoms: sexual problems, urinary complaints, vaginal dryness).

The sum scores for each of the dimensions (subscales or domains) are based on adding up the scores of the items of the respective dimensions. The composite score (total score) is the sum of the dimension scores. The three dimensions, their corresponding questions, and the evaluation are detailed and summarized in the evaluation scheme (Appendix 7.2).

Percentiles of the scores were calculated from a large population sample, i.e. for the total score, and for all three subscales (dimensions), separately. Normal values of the German population are available for comparison (Appendix 7.3).[18]

## International versions

The MRS had an excellent international response and acceptance. The first translation was into English.[22] Other translations followed, this way applying international methodological recommendations.[23] Currently, the following versions are available: Brazilian, Bulgarian, Belgium-French, Belgium-Dutch, Croatian, English, French, German, Indonesian, Italian, Mexican/Argentinean, Polish, Spanish, Swedish, Rumanian, Russian, Turkish, Ukrainian language. Some of these versions are available in a published form,[23] and all – including the unpublished ones – can be downloaded in PDF-format from the internet.[18,24]

## Psychometric characteristics

### Reliability

The assessment of scientific measurements depends first of all on their repeatability, i.e. consistency of results and test–retest reliability. In contrast to systematic and random variation, reliability gives an estimate of method-related measurement error, which should be low, so as not to hide or dilute intended systematic changes – due to treatment for example.

The internal consistency measured with Cronbach's alpha ranges between 0.6 and 0.9 across countries, for the total score as well the scores in the three domains (Table 7.1). This is a very acceptable consistency of the MRS. Moreover, there is no evidence that the scale works differently in so many different countries of four continents.[24]

The test–retest correlation coefficients (Pearson's correlation) support the suggestion of a good temporal stability of the total scale and its three domains. The test–retest coefficients of the total score range between (Pearson's correlation coefficient) $r = 0.8$ and $r = 0.96$ across Europe, North and Latin America, and Asia (Table 7.2).[25] This confirms earlier results.[26,27] When it comes to the subscales with much fewer items, the variation increased and some of the coefficients went down to 0.5 (e.g. urogenital domain in Indonesia). Altogether, the test–retest stability over a time period of two weeks aggregated at the international level supports the notion of a very acceptable test–retest reliability of the total scale and their three subscales.

Although there is an impressive set of information currently available concerning the reliability of the MRS, there are also limitations: small sample sizes prevent a final conclusion regarding test–retest reliability in some of the language transfers, and no information is currently available yet for several other languages.

### Validity

While reliability assesses the consistency of measurement, validity estimates whether or not a QoL scale really measures what it *intends* to measure. In contrast to reliability, which can be determined

Table 7.1 Internal consistency coefficients (alpha) for the MRS across countries: total score and scores for the psychological, somatic, and urogenital domain

| | International | Europe | | | | | N America | Latin America | | | | Asia |
| | Total | Overall | Sweden | Germany | France | Spain | US | Overall | Mexico | Brazil | Argentina | Indonesia |
|---|---|---|---|---|---|---|---|---|---|---|---|---|
| n | 9907 | 4465 | 1490 | 1050 | 941 | 984 | 1440 | 3002 | 1002 | 1000 | 1000 | 1000 |
| Total score | 0.83 | 0.86 | 0.85 | 0.84 | 0.86 | 0.86 | 0.88 | 0.86 | 0.87 | 0.86 | 0.83 | 0.84 |
| Psychological score | 0.87 | 0.88 | 0.88 | 0.86 | 0.89 | 0.86 | 0.90 | 0.85 | 0.86 | 0.87 | 0.81 | 0.79 |
| Somatic score | 0.66 | 0.64 | 0.65 | 0.64 | 0.64 | 0.61 | 0.70 | 0.66 | 0.65 | 0.69 | 0.64 | 0.69 |
| Urogenital score | 0.65 | 0.65 | 0.64 | 0.63 | 0.67 | 0.67 | 0.70 | 0.60 | 0.62 | 0.55 | 0.62 | 0.65 |

Data taken from Ref. 25.

Table 7.2 Test–retest coefficients (Pearson's correlation coefficient r) for the MRS across countries: total score and scores for the psychological, somatic, and sexual subscale — community samples

| | All | Europe | | | | | | | | Latin America | | | Asia | |
| | Overall | Overall | Germany | UK | France | Spain | Portugal | Sweden | Turkey | Overall | Argentina | Brazil | Overall | Indonesia |
|---|---|---|---|---|---|---|---|---|---|---|---|---|---|---|
| n | 349 | 259 | 73 | 30 | 36 | 30 | 30 | 30 | 30 | 60 | 30 | 30 | 30 | 30 |
| Total score | 0.90 | 0.92 | 0.82 | 0.80 | 0.89 | 0.93 | 0.96 | 0.90 | 0.90 | 0.81 | 0.78 | 0.82 | 0.84 | 0.84 |
| Psychological score | 0.84 | 0.87 | 0.76 | 0.72 | 0.88 | 0.92 | 0.91 | 0.79 | 0.82 | 0.72 | 0.66 | 0.76 | 0.71 | 0.71 |
| Somatic score | 0.89 | 0.90 | 0.80 | 0.85 | 0.82 | 0.88 | 0.97 | 0.95 | 0.93 | 0.85 | 0.86 | 0.85 | 0.81 | 0.81 |
| Urogenital score | 0.86 | 0.89 | 0.77 | 0.82 | 0.94 | 0.98 | 0.95 | 0.87 | 0.89 | 0.73 | 0.67 | 0.74 | 0.50 | 0.50 |

Data taken from Ref. 25.

straightforwardly with very few indicators, validation requires a continuing process (construct validation). It is a process of accumulating evidence for a valid measurement of what is intended.

There are many validity measures such as: internal structure, concurrent validity (criterion-oriented), discriminative, or predictive validity, and others.

## Internal structure of the MRS

Several analyses were performed since the first factor analysis in 1996 was applied to identify the dimensions of the scale. In three large samples studied until 2003, an astonishingly similar structure of the MRS was observed across time and different populations. Similar factor loadings (correlations) of the 11 items in the three domains – as can be seen in Table 7.3 – suggest that the scale constantly measures the same phenomenon across regions.[25]

One important issue relates to the independence of the three subscales from the aggregate total scale: theoretically, the correlations between subscales (supposed to be independent due to the statistical model) would be closer to 0 than the correlations with the total score to which all subscales should significantly contribute. But only a somewhat lower correlation among subscales ($r = 0.4$–$0.7$) was observed, when compared to the correlations of subscales with the total score ($0.7$–$0.9$). This suggests that the subscales are not as independent from each other as one would expect them to be – based on a factor analysis with assumed orthogonal factors. The situation was similar in the four regions analyzed,[25] and in the individual countries belonging to these regions. This needs to be considered when analyzing the results of the scale – often the total score might be preferred or utilized for interpretation.

## Compatibility of the MRS scores among countries

Currently, there are MRS population reference values for severity of complaints published (see Appendix 7.3 for the German population). Are these reference values applicable for other countries or cultures?

The data of our large, multinational survey would allow for some comparisons. The mean values (and standard deviations (SD)) of the MRS total score and the three domains are depicted in Table 7.4. These are not statistically significantly different between Europe and North America. Thus, there is no reason why MRS values between these regions may not be compared to each other.

However, the subscales seem to differ: total, psychological and somatic scores were systematically higher in Latin America and systematically lower in Asia (Indonesia) than in Europe or North America. The urogenital scores were significantly lower in Latin America or Indonesia than in Europe or the US. Obviously the perception of the prevalent symptoms depends on cultural factors – or the symptoms show real differences in prevalence. Thus, a direct comparison of MRS subscores between Europe or North America on the one side, and regions in Latin America and Asia on the other, should only be done with caution. This does not affect intra-individual comparisons (e.g. pre-/post-therapy), and it may have very little impact on the comparison of relative changes (pre-/post-treatment) among different countries. The latter is a working hypothesis and needs further research.

The prevalence of the complaint categories across the four regions studied is seen in Table 7.5. Apparently the above-mentioned differences between Europe or the US and Latin America or Indonesia very much depend on the severity of complaints. While the differences in the psychological domain were less impressive, the dissimilarity was most pronounced in the urogenital domain, and less so in the somatic domain. Whether this is due to different perception of identical symptoms, because of differences in the appearance of symptoms, or both, remains speculation. This, however, needs to be considered when direct comparisons among different cultures are intended. The prevalence of different 'degrees of severity' of menopausal symptoms measured with the MRS was found to be almost identical in the aggregate of Europe and North America.

## Concurrent validity: correlation with other scales

In order to further evaluate the MRS for scoring menopausal symptoms, it was compared with other instruments relevant for women in their menopausal transition: the Kupperman Index and the generic QoL scale SF-36.[28]

A comparison of the MRS with the Kupperman Index produced a high correlation of raw scores (Pearson's $r = 0.91$). The highest association of scores was found in the highest quartile (80%) of the MRS. The terms 'mild', 'moderate', and 'severe' for the degree of severity of menopausal

**Table 7.3**  Internal structure of the MRS across nine countries of four continents (2002) compared to the initial analysis of a German sample in 1996

| | n | Flushes (1) | Heart discomfort (2) | Sleep problems (3) | Joint and muscular discomfort (11) | Depression (4) | Irritability (5) | Anxiety (6) | Exhaustion (7) | Sexual problems (8) | Bladder problems (9) | Dryness of the vagina (10) |
|---|---|---|---|---|---|---|---|---|---|---|---|---|
| **Germany, 1996** | 479 | | | | | | | | | | | |
| somatic | | 0.8 | 0.7 | 0.6 | 0.5 | | | | | | | |
| psychological | | | | | | 0.8 | 0.7 | 0.8 | 0.6 | | | |
| urogenital | | | | | | | | | | 0.7 | 0.8 | 0.8 |
| **All countries, 2002** | 10297 | | | | | | | | | | | |
| somatic | | 0.7 | 0.8 | 0.5 | 0.5 | | | | | | | |
| psychological | | | | | | 0.8 | 0.8 | 0.8 | 0.7 | | | |
| urogenital | | | | | | | | | | 0.7 | 0.6 | 0.8 |
| **Europe, 2002** | 4791 | | | | | | | | | | | |
| somatic | | 0.7 | 0.7 | 0.6 | 0.6 | | | | | | | |
| psychological | | | | | | 0.8 | 0.9 | 0.8 | 0.6 | | | |
| urogenital | | | | | | | | | | 0.7 | 0.6 | 0.8 |
| **N America (US), 2002** | 1500 | | | | | | | | | | | |
| somatic | | 0.7 | 0.7 | 0.7 | 0.5 | | | | | | | |
| psychological | | | | | | 0.8 | 0.9 | 0.8 | 0.6 | | | |
| urogenital | | | | | | | | | | 0.8 | 0.6 | 0.8 |
| **Latin America, 2002** | 3006 | | | | | | | | | | | |
| somatic | | 0.5 | 0.9 | 0.5 | 0.4 | | | | | | | |
| psychological | | | | | | 0.8 | 0.8 | 0.8 | 0.7 | | | |
| urogenital | | | | 0.5 | | | | | | 0.6 | 0.7 | 0.8 |
| **Asia (Indonesia), 2002** | 1000 | | | | | | | | | | | |
| somatic | | 0.9 | 0.6 | 0.5 | 0.5 | | | | | | | |
| psychological | | | | | | 0.8 | 0.8 | 0.8 | 0.5 | | | |
| urogenital | | | | | | | | | | 0.8 | 0.5 | |

Principal component analysis, Varimax rotation. Complaints (item number in MRS), number of participants, and country groups. Factor loadings ≥0.5 only are presented. Data taken from Ref. 25.

**Table 7.4** Mean values and standard deviation of the MRS total score and its three domains: results from a large, multinational survey

|  | Total score | | Psychological score | | Somato-vegetative score | | Urogenital score | |
|---|---|---|---|---|---|---|---|---|
|  | n | Mean (SD) | n | Mean (SD) | n | Mean (SD) | n | Mean (SD) |
| Europe | 4246 | 8.8 (7.1) | 4453 | 3.4 (3.4) | 4465 | 3.6 (2.9) | 4465 | 1.9 (2.2) |
| N America (US) | 1376 | 9.1 (7.6) | 1426 | 3.4 (3.5) | 1440 | 3.8 (3.1) | 1437 | 2.0 (2.3) |
| Latin America | 3001 | 10.4 (8.8) | 3002 | 4.9 (4.5) | 3006 | 4.1 (3.6) | 3005 | 1.4 (2.2) |
| Asia | 1000 | 7.2 (6.0) | 1000 | 2.9 (2.9) | 1000 | 3.3 (2.7) | 1000 | 1.0 (1.6) |

Data taken from Ref. 25.

**Table 7.5** Degree of severity of the MRS and its domains

|  | Europe | North america | Latin America | Asia |
|---|---|---|---|---|
| **Total score** | | | | |
| no, little (0–4) | 28.8 (±1.3 ) | 28.0 (±2.3) | 31.0 (±1.7 ) | 40.2 (±3.0) |
| mild (5–8) | 21.9 (± 1.2) | 23.9 (±2.2) | 20.2 (±1.4 ) | 27.5 (±2.8) |
| moderate (9–16) | 25.1 (±1.2 ) | 25.7 (±2.2) | 26.2 (±1.6 ) | 22.8 (±2.6) |
| severe (17+) | 24.3 (± 1.2) | 22.5 (±2.1) | 22.7 (±1.5 ) | 9.5 (±1.8) |
| **Psychological domain** | | | | |
| no, little (0–1) | 35.4 (±1.4 ) | 36.8 (±2.4) | 36.8 (±1.6 ) | 41.3 (±3.1) |
| mild (2–3) | 21.8 (±1.2 ) | 21.9 (±2.1) | 21.9 (±1.4 ) | 25.4 (±2.7) |
| moderate (4–6) | 19.5 (±1.1 ) | 18.7 (±2.0) | 18.7 (±1.4 ) | 21.3 (±2.6) |
| severe (7+) | 23.4 (±1.2 ) | 22.5 (±2.1) | 22.5 (±1.7 ) | 12.0 (±2.0) |
| **Somato-vegetative domain** | | | | |
| no, little (0–2) | 39.5 (±1.4 ) | 37.9 (±2.4) | 42.1 (±1.8 ) | 46.8 (±3.1) |
| mild (3–4) | 22.6 (±1.2) | 25.6 (±2.2) | 19.4 (±1.4 ) | 27.0 (±2.8) |
| moderate (5–8) | 24.2 (±1.2 ) | 24.3 (±2.2) | 25.6 (±1.6 ) | 20.8 (±2.5 ) |
| severe (9+) | 13.7 (±1.0 ) | 12.1 (±1.7) | 12.9 (±1.2) | 5.4 (±1.4) |
| **Urogenital domain** | | | | |
| no, little (0) | 34.3 (±1.3 ) | 33.4 (±2.4) | 28.2 (±1.8 ) | 55.6 (±3.1) |
| mild (1) | 17.2 (±1.1 ) | 17.0 (±2.0) | 18.6 (±1.1 ) | 18.6 (±2.4) |
| moderate (2–3) | 23.0 (± 1.2) | 24.2 (±2.2) | 21.8 (±1.3 ) | 17.0 (±2.3) |
| severe (4+) | 25.6 (±1.2 ) | 25.4 (±2.2) | 31.4 (±1.3 ) | 8.8 (±1.8) |

Data given are percentage prevalence (95% confidence interval) of the regional population studied.
Data taken from Ref. 25.

symptoms reflect different contents in both scales, and are differently spread, i.e. they are not directly comparable.

There is a strikingly good association between the subscales of SF-36 and the MRS. The MRS correlates best in dimensions of the SF-36, which are highly relevant for women in the menopausal transition. For that reason, the MRS can be utilized as an age-/condition-specific QoL instrument.

The MRS is a valuable modern tool for the assessment of menopausal complaints. It combines in practice excellent applicability, good repeatability, and there are 'norm values for the population' available. The MRS could serve as an adequate diagnostic instrument for menopausal QoL.[25]

### The MRS as a clinical outcome measure

A recent report collected about 9300 women in a pre- and post-treatment experience with the MRS. This served as a basis to critically evaluate the capacity of the scale to measure the effect of hormone treatment independent from the severity of complaints.[29]

The absolute improvement of symptoms during treatment was 9.3 points of the MRS total score on average. This is equivalent to 36% of the baseline score, and was similar for all three subscales. Thus, the MRS was successful in detecting treatment effects.

Was the MRS also sufficient to detect treatment effects in women with only few or mild symptoms? An improvement of complaints or QoL was seen with increasing degree of symptom severity. Figure 7.1 shows that patients with few/no complaints before therapy improved by 11%; those

with mild complaints at entry by 32%; those with moderate complaints by 44%; and those with severe symptoms by 55%. The scale does detect treatment effects in women with few complaints, albeit to a lesser degree.

This can also be illustrated by a different approach – the comparison with norm values for the population (Figure 7.2). In the normal population, we find a higher percentage of women with no or few symptoms when compared to those with severe complaints. Women eligible for therapy, however, show a much lower proportion with few or mild complaints, in contrast to moderate or severe complainers. After 6 months of hormone treatment, however, the frequency distribution of patients with a certain severity of complaints returned towards a distribution that was similar to that observed in the general population. The extreme proportion of patients with no/few complaints after therapy should be interpreted with reservation because of the potential of patient selection and overestimated treatment effects (the MRS was completed in the physician's office). But,

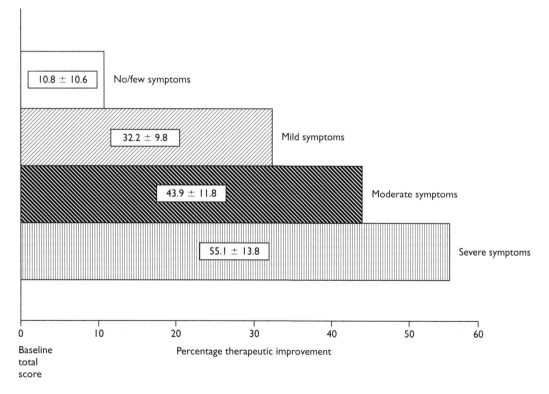

**Figure 7.1** Relative change of the MRS: mean values (SD) of the relative change (% improvement of complaints following HRT) in four categories of severity at baseline.

independent of such potential bias, the MRS is sensitive to detect treatment effects, and reference to population norms is another way of handling standardized scales. This procedure could assist (as in Table 7.3) in proper interpretation of results, but should not be used for formal statistical testing. Patient groups tend to be different from the general population, a difference that is hard to adjust for. As an example, women using HRT are more likely to be younger, have an earlier menarche and later menopause, be parous, have more benign breast disease, be better educated and have used oral contraceptives and progestogen before.

## SUMMARY

The MRS is one example out of a group of menopause-specific scales that do differ with respect to the vigor of evaluated reliability and validity. Most of the scales follow similar objectives as the MRS does, i.e. (1) to enable comparisons of the menopause-related symptoms among groups of women under different conditions; (2)

to compare severity of symptoms over time or across regions; and (3) to measure changes pre- and post-treatment.

The development of the MRS serves as an example for the extent of methodological safeguards necessary to establish a scale as a fully 'standardized instrument' (asymptotic approximation in the course of construct validation).

The currently available methodological evidence points to high-quality standards of the MRS to measure and to compare HRQoL of aging women in different regions and over time. Reliability measures (consistency and test–retest stability) were found to be good across countries. The internal structure of the MRS across countries was astonishingly similar, to allow for the fact that the scale really measures the same phenomenon in symptomatic women. Norm values from different populations document direct comparisons between Europe and North America. Small differences among other regions will not affect intra-individual comparisons within clinical trials.

The comparative evaluation of the Kupperman Index resulted in satisfying correlations, which

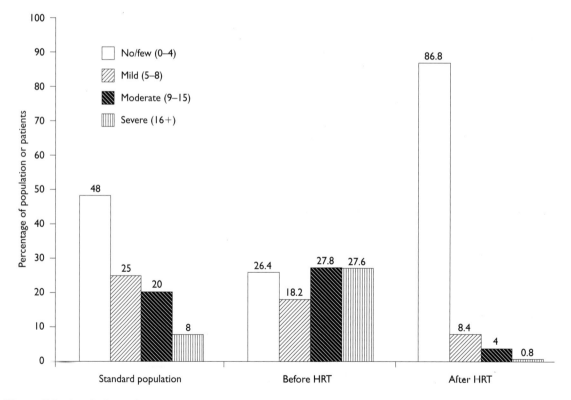

**Figure 7.2** Level of complaints in the population compared to women before and following HRT: frequency distribution before and after therapy compared with population normal values.

illustrates an adept criterion-oriented validity. The same holds true for the comparison with the generic QoL scale SF-36, where sufficiently close associations were documented.

As with other QoL scales, it is a challenge to satisfy the demands of clinical utility and outcomes measures. The MRS is well adapted to measure treatment effects on QoL across the full range of menopausal complaint severity.

The MRS has become internationally well accepted and is available in numerous languages. These versions are accessible in published form, or may be downloaded in PDF-format from the internet.[24]

## FUTURE DEVELOPMENTS

In view of the array of psychometrically sound scales available, such as the MRS, it is highly recommended that clinicians abstain from using ad hoc measures without scientific legitimacy. General QoL scales should only be applied in treatment studies of menopausal women to supplement the menopause-specific scales.

All of the introduced scales were developed to measure health-related problems and their impact on HRQoL based on a symptom profile (profile instruments). There is a new trend to develop instruments for health-economical evaluation (index instruments). This would enable us to estimate quality-adjusted life years (QALY) to be determined for all menopausal health states. Such an instrument would facilitate cost–utility evaluations of postmenopausal treatments based on empirical data, for example.[11]

Another application of HRQoL scales is emerging: the number of websites of organizations or individual physicians (groups) interested in educating the population on health issues increases, and thereby also the number of scales exhibited on websites. Behind this may simply be the objective to educate the population or subgroups in health-related issues. This may particularly apply to diseases or conditions with lesser awareness than for menopause and related issues, e.g. andropause. Another potential interest could be to encourage women to contact a certain medical service for diagnosis/therapy, to advertise certain remedies, or to offer self-testing of effects of drugs taken. Patients' self-assessment of symptoms (changes) and thereby learning about their own physical status might be a real motivation.

Finally, human beings are social individuals. If one changes the health status or QoL of an aging person, the partner might also be affected, sometimes strongly, and with positive or negative interaction. This is rarely considered in the development of tools to measure treatment. The awareness is increasing in the field of sexual dysfunction. Sexual function, as mentioned above, is an important variable which determines QoL. Treatments affecting sexual function such as hormone therapy (both in men and women) could be assessed in both partners (if available). There are already scales emerging to meet such needs.[30,32]

## REFERENCES

1. Kupperman HS, Blatt MHG, Wiesbader H et al. Comparative clinical evaluation of estrogen preparations by the menopausal and amenorrhoea indices. J Clin Endocrinol 1953; 13: 688–703.
2. Kupperman HS, Wetchler BB, Blatt MHG. Contemporary therapy of the menopausal syndrome. JAMA 1959; 171: 1627–37.
3. Greene JG. A factor analytic study of climacteric symptoms. Psychosom Res 1976; 20: 425–30.
4. Greene JG. Constructing a standard climacteric scale. Maturitas 1998; 29: 25–31.
5. Perz JM. Development of the Menopause Symptom Checklist. A factor analytic study of menopause associated symptoms. Women and Health 1997; 25: 53–69.
6. Hunter M. The Women's Health Questionnaire (WHQ): development, standardization and application of as measure of mid-aged women's emotional and physical health. Qual Life Res 2001; 9: 733–8.
7. Hunter M. The Women's Health Questionnaire: a measure of mid-aged women's perception of their emotional and physical health. Psychology and Health 1992; 7: 45–54.
8. Le Floch JP, Colau JC, Zartarian M. Réduction d'un questionnaire d'évaluation de la qualité de vie en ménopause. Contracept Fertil Sex 1996; 24: 238–45.
9. Zoellner YF, Oliver P, Brazier JE et al. Development of the 'QualiPause toolkit' to assess quality of life in climacteric and postmenopausal women. Gynecol Endocrinol 2001; 15 (Suppl 5): 56.
10. Zoellner YF, Oliver P, Brazier JE et al. Reliability and validity of a newly developed menopause-specific quality-of-life questionnaire, the QualiPause Inventory (QPI). Qual Life Res 2001; 10: 260.
11. Brazier JE, Roberts J, Platts M, et al. Estimating a preference-based index for a menopause specific health quality of life questionnaire. Health Qual Life Outcomes 2005; 3: 13. www.hqlo.com/content/3/1/13 (accessed 29 March 2006).
12. American Psychiatric Association. Diagnostic and statistical manual of mental disorders, 4th edn. Washington, DC: American Psychiatric Association, 1994.
13. Derogatis L, Rust J, Golombok S et al. Validation of the Profile of Female Sexual Function (PFSF) in surgically

and naturally menopausal women. J Sex Marital Ther 2004; 30: 25–36.

14. Genazzani AR, Schneider HPG, Panay N, Nijland EA. The European Menopause Survey 2005: women's perceptions on the menopause and postmenopausal hormone therapy. J. Gynaecol. Encrinol 2006; 22: 369–75.

15. Hogervorst E, Yaffe K, Richards M et al. Hormone replacement therapy for cognitive function in post-menopausal women. Cochrane Database Syst Rev 2002; CD003122.

16. Shumaker SA, Legault C, Rapp SR et al. WHIMS Investigators. Estrogen plus progestin and the incidence of dementia and mild cognitive impairment in post-menopausal women: the Women's Health Initiative Memory Study: a randomized controlled trial. JAMA 2003; 289: 2651–62.

17. Schneider HPG, Behre HM. Contemporary evaluation of climacteric complaints: Its impact on quality of life. In: Schneider HPG, ed. Hormone Replacement Therapy and Quality of Life. Boca Raton, London, New York, Washington: The Parthenon Publishing Group, 2002: 45–61.

18. Greene, JG. Measuring the symptom dimension of quality of life: general and menopause-specific scales and their subscale structure. In: Schneider HPG, ed. Hormone Replacement Therapy and Quality of Life. Boca Raton, London, New York, Washington: The Parthenon Publishing Group, 2002: 35–43.

19. Hauser GA, Huber IC, Keller PJ et al. Evaluation der klimakterischen Beschwerden (Menopause Rating Scale [MRS]). Zentralbl Gynakol 1994; 116: 16–23.

20. Schneider HPG, Doeren M. Traits for long-term acceptance of hormone replacement therapy – results of a representative German survey. Eur Menopause J 1996; 3: 94–8.

21. Potthoff P, Heinemann LAJ, Schneider HPG et al. Menopause-Rating Skala (MRS): Methodische Standardisierung in der deutschen Bevoelkerung. Zentralbl Gynakol 2000; 122: 280–6.

22. Schneider HPG, Heinemann LAJ, Thiele K. The Menopause Rating Scale (MRS): cultural and linguistic translation into English. Life and Medical Science Online 2002; 3.

23. Heinemann LAJ, Potthoff P, Schneider HPG. International versions of the Menopause Rating Scale (MRS). Health Qual Life Outcomes 2003; 1: 28. www.hqlo.com/articles/browse.asp (accessed 29 March 2006).

24. http://www.menopause-rating-scale.info (accessed 29 March 2006).

25. Heinemann K, Ruebig A, Potthoff P et al. The Menopause Rating Scale (MRS) scale: a methodological review. Health Qual Life Outcomes 2004; 2: 45. www.hqlo.com/content/2/1/45 (accessed 29 March 2006).

26. Heinemann K, Assmann A, Moehner S et al. Reliabilitaet der Menopause-Rating-Skala (MRS). Untersuchung fuer die Deutsche Bevoelkerung. Zentralbl Gynakol 2002; 124: 161–3.

27. Schneider HPG, Heinemann LAJ, Rosemeier HP et al. The Menopause Rating Scale (MRS): reliability of scores of menopausal complaints. Climacteric 2000; 3: 59–64.

28. Schneider HPG, Heinemann LAJ, Rosemeier HP et al. The Menopause Rating Scale (MRS): Comparison with Kupperman Index and Quality of Life Scale SF-36. Climacteric 2000; 3: 50–8.

29. Heinemann LAJ, DoMinh T, Strehlow F et al. Validity of the Menopause Rating Scale as outcome measure. A clinical outcome study. Health Qual Life Outcomes 2004; 2: 45. www.hqlo.com/content/2/1/67 (accessed 29 March 2006).

30. Heinemann LAJ, Potthoff P, Heinemann K et al. Scale for Quality of Sexual Function (QSF) as an outcome measure for both genders? J Sexual Med 2005; 2: 82–95.

31. Chevret M, Jaudinot E, Sullivan K et al. Quality of sexual life and satisfaction in female partners of men with ED: psychometric validation of the Index of Sexual Life (ISL) questionnaire. J Sex Marital Ther 2004; 30: 141–55.

## APPENDIX 7.1: MENOPAUSE RATING SCALE

Which of the following symptoms apply to you at this time? Please mark the appropriate box for each symptom. For symptoms that do not apply, please mark 'none'.

| Symptoms: | none | mild | moderate | severe | very severe |
|---|---|---|---|---|---|
| Score = | 0 | 1 | 2 | 3 | 4 |

1. Hot flushes, sweating (episodes of sweating)  ❑ ❑ ❑ ❑ ❑

2. Heart discomfort (unusual awareness of heart beat, heart skipping, heart racing, tightness)  ❑ ❑ ❑ ❑ ❑

3. Sleep problems (difficulty in falling asleep, difficulty in sleeping through, waking up early)  ❑ ❑ ❑ ❑ ❑

4. Depressive mood (feeling down, sad, on the verge of tears, lack of drive, mood swings)  ❑ ❑ ❑ ❑ ❑

5. Irritability (feeling nervous, inner tension, feeling aggressive)

     ❏       ❏       ❏       ❏       ❏

6. Anxiety (inner restlessness, feeling panicky)

     ❏       ❏       ❏       ❏       ❏

7. Physical and mental exhaustion (general decrease in performance, impaired memory, decrease in concentration, forgetfulness)

     ❏       ❏       ❏       ❏       ❏

8. Sexual problems (change in sexual desire, in sexual activity and satisfaction)

     ❏       ❏       ❏       ❏       ❏

9. Bladder problems (difficulty in urinating, increased need to urinate, bladder incontinence)

     ❏       ❏       ❏       ❏       ❏

10. Dryness of the vagina (sensation of dryness or burning in the vagina, difficulty with sexual intercourse)

     ❏       ❏       ❏       ❏       ❏

11. Joint and muscular discomfort (pain in the joints, rheumatoid complaints)

     ❏       ❏       ❏       ❏       ❏

## APPENDIX 7.2:  MENOPAUSE RATING SCALE (MRS) – EVALUATION FORM

Once the MRS questionnaire is completed by the respondent, the following form can be used if an evaluation on paper is intended. However, a computerized evaluation is recommended.

The scoring scheme of the MRS is simple: the questionnaire offers for each of the 11 items an option to check one of five degrees of severity of symptoms (severity 0 [none] to 5 [very severe] points). Put the scoring points of each of the items into the form below.

The composite scores for each of the three dimensions (subscales) are based on adding up the scores of the items of the respective dimensions. The composite score (total score) is the sum of the three dimension scores. The three dimensions, i.e. psychological, somato-vegetative, and urogenital subscale, and their corresponding question numbers are detailed in the form.

This form explains how the total sum-score and the sum-scores of the subscales are determined: add up the severity scoring points from each of items belonging to one of the subscales (indicated by a blank field) to get the sum-score for the respective subscale.

The 'total score' is the sum of the sum-scores of the three subscales.

| Question number | Score | Psychological subscale | Somatic subscale | Urogenital subscale |
|---|---|---|---|---|
| 1. | | | . . . . . | |
| 2. | | | . . . . . | |
| 3. | | | . . . . . | |
| 4. | | . . . . . | | |
| 5. | | . . . . . | | |
| 6. | | . . . . . | | |
| 7. | | . . . . . | | |
| 8. | | | | . . . . . |
| 9. | | | | . . . . . |
| 10. | | | | . . . . . |
| 11. | | . . . . . | | . . . . . |
| Sum of scores in | | subscales | Sum score | |
| | | PSYCH . . . . . | Sum score | |
| | | SOMAT . . . . . | Sum score | |
| UROGEN . . . . . | | | | |
| Total sum of scores of all subscales = total score: | | | | |

## APPENDIX 7.3: MRS – INTENSITY-CATEGORIES OF SYMPTOMS OR COMPLAINTS IN THE NORMAL FEMALE POPULATION OF GERMANY (45–60 YEARS)*

Data from a reference-sample of 479 women (45–60 years) who completed the questionnaire.[21]

Total score (sum of three subscales)

| Scores | Severity of symptoms | Percentage of the population |
|---|---|---|
| 0–4 | No (little) | 42 |
| 5–8 | Mild | 28 |
| 9–16 | Moderate | 24 |
| 17+ | Severe | 6 |

## Subscale 'somato-vegetative complaints'

| Scores | Severity of symptoms | Percentage of the population |
| --- | --- | --- |
| 0–2 | No (few) | 46 |
| 3–4 | Mild | 24 |
| 5–8 | Moderate | 24 |
| 9+ | Severe | 6 |

## Subscale 'psychological problems'

| Scores | Severity of symptoms | Percentage of the population |
| --- | --- | --- |
| 0–1 | No (few) | 48 |
| 2–3 | Mild | 23 |
| 4–6 | Moderate | 19 |
| 7+ | Severe | 10 |

## Subscale 'urogenital problems'

| Scores | Severity of symptoms | Percentage of the population |
| --- | --- | --- |
| 0 | No (few) | 61 |
| 1 | Mild | 16 |
| 2–3 | Moderate | 16 |
| 4+ | Severe | 7 |

# Section II

# Endocrinology of the menopause

# Chapter 8

# The sex hormonal continuum in the menopause and geripause

Bernard A Eskin

## INTRODUCTION

Menopause has been considered as that point in time when a total loss of estrogen function occurs in women. Since basic recognition in 1925, both analyses and syntheses of estrogen and its decreased biological action in menopause have generated a significant scientific literature which indicates that a reduction occurs, but never a total elimination. Menopause begins when the level of estrogen produced drops below a threshold required for specific endometrial growth and development. The decrease in quantity of estrogen differs for the onset of the various menopausal symptoms and signs. Clinical menopause is defined as beginning when menses have not occurred for one year and reproductive cycles cease.[1] Prior to the clinical menopause, related symptoms are already recognizable.

Immediately after the menopause, the post-menopause, both hormonal loss and biological aging become evident. The losses due to estrogen production are immediate compared with the gradual changes brought on by aging throughout the years. This chapter describes the changes acutely initiated by estrogen loss and attempts to distinguish them from the demographic processes seen in aging (Chapter 2).

## THE ESTROGEN CONTINUUM

Throughout this textbook the inevitable decreases in the production, secretion, and metabolism of estrogens and related sex hormones, androgens and progestogens, in women are described. Estrogen decreases in the late phases of reproductive life, and eventually is almost depleted by late geripause. The steroid sequence in the ovary shows a decreased pool of intermediate steroids, a reduction in aromitizing enzyme, and depressed estrogen synthesis and secretion. Inability of the hypothalamus to stabilize this loss by stimulating ovarian syntheses results in the continuous quantitative decrease of hormone. This reduction in estrogens leads to the onset of the menopause.

The devious onset of menopausal symptomatology interrupts the general daily vitality of active women in midlife. Her physiological and psychological reactions to it appear to be modified by the depressed levels of endogenous estrogen available and her personal responses to the changes that occur. Clinical laboratory tests of estrogen modulations during the last 50 years have not been able to predict accurately individual symptomatic responses.[2]

Estrogen function and metabolism at cellular levels are being successfully researched, a work still in progress. It has become evident that to initiate estrogen activity, complexing with estrogen receptor (ER) proteins is required.[3] Estrogens, particularly estradiol ($E_2$) functions throughout the brain and body. Estrogen locales can be recognized by distribution in microassays of intracellular ER proteins.[4] Activity occurs in the three estrogen receptors: α (ERα), and $β_1$ (ERβ) and $β_2$ (ERβ₂). Genomic responses in the cell are dependent on the estrogen metabolic pathway which initiates and stimulates protein activity. ER proteins can be recognized and quantified; they are highest in reproductive organs, but in variable amounts in almost all body structures and organs.[4] ERα appears to function best in reproductive tissues, while the β-receptors favor somatic tissue. The differences in activity are specific but quantitatively variable.[5]

Several authors have proposed that an added feature to estrogen loss is the decrease in binding affinity to receptors that occurs with aging.[6] The ligand (estrogen) is responsible for the level of biological effect, not the measure of affinity.[7,8] Thus, hormone replacement response is not only a matter of affinity to the ER, but also of the characteristic action of biological response provided by the ligand. ER action is described in Chapter 1. This provides a practical aspect for the level and form of estrogen most effective for the older women after certain biological losses. Significant advances have been made in recognizing which symptoms are most affected by a given chemical form of estrogen.[6]

Recent evidence has shown an exemplary finding occurs in the brain where ERα and ERβ are anatomically prevalent.[9] The studies involved are markedly complex, but there appears to be evidence that estrogen deficiency is involved in brain injury, neurodegeneration and cognitive decline predominantly shown by ERβ.[10–12] In the postmenopause, many intracellular effectors of ERs (down- and upregulators) appear also to be considerably responsive to the levels of the various other lost reproductive hormones.[13,14] Most of these are intermediate cyclic or reproductive steroids. There is an important loss in monamine control of cell transporters responsible for intracellular activity.[4,15]

From the multiple locations of the receptors in the brain (Figure 8.1), there has been speculation concerning the action of estrogen on the adjacent neurons.[9,14] For example, while much has been described for serotonin (5-HT) receptor activity and its link to estrogen, many neuron areas involved are not specific for expected reproductive action.[11,15] Several symptomatic conditions related to menopause are expressed instead in these brain areas in many women. Also, neurodegenerative diseases of aging that accompany the menopause and geripause may often overshadow those problems seen with aging.[16,17] It seems impossible to indicate what sources of complications exist, specifically from hormonal therapy, since no separation of the issues of hormones versus aging has been resolved.

Several other areas have been cited as possessing changes that are non-specific for ER action. These include the hair, skin, liver, and kidneys. Further concentration of basic changes on receptor activity may provide answers for these complex issues.

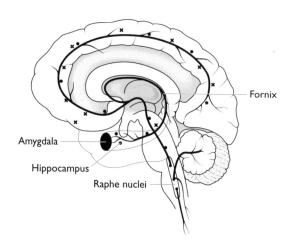

**Figure 8.1** Sagittal section of brain. Darkened lines and areas indicate serotonin receptors. Black dots signify estrogen receptor α (ERα); x represents ERβ locations. Note similarity of all of these receptors. (Reproduced from Figure 3 in Eskin. In: Schneider (ed.) Menopause: The State of the Art. Boca Raton: The Parthenon Publishing Group, 2003: 211–18.[18])

If estrogen deficiency is the main cause of menopausal symptoms, replacement would seem expeditious as used in other somatic hormone deficits. However, when using pharmacological estrogen in many forms and doses, the results remain inconsistent, and complete restoration of cellular loss unusual. Chapters 10 and 20 clarify and describe pharmacological use of estrogens. Increasing the doses of present replacement hormones may relieve several menopausal symptoms, but at the same time the higher dose level is often responsible for causing or enhancing complications and side-effects (Chapter 21). Recent clinical trials have shown that individual therapies may vary in specificity for each symptom and at reduced dosage.[19,20] Whether to use replacement steroids or other hormone activators (SERMS, agonists, etc.) is a decision that must be made by the well-informed patient and her physician, weighing the need against the risk.[21,22]

## Transitions of estrogen

Transitions are the result of the modifications in sex hormone levels that occur causing the major physiological events in a woman's reproductive life. The *thelarche* (age 8 years) introduces the onset of generalized estrogen activity; *menarche* (12.4 years) provides the first uterine bleed with cyclic menses following within two years. From the graph in Figure 8.2, it can be seen that a plateau appears in the early 20s with a decreasing slope beginning by 36 years. Irregularity and a steady fall follow from 42 years (premenopause), and an obvious downward slope at 50–52 years (*menopause*). The steep fall of estradiol perimenopausally is in contrast to the gradual decrease that begins at menopause and continues through *early postmenopause*.[23,24] A low point, *geripause* (<10 pg/ml) evolves at 65 years, with evidence of an extremely gradual decrease from there, since estrogen never completely disappears.[25] Studies beyond 80 years are limited and thus, difficult to interpret.[16]

With these changes several additional transitions have been defined. Presented earlier are the premenopausal changes that represent the endocrine responses between the brain-pituitary-ovary that downregulate the estrogen production and secretion from the ovary.[24] Adrenal estrogen accounts for both protective and problematical activity since it primarily provides the metabolized form of estrogen, estrone.[25,27] Figure 8.2 indicates some changes noted at this period causing irregular cycles and estradiol levels.

The sudden down-course of estradiol in the menopausal range once again indicates the unpredictable transition to menopause.[28] This range, representing the estrogen-endometrial threshold seems prolonged when compared with other transitional periods. The actual clinical result provides a difficult prognostication for the onset of menopause since the threshold is variable.[28,29] It is interesting to note that onset of endometrial menses at menarche appears at a lower level of estrogen than at menopause. The reason can easily be that the aging tissues of the pelvis and anterior pituitary require a higher level of estrogen for normal function. The reflex ovarian action shows prominent follicular losses and is a persistent casualty as the woman ages. The number of remaining follicles at menopause is below 1% of those seen at menarche.

### Graphical representation[26]

A major problem encountered throughout the postmenopause and geripause has been an inability to accurately measure the endogenous serum level of estrogen present.[13] Using age-designated estrogen levels could provide a better estimate of replacement dose requirements that would ideally suit the individual, and possibly alleviate undesirable complications. Theoretical ranges of estrogen through the many phases during a woman's lifetime have been recorded using appropriate clinical laboratory averages. Estradiol (17β) was employed as the essential estrogen, most capable of providing the required information. Estradiol

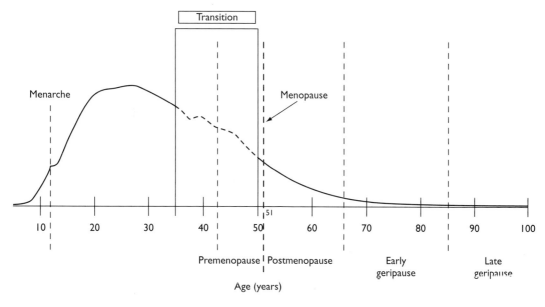

**Figure 8.2** Lifetime adjusted estrogen levels in a woman. (Reproduced from Eskin. Menopause: Comprehensive Management, 4th Edition. New York and London: Parthenon Press, 2000, 299.[26])

has both the highest affinity and greatest biological action for ERα, and is categorized as the active ovarian secretion. In studying estrogen throughout a woman's lifetime, as was anticipated, many modulations of the levels occur during reproductive cycles, as well as diurnally. To compensate for this, in this original study, medians were taken daily and averaged statistically for a 30-day cycle. Using these data from a large cohort of women, a lifetime theoretical representation of the graph was completed.

Considerably more effort was needed in this study for the post-reproductive woman because of the variability of the results. This graph (Figure 8.2) for laboratory-based estrogen levels at each age has been published in several books and journals.[26] It is useful as a significant teaching and clinical guide for defining serum estrogen changes during a woman's lifetime.

Since 2000, determinations of serum estrogen (pg/ml) show improved accuracy and acuity, and results as low as 1.7 pg/ml have been obtained.[30,31] This accuracy provides acceptable immediate measurement. Because of constant diurnal vacillations, especially in reproductive-aged women, median determination can only be obtained by multiple testing in younger women. In a recent review, these factors were considered when serum estrogens were statistically correlated and medians obtained on 30-day averages for each age during the woman's lifetime.[32] Using these data, a new presumptive graph of endogenous serum estradiol-17β medians and ages of women was constructed. Critical laboratory results for this basic graph were obtained from published results of several clinical laboratories using inter-laboratory data statistics. Estrogen serum tests differed in techniques and showed inter-laboratory differences, both of which were clarified by meta-analyses, so that the results might be equated statistically.

For this review, the serum levels from the perimenopause (premenopause through to one year after the last menstrual bleeding) and postmenopause were calculated.[32] Most numerical evaluations of each age appeared constant, probably due to reduced variability of hormone after the reproductive phase. The new graph appears similar to the original theoretical graph (Figure 8.2), but some interesting differences can be recognized, particularly in the geripause group. Figure 8.2 shows the overall changes that occur using earlier techniques for serum levels of estrogen, and represents the phases and transitions over a

woman's lifetime. Using more recent laboratory techniques, the new graph, Figure 8.3, presents serum estradiol levels using currently available techniques.[30,31] The methods used included double-antibody, radioimmunoassay, fluorescent immunoassay, electrochemo-luminescence immunoassay, enzyme-linked fluorescent assay, AxSym immunochemical automated analyzer, and automated chemiluminescence.

A value of the new graph (Figure 8.3) is that the data are from reproducible inter-laboratory estradiol levels obtained from a number of proficient laboratories specializing in patient care. Specific menopausal symptoms have been recognized by clinical trials from estrogen levels. Some evidence of both bone loss and hot flushes has been described in the literature, with each having a measurable estrogen relationship.[19,20,30] Clinical evaluation of all menopausal women, nevertheless, may be complicated by the effects of advancing age. Theoretically, the dose required would be a separation of physical results of estrogen deficiency from the complications of aging as described in Chapter 1. Information about estrogen level could be useful to assess whether a woman in the menopause or geripause who suffers severely from a particular menopausal-related problem should be started on estrogen therapy. However, determination of the actual dose needed would require individual observations, by trial and error, of results obtained.

Serum estrogen levels may serve to define other therapies that can be best utilized for treating midlife complaints. Patients should be given therapeutic dose levels of estrogen according to apparent need. However, it is necessary to take into account other diagnoses and symptoms not directly related to estrogen that the patient reports, and determine other treatment sources that could be used for those problems. In older patients, major medical conditions must be thoroughly treated before hormones are given to avoid complicating regular geriatric care.

While attention to the symptoms and problems related to menopause may be uppermost for estrogen therapy, the complications that have been described for such treatment must be considered.[21,22] As noted, the medical courses of conditions from non-estrogen diseases must be considered and dealt with first. Certainly, replacement or treatments that have the least side-effects or complications are used. Replacement with estrogen therapies for patients having minimal symptoms need to be maintained for only short

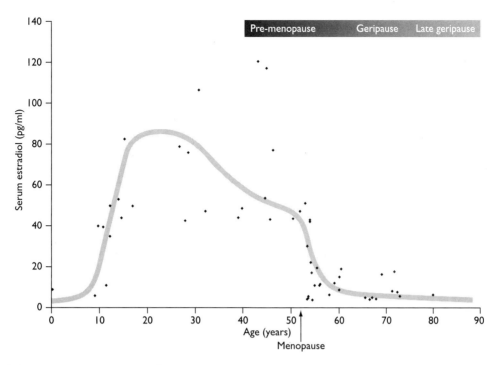

**Figure 8.3** Evaluation of estradiol-17β in women averaged every 30 days in pg/ml. (Reproduced from Eskin BA, Juhas EA, Brooks AR. Confirmation of 17β-estradiol serum levels in all phases of a woman's lifetime. Proc Discovery 2005; 5: 116–17.[32])

periods, and when necessary. Additional therapies that reduce or prevent complications of estrogen replacement can be considered concurrently for a limited period of time as well, when the symptoms from estrogen loss are particularly overwhelming (Chapter 21).

## Observations from the estradiol graphs

In collating overall results of the two graphs (Figures 8.2 and 8.3), some differences are evident. In the early perimenarchal phases, a steeper increase in estradiol is seen. Both show a plateau of estrogen by 25 years of age, with a descent by the early 30s. However, in Figure 8.3 transition occurs at 36 years with some linear flattening, and menopause is rapidly approached between the late 40s and 53 years of age. The evident rapid decline explains the difficulties of discerning where menopause can be diagnosed by an estrogen evaluation alone. Much of the determination of the onset of the menopause is the result of the many intermediate hormones in the biological chain responsible for cyclicity. Therefore, it seems generally unpredictable.

An estrogen plateau occurs again at 65 years, with the onset of a defined geripause in both graphs. For these women the use of medications, particularly estrogen, may be successful with a lower dosage, since the endogenous estrogen present should be exceedingly low. Recent research has confirmed that aromatase expression in adipose tissue is unaffected by menopausal estrogen loss, which indicates that estrogen metabolism may continue.[25] It has been shown already that estrogen is metabolized in fat to estrone in postmenopausal women, thus providing some women with available estrogen. However, since estrone dominance occurs, the overall value is questioned. Estrone studies in postmenopausal women indicate potential increases in malignancies in the breast or uterus. The effects of estrogens on receptor responses are not yet well established for elderly women, but preliminary studies in breast tissue culture cells show age-related reduced tissue responses. Unfortunately, the presence of increased adiposity remains a general health hazard that could reduce longevity.

## DIAGNOSES OF CONDITIONS ARISING FROM ESTROGEN LOSS

The many physical and mental dysfunctions seen in the menopause are described clinically in Section III. Estrogen loss and aging are often inseparable causes through the late post-menopause and geripause. Symptoms are concentrated at the end of the fourth and into the fifth decade. Menopausal conditions in the peri-menopause usually permit separation of these factors.

The hormonal consequences usually described as menopausal, subsequent to long-term studies such as the Study of Women's Health Across the Nation (SWAN), and the Women's Health Initiative (WHI) are listed in Table 8.1.[21,33] While many of these symptoms may be present earlier or later than indicated in some women, statistical averages show these time sequences. The clinician will find this chart useful in menopausal complaints.

While hot flushes do not occur in all women, they appear at some disturbing level in more than 90% of those who have attained the age of 80 years. The presence of these symptoms in young premenopausal women has caused numerous etiological hypotheses for a sympathetic nervous system dysfunction. While hot flushes are considered to be early signs, they seem to be caused by estrogen changes that are unrelated often to simply a lowered estrogen level. The potential causes are exposure to estrogen and sudden withdrawal, enhanced by a reduced predilection to withdrawal by its estrogen receptors.[5] Nevertheless, hot flushes are readily reduced by estrogen therapy.

Mental changes are an evident consequence of estrogen loss, resulting very early in insomnia, irritability and mood swings. As described earlier in this chapter, the presence of estrogen receptors in the brain has been generally considered as evidence of estrogen presence and activity.[3,4] Some localization of estrogen brain activity has been suggested by these discoveries. Trials for these conditions are difficult to interpret because of existing placebo effects.

After menopause occurs a number of gynecological effects are seen, since these are primarily controlled by the sex hormones. The most common sequence is initial loss of turgidity in the perineum, followed by endothelial atrophy of the vulva and vagina. Since the urethra is also dependent on estrogen for turgidity, urinary problems occur. Under parous conditions, trauma plus atrophy are considerably responsible for urinary incontinence (usually stress). Breasts lose contour as the lobules become more fibrotic, with less elasticity and the ducts diminish because of the atrophy that occurs to the lining cells.

This intermediate period also provides other problems, often more exasperating, of reduced sexual desire, and reduced cognition. Both estrogen loss and processes of aging are involved in these changes.

| Table 8.1 Consequences of estrogen loss – timeline of onset | | |
|---|---|---|
| **Time** | **Stage** | **Symptoms** |
| Early symptoms, 40–42 years | Perimenopause | Hot flushes |
| | | Insomnia |
| | | Irritability |
| | | Mood disturbances |
| Intermediate physical changes, 52–65 years | Menopause, immediate postmenopause | Vaginal and vulvular atrophy |
| | | Urinary (stress incontinence) |
| | | Delayed cognition |
| | | Reduced sexual desire |
| | | Breast cellular atrophy |
| | | Skin atrophy |
| | | Ostopenia |
| Late diseases, 65 + years | Late menopause – geripause, estrogen loss and aging | Osteoporosis |
| | | Colon and rectal cancer |
| | | Cardiovascular disease |
| | | Dementia of the Alzheimer's type |

After 65 years of age, geripause (defined as late postmenopause) becomes apparent and appears to accentuate losses incurred by both estrogen loss and aging. These issues have been described in Chapter 2. Enhancement of aging effects in non-reproductive tissues at this time have an interesting similarity to those seen in aging men. However, the similarity differs in that while estrogen remains extremely low, the male testosterone level, slowly descends at a regular rate.

## SUMMARY

This chapter shows interesting recent information that provides the basis for the menopause symptomatology. The use of replacement hormone for evident estrogen loss has had a difficult course. Section IV describes hormones and other treatment choices. Section II details the hormonal aspects of the menopause and geripause. These data indicate how the consequences of estrogen loss and other vital endocrine-affected tissues are changed and their physiological activity is modified. The culmination of many research studies and clinical trials are summarized in the following chapters.

The complexity of menopause is primarily caused by the admixture of hormonal changes and aging. Diagnosis and treatment aims should be towards caring for the losses incurred by both entities with resourceful therapies.

## REFERENCES

1.  McKinlay SM. The normal menopause transition: an overview. Maturitas 1996; 23: 137–45.
2.  Dennerstein L, Lahert P, Bruger H. The relative effects of hormones and relationship factors on sex function of women through natural menopause tradition. Fertil Steril 2005; 84: 174–80.
3.  Katzenellenbogen JA, O'Malley BW, Katzenellenbogen BS. Tripartate steroid hormone receptor pharmacology: interaction with multiple effector sites as a basis of the cell and – and promotor-specific action of these hormones. Mol Endocrinol 1996; 10: 119–31.
4.  Eskin BA, Stoddard IIF, Brooks AD. Microassay characterization of estrogen in iodine metabolic pathways in breast cancer. Proceedings of the 13th International Thyroid Congress, Buenos Aires 13 October–4 November 2005; 13: 131–2.
5.  Razandi M, Pedram A, Green GI. Cell membrane and nuclear estrogen receptors (ERs) originate from a single transcript. Mol Endocrinol 1999; 13: 307–19.
6.  McDonnell DP, Clemm DL, Hermann T, Goldman ME, Pike JW. Analysis of estrogen receptor function in vitro reveals three distinct classes of antiestrogens. Mol Endocrinol 1995; 9: 659–69.
7.  Shughrue PJ, Lane MV, Merchenthasler I. Comparative distribution of estrogen receptor α and β mRNA in the rat central nervous system. J Comp Neurol 1997; 388: 507–525.
8.  Beekman JM, Allan GF, Tsai SY, Tsai MJ, O'Malley BW. Transcriptional activation by the estrogen receptor requires a confirmational change in the ligand binding domain. Mol Endocrinol 1993; 7: 1266–74.
9.  Eskin BA, Aloyo VS. Chapter 36: Cellular senescence and estrogen. In: Schneider HPG. Menopause: The State of the Art. Boca Raton: CRC Press, 2002: 211–18.
10. McEwan B. Genome and hormones: gender differences in physiology, estrogen effects on the brain, multiple sites and molecular mechanisms. J Appl Physiol 2001; 91: 2785–801.
11. Gur RC, Mozley PD, Resnick S. Gender differences in age effect on brain atrophy measured by MRI. Proc Natl Acad Sci USA 1991; 88: 2845–9.
12. Dubal DB, Zhu H, Yu J. Estrogen receptor α not β is a critical link in estradiol-mediated protection against brain injury. Proc Natl Acad Sci USA 2001; 98: 1952–7.
13. Yasui T, Vemura H, Tezuka M, Yamada M. Biological effects of hormone replacement in relationship to serum estradiol levels. Horm Res 2001; 56: 38–44.
14. Eskin BA. Clinical considerations of age-related changes in serotonin and norepinephrine metabolism in reproductive function. Neurobiol Aging 1984; 5: 151–2.
15. Rance NE, Usurndi SV. GnRH gene expression is incurred in the medial basal hypothalamus of postmenopausal women. J Clin Endocrinol Metab 1996; 81: 3540–6.
16. Maneses A. Physiological, pathophysiological and therapeutic roles of 5–HT systems in learning and memory. Rev Neurosci 1998; 9: 275–289.
17. Blurton-Jones M, Tuszynslei MH. Reactive astrocytes express estrogen receptors in the injured primate brain. J Comp Neurol 2001; 443: 115–23.
18. Eskin BA. Cellular senescence and estrogen. In: Schneider HPG (ed.) Menopause: The State of the Art. Boca Raton: The Parthenon Publishing Group, 2003: 211–18.
19. Johnson SR, Ettinger B, Macer JL, Ensrud KE, Quan J, Grady D. Uterine and vaginal effects of unopposed ultralow-dose transdermal estradiol. Obstet Gynecol 2005; 105: 779–87.
20. Ettinger B, Pressman A, Sklarin P, Bauer DC, Canley JA, Cummings JR. Association between low levels of serum estradiol, bone density and fractures among elderly women; the study of osteoporetic fractures. J Clin Endocrinol Metab 1998; 83: 2239–43.
21. Anderson GL and the Steering Group WHI randomized control trial. Effects of conjugated equine estrogen in postmenopausal women with hysterectomy. JAMA 2004; 291: 1701–12.
22. Rossouw JE and the writing group for the WHI. Risks and benefits of estrogen plus progestin in health postmenopausal women: principal results from WHI. JAMA 2002; 288: 321–33.
23. Rannevik G. Jeppsson S, Johnell O. A longitudinal study of the perimenopausal transition. Maturitas 1995; 21: 103–13.
24. Eskin BA, Berger B. Dysfunctional uterine bleeding in the transitional woman: a definition. Female Patient 1993; 18: 23–6.

25. Misso ML, Jang C, Adams J, Tran J, Davis SR. Adipose aromatase gene expression is greater in older women and is unaffected by postmenopausal estrogen therapy. Menopause 2005; 12: 210–15.

26. Eskin BA. Epilogue. In: Eskin BA. Menopause: Comprehensive Management, 4th edn. New York and London: Parthenon Press 2000: 299.

27. Menozzi R, Cagnacci A, Zanni AL, Bondi M, Volpe A, Del Rio G. Sympathoadrenal response of post-menopausal women prior and during prolonged administration of estradiol. Maturitas 2000; 34: 275–81.

28. Dennerstein L, Dudley EC, Hopper JL. A prospective population-based study of menopausal symptoms. Obstet Gynecol 2000; 96: 351–8.

29. Freeman EW, Samuel MD, Gracia CR, Kapoor S, Lin H, Nelson DB. Follicular phase hormone levels and menstrual bleeding status in the approach to menopause. Fertil Steril 2005; 83: 383–92.

30. Aiello EJ, Tworoger SS, Yasui Y, Stanczyk FZ. Associations among circulating sex hormones, ILGF, lipids and mammographic density in postmenopausal women. Cancer Epidemiol, Biomarkers Prev 2005; 14: 1411–17.

31. England B, Parsons G, Possley R, McConnell D, Midgley A. Ultrasensitive semi-automated chemiluminescent immunoassay for estradiol. Clin Chem 2002; 48: 2584–6.

32. Eskin BA, Juhas EA, Brooks AR. Confirmation of 17β-estradiol serum levels in all phases of a woman's lifetime. Proc Discovery 2005; 5: 116–17.

33. Sowers MR, Finkelstein JS, Ettinger B, Bondarenko I, Sherman S. Study of Woman's Health Across the Nation. SWAN. Osteoporosis International 2003; 14: 44–52.

# Chapter 9

# Hormonal changes in the perimenopause and clinical consequences

Mason C Andrews

## INTRODUCTION

The term 'perimenopause' refers to the phase of the aging process of women preceding the menopause, during which ovarian function changes, fluctuates, and diminishes greatly, resulting in a variety of clinical consequences.

This chapter examines the specific hormonal changes, the clinical expression thereof, and management strategies. The average age of menopause is 51 years.[1] Measurable changes in ovarian pathophysiology occur during the preceding decade. Ovarian function as expressed by fecundity decreases gradually from age 19 years.[2] However, this gradual decrease begins to accelerate at age 37.5 years and, by age 40, results in sharply decreased spontaneous fecundity and decreased responsiveness to stimulation by exogenous gonadotropins.[3–5] After age 40 years, the rate of spontaneous abortions increases greatly.[5] Clinically observable changes generally begin to appear about five years before the final menstrual period.

## PATHOPHYSIOLOGY

Ovarian function from the standpoint of both estrogen support and reproductive function is completely dependent on the oocyte, which, surrounded by a small layer of epithelial cells, forms the primordial follicle.[6] The original seven million oocytes present in the seventh month of pregnancy decrease to two million by the time of birth. These proceed to atresia or ovulation until no more responsive primordial follicles remain. Generally by age 51 years, the number has been reduced to below 1000,[7] and there is cessation of estrogen production. Only four to five hundred

will have achieved, during a lifetime, the requisite set of conditions to produce ovulation (pituitary-ovarian sequences).

The rate of atresia monthly is relatively constant until age 37.5 years, when it accelerates.[7] Changes in ovarian cyclic function can be detected perhaps five years before clinical manifestations, as the number and quality of oocytes decline. An elevation in concentration of follicle-stimulating hormone (FSH) to or above 20 mIU/ml during the first three days of a clinically normal cycle can be detected,[4] indicating decreasing ovarian capacity and reserve. Similar results can be found in any of the conditions associated with premature menopause (endometriosis, ovarian resection, removal of a dominant ovary, or immunological disease).[8]

This increased FSH level causes a rapid follicular development, probably recruiting a larger cohort of less responsive oocytes, accelerating their rate of depletion, and results in a shorter follicular phase.[9,10] However, sufficient estrogen is still produced by this failing system for a while, to trigger a luteinizing hormone (LH) surge followed by a corpus luteum, as evidenced by normal serum progesterone and a 14-day cycle (Figure 9.1).[11]

Later in the perimenopause, the estradiol decreases sufficiently to fail to provide enough LH receptor induction and FSH synergy to trigger ovulation or, when ovulation does occur, to provide sufficient support to the granulose cells necessary to produce a normal luteal phase (Figure 9.2).[11–13]

The results are, first, frequently unopposed estrogen stimulating the endometrium, various degrees of endometrial hyperplasia, irregular and

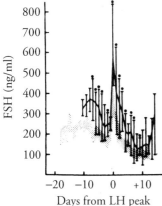

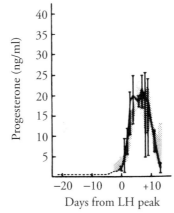

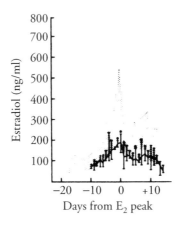

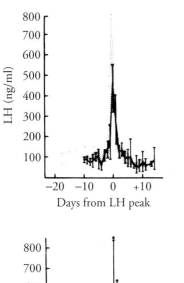

**Figure 9.1** Perimenopausal ovulatory cycles: mean values and range in six perimenopausal women; the follicular phase is shortened to 10 days while the luteal phase remains at 15 days; follicle-stimulating hormone (FSH) is higher and estradiol (E2) is lower than normal for younger ovulatory cycling women. LH, luteinizing hormone. (Reproduced from Sherman and Korneman. J Clin Invest 1975; 55: 699.[11])

excessive bleeding and, second, an additional impediment to fertility.

The sequence of events is quite variable during the four years immediately preceding the menopause, fluctuating over months and years, with ovulation and regularity appearing and disappearing. Since FSH fluctuates and ovarian responsiveness varies, a single measurement is only partially predictive.[14] FSH measured on day 3 of a cycle gives a most helpful indication of ovarian status. Values of 20 mIU/ml and above, with a normal estradiol level on that day are predictive of reduced ovarian capability and responsiveness and impending cessation of ovarian function.[5]

The erratic estrogen production is frequently higher during this period, on average, than during years of normal cycling,[15] producing clinically abnormal endometrial bleeding, and may be accompanied by vasomotor symptoms, breast soreness, and emotional stress-type symptoms. The failure of this increased estrogen to oppose

the rising FSH may be explained by consistently decreasing inhibin production by the failing follicular apparatus,[16] which is decreasing in quality and quantity at an accelerated rate.

An example of environmental influence on oocyte longevity may be the observation that smokers experience an earlier menopause than do non-smokers by 1.7 years.[17]

An example of genetic influence on oocyte longevity is that a woman having a mother or sister with menopause before age 46 years has herself an increased probability of menopause before age 46 years, from 5% to 25%.[18]

Experience with ovulation stimulation and in vitro fertilization (IVF) provides useful information about the diminishing ability of the ovary to respond to FSH during the 10 years preceding cessation of ovarian function, as the number and quality of oocytes is phased out. This diminished response results eventually in an inability to increase the number of follicles available for

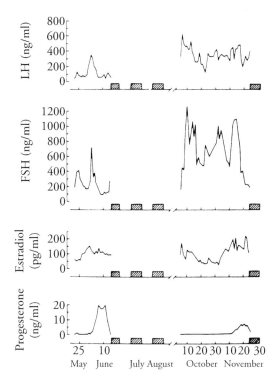

**Figure 9.2** Perimenopausal ovulatory and anovulatory cycles in a 50-year-old woman: hatched areas indicate bleeding episodes; first cycle shows a short follicular phase with a low estradiol and high follicle-stimulating hormone (FSH) and luteinizing hormone (LH) level; the second cycle which is assayed shows menopausal levels of FSH and LH and an inadequate luteal phase. (Reproduced from Sherman and Korneman. J Clin Invest 1975; 55: 699.[11])

oocyte retrieval, with any amount of stimulation. Of the eggs obtained and fertilized, fewer implant, compared to younger IVF patients.[19,20] Among the reduced number of pregnancies achieved, a much higher rate of pregnancy loss occurs. The rate of miscarriage due to diminishing steroidogenesis, which has been diminishing gradually since age 35 years, is lower, but that due to the quality of the aging oocytes in vivo, including a substantial increase in inappropriate chromosomes, is higher.[15]

For these reasons, the ability to achieve a pregnancy and carry it to viability diminishes drastically after age 39 years.[4]

## CLINICAL CONSEQUENCES

### Abnormal bleeding

The fluctuating, frequently elevated estrogen levels as cyclic ovarian function diminishes result in irregular and sometimes excessive vaginal bleeding. Also, as ovulatory cycles, and consequent progesterone secretion decrease in frequency, protracted unopposed estrogen stimulation of the endometrium results in increased endometrial thickness, endometrial hyperplasia, and occasionally endometrial carcinoma.[21] Coincidentally, endometrial polyps are most frequently encountered in women between 40 and 55 years of age.[22] The prevalence of menorrhagia was found by Ballinger and colleagues to be 45% in the early perimenopause, and 48% in the late perimenopause.[23]

### Vasomotor symptoms

It has been generally assumed that hot flushes, which are experienced by 80% of postmenopausal patients, are the result of deficient serum estrogen,[24] hypothalamic response to estrogen by the autonomic system, and catecholamine secretion. Estrogen replacement eliminates them.[25] Sleep disturbance and irritability in estrogen-deficient women respond similarly. Estrogen antagonists (tamoxifen, raloxifene and clomifene) produce hot flushes in a dose-related manner in varying proportions of women.

A generally accepted bioassay for physiologically adequate estrogen has been considered to be the ability of the endometrium to produce withdrawal bleeding after exposure to and withdrawal from progesterone, endogenous or exogenous. Menstruating women would seem to satisfy this test, and therefore not be at risk of hot flushes. However, Kronenberg found that significant hot flushes occur in 11–60% of menstruating perimenopausal women,[26] but specific estrogen levels in these women are not reported. Rannevik and associates found no correlation between the severity of vasomotor symptoms and levels of estradiol.[27] However, estrogen levels were found to be lower in premenopausal women having hot flushes than in those without hot flushes.[28,29] Most postmenopausal women have consistently low estrogen levels and have no hot flushes. Prepubertal girls have low estrogen levels and have no hot flushes after the initial transitional years. Postmenopausal women who have never had estrogen levels comparable to those of cycling women (gonadal dysgenesis) do not experience hot flushes unless they are first exposed to estrogen and subsequently withdrawn from it.[30] In view of the above, one must now conclude that a common denominator in the genesis of hot flushes is a diminution in circulating estrogen or its ability to bind to estrogen receptors. The withdrawal phase of erratically fluctuating high levels of estrogen during the perimenopause may explain the rather frequent occurrence of hot flushes and some affective disorders,[15] in women who are not yet estrogen deficient.

## Affective disorders

The complex personal and social changes prevalent at the time of perimenopause, compounded by the endocrine changes result in increased mood disturbances, including depression.[31,32] This is in contrast to previous reports,[33,34] but the methodology is now more precise. The mechanism of mood lability during the perimenopause appears to be independent of vasomotor symptoms.[31] The erratic fluctuating levels of estrogen may contribute to affective disorders in the menopause. Mood swings are reported in women with implant-related high estradiol levels and vasomotor symptoms.[35] Estradiol-medicated men show greater chemical evidence of stress than unmedicated men similarly exposed.[36] The perimenopause effect on mood appears to include a different, separate effect from estrogen withdrawal, probably related to fluctuating higher levels of estrogen.[15,31]

## Sexual function

Perimenopausal and menopausal women remain sexually active but at a lower frequency, and with an increased frequency and severity of sexual dysfunction.[37,38] These are often modifiable by hormone replacement and counseling by generalists or specialists. Prospective and retrospective studies show a gradual decline in sexual arousal, and decrease in coital frequency beginning in the perimenopause.[37,39] Lessening of sexual interest and desire, increased time required for arousal and vaginal lubrication, and decreased frequency of orgasm often begin during the perimenopause years.[40] Loss of lubrication and health of the vaginal mucosa related to decreased estrogen can contribute to dyspareunia.[41]

Estrogen deficiency may contribute to changes in sensory perception and central and peripheral nerve function.[42] Androgen reduction is a lesser factor in the perimenopausal years because the ovarian stroma continues its secretion at nearly previous levels. After oophorectomy at any age, the loss of testosterone may contribute to impaired libido. Androgens have an important role as sex-drive facilitators.[43,44] The contribution to sexual dysfunction resulting from deficient estrogen (dyspareunia, lack of vaginal moisture, thin vaginal mucosa, vulval atrophy) can be easily reversed by administration of systemic or local estrogen. The psychosocial contributions can be reduced by identifying and improving conditions, which can be modified, and by cultivating positive, supportive, appreciative interpersonal relationships. Results of serious efforts of this type can be enhanced by simultaneous supraphysiological testosterone administration (intramuscular or transdermal).[44,45] Transdermal testosterone patches offer a most convenient delivery route. Clinical studies show a significant improvement in sexual function and psychological wellbeing in patients treated with transdermal testosterone after oophorectomy.[41]

## Osteoporosis

A significant loss of bone density in the hip, vertebrae and forearm in patients experiencing continuing low levels of estrogen (menopausal values) is well documented.[46] This has been demonstrated in premenopausal patients whose serum estrogen level is reduced by medication with gonadotropin-releasing hormone (GnRH) agonists or antagonists.[47] Significant and possibly irredeemable bone loss may occur during six months of medication. Perimenopausal patients having protracted low estrogen levels may be expected to have similar bone loss, which can be prevented by estrogen replacement. Those having menstrual cycles would be expected not to share this risk, especially in view of the increased estrogen in some.[15] However, a series of studies suggests that, overall, in unmedicated patients the rate of spinal (and sometimes femoral) bone loss in the perimenopause exceeds that found in the early menopause.[15,48] Prior postulated that this difficult to understand, increased rate of bone loss may relate to elevated levels of cortisol, secondary to sleep disruption and emotional stress.[15]

## MANAGEMENT

A clear understanding by the patient of the range of symptoms she may encounter during the transition from cyclic ovarian function to actual menopause, and the physiological basis for them is useful to patients and may be therapeutic. In fact, this is a good time for general assessment of her health status and a plan for the future.

This includes reassurance, information concerning the basis for symptoms as they occur, and medication where appropriate. The relationship of affective and vasomotor symptoms to estrogen deficiency can be identified clinically (no menses for more than two months, vaginal appearance and cervical mucus) and by laboratory analysis (Pap smear maturation index, FSH > 20 mIU/ml and estradiol < 25 pg/ml), and treated by replacement. Other symptoms include hot flushes, impaired sleep, irritability, and depression. Antidepressant therapy has minimal efficacy if estrogen levels are inadequate.[49,50]

Estrogen doses (0.045 mg) equivalent to estradiol 0.05 mg/day transdermally, and conjugated estrogens 0.45 mg/day or estradiol 1 mg/day orally are generally appropriate for replacement therapy. If the uterus is intact, added progestin is indicated to protect the endometrium against hyperplasia and carcinoma. For patients who do not smoke and have no phlebitis, a low-dose birth control pill is convenient during the age period 40 to 50 years.

Oral synthetic progestins, most commonly medroxyprogesterone acetate 5 mg daily for 12 days each month of estrogen medication, achieve this goal with only occasional breakthrough bleeding. The alternative of 2.5 mg every day in the month has attained popularity because of convenience and the usual lack of bleeding after a few months of infrequent unscheduled bleeding. Since synthetic progestins oppose, to some extent, the beneficial effect of estrogen on high-density lipoprotein (HDL) and total cholesterol,[51] and since pure progesterone does not,[52] the use of progesterone for endometrial protection is appealing.[53] Micronized progesterone, 120 mg orally or vaginally each night for 12 days each month, is attractive when compared with medroxyprogesterone regimens.[54] Experiments analyzing the coronary arteries of menopausal monkeys show a strong beneficial effect from estrogen, which is reduced by medroxyprogesterone and unimpaired when pure progesterone is used instead.[45,55]

More progesterone reaches the endometrium when used vaginally. A dose of 200 mg micronized progesterone administered twice a week would be expected to protect the endometrium and result in no vaginal bleeding.

The affective and vasomotor symptoms present during the erratic, frequently elevated estrogen fluctuations (usually with some menstrual function) can be modified by estrogen replacement to reduce the depth of estrogen fall, but these are best addressed, in non-smokers, by low-dose estrogen (20 µg)-progestin birth control pills which can suppress the FSH driving the system. This gives an additional benefit by providing contraceptive reassurance. Continuous rather than cyclic estrogen–progestin medication appears to be preferable to prevent mood swings.[56] For patients who must smoke, the standard postmenopausal estrogen–progestin replacement is appropriate.

Excessive and irregular bleeding is the most common symptom of the perimenopause requiring treatment. This is usually the consequence of ovulatory failure resulting in protracted unopposed estrogen, erratic fluctuating estrogen levels, and estrogen withdrawal. Anatomical defects and carcinoma of the endometrium must be excluded before the above treatment options are considered.

Endometrial ablation or hysterectomy are last resorts, which can frequently be avoided by prophylactic treatment with a progestin-containing estrogen regimen, most conveniently a low-dose contraceptive pill.

## SUMMARY AND CONCLUSIONS

For about a decade before the final menstrual period, ovarian function is measurably different, although compensatory mechanisms generally prevent observable clinical changes during the first half of this time, except for a significant decrease in fertility.

The depletion of oocytes, which begins in utero, and finally terminates ovarian estrogen production at menopause, results in laboratory and, finally, clinical evidence of dysfunction during the perimenopause. In spite of serum estradiol levels sufficient to produce withdrawal endometrial bleeding with or without ovulation, hot flushes, sleep disorders, affective compromise, and even bone loss may occur prior to the menopause.

Unpredictable, irregular and/or heavy vaginal bleeding may occur without skipping menstrual periods. Appropriate diagnosis and treatment is important, not only to relieve these symptoms, but also to reduce the risk of endometrial hyperplasia and carcinoma. Tissue sampling by office endometrial biopsy and sonographic measurement of endometrial thickness are useful.

The absence of progesterone attenuation of the endometrium due to increasingly frequent ovulation failure is a common contributor. Also, the erratic, fluctuating, frequently higher than normal estradiol serum levels contribute to abnormal bleeding as well as hot flushes, sleep impairment, and affective compromise.

Replacing progesterone cyclically is a useful tool to combat abnormal bleeding. Providing a sufficient estrogen base for the endometrium makes intermenstrual bleeding less likely during the ever-changing peaks and valleys that characterize estrogen production during this time. Combination estrogen–progestin low-dose contraception (estrogen 20 µg) is an attractive option for non-smokers. This reduces the risk of bleeding and of endometrial carcinoma. It also eliminates hot flushes and most affective disorders attributable to estrogen fluctuations, and provides contraception, reduced though fertility may be.

Elimination of hot flushes in the perimenopause and early menopause may have other important long-term health implications. A part of the beneficial effect of estrogen replacement over all menopausal years is the reduction or delay of Alzheimer's disease.[57] The degree of benefit appears to be related to the length of replacement. In addition, evidence indicates that the replacement of estrogen in the months or years during which hot flushes would otherwise occur may be important in reducing irreversible damage to brain cells, which would contribute to impaired function during the years ahead.[58]

Another long-term health benefit of choosing low-dose estrogen–progestin contraceptive medication during the perimenopause to oppose hot flushes, abnormal bleeding, affective compromise, and osteoporosis is the significantly reduced risk of ovarian carcinoma during later years. This reduction, measurable after 6 months of use, is reported to be 40% overall, and reaches 80% reduction of risk of ovarian carcinoma after more than 10 years of use.[59]

The sharply reduced fertility during the perimenopause is accompanied by, and is apparently a result of the decreased quality of the oocytes, in spite of mobilizing larger cohorts by the increased level of FSH. These are more difficult to mobilize by exogenous FSH stimulation. They fertilize and implant less well, have a higher proportion of genetic imperfections, and result in a greatly increased proportion of abortions. Supporting the luteal phase may help some patients. However, a far more rewarding healthcare goal would be a lifestyle addressed to earlier reproduction.

## REFERENCES

1. Treloar AE, Boynton RE, Behn BG, Brown BW. Variation of the human menstrual cycle through reproductive life. Int J Fertil 1967; 12: 77–126.
2. Adashi E, Rock J, Rosenwaks Z. Reproductive Endocrinology, Surgery and Technology. Vol. 2. Philadelphia, PA: Lippincott Raven, 1996: 1901.
3. Muasher SJ, Oehninger S, Simonetti S et al. The value of basal and/or stimulated serum gonadotropin levels in prediction of stimulation response and in vitro fertilization outcome. Fertil Steril 1988; 50: 298–307.
4. Toner JP, Philput CB, Jones GS, Muasher SJ. Basal follicle-stimulating hormone level is a better predictor of in vitro fertilization performance than age. Fertil Steril 1991; 55: 784–91.
5. Jones GS, Muasher SJ, Rosenwaks Z, Acosta AA, Liu HC. The perimenopausal patient in in vitro fertilization: the use of gonadotropin-releasing hormone. Fertil Steril 1986; 46: 885–91.
6. O'Rahilly R, Muller F. Publication 637. Developmental Stages in Human Embryos. Washington, DC: Carnegie Institute, 1987.
7. Faddy MJ, Gosden RG, Gougeon A, Richardson SJ, Nelson JF. Accelerated disappearance of ovarian follicles in mid-life: implications for forecasting menopause. Hum Reprod 1992; 7: 1342–6.
8. Boutteville C, Muasher SJ, Acosta AA, Jones HW Jr, Rosenwaks Z. Results of in vitro fertilization attempts in patients with one or two ovaries. Fertil Steril 1987; 47: 821–7.
9. Vollman R. The menstrual cycle. In: Friedman E, ed. Major Problems in Obstetrics and Gynecology. Vol. 7. Toronto: WB Saunders, 1977: 11–193.
10. Collett ME, Wertenberger GE, Fiske VM. The effect of age upon the pattern of the menstrual cycle. Fertil Steril 1954; 5: 437–48.
11. Sherman BM, Korenman SG. Hormonal characteristics of the human menstrual cycle throughout reproductive life. J Clin Invest 1975; 55: 699–706.
12. Doring G. The incidence of anovular cycles in women. J Reprod Fertil 1969; (Suppl 6): 77–81.
13. Metcalf MG, Donald RA. Fluctuating ovarian function in a perimenopausal women. NZ Med J 1979; 89: 45–7.
14. Santoro N, Brown JR, Adel T, Skurnick JH. Characterization of reproductive hormonal dynamics in the perimenopause. J Clin Endocrinol Metab 1996; 81: 1495–501.
15. Prior JC. Perimenopause: the complex endocrinology of the menopausal transition. Endocr Rev 1998; 19: 397–428.
16. Seifer DB, Gardiner AC, Lambert-Messerlian G, Schneyer AL. Differential secretion of dimeric inhibin

in cultured luteinized granulosa cells as a function of ovarian reserve. J Clin Endocrinol Metab 1996; 81: 736–9.

17. McKinlay SM, Bifano NL, McKinlay JB. Smoking and age at menopause in women. Ann Intern Med 1985; 103: 350–6.

18. Cramer DW, Xu H, Harlow BL. Family history as a predictor of early menopause. Fertil Steril 1995; 64: 740–5.

19. van Kooij RJ, Looman CW, Habbema JD, Dorland M, te Velde ER. Age-dependent decrease in embryo implantation rate after in vitro fertilization. Fertil Steril 1996; 66: 769–75.

20. Andrews M, Gibbons W, Oehninger S et al. Optimizing use of assisted reproduction. Am J Obstet Gynecol 2003; 189: 327–32.

21. Seltzer VL, Benjamin F, Deutsch S. Perimenopausal bleeding patterns and pathologic findings. J Am Med Womens Assoc 1990; 45: 132–4.

22. Jutras ML, Cowan BD. Abnormal bleeding in the climacteric. Obstet Gynecol Clin North Am 1990; 17: 409–25.

23. Ballinger CB, Browning MC, Smith AH. Hormone profiles and psychological symptoms in peri-menopausal women. Maturitas 1987; 9: 235–51.

24. Prior J. Ovulatory disturbances: they do matter. Can J Diagn 1997: 64–80.

25. Meldrum DR, Shamonki IM, Frumar AM, Tataryn IV, Chang RJ, Judd HL. Elevations in skin temperature of the finger as an objective index of postmenopausal hot flashes: standardization of the technique. Am J Obstet Gynecol 1979; 135: 713–17.

26. Kronenberg F. Hot flashes: epidemiology and physiology. Ann NY Acad Sci 1990; 592: 52–86; discussion 123–33.

27. Rannevik G, Jeppsson S, Johnell O, Bjerre B, Laurell-Borulf Y, Svanberg L. A longitudinal study of the perimenopausal transition: altered profiles of steroid and pituitary hormones, SHBG and bone mineral density. Maturitas 1995; 21: 103–13.

28. Abe T, Furuhashi N, Yamaya Y, Wada Y, Hoshiai A, Suzuki M. Correlation between climacteric symptoms and serum levels of estradiol, progesterone, follicle-stimulating hormone, and luteinizing hormone. Am J Obstet Gynecol 1977; 129: 65–7.

29. Chakravarti S, Collins WP, Thom MH, Studd JW. Relation between plasma hormone profiles, symptoms, and response to oestrogen treatment in women approaching the menopause. BMJ 1979; 1: 983–5.

30. Casper RF, Yen SS, Wilkes MM. Menopausal flushes: a neuroendocrine link with pulsatile luteinizing hormone secretion. Science 1979; 205: 823–5.

31. Schmidt PJ, Roca CA, Bloch M, Rubinow DR. The perimenopause and affective disorders. Semin Reprod Endocrinol 1997; 15: 91–100.

32. Hay AG, Bancroft J, Johnstone EC. Affective symptoms in women attending a menopause clinic. Br J Psychiatry 1994; 164: 513–16.

33. Weissman MM, Leaf PJ, Tischler GL et al. Affective disorders in five United States communities. Psychol Med 1988; 18: 141–53.

34. Matthews KA. Myths and realities of the menopause. Psychosom Med 1992; 54: 1–9.

35. Gangar K, Cust M, Whitehead MI. Symptoms of oestrogen deficiency associated with supraphysiological plasma oestradiol concentrations in women with oestradiol implants. BMJ 1989; 299: 601–2.

36. Kirschbaum C, Schommer N, Federenko I et al. Short-term estradiol treatment enhances pituitary-adrenal axis and sympathetic responses to psychosocial stress in healthy young men. J Clin Endocrinol Metab 1996; 81: 3639–43.

37. Bachmann GA. Sexual function in the perimenopause. Obstet Gynecol Clin North Am 1993; 20: 379–89.

38. Hagstad A. Gynecology and sexuality in middle-aged women. Women Health 1988; 13: 57–80.

39. Cutler WB, Garcia CR, McCoy N. Perimenopausal sexuality. Arch Sex Behav 1987; 16: 225–34.

40. Sarrel PM. Sexuality in the middle years. Obstet Gynecol Clin North Am 1987; 14: 49–62.

41. Shifren JL, Braunstein GD, Simon JA et al. Transdermal testosterone treatment in women with impaired sexual function after oophorectomy. N Engl J Med 2000; 343: 682–8.

42. Punnonen R. Effect of castration and peroral estrogen therapy on the skin. Acta Obstet Gynecol Scand Suppl 1972; 21: 3–44.

43. Schreiner-Engel P, Schiavi RC, White D, Ghizzani A. Low sexual desire in women: the role of reproductive hormones. Horm Behav 1989; 23: 221–34.

44. Sherwin BB. Changes in sexual behavior as a function of plasma sex steroid levels in post-menopausal women. Maturitas 1985; 7: 225–33.

45. Andrews MC. Primary care for postreproductive women: further thoughts concerning steroid replacement. Am J Obstet Gynecol 1994; 170: 963–6.

46. Lindsay R, Hart DM, Clark DM. The minimum effective dose of estrogen for prevention of postmenopausal bone loss. Obstet Gynecol 1984; 63: 759–63.

47. Reproductive endocrinology, surgery and technology. In: Adashi E, Rock J, Rosenwaks Z, eds. Philadelphia, PA: Lippincott, 1996: 1666.

48. Nilas L, Christiansen C. The pathophysiology of peri- and postmenopausal bone loss. Br J Obstet Gynaecol 1989; 96: 580–7.

49. Page L. Menopause and Emotions: Making Sense of your Feelings when your Feelings Make no Sense. Vancouver: Primavera Press, 1994.

50. Schneider LS, Small GW, Hamilton SH, Bystritsky A, Nemeroff CB, Meyers BS. Estrogen replacement and response to fluoxetine in a multicenter geriatric depression trial. Fluoxetine Collaborative Study Group. Am J Geriatr Psychiatry 1997; 5: 97–106.

51. Hirvonen E, Malkonen M, Manninen V. Effects of different progestogens on lipoproteins during post-menopausal replacement therapy. N Engl J Med 1981; 304: 560–3.

52. Kim HJ, Kalkhoff RK. Changes in lipoprotein composition during the menstrual cycle. Metabolism 1979; 28: 663–8.

53. Wood PD, Kessler G, Lippel K, Stefanick ML, Wasilauskas CH, Wells HB. Physical and laboratory measurements in the PEPI Trial Postmenopausal Estrogen/Progestin Interventions. Control Clin Trials 1995; 16: 36S–53S.

54. Effects of estrogen or estrogen/progestin regimens on heart disease risk factors in postmenopausal women. The Postmenopausal Estrogen/Progestin Interventions (PEPI) Trial. The Writing Group for the PEPI Trial. JAMA 1995; 273: 199–208.

55. Adams MR, Kaplan JR, Manuck SB et al. Inhibition of coronary artery atherosclerosis by 17-beta estradiol in

ovariectomized monkeys. Lack of an effect of added progesterone. Arteriosclerosis 1990; 10: 1051–7.

56. Prior JC, Alojado N, McKay DW, Vigna YM. No adverse effects of medroxyprogesterone treatment without estrogen in postmenopausal women: double-blind, placebo-controlled, crossover trial. Obstet Gynecol 1994; 83: 24–8.

57. Gambrell RD Jr. The women's health initiative reports in perspective: facts or fallacies? Climacteric 2004; 7: 225–8.

58. Birge SJ. Hormones and the aging brain. Geriatrics 1998; 53 (Suppl 1): S28–30.

59. Centers for Disease Control Cancer and Steroid Hormone Study. The reduction in risk of ovarian cancer associated with oral-contraceptive use. The Cancer and Steroid Hormone Study of the Centers for Disease Control and the National Institute of Child Health and Human Development. N Engl Med 1987; 316: 650–5.

# Chapter 10

# Sex steroid hormone metabolism in the climacteric woman

Shira Varon, Jesse J Hade and Alan H DeCherney

## INTRODUCTION

Alterations in hormone production, metabolism and efficacy are of critical importance to the homeostasis of the climacteric woman. Imbalances in any of these processes can lead to problems involving irregular vaginal bleeding, osteoporosis, hirsutism and endometrial hyperplasia/cancer.

Menopause is defined by the World Health Organization as the complete cessation of menstruation due to the loss of ovarian follicular activity.[1] It occurs at a median age of 51.3 years and this age does not vary among different cultures or races.[2] Smoking is the only known factor that accelerates the onset of this event.[3] Variation in body size, parity, age of menarche and socioeconomic status do not influence the commencement of menopause. A total of 12 months of amenorrhea needs to elapse prior to establishing this diagnosis and labelling the woman as postmenopausal. Thus, menopause is a retrospective diagnosis.

The climacteric or 'change of life' is the term used to refer to the time interval immediately before the menopause, and includes the first year after the menopause. The term climacteric is colloquially known as the perimenopausal period, and is characterized by a change in the endocrine and biological capability of the aging female. It is during this time that the capacity to reproduce fails, and hormone production becomes markedly reduced. As a result, women undergo a physiological as well as a psychological transformation.

## THE OVARY

The ovaries contain a maximum number of oocytes during fetal life. At approximately 20 weeks' gestational age the ovaries contain about 7 million germ cells, and by birth only 1–2 million germ cells remain.[4] Upon entry into puberty, the number of oocytes is reduced to 300 000–400 000.[5] A process known as atresia is responsible for this reduction in oocyte number. Although a large number of primary oocytes remain at puberty, only a small fraction mature and undergo ovulation. From menarche to menopause it is estimated that only 300–500 oocytes mature and ovulate.

In a reproductive-age woman the ovary is responsible for secreting the majority of the estrogen found in the circulation. Estrogen, which is secreted by the granulosa cells of the ovary, is predominantly in the form of 17β-estradiol.[6] The production rate of estradiol varies throughout the menstrual cycle. In the early follicular phase the daily production of estradiol can be as low as 20–40 μg/day and as high as 1000 μg/day just prior to ovulation. Estrone, a less biologically active estrogen, is formed by the peripheral conversion of androgens into estrogens.[7] This process produces about 45 μg of estrone per day, and has minimal variation throughout the menstrual cycle. An insignificant amount of estradiol is produced by the peripheral conversion of dehydroisoandrosterone and testosterone.[8]

Estriol is a low-potency estrogen, and is the predominant estrogen found in the plasma during pregnancy. In non-pregnant women, estriol is derived from the metabolism of estrone and estradiol. During pregnancy, fetal adrenal dehydroepiandrosterone sulfate (DHEAS) is transported to the fetal liver and converted into 16α-OHDHEAS. This hormone then proceeds to the syncytiotrophoblast cells of the placenta where it is transformed into estriol and released into the maternal circulation.[9] Since the direct synthesis of estriol only occurs during pregnancy, the production of estriol and its influence on target organs is insignificant in both the non-pregnant, premenopausal, and postmenopausal woman.

The ovaries are also responsible for producing androgens and progesterone. Like estradiol, the production rates of these hormones vary during the menstrual cycle. All of these sex steroids are derived from cholesterol. They share a basic four-ring hydrocarbon skeleton, and are differentiated only by their various side-chains. The capacity to convert cholesterol into a progesterone, an androgen, or an estrogen depends on the ability of a target cell to accept a cholesterol molecule and then enzymatically alter its chemical configuration.

Variations in the production of these hormones occur as a result of cellular development and proliferation. During the follicular phase of the menstrual cycle, the proliferation of granulosa cells in both the dominant follicle and the cohort of developing follicles causes an increase in estradiol production. Prior to ovulation, the cohort of immature follicles undergoes atresia and provokes a decline in the production of estrogen. Upon ovulation, plasma levels of progesterone increase, and the production of estrogen declines. As the corpus luteum forms, the theca interna cells become responsible for the production of estradiol. The cells known as the zona granulosa cells of the corpus luteum are responsible for the production and secretion of progesterone.

Luteinizing hormone (LH) secreted by the cells of the anterior pituitary influences the corpus luteum to continue its production of progesterone. As the level of progesterone rises, the pituitary cells are negatively affected and cause a feedback inhibition of LH production. In the absence of fertilization, the corpus luteum involutes and stops producing both estrogen and progesterone within 14 days after ovulation.

## EFFECT OF AGE ON THE MENSTRUAL CYCLE

As a woman ages, her bleeding pattern and menstrual cycle length change. Initially, the cycle shortens, then gradually lengthens as anovulation occurs. Eventually, menses cease completely. Variation in cycle length can begin as early as 26 years of age.[10] However, the shortest menstrual cycles are most commonly observed 3–9 years before the menopause. The reduction in cycle length occurs as a result of a shortening of the follicular phase. These changes in menstrual pattern can last until the menopause, and are a result of follicular atresia and a reduced number of follicles.[11]

One of the primary changes associated with advancing age is the loss of regular ovulatory cycles and the reduced ability of maturing follicles to respond to circulating follicle stimulating hormone (FSH).[12] During the climacteric period, the cyclic secretion of estradiol from granulosa cells diminishes, and eventually ceases. Estrone produced from the peripheral conversion of androstenedione quickly becomes the predominant circulating estrogen. It is for this reason that older women have estradiol levels that are lower throughout all parts of the menstrual cycle, when compared with younger women.[13] Just prior to the cessation of bleeding, anovulatory cycles increase in frequency and result in a lengthening of the menstrual cycle. Despite abnormal bleeding patterns during this time, ovulation may infrequently occur and result in a pregnancy.

The source and rate of hormone production change as the number of years beyond the menopause increases. Women who are less than 4 years postmenopausal are capable of secreting testosterone and a small amount of estradiol from their ovaries. Women who are late in the natural menopause (more than 4 years postmenopausal) are unable to produce ovarian estradiol but do continue to secrete testosterone and, to a lesser extent, androstenedione from the ovaries.[14] However, it is important to realize that the major source of plasma estrogens is from extraglandular aromatization of precursors in all postmenopausal women, regardless of the number of years beyond the menopause.

## PRODUCTION OF ESTROGEN DURING THE CLIMACTERIC AND POSTMENOPAUSAL PERIOD

During the reproductive years there are two major sources of estrogen production. The primary source of circulating estrogen is estradiol, which is produced by the granulosa cells of the developing ovarian follicles. About 95% of circulating estradiol is produced by follicles in the ovary, and the remaining 5% is created through the conversion of estrone, testosterone and androstenedione in peripheral tissues.[15]

In reproductive-age women, the production of progesterone during the luteal phase of the menstrual cycle induces the enzyme estradiol 17β-hydroxysteroid dehydrogenase.[16] This enzyme is responsible for the conversion of estrone to estradiol and the metabolism of estradiol to estrone.[17] Since progesterone exerts a large influence upon this enzyme, the interconversion between estrone and estradiol is thought to decrease after the menopause. Despite the low progesterone levels during the postmenopausal period, the rate of conversion of estrone to estradiol, and the metabolism of estradiol to estrone do not change (Figure 1.4).[18]

### DHEAS and its metabolites inhibit the activity of 17β-hydroxysteroid dehydrogenase

Conditions such as liver failure and obesity result in elevated plasma levels of DHEAS and the inhibition of 17β-hydroxysteroid dehydrogenase.[19] Ultimately, this has a profound influence upon the interconversion between estrone and estradiol, and may account for some of the hormonal variation experienced by certain aging women.

The most prominent hormonal change associated with the cessation of ovarian function is the dramatic decline in estradiol production. For the first year after the menopause there is a gradual decline of both estrone and estradiol. After the first year, plasma levels of both estrogen hormones stabilize.[20] The majority of the circulating estradiol in the plasma of postmenopausal women is derived from the peripheral conversion of estrone.

The peripheral conversion of androstenedione and testosterone contributes minimally to the circulating estradiol pool in postmenopausal women.[21] Direct secretion of estradiol from the ovary is negligible. When an oophorectomy is performed on a postmenopausal woman, her circulating level of estradiol does not change.[22] This is further supported by studies which have demonstrated similar estradiol levels in both the ovarian and the peripheral veins of postmenopausal women.[23]

Direct glandular secretion of estrone by either the ovary or the adrenal gland is minimal during the postmenopausal years. Peripheral aromatization of androstenedione to estrone increases in women as they become postmenopausal.[7] Half of the estrone that is formed in postmenopausal women is metabolized into estradiol in extraglandular sites.[24] However, the majority of the estradiol that is formed by this process undergoes further metabolic conversion. Thus, only 5% of the original estrone enters the circulation as estradiol.[25]

A number of different tissues possess the capability of transforming androstenedione into estrone. These tissues include adipose tissue, bone, brain, breast, hair follicles, muscle, and skin.[26–31] It is speculated that estrone formation can occur in any tissue that is responsive to the actions of estrogen. Nevertheless, adipose tissue is the most important source of peripheral aromatization of androstenedione into estrone.[32]

The regulation of extraglandular estrone formation is based on the production rate of androstenedione, and also on the conversion rate of androstenedione to estrone. Since aromatase activity varies with the concentration of androstenedione in the plasma, extraglandular estrone formation is directly proportional to the amount of androstenedione produced.[33]

Aromatase activity in adipose tissue is present predominantly in the stromal cells and not in the adipocytes. As an individual gains weight and becomes obese, the number of stromal cells in the adipose tissue increases.[34] In contrast, when an obese individual loses weight, the number of stromal cells does not decrease.[35] The rate of aromatase activity is also controlled by hormonal factors. It has been shown that treatment of adipose tissue with glucocorticosteroids or cyclic adenosine monophosphate (AMP) analogs can increase the rate of aromatase activity as much as 50-fold.[36]

With advancing age, there is an increase in the amount of androstenedione converted into estrone.[7] The portion of androstenedione converted to estrone is two to three times greater in postmenopausal woman than it is in premenopausal women. Age and obesity appear to work synergistically in promoting the extraglandular formation of estrone.

Liver disease and failure can also increase extraglandular formation of estrone. The liver is responsible for irreversibly clearing about 90% of the circulating androstenedione.[37] When the liver is incapable of performing this function, a larger fraction of androstenedione continues to circulate in the blood plasma. Thus, a larger amount of precursor (androstenedione) is available for peripheral conversion into estrone. Hyperthyroidism has also been shown to increase the extraglandular formation of estrone.[38]

The clearance of estrogen from the circulation begins in the liver. Estrogen is excreted from the body by hepatic conjugation to glucuronides and sulfates.[39] Nearly 80% of these products are then excreted in the urine, and the remaining 20% in the bile. Any process that interferes with the clearance of estrogen could result in elevated levels of circulating estrogen. As a consequence, continuous unopposed estrogen stimulation may cause deleterious end-organ effects and ultimately cancer.

## CHANGE IN OVARIAN AND ADRENAL ANDROGEN PRODUCTION WITH ADVANCING AGE

### The ovary

In reproductive-age women, androstenedione is the major androgen produced by the ovary.[40] The mean plasma concentration is approximately 150 ng/dl, and rises during mid-cycle by about 15%.[41] After the menopause, the plasma level of androstenedione declines by 50%. This decline in androstenedione in the postmenopausal period is comparable to that observed in younger women after bilateral oophorectomy.[42]

Ovarian secretion of androstenedione continues after the menopause but is responsible for only a small fraction of the circulating androstenedione. When a bilateral oophorectomy is performed on a postmenopausal woman, the concentration of androstenedione in the peripheral circulation decreases by only 20%.[42] This is in contrast to a menstruating woman, whose ovaries are responsible for producing 50% of the plasma levels of androstenedione. Since the metabolic clearance rate for androstenedione is not altered by age or by ovarian function, the 30% difference in androstenedione production between pre- and postmenopausal ovaries reflects the declining ability of the aging ovary to produce a androstenedione.[43]

During the reproductive years, approximately 50% of the circulating testosterone is derived from the peripheral conversion of androstenedione.[44] The remainder of the circulating testosterone is secreted directly by both the ovaries and the adrenal glands. Each of these glands secretes approximately 25% of the total circulating testosterone. Nearly 14% of the total circulating pool of androstenedione is converted to testosterone in normal premenopausal women.

After the menopause, the levels of androstenedione and testosterone fall, and then stabilize and remain constant.[20] The ovary becomes the major source of testosterone production and secretes more than 60% of the circulating testosterone. Still, the concentration of testosterone in postmenopausal women is 40% less than that found in the circulation of younger women.[45]

Although the total plasma concentration of testosterone is decreased in postmenopausal women, the secretion of testosterone by the ovaries may in actuality increase. The increase in testosterone production may be attributed to the elevation of circulating gonadotropins. Elevated levels of gonadotropins can in turn stimulate the hilus cells and luteinized stromal cells of the ovary to secrete more androgens. Ultimately, the increase in testosterone production combined with a markedly reduced estrogen production can cause symptoms of defeminization in some women.[46]

### The adrenal gland

In normal menstruating women, the ovary and the adrenal cortex contribute nearly equal amounts of testosterone, dihydrotestosterone and androstenedione to the peripheral circulation. Alternatively, DHEAS is almost exclusively produced by the adrenal cortex.[47] In postmenopausal women, androstenedione is secreted almost exclusively by the adrenal glands. Androstenedione levels decrease by almost 45–50% after the menopause, and remain constant even when the ovaries are removed.[48]

Plasma levels of dehydroepiandrosterone (DHEA) and DHEAS gradually decline with increasing age.[49] By the time a woman becomes menopausal, her circulating levels of DHEA, DHEAS and adrenal androgens decrease by approximately 20–40%.[50] By age 60 years, these levels drop by nearly 70% of their peak values.[51] Despite this decline in adrenal androgen production, the secretion of cortisol by the zona fasciculata remains unchanged in elderly women. The central control of cortisol production by both the hypothalamus and anterior pituitary remains unaffected by advancing age. This is reflected by findings of comparable circulating plasma levels of adrenocorticotropic hormone (ACTH) and cortisol in both young and elderly patients. Therefore, the decline of both DHEA and DHEAS production is caused not by a decrease in the central regulatory process of these hormones, but rather by a selective reduction in the number of functional zona reticularis cells in the adrenal cortex.[52]

The adrenal glands produce more dihydrotestosterone than do the ovaries in both pre- and postmenopausal women.[53] The adrenal cortex is also the predominant source of 17-hydroxy-pregnenolone production.[45] The activity of the enzyme 17,20-desmolase is reduced in postmenopausal women. As a result, the adrenal glands' ability to convert C-21 progestins into C-19 androgens is diminished.[54]

## PROGESTERONE PRODUCTION

In reproductive-age women, the concentration of progesterone rises sharply after ovulation. The granulosa cells or the corpus luteum are responsible for the secretion of progesterone. However, in the follicular phase, the majority of the progesterone is derived from extraglandular conversion of adrenal pregnenolone and pregnenolone sulfate. The contribution of the ovaries to the plasma levels of progesterone is small during this phase of the menstrual cycle.

In postmenopausal women, the site of progesterone production is controversial. Some authorities contend that the ovaries produce a small portion of the total progesterone, while others refute this notion.[55] Postmenopausal women who have undergone a bilateral oophorectomy will display a sustained progesterone level that is consistent with that of postmenopausal women who have both ovaries. The administration of dexamethasone to postmenopausal women can reduce the level of circulating progesterone to an undetectable concentration. In addition, the administration of ACTH can stimulate progesterone production in these women by as much as 500%.[56] However, human chorionic gonadotropin (HCG) administration does not alter the concentration of progesterone in postmenopausal women with intact ovaries. Therefore, the ability of the ovary to produce progesterone is limited, at best.

In menstruating women, the source of 17-hydroxyprogesterone (17-OHP) is both the ovaries and the adrenal glands. The circulating level of 17-OHP during the follicular phase is low. It rises after ovulation and then peaks during the mid-luteal phase.[57] When measured in the plasma of postmenopausal women, the concentration of 17-OHP is similar to the values observed during the follicular phase of menstruating women. Like progesterone, 17-OHP appears to be secreted predominantly by the adrenal glands in postmenopausal women.[58]

## INHIBIN PRODUCTION

Inhibin is a glycoprotein hormone that is produced by the granulosa cells of a pre-ovulatory follicle. The corpus luteum also produces and secretes inhibin. During the mid-luteal phase, inhibin levels rise and quickly reach its maximum concentration. This mid-luteal rise in circulating inhibin is believed to prevent other follicles from precocious maturation.[59]

Inhibin can act directly on the cells of the anterior pituitary and inhibit the synthesis and release of FSH.[60] As the total number of follicles diminishes throughout the span of a woman's life, concentrations of inhibin diminish and cause an elevation in the serum levels of FSH. Elevated levels of FSH may thus be a marker of declining follicular numbers.[61]

During the climacteric period, some women will demonstrate regular menstrual periods despite having persistently elevated FSH levels. These FSH levels remain high as a result of reduced inhibin levels. Unlike younger women, perimenopausal women tend to have reduced levels of inhibin in all phases of the menstrual cycle. However, after the menopause, inhibin becomes undetectable in the circulation, and only high levels of FSH can be found.[62]

Two forms of inhibin exist: inhibin B, which is primarily produced by granulosa cells during the early follicular phase, and inhibin-a, which is produced late in the follicular phase, and also by the corpus luteum. The rise in the day-3 FSH noted in older women is associated with a decrease in inhibin B production but not of inhibin-a.[63] As ovaries age, there is a decrease in both inhibin-a and inhibin B production. This decline of dimeric inhibin production is associated with an elevation of follicular phase FSH levels. In fact, a decline in luteal phase inhibin-a and follicular phase inhibin B values correlates more consistently with chronological age than does a day-3 FSH value.[64]

## THE HYPOTHALAMUS AND PITUITARY

In ovulatory women, there is a co-ordinated pulsatile release of both FSH and LH. This pulsatile release is mediated by factors modulating both the hypothalamus and the ovary. In response to the pulsatile release of the gonadotropins, the ovary undergoes monthly synthesis and secretion of estrogen and progesterone, which ultimately feed back and alter the stimulation of the hypothalamus and pituitary.

The hypothalamus is responsible for the pulsatile release of gonadotropin-releasing hormone (GnRH) and the overall regulation of the menstrual cycle in reproductive-age women. Pulsatile release of GnRH is controlled by a combination of neurotransmitters and neuromodulators within the central nervous system. Neuromodulators, such as opioids, influence control over the hypothalamus by decreasing the rate of GnRH pulsation. The hypothalamus is able to communicate with the anterior pituitary via the portal circulation to stimulate the secretion of both LH and FSH. This relationship between the hypothalamus and the pituitary is represented in Figure 10.1.

Each month, FSH influences a select cohort of primordial follicles to mature into secondary follicles. As these follicles mature, they undergo cellular changes to form a granulosa cell layer. The theca cell layer configures into two layers of cells called the theca interna and the theca externa. The theca externa consists of vascularized connective tissue and has no endocrinological role. The theca interna, which contains LH receptors, allows cho-

lesterol to enter into these cells and then metabolize into androstenedione. This androgen then passes from the theca interna cells into the granulosa cells. The granulosa cells contain the aromatase enzyme and convert androstenedione into estradiol.

As women age and enter into the climacteric period, the levels of FSH and estradiol change. Initially, there is an early rise in both FSH and estradiol in the menstrual cycle, reflecting a decline in the number of functional ovarian follicles. With further aging and follicular depletion, levels of ovarian inhibin decline, resulting in elevated levels of FSH coupled with low estradiol levels. Climacteric women can also have elevated levels of FSH during the luteal phase. This causes premature follicular recruitment and development, and ultimately inadequate estradiol production in the dominant follicle.[65] However, the ovulatory capacity of these women is maintained, and the luteal phase length and secretion of progesterone from the corpus luteum are similar to those of a younger woman.

In the late climacteric period, FSH levels can increase as high as ten to 20-fold above baseline. LH levels, however, do not fluctuate during the climacteric period, and only become elevated after the menopause. Despite a nearly 20-fold rise in

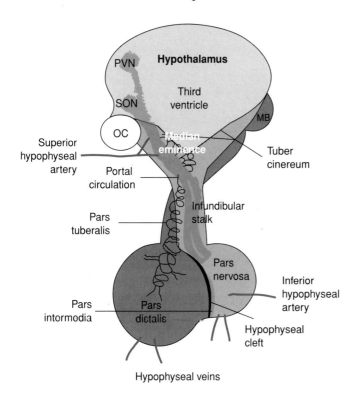

**Figure 10.1**  Relationship between the hypothalamus and the pituitary. MB, mannary body; PVN, paraventricular nucleus; SON, supraoptic nucleus; OC, optic chiasma.

FSH levels, LH rises only three- to five-fold after the menopause.[66] Women who are 15 or more years postmenopausal experience a decline in LH level to below that of a premenopausal women.[67] Alone, levels of gonadotropins are not useful in determining whether a woman is menopausal or not. Hormonal events are too unpredictable during the climacteric period, and thus cannot be used to determine the true ovulatory status of a woman.

## SEX HORMONE TRANSPORT WITHIN THE CIRCULATION

Sex hormones are transported in the bloodstream either bound to a carrier protein, or free in the circulation. Carrier proteins include sex hormone-binding globulin (SHBG) and albumin. These proteins bind to the different sex steroids and make them water-soluble for transport. Only the unbound free-floating hormones can enter the cell and bind to specific receptors on the nuclear membrane. The various tissues that contain specific estrogen receptors include the brain, uterus, vagina, vulva, skin, urethra, bladder trigone, bones, breasts, liver, and elastic arteries.[68]

The main factor that influences the concentration of circulating free hormones is the serum concentration of SHBG. There is a strong negative correlation between body mass index and SHBG levels.[69] As the body mass index increases, the production of SHBG decreases and, therefore, allows more free hormones to circulate within the bloodstream. Older women in general have a higher body mass index than do younger women, and thus lower SHBG levels and more circulating free hormones.

## PERIPHERAL HORMONE CONVERSION

Aromatase in fat tissue is responsible for converting androstenedione to estrone. Other tissues that are capable of doing this include bone, muscle, hair, and brain. Factors that increase aromatase activity include obesity, liver disease, hyperthyroidism, compensated congestive heart failure, and starvation.

In postmenopausal women, the production of estrogen is almost exclusively from extraglandular aromatization of androstenedione to estrone.[43] Little, if any, estrogen is secreted directly by the adrenals or ovaries. The biologically weaker estrogen, estrone, is produced at a much greater rate than the more potent estrogen, estradiol. The preponderance of circulating estradiol in postmenopausal women is derived from the peripheral conversion of estrone.[21] The metabolic clearance rate of estradiol does not differ between premenopausal and postmenopausal women.[21] In non-obese women, the production of estrone is 40–50 μg/day. However, when the daily production rate of estrone exceeds 70–75 μg/day, uterine bleeding usually occurs.[70]

## ESTRADIOL AND CORONARY PLAQUE FORMATION

Over the past seven years there has been a paradigm shift in prescribing estrogen therapy for postmenopausal women. In premenopausal women, estradiol has been shown to protect against coronary plaque formation by enhancing endothelial nitric oxide synthesis and reducing oxidative stress and nitric oxide breakdown. This theory was confirmed by observational studies, and led to the idea that estrogen was a cardioprotective hormone and should be replaced during menopause to prevent progression and formation of coronary artery disease. However, inflammation plays an integral role in the evolution of atherosclerosis and acute ischemic events, and estradiol may be a pro-inflammatory hormone via C-reactive protein and other acute-phase proteins. More recent data show that estrogen therapy may increase a woman's risk of having a cardiovascular event.[71,72]

In 1998, results from the randomized, blinded, placebo-controlled Heart and Estrogen/Progestin Replacement Study (HERS) on clinical endpoints demonstrated that daily supplementation with 0.625 mg of conjugated equine estrogen (CEE) plus 2.5 mg of medroxyprogesterone acetate (MPA) increased the rate of cardiovascular events during the first year of treatment in postmenopausal women with established coronary heart disease, followed by a subsequent decrease in the rate of events.[72,73] In addition, data from the Women's Health Initiative (WHI), which was designed to investigate primary prevention of cardiovascular disease, revealed that combined therapy with CEE and MPA increased the rate of non-fatal myocardial infarction or death due to coronary heart disease (CHD) by 24% (39 versus 33 events per 10 000 person years).[74] The arm of WHI with unopposed CEE versus placebo was discontinued in February 2004 due to an increased risk of stroke.[75,76]

The type of estrogen used in these trials may be important in determining risk. Both the WHI and HERS used CEE. In comparison, the Estrogen in Prevention of Atherosclerosis trial (EPAT) used 17β-estradiol. In this trial, 222 healthy postmenopausal women were randomly assigned to unopposed 17β-estradiol or placebo. Estradiol therapy was associated with a decreased risk of atherosclerosis, measured by carotid artery intima–media thickness.[75,77]

Adams et al studied the effects of 17β-estradiol on the progression of atherosclerosis in ovariectomized monkeys.[78,79] This trial showed that estradiol alone reduces atherosclerosis when the endpoint is coronary plaque size. But estrogen's beneficial effect may be negated depending on which progestin is added. In this study, the combination of estradiol and MPA had no beneficial effect on atherosclerosis, but the combination of estradiol and natural progesterone produced a beneficial effect equivalent to estradiol alone. These data implies that the outcomes measured in WHI and HERS may be related to MPA.[76]

## CONCLUSION

Women go through many biological changes throughout their lives. A delicate balance of hormone production and clearance exists throughout these various stages. When an imbalance occurs, problems may arise. However, exogenous estrogens, progesterones, and androgens can correct these imbalances and restore the natural steady state. Future studies of estradiol and different progestins will hopefully elucidate the safety and efficacy of hormone replacement therapy in postmenopausal women.

## REFERENCES

1. WHO Scientific Group. Research on the menopause. WHO Tech Rep Ser 1981: 670.
2. McKinlay SM, Brambilla DJ, Posner JG. The normal menopause transition. Maturitas 1992; 14: 103–15.
3. Richardson SJ. The biological basis of the menopause. Baillière's Clin Endocrinol Metab 1993; 7: 1–16.
4. Baker TG. A quantitative and cytological study of germ cells in the human ovaries. Proc R Soc London B (Biol) 1963; 158: 417–33.
5. Ohno S, Klinger HP, Atkin NB. Human oogenesis. Cytogenetics 1962; 1: 42.
6. Zhang Y, Word A, Fesmire S et al. Human ovarian expression of 17β-hydroxysteroid dehydrogenase types 1, 2, and 3. J Clin Endocrinol Metab 1996; 81: 3594–8.
7. Hemsell DL, Grodin JM, Brenner PF et al. Plasma precursors of estrogen. II. Correlation of the extent of conversion of plasma androstenedione to estrone with age. J Clin Endocrinol Metab 1974; 38: 476–9.
8. MacDonald PC, Edman CD, Kerber IJ et al. Plasma precursors of estrogen. III. Conversion of plasma dehydroisoandrosterone to estrogen in young nonpregnant women. Gynecol Invest 1976; 7: 165–75.
9. Pepe GJ, Albrecht ED. Transutero placental metabolism of cortisol and cortisone during mid and late gestation in the baboon. Endocrinology 1984; 115: 1946–51.
10. Treloar AE, Boynton RE, Behn BG, Brown BW. Variation of the human menstrual cycle through reproductive life. Int J Fertil 1967; 12: 77–126.
11. Barbo DM. The physiology of the menopause. Med Clin North Am 1987; 71: 11–22.
12. Sherman BM, West JH, Korenman SG. The menopause transition: analysis of LH, FSH, estradiol, and progesterone concentrations during menstrual cycles of older women. J Clin Endocrinol Metab 1976; 42: 629–36.
13. Sherman BM, Korenman SG. Hormonal characteristics of the human menstrual cycle throughout reproductive life. J Clin Invest 1975; 55: 699–706.
14. Vermeulen A. Sex hormone status of the postmenopausal woman. Maturitas 1980; 2: 81–9.
15. Hammond CB. Climacteric. In Scott JR, DiaSaia PJ, Hammond CB et al., eds. Danforth's Obstetrics and Gynecology, 7th edn. Philadelphia: JB Lippincott, 1994: 771–90.
16. Tseng L, Gurpide E. Induction of endometrial estradiol dehydrogenase by progestins. Endocrinology 1975; 97: 825.
17. Labrie F, Luu-The V, Lin SX et al. The key role of 17β-HSDs in sex steroid biology. Steroids 1997; 62: 148–58.
18. Reed MJ, Beranek PA, Ghilchik MW, James HT. Conversion of estrone to estradiol and estradiol to estrone in postmenopausal women. Obstet Gynecol 1985; 66: 361–5.
19. Bonney RC, Reed MJ, James VHT. Inhibition of 17β-hydroxysteroid dehydrogenase activity in human endometrium by adrenal androgens. J Steroid Biochem 1983; 18: 59.
20. Longcope C, Franz C, Morello C, Baker R, Johnston CC. Steroid and gonadotropin levels in women during the peri-menopausal years. Maturitas 1986; 8: 189–96.
21. Judd HL, Shamonki JM, Frumar AM et al. Origin of serum estradiol in postmenopausal women. Obstet Gynecol 1982; 59: 680–6.
22. Judd HL, Lucas WE, Yen SSC. Serum 17β-estradiol and estrone levels in postmenopausal women with and without endometrial cancer. J Clin Endocrinol Metab 1976; 43: 272–8.
23. Judd HL, Lucas WE, Yen SSC. Effect of oophorectomy on circulating testosterone and androstenedione levels in patients with endometrial cancer. Am J Obstet Gynecol 1974; 118: 793–8.
24. MacDonald PC, Madden JD, Brenner PF et al. Origin of estrogen in normal men and in women with testicular feminization. J Clin Endocrinol Metab 1979; 49: 905–16.
25. Gurpide E. Hormones and gynaecologic cancer. Cancer 1976; 38 (Suppl 1): 503–8.

26. Frisch RE, Canick JA, Tulchinsky D. Human fatty marrow aromatizes androgen to estrogen. J Clin Endocrinol Metab 1980; 51: 394–6.

27. Naftolin F, Tyan K, Petro Z. Aromatization of androstenedione by the diencephalon. J Clin Endocrinol Metab 1971; 33: 368–70.

28. Perel E, Wilkins D, Killinger DW. The conversion of androstenedione to estrone, estradiol and testosterone in breast tissue. J Steroid Biochem 1980; 13: 89–94.

29. Schweikert HU, Milewich L, Wilson JD. Aromatization of androstenedione by isolated human hairs. J Clin Endocrinol Metab 1975; 40: 413–17.

30. Longcope C, Pratt JH, Schneider SH et al. Aromatization of androgens by muscle and adipose tissue in vivo. J Clin Endocrinol Metab 1978; 46: 146–52.

31. Schweikert HU. Conversion of androstenedione to estrone in human fibroblasts cultured from prostate, genital and nongenital skin. Horm Metab Res 1979; 11: 635–40.

32. Perel E, Killinger DW. The interconversion and aromatization of androgens by human adipose tissue. J Steroid Biochem 1979; 10: 623–7.

33. Aiman EJ, Edman CD, Worley RJ et al. Androgen and estrogen formation in women with ovarian hyperthecosis. Obstet Gynecol 1978; 51: 1–9.

34. Klyde BJ, Hirsch J. Increased cellular proliferation in adipose tissue of adult rats fed a high fat diet. J Lipid Res 1979; 20: 705–15.

35. Siiteri PK, Williams JE, Takaki NK. Steroid abnormalities in endometrial and breast carcinoma: a unifying hypothesis. J Steroid Biochem 1976; 7: 897–903.

36. Mendelson CR, Cleland WH, Smith ME et al. Regulation of aromatase activity of stromal cells derived from human adipose tissue. Endocrinology 1982: 1077–85.

37. Rivarola MA, Singleton RT, Mignon CJ. Splanchnic extraction and interconversion of testosterone and androstenedione in man. J Clin Invest 1967; 46: 2096–100.

38. Southern AL, Olivo J, Gordon GG et al. The conversion of androgens to estrogens in hyperthyroidism. J Clin Endocrinol Metab 1974; 38: 207–14.

39. Stumpf PG. Pharmacokinetics of estrogen. Obstet Gynecol 1990; 75: 9s–14s.

40. Bardin CW, Lipsett MB. Testosterone and androstenedione blood production rates in normal women and women with idiopathic hirsutism or polycystic ovaries. J Clin Invest 1967; 46: 891–902.

41. Judd HL, Yen SSC. Serum androstenedione and testosterone levels during the menstrual cycle. J Clin Endocrinol Metab 1973; 36: 475–81.

42. Judd GE, Lucas WE, Yen SSC. Endocrine function of the postmenopausal ovary: concentrations of androgens and estrogens in ovarian and peripheral vein blood. J Clin Endocrinol Metab 1974; 39: 1020–4.

43. Grodin JM, Siiteri PK, MacDonald PC. The source of estrogen production in postmenopausal women. J Clin Endocrinol Metab 1973; 36: 207–14.

44. Horton R, Tait JF. Androstenedione production and interconversion rates measured in peripheral blood and studies on the possible site of its conversion to testosterone. J Clin Invest 1966; 45: 301–13.

45. Maroulis GB, Abraham GE. Ovarian and adrenal contributions to peripheral steroid levels in postmenopausal women. Obstet Gynecol 1976; 48: 150–4.

46. Judd HL, Fournet N. Change of ovarian hormonal function with aging. Exp Gerontol 1994; 29: 285–98.

47. Abraham GE. Ovarian and adrenal contribution to peripheral androgens during the menstrual cycle. J Clin Endocrinol Metab 1974; 39: 340.

48. Chang RJ, Judd HL. The ovary after menopause. Clin Obstet Gynecol 1981; 24: 181–91.

49. Ravaglia G, Forti P, Maidi F. The relationship of dehydroepiandrosterone sulfate (DHEAS) to endocrine-metabolic parameters and functional status in the oldest-old. J Clin Endocrinol Metab 1996; 81: 1173.

50. Belanger A, Candas B, Dupont A et al. Changes in serum concentrations of conjugated and un-conjugated steroids in 40- to 80-year-old men. J Clin Endocrinol Metab 1994; 79: 1086–90.

51. Labrie F, Belanger A, Cusan L, Candas B. Physiological changes in DHEA are not reflected by the serum levels of active androgens and estrogens but of their metabolites: intracrinology. J Clin Endocrinol Metab 1997; 82: 2403–9.

52. Herbert J. The age of dehydroepiandrosterone. Lancet 1995; 345: 1193.

53. Coyoputa J, Parlow AF, Abraham GE. Simultaneous radioimmunoassay of plasma testosterone and dihydrotestosterone. Anal Lett 1972; 5: 329–40.

54. Meldrum DR, Davidson BJ, Tataryn IV, Judd HL. Changes in circulating steroids with aging in postmenopausal women. Obstet Gynecol 1981; 57: 624–8.

55. Dennefors BL. Hilus cells from human postmenopausal ovaries: gonadotropin sensitivity, steroid and cyclic AMP production. Acta Obstet Gynecol Scand 1982; 61: 413–16.

56. Vermuelen A, Verdonck L. Sex hormone concentration in postmenopausal women. Clin Endocrinol 1978; 9: 59–66.

57. Abraham GE, Odell WD, Swerdloff RS, Hopper K. Simultaneous radioimmunoassay of plasma FSH, LH, progesterone, 17-hydroxyprogesterone, and estradiol-17β during the menstrual cycle. J Clin Endocr 1972; 34: 312–18.

58. Vermeulen A. The hormonal activity of the postmenopausal ovary. J Clin Endocrinol Metab 1976; 42: 247–53.

59. McLachlan RI, Robertson DM, Healey DL, Burger HD, Kretser DM. Circulating immunoreactive inhibin levels during the normal human menstrual cycle. J Clin Endocrinol Metab 1987; 65: 954–61.

60. McLachlan RI, Robertson DM, De Krestser DM, Burger HG. Advances in the physiology of inhibin and inhibin-related peptides. Clin Endocrinol 1988; 29: 77–101.

61. Burger HG. Diagnostic role of follicle-stimulating hormone (FSH) measurements during the menopausal transition – an analysis of FSH, estradiol and inhibin. Eur Endocrinol 1994; 130: 38–42.

62. Buckler HM, Evans CA, Mamtora H, Burger HG, Anderson DC. Gonadotropin, steroid, and inhibin levels in women with incipient ovarian failure during anovulatory and ovulatory rebound cycles. J Clin Endocrinol Metab 1991; 72: 116–21.

63. Klein NA, Illinworth PJ, Groome NP, McNeilly AS, Bataglia DE, Soules MR. Decreased inhibin B secretion is associated with the monotropic FSH rise in older, ovulatory women: a study of serum an follicular fluid

levels of dimeric inhibin A and B in spontaneous menstrual cycles. J Clin Endocrinol Metab 1996; 81: 2742–5.

64. Danforth DR, Arbogast LK, Mroueh J et al. Dimeric inhibin: a direct marker of ovarian aging. Fertil Steril 1998; 70: 119–23.

65. Metcalf MD, Livesey JH. Gonadotropin excretion in fertile women: effect of age and the onset of the menopausal transition. J Endocrinol 1985; 105: 357–62.

66. Wide L, Nillus JS, Gemzell C et al. Radioimmunosorbent assay of follicle-stimulating hormone and luteinizing hormone in serum and urine from men and women. Acta Endocrinol 1973; 174 (Suppl): 7–58.

67. Chakravarti S, Collins WP, Forecast JD et al. Hormonal profiles after the menopause. BMJ 1976; 2: 281–6.

68. Bolognia JL, Braverman IM, Rousseau ME et al. Skin changes in menopause. Maturitas 1989; 11: 295–304.

69. Rannevik G, Jeppsson S, Johnell O, Bjerre B, Laurell-Borulf Y, Svanberg L. A longitudinal study of the perimenopausal transition: altered profiles of steroid and pituitary hormones, SHBG and bone mineral density. Maturitas 1995; 21: 103–13.

70. MacDonald PC, Grodin JM, Siiteri PK. The utilization of plasma androstenedione for estrone production in women. In: Progress in Endocrinology. Proceedings of the Third International Congress of Endocrinology. Amsterdam: Excerpta Medica Int Congress Series 184, 1969: 770–6.

71. Ganz P. Vasomotor and vascular effects of hormone replacement therapy. Am J Cardiol 2002; 90: 2218–24.

72. Hulley S, Grady D, Bush T et al for the Heart and Estrogen/progestin Replacement Study (HERS) Research Group. Randomized trial of estrogen plus progestin for secondary prevention of coronary heart disease in postmenopausal women. JAMA 1998; 280: 605.

73. Grady D, Herrington D, Bittner V. Cardiovascular disease outcomes during 6.8 years of hormone therapy. Heart and Estrogen/progestin Replacement Study follow-up (HERSII) JAMA 2002; 288: 58.

74. Risks and benefits of estrogen plus progestin in healthy postmenopausal women: principal results from the Women's Health Initiative randomized controlled trial. JAMA 2002; 288: 321.

75. Herrington DM, Reboussin DM, Brosnihan KB. Effects of estrogen replacement on the progression of coronary-artery atherosclerosis. N Engl J Med 2000; 343: 522.

76. Anderson GL, Limacher M. Assaf AR. Effects of conjugated equine estrogen in postmenopausal women with hysterectomy: the Women's Health Initiative randomized controlled trial. JAMA 2004; 291: 1701.

77. Hodis HN, Mack WJ, Lobo RA. Estrogen in the prevention of atherosclerosis. A randomized, double-blind, placebo-controlled trial. Ann Intern Med 2001; 135: 939.

78. Adams MR, Kaplan JR, Manuck SB, Koritnik DR, Parks JS. Inhibition of coronary artery atherosclerosis by 17-beta estradiol in ovariectomized monkeys lack of an effect of added progesterone. Arteriosclerosis 1990; 10: 1051–7.

79. Adams MR, Rester TC, Golden DL, Wagner JD, Williams JK. Medroxyprogesterone acetate antagonizes inhibitory effects of conjugated equine estrogens on coronary artery atherosclerosis. Arterioscler Thromb Vasc Biol 1997; 17: 217–21.

# Chapter 11

# Infertility in the older woman

Brian M Berger

## INTRODUCTION

A dramatic increase in the numbers of US women with impaired fecundity has occurred over the past decade. This is largely due to the baby-boom cohort of women, many of whom delayed child-bearing, reaching their later and less fecund reproductive years.[1] A recent study projected that the number of women experiencing infertility will range from 5.4 to 7.7 million in 2025, with the most likely number being just under 6.5 million.[2] This is a substantial revision (upwards) in the number of infertile women, largely a result of the increase in the observed percentage of infertile women in 1995.[3] This increase in both rates and numbers has made advanced age the leading cause of infertility in the US.

Aging, in particular the effect of decreased ovarian reserve and possibly uterine senescence, causes a decreased natural fecundity rate, and adversely affects the success rates of fertility therapy in women over the age of 35 years. Prestimulation testing has become an important part of infertility management in older women, along with preconceptual counseling on the likelihood of achieving a live birth and the risks of pregnancy at advanced maternal age. Many strategies have been devised in order to improve the chances of achieving a live birth in older women, using their own oocytes. In addition, oocyte donation is a highly successful alternative treatment for patients with reduced ovarian function. Finally, new experimental technologies show great promise and may change the spectrum of fertility care in the 21st century.

## AN OVERVIEW OF FERTILITY

Female life expectancy is higher at birth and at age 65 years than the corresponding male life expectancies in the US – and in most developed countries.[4] Current estimates project that women will live an average of 90 years by the year 2020.[5] However, while women are living longer than ever before, the age of menopause has not changed, occurring at approximately 51 years in the US.[6–8] The age of menopause and of the preceding reproductive events such as the beginning of subfertility and infertility are likely to be dictated by the process of follicle depletion, leading to loss of oocyte quantity and quality. To some extent this process is influenced by lifestyle factors such as smoking, and possibly also by the use of oral contraceptives.[7,9]

Women can expect to live one-half of their adult lives beyond the menopause, and experience a decline in fertility that precedes the menopause by several years. Therefore, women are infertile for over half of their life expectancy. The advent of assisted reproductive technology (ART) has allowed many women to conceive in situations that were unimaginable only a few years ago. This, in turn, has created numerous medical and ethical dilemmas that we will continue to address well into the next century.

## OVARIAN FUNCTION WITH AGING

Whether reproductive aging is an intrinsic ovarian process, or the ovary is simply responding to exogenous influences, the ovary in general and its follicles in particular are the primary site of the effects of aging. Ovarian follicles in older ovulatory women have some unique features:

1. the follicles are the same size as those in younger women, but form more rapidly
2. secretion of estradiol and inhibin is not compromised
3. the concentrations of steroids in the follicular fluid are indicative of a healthier follicle, i.e. increased progesterone levels and higher estrogen/androgen ratio
4. serum and follicular fluid levels of insulin-like growth factor-I (IGF-I) are decreased, but there are no differences in IGF-II levels.[10]

Older reproductive-age women also have accelerated development of a dominant follicle in the presence of a monotropic follicle-stimulating hormone (FSH) rise.[11] This is manifested as a shortened follicular phase and elevated follicular phase estradiol level.[12] The fact that ovarian steroid and inhibin secretion are similar to those in younger women suggests that elevated FSH in women of advanced reproductive age may represent a primary neuroendocrine change, in addition to the ovarian changes associated with reproductive aging.

## FEMALE FECUNDITY

Female fertility, in sharp contrast to male fertility,[13] is known to decline as early as the third decade of life, with a steep decline after the age of 35 years.[14] Age as an independent prognosticator of infertility has been clearly demonstrated.[15] Fertility becomes significantly compromised long before overt clinical signs occur, such as cycle irregularity. The FSH level has been shown to increase sharply with age.[16] Although women are not considered to be menopausal until the cessation of menses for at least 6 months, the FSH level begins to rise at least 5–10 years prior to the menopause. Scott and colleagues showed that FSH measured on the third day of the menstrual cycle was a strong predictor of success rates associated with in vitro fertilization (IVF), with levels over 15 mIU/ml predicting poor pregnancy rates.[17] Older women have a significantly shorter follicular phase length associated with an early acute rise in follicular phase estradiol, reflecting accelerated development of a dominant follicle. This is manifested as a shortened follicular phase and elevated FSH and estradiol levels.[18] Investigators have shown that an estradiol measurement on day 3 of the menstrual cycle combined with the day 3 FSH level improves upon the prognostic ability of the measurement of either of these hormones alone.[19]

## MISCARRIAGE AND ANEUPLOIDY

Genes and exposures affecting pool size, hormonal homeostasis, and interactions between oocytes and their somatic compartment have the potential to influence chromosome distribution critically in female meiosis, and affect fertility in humans and other mammals. Much of the decline in fecundity can be attributed to an increasing risk of fetal loss with maternal age.[20] Most of this fetal loss is a result of chromosomal abnormalities: a consequence of aging oocytes. Errors in chromosome segregation are most frequent in meiosis I of oogenesis in mammals, and predominantly predispose specific chromosomes and susceptible chiasmate configurations to maternal age-related non-disjunction.[21] Baseline serum FSH and/or estradiol concentrations may be valuable as predictors of fetal aneuploidy.[22] In morphologically and developmentally normal human embryos, cleavage-stage aneuploidy significantly increases with maternal age.[23] The results suggest that implantation failure in older women is largely due to aneuploidy.

One study analyzed 201 clinical pregnancies in which cardiac activity had been documented by transvaginal ultrasound, 35–42 days after ovulation in a previously infertile population treated at a tertiary fertility center.[24] A profound increase in spontaneous abortion rates occurred as a function of maternal age in this population ($\chi^2$ for trend = 15.1). A spontaneous abortion rate of 2.1% was observed for maternal ages $\leq$35 years, but this rate increased to 16.1% for patients $\geq$36 years (odds ratio 8.72; 95% confidence interval (CI) 2.3–32.9). A five-fold increase in spontaneous abortion rate was observed in women $\geq$40 years, compared to women 31–35 years (3.8% versus

20.0%). The incidence of pregnancy loss after confirmation of early fetal cardiac activity by transvaginal ultrasound is substantially greater in infertile patients than previously reported, when considered as a function of maternal age. In particular, patients ≥36 years should be counseled that their risk of spontaneous abortion is significant, even after fetal heart motion is detected on transvaginal ultrasound.

## FERTILITY TREATMENT

The effectiveness of controlled ovarian hyperstimulation together with intrauterine insemination has been established in a meta-analysis,[25] and recently in a large prospective study. Guzick and colleagues found that, among infertile couples, treatment with induction of superovulation and intrauterine insemination is three times as likely to result in pregnancy as is intracervical insemination, and twice as likely to result in pregnancy as is treatment with either superovulation and intracervical insemination or intrauterine insemination alone.[26] The treatment, however, appears to be less effective in women over 40 years. Pearlstone and coworkers showed, in a prospective analysis of 402 cycles in 85 women age 40 years and older, a clinical pregnancy rate of 3.5% per cycle (95% CI 1.7–5.3%).[27] The live-birth rate was 1.2% per cycle (95% CI 0.1–2.3%). Women with a basal FSH level <25 mIU/ml and age <44 years had a clinical pregnancy rate of 5.2% per cycle (95% CI 2.5–7.9%), compared with 0.0% per cycle (95% CI 0.0–2.1%) in cases in which either basal FSH was ≥25 mIU/ml or age was ≥44($P$ <0.005).

The IVF data are slightly better for women over 40 years; however, the data for women over age 42 years are only marginally improved. Lass and colleagues studied 471 women over 40 years undergoing 1087 cycles of IVF.[28] A total of 842 cycles reached oocyte retrieval (77.5%), and 702 had embryos transferred (64.6%). The pregnancy rate was significantly lower in women ≥40 years of age than in a control group of women <40 years of age (11.3% versus 28.2%). It decreased sharply in women >42 years of age, and no women >45 years of age had a child. In addition, women ≥40 years of age were more likely to miscarry (27% versus 12.7%). Yaron and coworkers studied 31 patients over age 45 years, who underwent 52 treatment cycles in standard IVF.[29] Of the 52 standard IVF cycles, oocytes were retrieved successfully in only 32. Of these, fertilization and embryo transfer were performed in 21 cycles. None of these treatment cycles resulted in a clinical pregnancy.

## STRATEGIES TO INCREASE RESPONSE IN POOR RESPONDERS UNDERGOING IVF

Poor responders are defined as patients who fail to achieve an estradiol level greater than 500 pg/ml on the day of human chorionic gonadotropin (HCG) administration (luteinizing hormone, LH surge simulation), and in whom no more than three oocytes are obtained. Currently, most IVF cycles are carried out using a long protocol of gonadotropin-releasing hormone (GnRH) downregulation, using GnRH analogs prior to stimulation with gonadotropins.[30] Because pregnancy rates in patients over age 40 years have been correlated with the response to gonadotropin stimulation, and therefore the number of embryos transferred,[31] the standard IVF protocol regimen has been modified to increase the number of oocytes retrieved and thereby increase success rates in poor responders.

One of the most successful regimens uses downregulation with oral contraceptives combined with microdose GnRH-analog (GnRH-a) administration.[32] Surrey and associates found that a low-dose oral contraceptive (for 21 days) followed by a GnRH-a (leuprolide acetate, 40 μg subcutaneously twice a day) flare, and gonadotropin, initiated on day 3 of GnRH-a administration statistically increased maximal estradiol levels as well as clinical and ongoing pregnancy rates.[33] Using the same regimen, Scott and Navot found that the patients had a more rapid rise in estradiol levels, much higher peak estradiol levels, the development of more mature follicles, and the recovery of larger numbers of mature oocytes at the time of retrieval.[34] Although these data are encouraging, the effect of this regimen on pregnancy rate and live-birth rate has not conclusively been shown to be statistically different.

A more recent and popular regimen for low responders consists of high-dose gonadotropin treatment combined with a GnRH antagonist.[35] This regimen is usually preceded by oral contraceptive pretreatment which downregulates the ovarian function, and also helps to assure follicle 'synchronization' during the stimulatory part of the cycle. Direct comparisons of these two protocols are few, and it remains to be determined which of the protocols are superior.[36] Lastly, a newer protocol called the Agonist–Antagonist Protocol has been reported by our group with some degree of success.[37]

## OOCYTE DONATION

Over the past 20 years, the use of assisted reproductive technologies has changed the choices available for older women. These choices include donor egg in vitro fertilization (DE IVF) which is now a standard treatment in most IVF centers. Patients who might benefit from DE IVF include women with premature ovarian failure, ovarian failure due to either chemotherapy or radiation, and women with gonadal dysgenesis. A second and much larger group includes women with diminished ovarian function, and today, the predominant indication for egg donation at most IVF centers is diminished ovarian reserve in women with functioning ovaries. Other candidates are women who have previously failed multiple IVF attempts, and women carrying transmittable genetic abnormalities that could affect their offspring.

Lutjen and colleagues first reported egg donation to a recipient with premature ovarian failure in 1984.[38] They used a steroid replacement regimen consisting of estrogen valerate (Progynova; Schering, Sydney, Australia) and progesterone suppositories (Utrogestan; Piette, Brussels, Belgium). Since then, many different regimens of estrogen and progesterone replacement have been tried successfully, differing in both the method of administration and timing.[39–41]

When oocytes from young women are used to create embryos for transfer to older recipients, implantation and pregnancy rates mimic those seen in younger individuals.[42] Furthermore, following oocyte donation, the number of miscarriages and chromosomal anomalies dramatically decreases. These results strongly suggest that the pregnancy wastage experienced by older women is largely a result of degenerative changes within the aging oocyte. There are data to suggest that pregnancy rates do not depend merely on oocyte age and quality, but also depend on senescent changes in the uterus, for example diminished endometrial receptivity.[43] Whether or not the uterus plays a role in success rates, the poor prognosis for fertility in older women can largely be reversed through oocyte donation from younger individuals.

## NEW TECHNOLOGIES

One of the effects of aging is a thickening of the zona pellucida resulting in a failure to hatch and implant. Assisted hatching (AH), probably the most frequently applied clinical embryo micromanipulation procedure, may enhance embryo implantation not only by mechanically facilitating the hatching process, but also by allowing earlier embryo–endometrium contact. However, considerable heterogeneity of the studies that have examined the effects of AH does not permit definitive conclusions to be drawn regarding its efficacy. The method usually employed involves the release of acidified Tyrode's medium against the zona pellucida to create an opening approximately 20 µm in diameter. According to one study, the outcome of AH is largely dependent on the mode by which the zona pellucida is breached, the size of the artificial gap and the thickness of the zona pellucida, as embryos with zonae thicker than 17 µm rarely implant.[44]

Schoolcraft and colleagues showed that the delivery rate per oocyte retrieval was significantly higher in the AH group (18/38, 48%), compared to the non-hatched controls (3/28, 11%; $P = 0.0003$).[45] Magli and associates showed that with AH, the percentage of clinical pregnancies per cycle was significantly higher in patients over 38 years old than in controls (31% versus 10% in controls; $P < 0.05$), and in patients with more than three IVF failures than in controls (36% versus 17% in controls; $P < 0.05$).[46] Tucker and coworkers showed that in female patients aged ≥35 years, AH appeared to convey a marginally significant benefit in terms of both the viable pregnancy rate (35.5% AH versus 11.1% controls) and the embryonic implantation rate (10.3% AH versus 3.1% controls).[47] Hellebaut and colleagues showed that pregnancy and implantation rates in the groups with and without AH were, respectively, 42.1% versus 38.1%, and 17.9% versus 17.1%, concluding that AH through partial zona dissection prior to embryo transfer does not improve pregnancy and embryo implantation rates in unselected patients undergoing IVF with or without intracytoplasmic sperm injection (ICSI).[48] Lanzendorf and associates also showed no significant differences in the rates of implantation (11.1% versus 11.3%), clinical pregnancy (39.0% versus 41.7%), and ongoing pregnancy (29.3% versus 35.4%) between the hatched and control groups, respectively.[49] These results suggest that AH may have a significant impact on IVF success rates only in a select subset of older patients.

## Preimplantation genetic diagnosis

As a woman ages her fertility diminishes.[50] The mean age for the birth of the last child in so-called natural fertility populations is 40–41 years.[51,52] This age can be regarded as the mean age at which female fertility comes to an end, although most women have still seemingly normal, regular ovulatory menstrual cycles. The same picture emerges from IVF; the probability of pregnancy and live birth sharply decreases from age 37–38 years onward.[53] Chromosomal aneuploidy of the embryos is a cause of this age-related decline, although other unknown factors might also play an important role. Previous investigations into the chromosomal status of IVF embryos confirmed that the majority of embryos derived from women older than 37 years are chromosomally abnormal.[53,54] By selecting chromosomally normal embryos for replacement, preimplantation genetic diagnosis (PGD) for aneuploidy can (1) increase implantation rates; (2) reduce spontaneous abortion rates; and (3) avoid aneuploid conceptions. PGD is also found to significantly reduce the incidence of spontaneous abortion and chromosomally abnormal conceptions. PGD for patients of advanced maternal age with an adequate number of embryos will improve their chances of childbirth, via improved implantation and sustained gestation.[54]

## EXPERIMENTAL TECHNOLOGIES

Some oocytes are unable to fertilize and/or develop into normal embryos. It may be possible that the problem is with the machinery of cytoplasm of the oocyte.[55] Therefore, cytoplasmic transfer from a normal oocyte to an abnormal oocyte may overcome the problem. Thus far, only two deliveries have been reported using this technique.[56]

Mitochondrial transfer may be another way of enhancing the reproductive potential of older oocytes. Mitochondrial dysfunctions resulting from a variety of intrinsic and extrinsic influences, including genetic abnormalities, hypoxia and oxidative stress, can profoundly influence the level of adenosine triphosphate (ATP) generation in oocytes and early embryos, which in turn may result in aberrant chromosomal segregation or developmental arrest. The developmental competence of mouse and human early embryos appears to be directly related to the metabolic capacity of a finite complement of maternally inherited mitochondria that appear to begin to replicate after implantation. Van Blerkom and coworkers have demonstrated the feasibility of isolating and transferring mitochondria between oocytes, an apparent increase in net ATP production in the recipients, and the persistence of activity in the transferred mitochondria.[57]

## CONCLUSION

Age is the major determinant of female fertility potential. Ovarian aging begins to impact on fecundity rates at age 30 years, and has a profound effect after age 35 years, over 10 years before the menopause. Assisted reproductive technology offers tremendous opportunities for older patients seeking fertility treatment today. The development of new fertility treatment modalities continues to enlarge the armamentarium of reproductive endocrinologists, and will continue to offer new hope well into the next millennium.

## REFERENCES

1. Chandra A, Stephen EH. Impaired fecundity in the United States: 1982–1995. Fam Plan Perspect 1998; 30: 34–42.
2. Stephen EH, Chandra A. Updated projections of infertility in the United States: 1995–2025. Fertil Steril 1998; 70: 30–4.
3. Anonymous. Assisted reproductive technology in the United States and Canada: 1995 results generated from the American Society for Reproductive Medicine/ Society for Assisted Reproductive Technology Registry. Fertil Steril 1998; 69: 389–98.
4. Manton KG. Demographic trends for the aging female population. J Am Med Women's Assoc 1997; 52: 99–105.
5. Murray CJ, Lopez AD. Alternative projections of mortality and disability by cause 1990–2020: Global Burden of Disease Study. Lancet 1997; 349: 1498–504.
6. Brambilla DJ, McKinlay SM. A prospective study of factors affecting age at menopause [Published erratum appears in J Clin Epidemiol 1990; 43: 537]. J Clin Epidemiol 1989; 42: 1031–9.
7. McKinlay SM, Bifano NL, McKinlay JB. Smoking and age at menopause in women. Ann Intern Med 1985; 103: 350–6.
8. Bromberger JT, Matthews KA, Kuller LH, Wing RR, Meilahn EN, Plantinga P. Prospective study of the determinants of age at menopause. Am J Epidemiol 1997; 145: 124–33.
9. van Noord P, Dubas JS, Dorland M, Boersma H, te VE. Age at natural menopause in a population-based

screening cohort: the role of menarche, fecundity, and lifestyle factors. Fertil Steril 1997; 68: 95–102.

10. Klein NA, Battaglia DE, Miller PB, Branigan EF, Giudice LC, Soules MR. Ovarian follicular development and the follicular fluid hormones and growth factors in normal women of advanced reproductive age. J Clin Endocrinol Metab 1996; 81: 1946–51.

11. Klein NA, Battaglia DE, Fujimoto VY, Davis GS, Bremner WJ, Soules MR. Reproductive aging: accelerated ovarian follicular development associated with a monotropic follicle-stimulating hormone rise in normal older women. J Clin Endocrinol Metab 1996; 81: 1038–45.

12. Klein NA, Soules MR. Endocrine changes of the perimenopause. Clin Obstet Gynecol 1998; 41: 912–20.

13. Gallardo E, Simon C, Levy M, Guanes PP, Remohi J, Pellicer A. Effect of age on sperm fertility potential: oocyte donation as a model. Fertil Steril 1996; 66: 260–4.

14. Hull MG, Fleming CF, Hughes AO, McDermott A. The age-related decline in female fecundity: a quantitative controlled study of implanting capacity and survival of individual embryos after in vitro fertilization. Fertil Steril 1996; 65: 783–90.

15. van Noord-Zaadstra BM, Looman CW, Alsbach H, Habbema JD, te VE, Karbaat J. Delaying childbearing: effect of age on fecundity and outcome of pregnancy. BMJ 1991; 302: 1361–5.

16. Sherman BM, West JH, Korenman SG. The menopausal transition: analysis of LH, FSH, estradiol, and progesterone concentrations during menstrual cycles of older women. J Clin Endocrinol Metab 1976; 42: 629–36.

17. Scott RT, Toner JP, Muasher SJ, Oehninger S, Robinson S, Rosenwaks Z. Follicle-stimulating hormone levels on cycle day 3 are predictive of in vitro fertilization outcome. Fertil Steril 1989; 51: 651–4.

18. Toner JP, Philput CB, Jones GS, Muasher SJ. Basal follicle-stimulating hormone level is a better predictor of in vitro fertilization performance than age. Fertil Steril 1991; 55: 784–91.

19. Licciardi FL, Liu HC, Rosenwaks Z. Day 3 estradiol serum concentrations as prognosticators of ovarian stimulation response and pregnancy outcome in patients undergoing in vitro fertilization. Fertil Steril 1995; 64: 991–4.

20. O'Connor KA, Holman DJ, Wood JW. Declining fecundity and ovarian ageing in natural fertility populations. Maturitas 1998; 30: 127–36.

21. Eichenlaub-Ritter U. Genetics of oocyte ageing. Maturitas 1998; 30: 143–69.

22. Nasseri A, Mukherjee T, Grifo JA, Noyes N, Krey L, Copperman AB. Elevated day 3 serum follicle stimulating hormone and/or estradiol may predict fetal aneuploidy [in Process citation]. Fertil Steril 1999; 71: 715–18.

23. Munné S, Alikani M, Tomkin G, Grifo J, Cohen J. Embryo morphology, developmental rates, and maternal age are correlated with chromosome abnormalities. Fertil Steril 1995; 64: 382–91.

24. Smith KE, Buyalos RP. The profound impact of patient age on pregnancy outcome after early detection of fetal cardiac activity. Fertil Steril 1996; 65: 35–40.

25. Hughes EG. The effectiveness of ovulation induction and intrauterine insemination in the treatment of persistent infertility: a meta-analysis. Hum Reprod 1997; 12: 1865–72.

26. Guzick DS, Carson SA, Coutifaris C et al. Efficacy of superovulation and intrauterine insemination in the treatment of infertility. National Cooperative Reproductive Medicine Network. N Engl J Med 1999; 340: 177–83.

27. Pearlstone AC, Fournet N, Gambone JC, Pang SC, Buyalos RP. Ovulation induction in women age 40 and older: the importance of basal follicle-stimulating hormone level and chronological age. Fertil Steril 1992; 58: 674–9.

28. Lass A, Croucher C, Duffy S, Dawson K, Margara R, Winston RM. One thousand initiated cycles of in vitro fertilization in women ≥40 years of age. Fertil Steril 1998; 70: 1030–4.

29. Yaron Y, Amit A, Brenner SM, Peyser MR, David MP, Lessing JB. In vitro fertilization and oocyte donation in women 45 years of age and older. Fertil Steril 1995; 63: 71–6.

30. Meldrum DR, Wisot A, Hamilton F, Gutlay AL, Kempton WF, Huynh D. Routine pituitary suppression with leuprolide before ovarian stimulation for oocyte retrieval. Fertil Steril 1989; 51: 455–9.

31. Widra EA, Gindoff PR, Smotrich DB, Stillman RJ. Achieving multiple-order embryo transfer identifies women over 40 years of age with improved in vitro fertilization outcome. Fertil Steril 1996; 65: 103–8.

32. Schoolcraft W, Schlenker T, Gee M, Stevens J, Wagley L. Improved controlled ovarian hyperstimulation in poor responder in vitro fertilization patients with a microdose follicle-stimulating hormone flare, growth hormone protocol. Fertil Steril 1997; 67: 93–7.

33. Surrey ES, Bower J, Hill DM, Ramsey J, Surrey MW. Clinical and endocrine effects of a microdose GnRH agonist flare regimen administered to poor responders who are undergoing in vitro fertilization. Fertil Steril 1998; 69: 419–24.

34. Scott RT, Navot D. Enhancement of ovarian responsiveness with microdoses of gonadotropin-releasing hormone agonist during ovulation induction for in vitro fertilization. Fertil Steril 1994; 61: 880–5.

35. Akman MA, Erden HF, Tosun SB, Bayazit N, Aksoy E, Bahceci M. Addition of GnRH antagonist in cycles of poor responders undergoing IVF. Hum Reprod 2000; 15: 2145–7.

36. Akman MA, Erden HF, Tosun SB, Bayazit N, Aksoy E, Bahceci M. Comparison of agonistic flare-up-protocol and antagonistic multiple dose protocol in ovarian stimulation of poor responders: results of a prospective randomized trial. Hum Reprod 2001; 16: 868–70.

37. Berger BM, Ezcurra D, Alper MM. The Agonist–Antagonist Protocol: a novel protocol for treating the poor responder. Fertil Steril 2004; 82: S126.

38. Lutjen P, Trounson A, Leeton J, Findlay J, Wood C, Renou P. The establishment and maintenance of pregnancy using in vitro fertilization and embryo donation in a patient with primary ovarian failure. Nature 1984; 307: 174–5.

39. Yaron Y, Amit A, Mani A et al. Uterine preparation with estrogen for oocyte donation: assessing the effect of treatment duration on pregnancy rates. Fertil Steril 1995; 63: 1284–6.

40. Borini A, Violini F, Bianchi L, Bafaro MG, Trevisi MR, Flamigni C. Improvement of pregnancy and implantation rates in cyclic women undergoing oocyte donation after long-term down-regulation. Hum Reprod 1995; 10: 3018–21.

41. Navot D, Scott RT, Droesch K, Veeck LL, Liu HC, Rosenwaks Z. The window of embryo transfer and the efficiency of human conception in vitro. Fertil Steril 1991; 55: 114–18.

42. Sauer MV, Paulson RJ, Lobo RA. A preliminary report on oocyte donation extending reproductive potential to women over 40. N Engl J Med 1990; 323: 1157–60.

43. Borini A, Bianchi L, Violini F, Maccolini A, Cattoli M, Flamigni C. Oocyte donation program: pregnancy and implantation rates in women of different ages sharing oocytes from single donor. Fertil Steril 1996; 65: 94–7.

44. Cohen J, Alikani M, Liu HC, Rosenwaks Z. Rescue of human embryos by micromanipulation. Baillière's Clin Obstet Gynaecol 1994; 8: 95–116.

45. Schoolcraft WB, Schlenker T, Jones GS, Jones HWJ. In vitro fertilization in women age 40 and older: the impact of assisted hatching. J Assist Reprod Genet 1995; 12: 581–4.

46. Magli MC, Gianaroli L, Ferraretti AP, Fortini D, Aicardi G, Montanaro N. Rescue of implantation potential in embryos with poor prognosis by assisted zona hatching. Hum Reprod 1998; 13: 1331–5.

47. Tucker MJ, Morton PC, Wright G et al. Enhancement of outcome from intracytoplasmic sperm injection: does co-culture or assisted hatching improve implantation rates? Hum Reprod 1996; 11: 2434–7.

48. Hellebaut S, De SP, Dozortsev D, Onghena A, Qian C, Dhont M. Does assisted hatching improve implantation rates after in vitro fertilization or intracytoplasmic

sperm injection in all patients? A prospective randomized study. J Assist Reprod Genet 1996; 13: 19–22.

49. Lanzendorf SE, Nehchiri F, Mayer JF, Oehninger S, Muasher SJ. A prospective, randomized, double-blind study for the evaluation of assisted hatching in patients with advanced maternal age. Hum Reprod 1998; 13: 409–13.

50. O'Connor KA, Holman DJ, Wood JW. Declining fecundity and ovarian ageing in natural fertility populations. Maturitas 1998; 30: 127.

51. Spira N, Spira A, Schwartz D. Fertility of couples following cessation of contraception. J Biosoc Sci 1985; 17: 281.

52. Wood JW. Fecundity and natural fertility in humans. Oxf Rev Reprod Biol 1989; 11: 61.

53. Verlinsky Y, Cohen J, Munne S et al. Over a decade of experience with preimplantation genetic diagnosis: a multicenter report. Fertil Steril 2004; 82: 292–4.

54. Munné S. Preimplantation genetic diagnosis and human implantation – a review. Placenta 2003; 24 (Suppl B): S70–6.

55. St John J, Barratt CL. Use of anucleate donor oocyte cytoplasm in recipient eggs [Letter; Comment]. Lancet 1997; 350: 961–2.

56. Cohen J, Scott R, Alikani M et al. Ooplasmic transfer in mature human oocytes. Mol Hum Reprod 1998; 4: 269–80.

57. Van Blerkom J, Sinclair J, Davis P. Mitochondrial transfer between oocytes: potential applications of mitochondrial donation and the issue of heteroplasmy. Hum Reprod 1998; 13: 2857–68.

# Chapter 12

# The thyroid in the menopause

Bernard A Eskin

## INTRODUCTION

The menopause is known to cause many associated endocrine changes. Compounded with estrogen deprivation are those related to abnormal thyroid function. Common menopausal complaints of lethargy, tiredness, and weight gain are often blamed on thyroid hormone dysfunction. Because there is a possibility, menopausal women should have full thyroid evaluation and function tests, at least once, when menopause begins. If hypothyroidism exists, it can cause some of the symptoms and complaints initially described by premenopausal phase women. Similarly, hyperthyroidism can result in general exhaustion following the overactivity that becomes evident. In addition, usual treatments for hyperthyroidism, such as antithyroid drugs, radioactive iodine and subtotal (or total) thyroidectomy may lead to hypothyroidism as well. Thyroiditis routinely begins with hyperthyroid symptoms and eventuates, after thyroid damage and inflammation, into clinical hypothroidism. Thyroid carcinoma occurs very frequently in the perimenopause, and treatment may lead to cellular thyroid hormone exhaustion, with profound hypothyroidism.

Thyroid functional diseases occur more often in women than men, and this is particularly true in older women, especially after the menopause. Screening for these hormonal conditions is important for all physicians who treat menopausal and geripausal women, since they are the highest population cohort for thyroid pathology. Multiple etiological factors have been recognized, and genetic testing and therapies for abnormal thyroid metabolism have become more useful clinically. Autoimmune thyroid diseases have recently been classified for diagnosis and treatment protocols.[1]

The thyroid gland in adult women normally weighs about 12–20 g, but is responsible for providing an extraordinary metabolic activity. In general, thyroid gland activities vary according to sex, age, reproductive function, climate and nutritional status. The thyroid is essential to women's general health, and diagnoses of abnormal thyroid states occur five times more often in women than in men. During the menopause, as with all endocrine glands the thyroid gland tissue ages with evident functional changes.

The thyroid gland shows cyclic modifications during menstrual cycles. It enlarges during the luteal phase and is small and difficult to examine immediately after menses. During pregnancy the thyroid enlarges to 30–40 g in size (small plum), and may cause speculation that a goiter is present. When a woman enters the perimenopause (onset of the premenopause) chronic damage caused by the persistent reproductive changes may be a reason for differences in size, histology and secretion in many women. The histopathological events may cause alterations in activity in the premenopausal transition, and irregularities in thyroid hormone secretions as the ovary wanes.

These thyroid modifications in early perimenopause are frequently overlooked because of the symptomatic guises that they take. The clinical presentations of thyroid endocrinopathies are subtle, non-specific, and confusing. The presenting signs and symptoms may be rightly attributed to normal aging or other acute and chronic diseases seen in the mature individual.[2] Thus, thyroid function tests, which have become more sensitive, are desirable in early menopause (Table 12.1). A compendium of the basic and essential aspects, clinical diseases, and therapies of the thyroid gland seen in women as they age, will be presented in this chapter. Comparisons with reproductive-aged women will be described.

## ANATOMY

The thyroid gland is located in the anterior portion of the trachea. It consists of two lobes with a thin isthmus between (Figure 12.1). The isthmus lies just below the cricothyroid cartilage, which is a convenient clinical landmark on examination. The right lobe is generally larger, and more vascular than the left. Both lobes diffusely enlarge with functional disorders.

The thyroid gland is extremely vascular, receiving its blood supply directly from the carotid artery through two major arteries, the superior and inferior thyroid. It is larger in men than women, although the size and weight rely on the height and weight of the individual. Reports of an increase in size in aging have been noted; nevertheless, the gland is more nodular with advancing age. Most clinical examinations describe the thyroid by size on the basis of weight (i.e. grams) as well as regularity, pulsations, similarity of lobes by size and weight, and relative size of the isthmus. Thus, examination and estimation of the size of the thyroid gland in menopausal women is more difficult because of arthritic changes in the neck, obesity, or pulmonary diseases. For this reason, most physicians have come to rely on ultrasound studies of the gland whenever thyromegaly is encountered.

## PHYSIOLOGY

### Thyroid hormones

The thyroid gland secretes the thyronines, thyroxine ($T_4$), triiodothyronine ($T_3$), and reverse $T_3$ ($rT_3$) which appear to be synthesized from simple substrates of tyrosine and iodine (Figure 12.2). All of these exist in plasma. $T_4$ is highest in concentration and appears to be the only one that arises exclusively from the thyroid gland. Under normal conditions, $T_3$ is secreted to a slight extent from the thyroid, but most $T_3$ is obtained from peripheral metabolism in several extrathyroidal sites by the removal of a single iodine atom from $T_4$. The evaluation and study of iodine-influenced tissue has become an interesting and fruitful research entity in recent years. Present in infants and aging patients, $rT_3$ and secondary thyronines are derived from peripheral conversion of $T_4$.[3]

Restricted anatomically to the follicles of the thyroid gland is thyroglobulin, a large molecule which contains tyrosyl residues and the amino acid tyrosine (designated in Figure 12.3 as 3). Tyrosyls are proteins which are iodinated directly in the thyroid gland from iodine or iodides in the blood. These primary thyroid hormones, generated in the thyroglobulin, can be released only from various foods, water supplies and iodine therapies. Generally, the thyroid gland removes the greatest portion of the iodines as iodide in the blood, an important clinical fact. Non-thyroidal tissues that accept major iodine forms in women are salivary glands, stomach mucosa, mammary tissues (particularly in the terminal ducts), and the

| Table 12.1   Screening recommendations | |
|---|---|
| **Organization** | **Recommendation** |
| American Association of Clinical Endocrinologists | Measure thyroid-stimulating hormone in women of childbearing age before pregnancy or during the first trimester. |
| American Academy of Family Physicians | Do not routinely screen asymptomatic patients younger than 60 years. |
| American College of Obstetricians and Gynecologists | Evaluate patients with risk factors or symptoms of postpartum thyroid dysfunction. |
| American College of Physicians | Screen women older than 50 years, who have one or more symptoms that could be caused by thyroid disease. |
| American Thyroid Association | Measure thyroid function at least every five years in all adults, beginning at age 35 years. |

Adapted from US Preventive Services Task Force. Ann Intern Med 2004; 140: 125–7.[13]

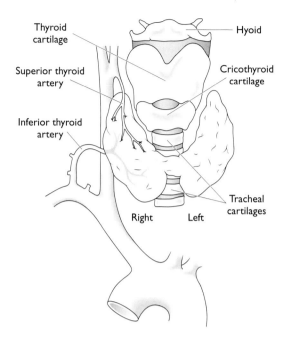

**Figure 12.1** Anatomy of the thyroid gland. Note relationship of the thyroid gland to the trachea and major arterial supply of the neck.

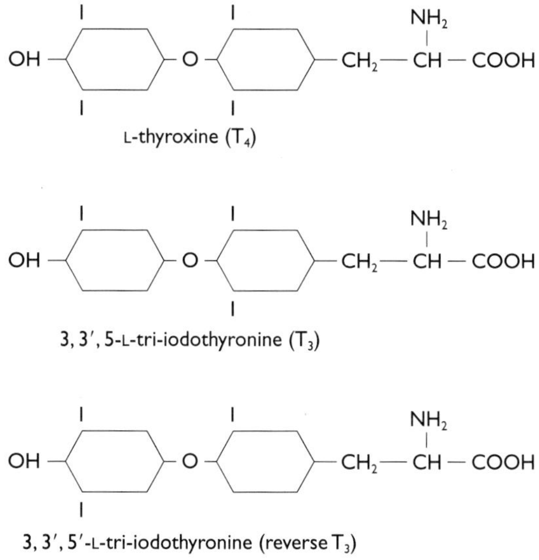

**Figure 12.2** Major thyroid hormones.

ovaries.[4,5] The mechanics involved in iodine trapping by these extrathyroidal organs appear to follow the general scheme of the thyroid metabolic pathways. The differential action within the specific tissue shows particular variations in the utilization of iodine, as a major transporter and intermediate mechanism, for cell metabolism.[6,7]

Upon reaching the thyroid cell membranes, iodides are introduced into the cell in the membrane mostly by the sodium/iodine symporter (NIS). While iodides are most commonly seen in the thyroid, iodine ($I_2$) can in itself enter the thyroid and participate. Once within the cell iodide ($I^-$) is converted to iodine ($I_2$) by a thyroid peroxidase (designated in Figure 12.3 as 2). After the $I_2$ enters the lumen of the follicle, it is incorporated into the organic combinations with proteins and lipids (designated in Figure 12.3 as 4). Organic iodinations are generally under the control of thyroid-stimulating hormone (TSH) stimulation. Iodine ($I_2$), which can be carried in the blood, appears to enter directly through another means in the cell and is readily oxidized to the iodoprotein form.[6]

Lipid transformations with iodine are most important in the breast for lactation. However, in the thyroid, the iodination of proteins, particularly tyrosine, is essential for the formation of the thyroid hormones, and is clinically functional for tissue maintenance. The formation of mono-iodotyrosine (MIT) and diiodotyrosine (DIT) occurs in approximately equal amounts. Since non-iodinated thyronine has not been demonstrated, the intracellular thyroproteins $T_4$ and $T_3$

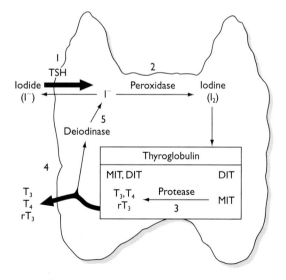

**Figure 12.3** Intrathyroid pathways. Thyroid hormone synthesis as described in the text. TSH, thyroid-stimulating hormone; DIT, diiodotyrosine; MIT, monoiodotyrosine; $T_3$, triiodothyronine; $T_4$, thyroxine; $rT_3$, reverse $T_3$.

must arise from iodotyrosines. $T_4$ would arise from doubling of two DIT molecules, while $T_3$ would be the result of DIT and MIT moieties (designated in Figure 12.3 as 4). This is the 'coupling reaction'.

## Transport of thyroid hormones: binding proteins

Thyroid hormones, $T_4$ and $T_3$, as well as other iodinated tyrosyls are transported in the blood bound firmly, although chemically reversibly, to the serum proteins: thyroid binding globulin (TBG), thyroid binding prealbumin (TBPA), and albumin. The biological activities, and transport throughout the body are dependent on the state of binding of the thyroid to these proteins. Degradation of the thyroid hormones is influenced by the binding affinities of these proteins to the hormones and deiodination may often occur within the thyroid itself (designated in Figure 12.3 as 5). The binding procedures have been carefully studied, and many physical conditions change the concentration of TBG. These changes modify the final reactions at the target cells. Generally, clinical responses are most dependent on the quantity of free thyroid hormones available in the serum.

$T_4$ is the primary secretory thyronine from the thyroid gland, and is derived by direct secretion. $T_3$ and $rT_3$ are present in greater quantities in the blood than can be assigned to thyroid gland secretion only, and therefore $T_4$ performs generalized action throughout the body. Peripheral synthesis from $T_4$ is apparent quantitatively, and under these circumstances, the formation of $T_3$ occurs in peripheral locations in such diverse places as nervous tissues (including CNS), liver, kidney, and generalized fat.

$rT_3$ is found in greater amounts in perimenopausal through geripausal women, but appears to be biologically inactive.[3] It may be involved in receptor response in some tissues, thus, when $rT_3$ is formed, the parent $T_4$ shares the receptor pool. This reduction in thyroid hormone response may be a controlling factor when thyroid hormone overactivity is present, and thus prevents hyperthyroid disease at the target tissues in patients aged over 50 years.

## Metabolism and degradation of thyroid hormones

Degradation of $T_4$ and $T_3$ is influenced by the available binding proteins, TBG, TBPA and albumin. About 10% of the $T_4$ secreted daily is excreted in bile as free $T_4$. In the liver, intracellular breakdown seems to take place in the endoplasmic reticulum of the liver cells. The rest of degradation of the thyroid hormones apparently takes place in kidney and muscle. Cellular degradation, which includes deiodination, takes place in the target organs; deamination, transamination and decarboxylation occur immediately after deiodination.

## Regulation of thyroid activity

Three major regulatory mechanisms are known to exist for thyroid gland activity. These are: (1) the hypothalamic-pituitary-thyroid axis; (2) intrathyroidal autoregulation; and (3) peripheral synthesis and cellular regulation.

### The hypothalamic-pituitary axis

Iodine transport, hormone synthesis and hormone secretion in the thyroid gland are controlled by TSH secreted by the anterior pituitary. Further, it appears that TSH influences both thyroid structure and function and is involved in the amount and response of the vascularity, the changes in the epithelial cells, especially their height, and the total amount of stored colloid that occurs in the thyroid gland. TSH is able to control peripherally the intrathyroidal metabolic processes which include glucose oxidation, phospholipid synthesis and RNA synthesis. The release of TSH from the pituitary is caused by the feedback on the pituitary by the free (unbound) forms of both $T_4$ and $T_3$ (Figure 12.4). The specific effect of reverse $T_3$ remains questionable.

Unlike several other endocrine systems, the pituitary secretion (TSH) has the primary control of thyroid metabolism. While the hypothalamus secretes thyrotropin-releasing hormone (TRH), it does not appear to be the major regulator of the thyroid through feedback control. The hypothalamus has a modulating influence on the pituitary and resulting TSH secretion. Since there are other factors evident which control pituitary secretions, the final result is often unpredictable (Figure 12.4). The mechanisms involved have not yet been totally defined. It appears that TRH acts to stimulate first the release and later the synthesis of TSH, while thyroid hormones act to inhibit these functions. Thyroid hormones seem to mediate the feedback regulation of TSH secretion, while TRH determines its set-point. Receptor systems for both $T_4$ and $T_3$ are present in the pituitary, although binding affinity varies.

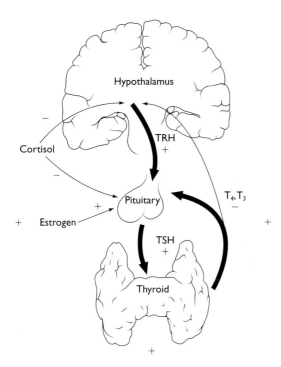

**Figure 12.4** Endocrine control of thyroid hormone secretion. TRH, thyroid-releasing hormone; TSH, thyroid-stimulating hormone; $T_4$, thyroxine; $T_3$, triiodothyronine.

Some mechanisms that regulate TSH secretion have been seen to affect TRH receptors which are located on pituitary thyrotrophin surfaces. These are modified also by both thyroid and steroid hormones (Figure 12.4). Small doses of thyroid hormone reduce the clinical effectiveness of exogenous TRH on pituitary secretion of TSH. Iodides cause the reverse. TRH also has an influence on extrathyroidal iodine metabolic tissues, particularly the breast. In the breast, TRH has been shown to act similarly to prolactin (PRL) secretion from the anterior pituitary. The interactions of this releasing hormone have vacillated during the last several years showing the universality of thyroid action.

### Intrathyroidal autoregulation

A basic quantity of hormone must remain stored within the thyroid gland. This constant amount of hormone operates independently of the external secretions and stimulus from the hypothalamus or pituitary. When the synthesis of thyroid hormone decreases, as reflected by a reduction of glandular thyroid hormones, it brings about biochemical changes which increase the synthesis of thyroid hormone. On the other hand, when hormone stores increase there is an inhibition of TSH release, with a suppression of the biosynthetic pathways.

### Peripheral synthesis and cellular regulation

It has become apparent that extrathyroidal metabolism maintains the level and type of thyroid hormone available. Peripheral metabolism consists of (1) synthesis of thyroid hormones, and (2) peripheral action at the other target cells.

## Metabolic effects of thyroid hormones

The thyroid hormones that are effective (i.e. free $T_4$ and $T_3$) stimulate several metabolic functions at the target tissues. The iodine on the $T_4$ and $T_3$ structures (Figure 12.2) are considered as a means of stereotypically stabilizing the iodothyronine molecule, since the iodine prevents the free rotation around either oxygen. This configuration is necessary for its attachment to the target receptors.

Thyroid hormones cause:

1. an increase in oxygen consumption and calorogenesis in the heart, liver, kidney, and skeletal muscle
2. an increase in the activities of mitochondria
3. conversion of carotene to vitamin A
4. an increase in the incorporation of amino acids in the ribosomes
5. an increase in bond turnover
6. an increase in carbohydrate absorption from the GI tract with a decrease in glycogen synthesis
7. an increase in RNA plasma flow in glomerular filtration rate
8. an increase in the excretion of cholesterol into the biliary tract
9. an increase in hepatic cholesterologenesis
10. an increase in lipolysis and support actions of catecholamines on this activity.

These biochemical actions result in:

1. an increase in basal metabolism rate and oxygen consumption ($T_3$ is three to four times greater than $T_4$ in increasing oxygen consumption, while $T_4$ has a much faster action)
2. stimulation and growth processes in various organs and tissues, such as the mammary glands and reproductive system

3.  enhanced maturation of the nervous system
4.  increased oxygen consumption by the myocardium
5.  increased gastrointestinal motility and decreased production of mucoid substance by the mucosa cells
6.  increased blood flow to the skin. Because of these many physiological effects, a remarkable series of clinical responses result.

## CLINICAL ASPECTS OF THE THYROID

Thyroid dysfunction may generate overall abnormal metabolic and hormonal states. Thyroid disturbances occur more commonly in women, due to the repetitive perturbations of reproductive hormone during regular cyclicity, and irregularities of menstruations prior to menopause. During the transitional years these aberrations occur when either sex hormone or thyroid hormone homeostasis breaks down.[8] The effect on the other axis is seen when thyroid diseases (both hypo- and hyperthyroidism) cause gynecological irregularities, and inversely, when irregular ovarian hormone secretions are responsible for thyroid dysfunction. The menopause results when there is reduced estrogen synthesis and release from the ovary, and thus, inadequate endometrial stimuli for menstrual flow. Simultaneously the thyroid has aged and has been modified throughout reproductive life. In the menopause, the thyroid is associated with a number of morphological and functional changes, such as decreased serum $T_3$ and mean TSH concentrations that are to some extent independent of intercurrent non-thyroidal illnesses.[9] The result is an endocrine pattern in the thyroid that is unpredictable.[10] There are specific changes which are seen in menopausal women and which are responsible for the increasing morbidity seen (Table 12.2).

Thyroid diseases in women occur often later in life. Evaluation of function and clinical examination of the thyroid are a priori requirements of the complete evaluation in the pre- and postmenopause. The clinical symptoms manifested are more subtle because it is anticipated than an aging patient will show energy loss, lethargy, sexual dysfunction, mild depression, and other non-definitive incapacitations are brought on by time (perhaps a fallacy for this millenium).

Hypothyroidism, hyperthyroidism, thyroid malignancies, and the sick euthyroid syndrome

| Table 12.2   Menopausal changes in thyroid physiology |
|---|
| **Decreased:** |
| • renal iodide clearance |
| • thyroid iodide clearance |
| • total $T_4$ production |
| • serum TBG concentration |
| • $T_3$ concentration |
| • TSH response to TRH |
| • diurnal variation of TSH |
| **Increased:** |
| • $T_4$ degradation |
| • reverse $T_3$ concentration |
| **Same:** |
| • serum $T_4$ concentration |

are more common in the menopause. While men also have an increased risk for thyroid disease as they age, the resulting numbers characteristically still favor the women by at least five to one.

## MENOPAUSAL SCREENING FOR THYROID DISEASE

In light of the changes occurring, it is advisable to screen perimenopausal women, generally at 35–40 years, 40–45 years, and again at 45–50 years of age. However, very definitive screening recommendations have been suggested by several groups and are included in Table 12.1. Obviously, testing is done whenever thyroid disease is suspected at any time, particularly after menopause, since a number of pathophysiological changes occur in thyroid tissues at the time of the menopause, so a thyroid evaluation has become routine in many quarters. Often when positive tests appear, there are no immediate medical abnormalities or concerns visible (Table 12.2). A significant decrease of FSH levels was observed in hyper- and hypothyroid (−52% and −43%, respectively) postmenopausal women. The FSH levels remain elevated in the postmenopausal range until late geripause. Under this circumstance an altered thyroid function affects serum inhibin B levels in postmenopausal women.[11] All thyroid function tests are not accurate for patients with acute psychiatric problems or on medications for medical illnesses because of laboratory interference.[12] Patients with symptoms of failure to thrive, depression, and disability benefit from physician examination and screening for thyroid disease. Subtle evidences of early thyroid problems can be easily treated as needed. The quality of life is greatly improved, and conditions such as elevated cholesterol, apathy and anxiety can be relieved. Screening is easily performed by measuring either TSH alone or TSH with reference to free thyroxine ($FT_4$).

## SUBCLINICAL THYROID DISEASE

There has been added a good deal of literature concerning factitious use of thyroid hormone. Clearly available for weight-loss treatment and cholesterolemia, media advertising has impacted a heavy notion for the unwarranted use of the hormone. For several years subclinical thyroid disease has been considered because testing systems are not always reliable and a symptom mantra similar to hypo- or hyperthyroidism is apparent. Recent correlated reports show that observational data alone may be questionable. Recommended laboratory evaluations that should be used are summarized by the US Preventive Service Task Force (USPSTF) from several prime sources (Table 12.1).[13,14]

### Identifying subclinical disease

Subclinical thyroid disease is most often found in women older than 60 years, and has been linked to atrial fibrillation, dementia, poor obstetric outcomes, and, possibly, osteoporosis. Evidence of increased serum TBG is seen with estrogen and relaxifene therapies, but estrogen alone can change the results seen with $FT_4$ and TSH concentrations as well.[15] There is little evidence that overt hyperthyroid disease develops in patients found by screening to have a low TSH level and no symptoms. In contrast, there is good evidence that subclinical disease progresses to overt hyperthyroidism in patients with a goiter or nodule, and that subclinical hypothyroidism is a risk factor for overt hypothyroidism. Good-quality cohort studies have shown that screening programs are able to detect subclinical thyroid dysfunction. The USPSTF noted, however, that when TSH only is used to screen primary care patients, its positive predictive value becomes low.[13,14] Suggestions have been made to have a radioimmunoassay (RIA) free thyroxine ($FT_4$) as a reference for clarification. Thus TSH with reference to $FT_4$ has become a standard testing for diagnoses and follow-up in most thyroid centers.

### Treating subclinical disease

Minimal data exist regarding the efficacy of treating subclinical thyroid dysfunction detected by screening.[16] Treatment trials of patients with subclinical hyperthyroidism have not been performed; trials of subclinical hypothyroidism have been small and yielded inconclusive results. Moreover, the adverse effects of broader L-thyroxine (levothyroxine) use have not been fully evaluated either. 'The main gap in the evidence' noted the author of the USPSTF review, 'is the lack of convincing data from controlled trials that early treatment reduces lipid levels, symptoms, or the risk for cardiovascular disease in patients with mild thyroid dysfunction detected by screening'.[13,14]

## HYPOTHYROIDISM

Hypothyroidism is a condition caused by thyroid failure where there is a deficient supply of thyroid hormone available to peripheral tissues. The range of the thyroid deficiency is extensive; however, it may be only present minimally or it may exist as myxedema. Myxedema is the term applied to the most severe expression of hypothyroidism, and may follow thyroid surgery or radioactive iodine treatment for hyperthyroidism. It occurs spontaneously as so-called idiopathic myxedema (Gull's disease). This is considered as the end result of an autoimmune process which is expressed as similar or identical to that in Hashimoto's thyroiditis. Other origins include drug induction, goiters, or hypothalamic and pituitary abnormalities.

### Prevalence

The prevalence of hypothyroidism has been reported to increase with age, and is up to 10% in menopausal women.[17] Almost one-third of these cases are of iatrogenic origin (Table 12.3). This disease is infrequently a cause of hospital admissions, since full-blown myxedema is rare. In menopausal women, the pathogenesis seems to be almost entirely explicable on the basis of a chronic autoimmune (Hashimoto's) thyroiditis. However, several causes have been described by thyroidologists in characterizing the disease (Table 12.3). Chronic autoimmune thyroiditis is characterized by a focal or diffuse lymphocytic infiltration of thyroid parenchyma, damaged or atrophic follicles, and the presence of autoantibodies in the serum. Postmenopausal women have been shown to have an increase in thyroid autoimmunity due to estrogen loss.[18] The presence of thyroid antibodies may be associated with lower total and low-density lipoprotein (LDL) cholesterol.[19]

## Diagnosis

Prominent clinical features include a puffy face, a pleasant personality, non-pitting myxedema, marked cold intolerance, and coarse, dry skin and hair.[20] Clinical features of hypothyroidism in the menopause are listed in Table 12.4. Enlargement of the heart shadow is frequently due to a pericardial effusion. Adrenal function is decreased with 17-ketosteroid and hydroxycorticoid excretion reduced, serum cortisol and corticoid serum levels lowered. Cardiac output is decreased, and the body is less sensitive to catecholamines. Certain signs are readily seen, such as reflex relaxation time, which is markedly prolonged, decreased metabolic rate and blood cholesterol, and increases in other lipid fractions.

The signs and symptoms of hypothyroidism in the menopause tend to be non-specific because of the insidious onset of the disease and its long progression.[21] The diagnosis of primary hypothyroidism is confirmed by finding an elevation of serum TSH accompanied by a reduced free $T_4$ while total $T_4$ is adequate.[12] The hypothalamic-pituitary axis is so sensitive that it is often possible to detect TSH elevation indicating thyroid damage before the patient notices symptoms. This is

**Table 12.3** Causes of hypothyroidism in the menopause

**Primary hypothyroidism**
- Chronic autoimmune thyroiditis
- Radiation:
  - $^{131}I$ therapy for hyperthyroidism
  - radiation therapy for head and neck cancer
- Surgical thyroidectomy
- Drugs:
  - iodine-containing drugs – amiodarone, iodinated glycerol
  - antithyroid drugs: propylthiouracil, methimazole lithium

**Secondary hypothyroidism**
- Hypothalamic tumors or granuloma
- Pituitary tumors
- Pituitary surgery
- Radiation

**Table 12.4** Clinical features of hypothyroidism in the menopausal woman

**Cutaneous**
- Dry skin
- Hair loss
- Edema of the face and eyelids
- Cold intolerance

**Neurological**
- Parasthesia (carpal tunnel syndrome)
- Ataxia
- Dementia

**Psychiatric and behavioral**
- Depression
- Apathy or withdrawal
- Psychosis
- Cognitive dysfunction

**Metabolism**
- Weight gain
- Hypercholesterolemia
- Hyperglyceridemia
- Peripheral edema

**Musculoskeletal**
- Myopathy
- Arthritis/arthralgia

**Cardiovascular**
- Bradycardia
- Pericardial effusion
- Congestive heart failure

uncommon, but is often the cause of the diagnosis of subclinical hypothyroidism.

When working with functional changes of thyroid disease, it is important to take into consideration several similar symptoms seen in both hypo- and hyperthyroidism. For this reason several algorithms have been suggested in textbooks. These have been modified and presented in Figure 12.5. Using these tests, differentiation in the menopausal woman is reasonably evident.[22]

## Therapy

Therapy of primary hypothyroidism should be instituted with levothyroxine at a dose that takes into account the age of the patient, the severity and duration of the hypothyroidism, and the presence of coexisting medical conditions, particularly

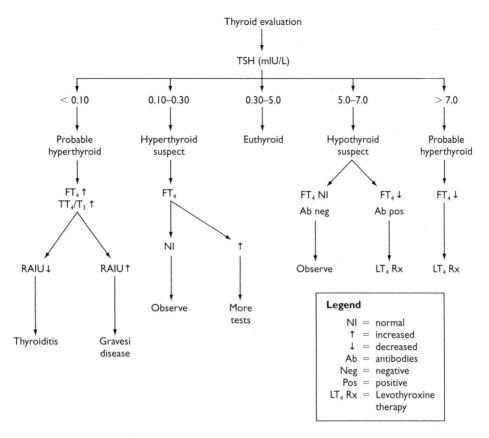

**Figure 12.5** Suggested algorithm for evaluation, management and treatment of thyroid diseases using TSH as an initial diagnostic test. (Reproduced from Kane and Gharib. Thyroid Testing in Contemporary Endocrinology. In: Braverman LE, ed. Diseases of the Thyroid. Totowa, NJ: Humana Press, 2004: 41–4.[22]

symptomatic coronary artery disease. Partial substitution of $T_3$ for $T_4$ may improve mood and neuropsychological function in older women. This finding suggests a specific effect of $T_3$ normally secreted by the thyroid gland.[23] An important consideration is whether therapy should be instituted slowly at a lower dose, and increasing after treatment observation. In the premenopausal patient, with no complicating illnesses, a starting levothyroxine replacement dose of 0.6 to 0.7 μg/kg ideal body weight 91.6 to 1.8 μg/kg) can be given immediately. However, lower doses should be instituted in the older menopausal or geripausal patients and those with illnesses that may compromise the capacity of the cardiorespiratory system to respond to an increased metabolic demand.[24]

Patients who present with hypothyroidism and symptomatic angina should be evaluated prior to treatment for the presence of a readily treated obstructive lesion of the coronary arteries.[25] The

biochemical endpoint of therapy is normalization of the serum TSH, and should be done cautiously even if it requires several months to achieve the euthyroid state. Chronic therapy should be monitored at first, at least semiannually, by measurements of TSH using a third-generation assay capable of accurately measuring the lower limit of the normal range (usually 0.3 to 0.5 μU/l).

Patients with hypothyroidism due to pituitary or hypothalamic causes can be evaluated for deficiencies of other trophic hormones, especially adrenocorticotrophic hormone (ACTH) and prolactin (PRL). The availability (1999) of thyrotropin α for injection (Thyrogen[R]) provides a direct method for testing pituitary release diagnostically. Glucocorticoid replacement may be required prior to instituting levothyroxine treatment to stabilize the condition. Appropriate imaging of the hypothalamic-pituitary region may yield neuroanatomical lesions which require attention first. In these cases, the biochemical endpoint of levothyroxine replacement would be a free $T_4$ (preferably $FT_4$ by RIA), or calculations which are in the high normal range.

Malabsorption and old age will increase levothyroxine requirements.[26] Administration of cholesterol or potassium-binding resins, $FeSO_4$, anticonvulsants, certain antacids, and amiodarone will decrease the test results. Women who also receive androgens in the menopause (including replacement medications) do not require as much levothyroxine replacement. Appropriate adjustments and more frequent monitoring are necessary when any of these conditions are seen.

A serious complication, myxedema coma, represents the ultimate expression of progressively lowered body metabolism due to a severe lack of thyroid hormone. It occurs only in the elderly. Whether massive or minute doses of hormone should be used in the institution of therapy is not clear. Large doses are favored, but the conditions described previously should be considered. Steroids are always given concurrently, and if the circulation and oxygenation are not well maintained, vasopressor drugs with intubation should be used. Ancillary measures include internal readministration of fluids while keeping in mind the impaired free kidney clearance of the hypothyroid patient.

## HYPERTHYROIDISM

The clinical syndrome of hyperthyroidism is usually caused by Graves' disease or diffuse toxic goiter. Thyroiditis is much less common in menopausal than in premenopausal women.[27] Thyrotoxicosis (symptomatic hyperthyroidism) may also be produced by toxic multinodular goiter, toxic adenomas, excessive thyroid hormone ingestion, and several rare syndromes. In older patients, toxic multinodular goiter is more common, reaching as many as one-half of these patients, especially in areas of iodine deficiency. Graves' disease includes thyrotoxicosis, goiter, exophthalmos, and pretibial myxedema when fully expressed, but can occur with one or more of these features (Table 12.5).

Graves' disease, a disease of autoimmunity, shows strong hereditary tendency. Inheritance of specific human leukocyte antigen (HLA) antigens has been shown to predispose to Graves' disease. Psychic trauma, sympathetic nervous system activation, strenuous weight reduction, and iodide

**Table 12.5**  Clinical features of hyperthyroidism in the menopause

**Cardiovascular**
- Palpitation
- Chronic or intermittent atrial fibrillation
- Congestive heart failure

**Psychiatric and behavioral**
- Depression
- Apathy
- Lethargy
- Irritability

**Gastrointestinal**
- Decreased appetite
- Weight loss
- Nausea
- Constipation

**Musculoskeletal**
- Proximal muscle weakness
- Muscle atrophy

administration have been associated also with the initiation of hyperthyroidism.

Immune response is characterized by the presence of abnormal antibodies directed against specific thyroid tissue antigens that particularly bind with the thyrotrophin receptor. These antibodies act either as agonists or antagonists, thus stimulating or blocking TSH. Antibodies of this type can be measured in 80–100% of untreated patients with Graves' disease. The serum factor TSAb (LATS) is measurable and most commonly involved. Serum TSH is typically suppressed, and may be near zero.

The thyroid gland is hyperfunctioning in Graves' disease, and its activity is not suppressed when exogenous $T_3$ is administered. The pituitary response to TRH is also suppressed. The gland is unusually responsive to iodide, which both blocks further hormone synthesis and inhibits release of hormone from the gland.

### Prevalence

In studies, the incidence of Graves' disease varies from 3.4% to 6.8% of menopausal women. Approximately 10–17% of all hyperthyroid patients are over the age of 60 years. The frequency in women is always greater than in men.

Thyrotoxicosis itself is associated with pathological changes, including damage to muscles and mild damage to the liver. Graves' disease is associated with thyroid hyperplasia with lymphoid infiltration, generalized lymphoid hyperplasia, and the specific changes of infiltrative ophthalmalopathy and pretibial myxedema.

## Diagnosis

The classic features of thyrotoxicosis are described as nervousness, diminished sleep, tremulousness, tachycardia, increased appetite, weight loss, and increased perspiration.[28] Graves' disease shows specific symptoms and signs which are associated with goiter, occasionally with exophthalmos, and, rarely, with pretibial myxedema. Physical findings include fine skin and hair, tremulousness, a hyperactive heart, Plummer's nails, muscle weakness, accelerated reflex relaxation, occasional splenomegaly, and often peripheral edema. Thyroid changes seen in menopausal Graves' disease are seen in Table 12.5. Skin changes that are seen are probably autoimmune vitiligo or hives. The extent and degree of hyperthyroid bone diseases, particularly osteoporosis, surpass the effects of menopause on the bone mass.[29]

Absence of some of the typical manifestations of hyperthyroidism in the menopause and geripause was called 'apathetic hyperthyroidism' because there were only slight evidence of hypermetabolism. The diagnosis of hyperthyroidism may be overlooked because of apathy, or the dominant clinical findings may be weight loss, cardiac or gastrointestinal manifestations. The prevalence of subclinical hyperthyroidism is higher than that of subclinical hypothyroidism in older women, and it might relate to non-autoimmune factors.[30]

The disease typically begins gradually in adult (premenopausal) women, and progressively worsens unless treated. Muscle weakness is frequent, myasthenia may coexist, and hypokalemic periodic paralysis may be induced by thyrotoxicosis. Hypercalcuria is frequent, but kidney stones rarely occur. Thyrotoxicosis can cause congestive heart failure, mitral valve prolapse, atrial tachycardia, and cardiac fibrillation. Other medical findings may include normocytic anemia, diarrhea without malabsorption, minimal liver damage and hyperbilirubinemia.

The laboratory tests that are most effective for evaluating the status of thyroid function are the sensitive TSH assay, or any technique measuring free $T_3$. As an initial single test, a sensitive TSH assay may be most cost-effective and specific. Although this may range slightly according to the kit or technique, the sensitive TSH test should yield 0–0.1 µU/ml in thyrotoxicosis. In menopausal women a range of 0.1 to 0.25 µU/ml is sometimes seen, especially with the toxic form of multinodular goiters, more common in this group.

A variety of free thyroxine techniques have become available, and are often suitable as a single testing system as well. However, if clinical judgment places considerable doubt on a normal result, an additional test may be employed – serum $T_3$ level determined by RIA. It is almost always elevated in thyrotoxicosis. Interpretations can be made without correcting for protein binding. The serum $T_4$ level is elevated in 86% of menopausal hyperthyroid patients, providing a reasonably sensitive alternative for hyperthyroidism. However, there are hyperthyroxinemic patients without hyperthyroidism, indicating low specificity of the serum total $T_4$ assay.

## Treatment

In general, the choice of treatment of all forms of thyrotoxicosis requires full patient participation. Thyrotoxicosis in untreated cases leads to cardiovascular damage, bone loss and fractures, or inanition, and can be fatal. The long-term history also includes spontaneous remission in some cases, and eventual spontaneous development of hypothyroidism if autoimmune thyroiditis coexists and destroys the thyroid gland.

Primary treatment of Graves' disease has essentially fallen into three forms:

1. blocking of thyroid hormone synthesis in the thyroid by the use of antithyroid drugs
2. complete destruction of the thyroid tissues by radioactive iodine
3. partial or complete surgical ablation of the thyroid.

In women of childbearing age, antithyroid drugs are used, primarily, unless persistent failure of the medication is apparent. Women in the menopause often do very well on antithyroid medications given for six months to a year and then discontinued.[31] This may require longer periods of time or repetitive therapy after an unsuccessful hiatus. The spontaneous successes from medical therapy are satisfying since both radiation and surgery may induce damage to the thyroids, parathyroids, or recurrent nerves. However, side-effects and complications by the medications to the individual must be weighed up in each case.

Radioactive ablation, which is commonly used in menopausal women, may cause some damage to the peripheral tissues and most often results in hypothyroidism with a need for treatment. A population-based study (1999) resulted in a decrease in overall cancer incidence and mortality in those treated for hyperthyroidism with radioiodine.[32] The absolute risk of cancers of the small bowel and thyroid remained low, but an increased relative risk was considered a problem requiring long-term vigilance. However, the simplicity of the treatment is useful where the older patient cannot tolerate long-term medical therapy.

Surgery, the usual therapy until 1950, is minimally used for hyperthyroidism. It is generally resorted to when the patient chooses not to have radioactive treatment, and is unsuccessful with medical treatment.

## THYROID TUMORS AND MALIGNANCY

### Adenomas

Thyroid adenomas occur in the United States in approximately 2% of the total population. Women have six times as many nodular thyroidal conditions as men. Histological types include embryonal, fetal, follicular adenomas, and colloid nodules. Adenomas are neoplasms, and possibly arise from the same types of stimuli that cause carcinomas. There are two types: adenomas which grow slowly and, if non-functioning, produce symptoms because of distortion of local anatomy; and hyperfunctioning adenomas which may suppress the remainder of the gland or induce thyrotoxicosis. Bleeding into an adenoma causes sudden painful enlargement, often with destruction of the lesion. Very rarely, adenomas appear to progress to carcinomas.

### Diagnosis

Thyroid nodules are evaluated by a review of features that may suggest malignancy, such as an increase in size, pain, undue firmness or fixation, and the presence of local adenopathy. A basic ultrasound of the thyroid is sometimes useful in determining the size of the lesion and the consistency – fluid or solid – of the lesions. Isotope scintiscans and thyroid uptake studies are of some value as well, since the information they provide may suggest an alternative diagnosis, such as multinodular goiter or Hashimoto's thyroiditis, or may show hyperfunction of the adenoma, suggesting that it is a benign lesion.[33] Currently, emphasis is placed upon fine needle aspiration (FNA) cytology for evaluation of the possibility of malignancy (Figure 12.6). This diagnostic procedure appears to be 90–95% accurate in experienced hands.[34] In recent studies researchers have evaluated the accuracy of molecular diagnosis of residual and recurrent thyroid cancer by amplifi-

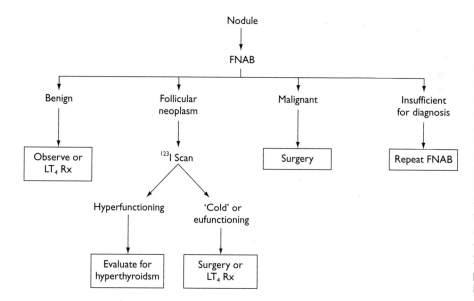

**Figure 12.6**
Suggested algorithm for management of the solitary thyroid nodule.[37] LT$_4$ Rx, levothyroxine therapy; FNAB, fine needle aspiration biopsy. (Reproduced from Singer PA. Evaluation and management of the solitary thyroid nodule. Otolaryngol Clin North Am 1996; 29: 577–91[37] with permission from Elsevier.)

cation of thyroglobulin messenger RNA (mRNA) in peripheral blood.[35]

Nodules that on FNA cytology (Figure 12.6) are benign may be treated conservatively by administration of thyroid hormone replacement therapy to suppress TSH and prevent further growth. Lesions that have suspicious clinical or physical signs, from which it is impossible to obtain adequate cytologial findings, or that have an abnormal cytology, should be resected.[36] Hyperfunctioning solitary thyroid nodules can be destroyed by administration of large doses of radioactive iodine or resected.

### Carcinoma

Thyroid cancer accounts for 0.6–1.6% of all cancers. Mortality is less than 0.4% of all cancer deaths. An increase in thyroid cancer has been seen since 1999 due to improved diagnosis; however, mortality has decreased due to early detection.

### Prevalence

Thyroid carcinomas occur with an incidence of 30 to 60 new cases per million population per year, and a mortality of approximately 4.5 per million population per year.[36,37] Thyroid neoplasia has been shown to be caused by prior irradiation of the thyroid. Even small doses such as 7 to 20 rads have adverse effect. Doses of several hundred rads may increase the incidence of malignancy over 100-fold. Chronic stimulation by TSH can also produce malignant change in the human thyroid. Occult cancers that are generally less than 0.5 cm in their greatest diameter occur in up to 6% of adult thyroids, but rarely appear to change into clinically significant thyroid tumors.

Papillary thyroid carcinomas grow very slowly, metastasizing primarily to cervical nodes and later to the lungs. Many persons survive for two to four decades with extensive metastatic disease. Follicular carcinomas invade more aggressively, and are prone to metastasize to soft tissues and bones. Their mortality is 30–50% over 10 to 20 years. Medullary thyroid carcinomas develop from thyroid C cells and may occur sporadically or as part of familial syndromes associated with multiple endocrine tumors. These tumors secrete calcitonin, which aids in their detection and management. Undifferentiated or anaplastic thyroid carcinomas are extremely malignant. The vast majority cause death within four months to one year.

### Therapy

The basic therapy for thyroid carcinoma remains surgical resection. The minimum desirable operation is a lobectomy on one side complemented by subtotal thyroidectomy on the opposite side. Many surgeons prefer a near-total thyroidectomy for any tumor larger than 1 cm in size. Modified neck dissection is done if local adenopathy is present. In most instances, residual thyroid tissue is destroyed by administration of [131]I. Metastatic thyroid disease that can be shown to accumulate isotope is treated by administration of large doses of [131]I on one or more occasions.

Radiotherapy is probably advisable in differentiated thyroid carcinoma that is invasive into the tissue of the neck, in menopausal patients and in recurrences resistant to [131]I therapy. Radiotherapy to the thyroid bed is probably advisable in all anaplastic thyroid cancers.

Chemotherapy, depending primarily upon adriamycin, is occasionally valuable in some progressive differentiated, medullary, and anaplastic thyroid carcinomas.

## CONCLUSIONS

Women are more subject to thyroid pathology. Hypothyroidism is particularly prevalent in menopausal women. Examination of the patient should include diagnostic examination and testing when even subtle symptoms are described. Treatment of thyroid disease should be personalized. Nodular changes should be carefully followed by ultrasound and palpation. Biopsy is indicated when the findings are confusing, or the disease is rapidly changing. Difficulty often arises with diagnosing thyroid cancer, which requires specialized care. Fine needle aspiration, now available, has made diagnosis somewhat easier, although diagnostic difficulty remains because of the small sample obtained. Several new methods have become available or are in an experimental status.

Menopausal women should be routinely studied for thyroid disease by a screening test sensitive to TSH (sTSH), preferably sTSH referred to $FT_4$, and neck palpation annually from the age of 40 years. Because of the accessibility of the thyroid, an annual or semi annual examination should be routine. Where there is doubt, the woman should be referred for an endocrine evaluation of her thyroid.

# REFERENCES

1. Braverman LE. Diseases of the Thyroid, 2nd edn. Totowa, New Jersey: Humana Press, 2003.
2. Wong TK, Hershman JM. Changes in thyroid function in nonthyroid illness. Trends Endocrinol Metab 1992; 3: 8.
3. Nishikawa M, Inada M, Naito K et al. Age related changes of serum 3,3-diiodothyronine, 35-diiodothyronine, and 3,5-diiodothyronine concentrations in man. J Clin Endcrinol Metab 1981; 52: 517.
4. Ghent WR, Eskin BA, Low DA, Hill LP. Iodine replacement in fibrocystic disease of the breast. Canad J Surg 1993; 36: 453.
5. Dunn JT. What's happening to our iodine [editorial]? J Clin Endocrinol Metab 1998; 83: 3398–400.
6. Eskin BA, Grotkowski CE, Connolly CP, Ghent WR. Different tissue responses for iodine and iodide in rat thyroid and mammary glands. Biol Trace El Res 1995; 49: 9–19.
7. Venturi S, Donati EM, Venturi M, Venturi A. Role of iodine in evaluation and carcinogenesis of thyroid breast and stomach. Adv Clin Path 2000; 4: 11–17.
8. Bagchi N, Brown TR, Parish RF. Thyroid dysfunction in adults over age 55 years. Arch Intern Med 1990; 150: 785.
9. Chrovato L, Minotti S, Pinchera A. Thyroid diseases in the elderly. Baillières Clin Endocrinol Metab 1997; 11: 251–70.
10. Hershman JM, Pekary AE, Berg L et al. Serum thyrotropin and thyroid hormone levels in elderly and middle-aged euthyroid persons. J Am Geriatr Soc 1993; 41: 823.
11. Viceconti N, Luisi S, Nardo S et al. Increased serum inhibin B levels in postmenopausal women with altered thyroid function. Horm Metab Res 2003; 35: 498–501.
12. Brent GA, Hershman JM. Effects of nonthyroidal illness on thyroid function tests. In: L Van Middlesworth L, ed. The Thyroid Gland. Chicago: Year Book Medical Publishers, 1986, 83.
13. United States Preventative Services Task Force. Screening for thyroid disease: recommendation statement. Ann Intern Med 2004; 140: 125–7.
14. Helfand M. Screening for subclinical thyroid dysfunction in non-pregnant adults: a survey of the evidence of the US Preventive Services Task Force (USPSTF). Ann Intern Med 2004; 140: 128–41.
15. Ceresini G, Morganti S, Rebecchi I et al. A one-year follow-up on the effects of raloxifene on thyroid function in postmenopausal women. Menopause 2004; 11: 176–9.
16. Figge J, Leinung M, Goodman AD et al. The clinical evaluation of patients with subclinical hyperthyroidism and free triiodothyronine toxicosis. Am J Med 1994; 96: 229.
17. Faughnan M, LePage R, Fugere P, Bissonnette F, Brossard JH, D'Amour P. Screening for thyroid disease at the menopausal clinic. Clin Invest Med 1995; 18: 11–18.
18. Lotz H, Salabe GB. Lipoprotein(a) increase associated with thyroid autoimmunity. Eur J Endocrinol 1995; 136: 87–91.
19. Massoudi MS, Meilahn EN, Orchart TJ et al. Thyroid function and perimenopausal lipid and weight changes: the thyroid study in healthy women. J Womens Health 1997; 6: 553–8.
20. Doucet J, Trivalle C, Chassagne P et al. Does age play a role in clinical presentation of hypothyroidism? Am J Geriatr Soc 1994; 42: 984.
21. Bemben DA, Winn P, Hamm RM et al. Thyroid disease in the elderly: I. Prevalence of undiagnosed hypothyroidism. J Fam Pract 1994; 38: 577.
22. Kane LA, Gharib H. Thyroid Testing in Contemporary Endocrinology. In: Braverman LE, ed. Diseases of the Thyroid. Totowa, NJ: Humana Press, 2004: 41–4.
23. Buneorcius R, Kazanavicius G, Zalinkaviciars R, Prange AJ Jr. Effects of $T_4$ as compared with $T_4$ and $T_3$ in patients with hypothyroidism. N Engl J Med 1999; 340: 424–9.
24. Biondi B, Fazio S, Carella C et al. Cardiac effects of long term thyrotropin-suppressive therapy with levothyroxine. J Clin Endocrinol Metab 1993; 77: 334.
25. Shapiro LE, Sievert R, Ong L et al. Minimal cardiac effects in asymptomatic athyreotic patients chronically treated with thyrotropin-suppressive doses of L-thyroxine. J Clin Endocrinol Metab 1997; 82: 2592.
26. Mariotti S, Barbesino G, Caluregli P et al. Complex alteration of thyroid function in healthy centenarians. J Clin Endocrinol Metab 1993; 77: 1130.
27. Davis PJ, Davis FB. Hyperthyroidism in patients over the age of 60 years. Medicine 1974; 53: 161.
28. Trivalle C, Doucet J, Chassagne P et al. Differences in the signs and symptoms of hyperthyroidism in older and younger patients. J Am Geriatr Soc 1996; 44: 50.
29. Jodar E, Mung-Jones M, Escobar-Jimenez F, Quesada-Charueco M, Lund del Castillo JD. Bone loss in hyperthyroid patients: influence of aetiology and menopause. Clin Endocrinol 1997; 47: 279–85.
30. Chuang CC, Wang ST, Wang PW, Yu ML. Prevalence study of thyroid dysfunction in the elderly of Taiwan. Gerontology 1998; 44: 162–7.
31. Yamada T, Aizawa T, Koizumi Y et al. Age-related therapeutic response to antithyroid drugs in patients with hyperthyroid Graves' disease. J Am Geriatr Soc 1994; 42: 513.
32. Franklyn JA, Maisoneuve P, Sheppard M, Betteridge J, Boyle P. Cancer incidence and mortality after radioiodine treatment for hyperthyroidism: a population-based cohort study. Lancet 1999; 353: 2111–15.
33. Belfiore A, LaRosa GL, LaPorta GA et al. Cancer risk in patients with cold thyroid nodules: relevance of iodine intake, sex, age, and multinodularity. Am J Med 1992; 93: 363–9.
34. Gharib H, Goellner JR. Fine needle aspiration biopsy of the thyroid: an appraisal. Ann Intern Med 1993; 118: 282.
35. Ringel MD, Ladenson PW, Levine MA. Molecular diagnosis of residual and recurrent thyroid cancer by amplification of thyroglobulin messenger ribonucleic acid in peripheral blood. J Clin Endocrinol Metab 1998; 83: 4435–42.
36. Mazzaferri EL. Management of a solitary thyroid nodule. N Engl J Med 1993; 328: 553.
37. Singer PA. Evaluation and management of the solitary thyroid nodule. Otolaryngol Clin North Am 1996; 29: 577–91.

# Section III

# Clinical problems in the menopause

# Chapter 13

# Surgical care in the menopause

Hugh RK Barber and Martin A Martino

The word menopause and climacteric may have been considered similar in the past, but with an increased understanding of the hormonal milieu that accompanies this time period, we now know these two terms are distinctly different. Moreover, with the increased life expectancy of females in the 21st century, a new time period has emerged, that time period is the geripause, or the time after menopause from years 65 and on. Strictly speaking, the word menopause means the final cessation of menstruation. In its broadest sense, it gives a grossly erroneous idea that yesterday all was well, but today everything has changed and this will continue indefinitely. It also implies that a hysterectomy causes a menopause. This is not necessarily true. Menopause occurs when the ovaries are removed or cease to function. Climacteric, meaning a period of change, is a better word because it expresses the all-important concept of a time-scale, but is not in common use. Therefore, it is important to stick to the word menopause and define it as it is used in this chapter.

The menopause is centered on the ovary and its end-built obsolescence. The events of the menopause start when the active ovary begins to fail, and ends with the final lapse of the ovary into inactivity. The duration of these events is extremely variable, and can cause as much trouble before menstruation ceases as after the last period. The end of the menopause merges into the geripause.

The climacteric is that phase in the life of a woman which marks the interval of transition from reproductive age to the age at which reproductive function is lost. This stage is characterized by progressive endocrine changes that lead to the menopause, the final menstrual period that signals the end of cyclic ovarian function. The peri-

menopause is defined arbitrarily to include the last few years of the climacteric and the first year after the menopause.

It is to be emphasized that menopause is a natural physiological process and only rarely is it a pathological state. The menopause usually occurs at about age 50–52 years, and may be abrupt, or gradual, over a period of months. With age, there is resistance of the follicle to follicle-stimulating hormone (FSH) and luteinizing hormone (LH), and thus an increase in the levels of blood circulation. This leads to stromal stimulation, an increase in estrone levels, and a decrease in estradiol levels. During this time, we also notice a decrease in the level of inhibition due to negative feedback from elevated FSH levels. The symptoms associated with menopause are due to the loss of circulating estrogen levels. In summary, there is an increased level of FSH and a decrease in circulating estrogen levels. The predominant estrogen becomes the aromotization of androgens to estrone in the periphery. An FSH level over 20 mg/ml is often associated with a decrease in fertility most likely secondary to loss of normal ovulatory function. It is the events underlying the changes that are responsible for most of the clinical features. These include the loss of estrogen support to the secondary sex organs and, to a lesser extent, to other structures, such as bone, urinary tract, skin, and hair. It is the consequent release from feedback inhibition of the hypothalamic-pituitary complex.

There are two types of menopause classified according to cause. One, physiological menopause occurs at about age 51 years and results when the oocytes (follicles) responsive to gonadotropins disappear from the ovary and, second, the few remaining oocytes do not respond to gonadotropins. Spontaneous cessation of menses before age 40 years is called premature menopause or premature ovarian failure. Cessation of menstruation and the development of climacteric symptoms and complaints can occur as early as a few years after menarche. The reasons for premature ovarian failure are largely unknown. However, autoimmune disorders and certain viral diseases, as well as genetics, may play a role in ovarian failure.

Surgical menopause is the permanent cessation of ovarian function brought about by removal of the ovaries or by radiation therapy. Irradiation to ablate ovarian function is rarely used today. Artificial menopause is employed as a treatment for endometriosis and estrogen-sensitive neoplasms of the breast and endometrium. More frequently, surgical menopause is a side-effect of treatment of intra-abdominal disease, that is, ovaries are removed in premenopausal women because the gonads have been damaged by infection or neoplasia, or replaced beyond salvage by endometriosis.

## SYMPTOMS IN GERIATRIC GYNECOLOGICAL PATIENTS

The most frequent symptoms that occur among inpatient admissions include genital bleeding, and this is present even in the very elderly. A rule of thumb that has been useful in discussing the problem of bleeding in the postmenopausal woman is that, among those with vaginal bleeding, one-third will have a neoplasm, one-third will have a benign process, and in one-third the cause will not be able to be determined. It must be emphasized that in this age group vaginal bleeding must be looked upon as a malignancy until it is ruled out. Genital displacement in elderly women is very common. Urinary incontinence is frequently associated with genital displacements, and constitutes not only a medical, but also a social, nursing, and sociological problem, especially in very old women. Pruritus vulvae is a very frequent symptom. The genital disorders most likely to affect the menopausal patient include those resulting from the cessation of ovarian function with consequent hypoestrogenism, dermatological diseases of the vulva, uncertainties concerning sexual activities, neoplasms that are more common after the menopause, and symptomatic relaxation of the pelvic supporting structures. The genitalia of the menopausal patient are less likely to develop benign neoplasms. Sexually transmitted diseases are less frequently encountered in the older patient, but are being diagnosed with increasing frequency in recent times, especially with the increased usage of male erectile dysfunction medications such as viagra and the use of female sexual stimulants that are under development.

## HISTORY AND PELVIC EXAMINATION

The setting for a meeting with the patient must be well structured. The medical evaluation and examination should be conducted in a relaxed and unhurried manner, and the patient given as much privacy and personal attention as possible. Ideally, a multidisciplinary team, consisting of a social worker, nurse clinician, and nutritionist, together with a physician, should work with the patient to institute the necessary medical care and support services. The confidence of the patient must be gained, a relaxed and friendly atmosphere created, and the practitioner must be prepared to be unhurried as he or she starts to take a history from the menopausal patient. The word menopause has been shrouded in the mystery of silence. Many patients are upset by hearing the word. It is the responsibility of the physician to explain carefully that the menopause is just one part of an overall life process.

Patients in the early geripausal period are able to give a useful history of their obstetric and gynecological experience or the age at which menopause occurred. However, in the late menopausal period, it may be difficult to obtain this information directly from the patient. It is important, therefore, to have a relative or a close friend available, but often this is not possible. Some elderly patients may present or be referred for so-called vaginal bleeding, but on close questioning they are uncertain whether the bleeding is coming from the urethra, vagina or the anal area.

It is important to obtain a careful obstetric, menstrual, postmenopausal and gynecological history. The patient should be asked about drug ingestion, particularly whether she has ever taken any type of hormone or is currently taking hormones. The patient must be questioned about the use of over-the-counter drugs (OTC), or the use of herbal medicines. The eating habits and nutrition of these patients are most important to explore. The elderly woman living alone may live on tea and toast and develop an anemia.

The most recent epidemiological data suggest that anxiety disorders are exceedingly common, occurring more frequently in women than in men across all age groups. It is estimated that approximately 5% of all women, at some time in their lives, will have an anxiety disorder of sufficient severity to interfere with their ability to function in their usual roles. An estimated 10–15% of females over the age of 65 years experience anxieties sufficiently severe to warrant medical intervention. The prevalence of anxiety disorders in the elderly demands a basic understanding by the physician of the numerous ways in which these disorders may present: anxiety in the elderly may present as neurological, gastrointestinal, cardiovascular and respiratory symptoms. The most common genitourinary symptoms are pruritus vulvae/vaginae, or pruritus ani, or the occurrence of dyspareunia.

The Victorian concept that all sexual activity ends at the time of the menopause has been shown to be totally inaccurate. Many studies have shown that women are able to function sexually very late in their lives. Therefore, it is very important to ask about sexual function. The way in which the inquiry about sexuality is approached confirms and supports the patient's feelings that she is still considered a woman and, if carried out in an open but discerning manner, reinforces the patient's regard for the physician. Sexuality and sexual function in the menopausal and postmenopausal years is now receiving a great deal of attention in the literature.

In 1953, Kinsey reported that the sexual activity of an unmarried woman remains relatively constant until age 55 years, whereas that of an unmarried man declines progressively from adolescence.[1] Kinsey concluded that, in women, age has no effect on sexual activity until late in life, and he suggested that the subsequent reduction in sexual activity may be due primarily to diminution in the sexuality of the male partner.

By this time in the history taking, the patient should relate well to the responsible physician and, having gained the patient's confidence, it is time to ask if there is any sexual dysfunction. Disinterest in intercourse is often a result of dyspareunia secondary to an atrophic vaginal mucosa, introital stricture, or decreased vaginal distensibility resulting from estrogen deficiency or inability to lubricate. Although the true significance of sexual dysfunction in the menopause is difficult to measure, it is important for the physician to work with the patient in an attempt to find reasons for the dysfunction. Some patients often ask for a consultation with a sex counselor and

the physician should co-operate by making this referral.

When the significance of a complaint is not readily apparent, the physician should listen carefully and question the patient further. The history is most important in establishing a good patient–physician relationship.

## GYNECOLOGICAL EXAMINATION

The findings on physical examination vary greatly, depending on the time elapsed since menopause and the severity of estrogen deficiency. Older women often question the need for periodic gynecological examinations after the menopause. It is important to impress upon the patient that they should continue to protect their health. Recently, newspaper articles have alluded that elderly women do not need to follow-up for annual checks. Age does not prevent the development of cancer of the genitalia or breast. Although the incidence of some genital malignancies may plateau after the menopause, that of some other cancers, particularly of the endometrium, vagina, vulva, and ovary, actually increases.

Many menopausal patients recognize that they have atrophic vaginal and vulvar tissue, and that examination may be painful. Therefore, they are inclined to avoid routine examinations. It is important that the patient undergoes as little discomfort and pain as possible during the examination. An explanation about the examination often dispels some of the anxiety and may put the patient at ease.

The examining physician should carefully observe the vulva, urethra and Bartholin's and Skene's glands, and it is important to palpate the texture of these structures. Since menopausal women may have atrophic vaginal or vulvar tissue resulting from hypoestrogenism, it is important to use a small speculum or Peterson's speculum. The speculum should be inserted by holding the blades parallel to the introitus, slowly turning the speculum so that the posterior blade rests against the posterior wall of the vagina and, with gentle pressure downwards, opening the vagina without disturbing the sensitive organs that lie anteriorly.

Once the speculum is in place and the cervix is identified, any vaginal secretion should be removed and a careful Pap smear taken, attempting to get into the cervical canal, if possible, also taking a smear of the posterior fornix. It is most important to sample the endometrium if there are any signs of vaginal spotting or complaints of vaginal bleeding.

A one-finger vaginal examination should be carried out at the beginning, and the finger should be very carefully directed around the entire length and breadth of the vagina, in addition to exploring the fornices and the area under the urethra. Having done this, the uterus should be outlined as to size, shape and mobility, and then the adnexal area is carefully examined. It is important to explain each step of the examination to the patient and to assure the patient that, if there is any pain, the examination will be stopped immediately. Unfortunately, in the elderly, the vagina is often conical and inelastic, limiting a proper adnexal examination.

Rectovaginal bimanual examination is often preferable to vaginal abdominal bimanual examination in the menopausal patient. This allows the rectovaginal septum, cardinal ligaments, and uterosacral ligaments to be carefully examined. A rectal examination should be carried out and any blood on the finger identified, and, in those patients in whom blood is not identified, one of the tests for occult blood should be carried out.

Having completed the routine examination, if a patient notes vaginal bleeding, the physician must make a judgment about whether to attempt an endometrial aspiration at this particular examination, or to have the patient return at another time for the endometrial aspiration. Either way, it is important to be as gentle as possible. Using ultrasound to evaluate the endometrium is still controversial. It is possible to measure the thickness of the endometrium and, when significantly over the baseline level, curettage or endometrial biopsy is probably indicated.

In addition to the physical and pelvic examinations, a Pap smear, colposcopy and biopsy must be carried out to establish the diagnosis of any early lesion if indicated. The breasts are considered a part of the upper genital tract and should be carefully examined. The examination must be done in an unhurried manner and all quadrants should be examined. The patient should be examined while lying down, as well as sitting up. The American Cancer Society has published pamphlets demonstrating the ideal breast examination to be carried out by the physician. During the examination, it is important for the physician to teach the patient breast self-examination. This is the 1–2–3 method: first while taking a shower, then in front of a mirror and, last, while lying down.

## CYSTOURETHROCELE AND UTERINE DESCENSUS

It is generally agreed that the support of pelvic structures depends on the endopelvic fascia, the uterosacral and cardinal ligaments, and the levator muscles. This intact fascial system with its attachments to the vaginal fornices and upper two-thirds of the lateral vagina provides a well-supported vaginal tube, which in turn is the most important supporting structure for the uterus and vaginal vault. Traumatic (obstetric) stretching, wear and tear of living, occupational and unusual athletic endeavors, heredity, and postmenopausal attenuation of the pelvic and perianal muscles all contribute in varying degrees to the development of pelvic relaxation. Additional contributing factors that promote uterine descensus are chronic obstructive pulmonary disease (COPD), and asthma and other chronic lung diseases. These are commonly associated with cystocele and occur in women who have urinary stress incontinence. However, urethrocele is not a cause of urinary incontinence. It is interesting that in women with large cystoceles there is seldom any stress incontinence. However, these patients often have repeated bouts of cystitis. Patients with large cystoceles often have to put their finger in their vagina and push the bladder upward in order to empty their bladder. The patient with a large cystocele may pull on the trigone of the bladder and, as a result, have a constant urge to pass urine. Nothing short of surgery will correct this condition.

The essentials of diagnosis include:

1. sensation of vaginal fullness, pressure of falling out
2. feeling of incomplete emptying of the bladder, urinary frequency, and perhaps the need to push the bladder up in order to empty the bladder completely
3. the presence of soft, reducible mass bulging into the anterior vagina and distending the vaginal introitus
4. with straining or coughing, increased bulging and descent of the anterior vaginal wall as well as the urethra.

Although a degree of cystocele is demonstrable in virtually all parous women during the childbearing years, their condition may not progress and may not cause symptoms.

The importance of physiological and anatomical factors in the problems of prolapse and incontinence has led to the adoption of the term 'pelvic floor dysfunction'. When examining living persons, the pelvic floor is a convex, dynamic structure that must continually expand and contract in response to different stimuli and conditions. It must contract to help maintain urinary and fecal continence, yet it must relax to allow the expulsion of urine and feces. It has a role in normal sexual responsiveness in females, and may play a role in the generation of an orgasm at the peak of sexual excitement.

Treatment in such cases is not usually required until after the menopause, when the pelvic fascial and muscular supports become attenuated by slowly progressive involutional changes. The cystocele requires surgical repair if there are repeated bouts of cystitis or trigonitis, or if the cystocele becomes so large that the patient cannot adequately empty her bladder, with repeated bouts of cystitis, or the cystocele protrudes outside the vaginal introitus and causes an ulceration of the vaginal wall. A large cystocele may result in pulling on the trigone, giving rise to a constant urgency. The various types of pessaries do not usually help cystoceles, and very often create stress incontinence. Many older women tolerate large cystourethroceles and some degree of descensus without complaint, but massive procidentia (complete prolapse) is always disabling, and is occasionally associated with trophic ulceration of the exposed vaginal mucosa, or with kidney dysfunction caused by kinking from displacement of both ureters. The uterus gradually descends from the axis of the vagina, taking the vaginal wall with it. It may present clinically at any level, but is usually classified as one of three degrees: first, the cervix is still inside the vagina; second, the cervix appears outside the vulva, the cervical lips become congested and ulcerated; and third, complete prolapse. This is sometimes called complete procidentia. (Procidentia means 'parts of the body falling out of place'.) The uterovaginal prolapse represents the herniation of the genital tract through the pelvic diaphragm. The uterus and vagina are held in the pelvis by the cardinal and uterosacral ligaments, and by the pelvic floor musculature, mainly the levator ani. When these ligaments and muscles become ineffective, the uterus and vagina descend (prolapse) through the gap between the muscles. The causes of prolapse are:

1.  stretching of muscle and fibrous tissue which occurs with repeated childbirth
2.  increased intra-abdominal pressure which occurs in women with a chronic cough or asthma, and in women who undertake heavy industrial work. It is a constitutional predisposition to stretching of the ligaments as a response, presumably, to years in the erect position.

Thus, nulliparous women can develop prolapse. However, in those that do, a thorough neurological examination should be carried out, as well as careful metabolic and endocrine studies as indicated. It is often reported that obesity might increase the load on the pelvic floor; however, this is probably not the case, because the abdominal viscera present essentially a fluid-like mass, and the pressure at the bottom of a column of fluid is related only to the height of the column, and not to its overall diameter.

*Management*

These conditions are probably best treated surgically, and even the most elderly can tolerate the surgery fairly well. However, there are some women for whom it is well advised not to perform surgery, and a vaginal pessary of the Gellhorn, disc type or Smith–Hodge type may support the uterus and bladder. Although the patient will require scheduled visits for removal and cleansing of the pessary, it decreases the need for an operation. The pessary is usually considered as the last resort measure. However, when indicated, it can be a great comfort to a very sick old woman with severe heart disease, emphysema, and the presence of a procidentia.

## RECTOCELE

Bulging of the posterior vaginal wall and underlying rectum through the rectovaginal fascia results in a rectocele. If the prolapse is at the level of the middle third of the vagina, the rectovaginal septum is often involved, and the rectum prolapses with the vaginal wall. This is called a classic rectocele. If the lowest part of the vagina is prolapsed, the perianal body is involved rather than the rectum.

A mild degree of rectocele (rarely causing symptoms) is usually present in all multiparous patients. A large rectocele may cause a sense of pelvic pressure, rectal fullness or incomplete evacuation of stool. Occasionally a patient may find it necessary to reduce the posterior vaginal wall manually in a backward direction to evacuate stool effectively from the lower rectum. Distinguishing a high rectocele (involving the entire rectovaginal septum) from an enterocele may sometimes be difficult. Generally, with the patient straining, a rectovaginal examination will confirm the presence of abdominal contents sliding into the enterocele sac, so that an enterocele, as opposed to rectocele, presents as a true hernia. Since pessaries are not helpful for either a rectocele or an enterocele, surgical repair is indicated when symptoms interfere with the quality of life.

## ENTEROCELE

An enterocele results when the small bowel pushes the peritoneum between the rectum and the vagina. Large enteroceles occasionally give upper abdominal distress because of the pull on the mesentery of the bowel. If the upper part of the posterior vaginal wall prolapses, the pouch of Douglas is elongated, and small bowel or omentum may descend, pushing the peritoneum in front of it. This has been called the classic enterocele. Enterocele is usually associated with uterine prolapse and is sometimes called vault prolapse, or hernia of the pouch of Douglas. The diagnosis is made from the following:

1.  an uncomfortable pressure and a 'falling out' sensation of the vagina
2.  association with uterine prolapse or subsequent to hysterectomy in any age group, most commonly in postmenopausal women
3.  demonstration of a mass bulging into the posterior fornix and upper posterior vaginal wall
4.  occasionally the enterocele will put traction on the mesentery of the small bowel, causing upper abdominal discomfort.

The diagnosis is made by having the patient stand and by inserting the index finger into the rectum and the thumb into the vagina, and asking the patient to strain or cough. An impulse of the small bowel against the examining fingers is almost certain to be an enterocele. If the enterocele is large and bulges through the introitus, or if there is a great deal of abdominal discomfort, the enterocele should be repaired surgically. It is important in repairing an enterocele to have a high ligation of the peritoneal sac and closure of the transversalis fascia, and an additional insurance against recurrence is to bring the uterosacral ligaments together and to close off the cul-de-sac.

## STRESS INCONTINENCE

Urinary incontinence and lower genital tract disorders become more frequent after the menopause. The lower urinary tract and the lower genital tract are of the same embryonic origin and influence each other in physiological and pathophysiological conditions.

Stress incontinence is defined as involuntary loss of urine due to a sudden increase in intra-abdominal pressure such as occurs with laughing, coughing or sneezing. About 50% of parous women occasionally experience stress incontinence. It must be distinguished from overflow incontinence, urgency incontinence, enuresis, and incontinence resulting from a neurological disorder.

The causes of genuine stress incontinence are urethral sphincter incompetence, or anatomical scarred urethra (iatrogenic or traumatic), or urethral denervation. During the stress of coughing, the proximal portion of the urethra drops below the pelvic floor. An increase in intra-abdominal pressure induced by coughing transmits to the bladder, but not to the urethra. Since the urethral resistance is overcome by the increased bladder pressure, leakage of urine results. On urodynamic evaluation, there is a decrease in the functional length of the urethra, decreased urethral closure pressure, and abnormal response of the sphincteric mechanism in reaction to stress. Stress incontinence occurs when the urethra sags away from its attachments to the symphysis. It may appear before the menopause, but for many women it becomes increasingly distressing after the age of 60 years. Loosening of the pelvic supporting tissue, damaged years earlier by vaginal delivery, and aggravated by years of standing and straining, becomes more marked after estrogen secretion decreases following the menopause.

The function of the levator ani muscles can be compromised in two ways: first, there can be direct injury to the muscle, resulting in mechanical disruption of the entire muscle; second, damage to nerves supplying the muscles could lead to their inability to contract, even though they themselves remain intact. Damage to the nerve supply of the muscle probably explains why the Kegel exercises fail to control stress incontinence in some women.

Urodynamic studies are important for correct diagnosis. This procedure is favored over others for differentiating bladder instability due to cystitis and nerve or muscle dysfunction. Urodynamics means the determination of bladder tone and its response to gradual distention with normal saline. This will provide a measurement of capacity (the normal bladder can hold about 700 ml), and of any residual urine after voiding (as with cystocele). About 50 ml are instilled at a time, and the bladder wall given time to accommodate. The manometer indicates detrusor contractions and, if they are frequent and occur early on, an irritable bladder is diagnosed. Cystometry cannot determine the cause.

Half the women with stress incontinence can avoid surgery if they have good pubococcygeal tone and faithfully practice pubococcygeal exercises (puckering the vagina and urethral supporting tissue in a manner comparable to stopping a stream of urine). This is called a Kegel perineal exercise. The patient is advised to carry out this exercise for 2 minutes at least four times a day. It takes approximately 2 months before any positive results are seen in a great number of cases. Incontinence will recur if the exercises are not continued. If the Kegel exercises are done properly, and there is absolutely no response, it probably represents damage to the nerve supply of the muscles which leads to their inability to contract, even though they themselves remain intact.

Three-quarters of women with stress incontinence are asymptomatic after surgery that is carried out to repair a cystourethrocele and return the urethra to its normal position above and behind the symphysis. The most commonly employed operation to restore the urethrovesicle angle was the Marshall–Marchetti–Krantz operation or the Burch operation, however these procedures have been replaced by the transvaginal tape and trans-obturator tape procedures. Both approaches employ the positioning of a pubovaginal sling that appears to have decreased morbidity compared to older procedures with equivalent efficacy.

Loss of urine control or urinary incontinence is especially common in postmenopausal women, but occurs in men as well. At least one in ten patients aged 65 or older has a problem with this.

Incontinence can range from the discomfort of slight losses of urine to the disability and shame of severe frequent wetting. Persons who are incontinent often withdraw from social life and try to hide their problem from their family, friends, and even their doctors. Relatives of an incontinent person often do not know about the choices of treatment and are made to believe that nursing-home care is the only option. These reactions are unfortunate, because in many cases incontinence can be treated and controlled, if not cured. Incontinence is not an inevitable result of aging. It is caused by specific changes in bodily function which often result from disease or use of medication. If untreated, incontinence can increase the risk of skin irritation, and might raise the risk of developing bed-sores. Some patients are put in a nursing home for incontinence and not incompetence.

Incontinence may be brought on by illness that is accompanied by fatigue, confusion and hospital admission. Incontinence is sometimes the first and only symptom of urinary tract infection. Curing the infection will usually relieve or clear up the incontinence. It is important to differentiate stress incontinence, urgency incontinence, and overflow incontinence. They all have different etiologies and treatment. In the rare instance in which the incontinence cannot be totally cured, specially designed absorbent underclothing is available. Many of these garments are no more bulky than normal underwear, can be worn under everyday clothing, and free a person from the discomfort and embarrassment of incontinence. It is important to remember that incontinence can be treated and often cured. Even incurable problems can be managed to reduce complications, anxiety, and family stresses.

## EXOGENOUS ESTROGENS AND ENDOMETRIAL CANCER

It has been estimated that approximately 25% of women of menopausal age have symptoms of such severity as to warrant estrogen therapy. Although the evidence is not conclusive, it is suggested that estrogen replacement therapy has long-term metabolic benefits by reducing the incidence of stroke, heart disease (age 50–59), osteoporosis, and fractures, and by slowing aging of the brain. Those that have been receiving estrogen replacement for five or more years have a decrease of Alzheimer's disease by 60%. A number of case–control studies, however, have indicated that this form of treatment is associated with an increased incidence of endometrial cancer, with a risk ratio ranging between 5 and 15. These studies were based on case–control studies that are cheap, quick and easy to perform because they are retrospective. The problem involves an accurate and rigid selection of the case controls and, without this, the study has very little value. Although there is still slight concern about the relationship of exogenous estrogens to carcinoma of the endometrium, the physician should not be discouraged from using estrogen therapy when indicated. The recent results of the Women's Health Initiative trial (WHI) for the estrogen only arm has conclusively demonstrated that estrogen does NOT cause breast cancer. Interestly, there was a decreased hazard ratio demonstrated of nearly 23%, but this was not statistically significant.[2] The judicial use of progesterone when giving estrogen replacement therapy will cut the incidence of carcinoma of the endometrium almost to zero.

The common symptoms that can be helped by estrogen replacement therapy include flushes, flashes, sweats, insomnia and dry vagina. As the patient gets older, the flushes and sweats disappear, but the dry, atrophic vagina becomes worse. Since osteoporosis is usually seen in the postmenopausal period, the issue of estrogen replacement therapy as a preventive treatment or a method of preventing the progress of osteoporosis is raised. Therefore, although the risk of endometrial cancer is increased, the physician must treat the symptomatic patient. The protection provided to the cardiovascular system by estrogen therapy is an indication to continue estrogen therapy for the duration of the patient's lifetime. The use of low-dose progesterone when giving estrogen replacement therapy does not seem to affect the lipid profile, but does protect the endometrium.

Occasionally this will cause vaginal bleeding, but, if the patient is monitored and has endometrial screening, it should not be a deterrent to keeping these women comfortable. Some women who have atrophic vulvitis and vaginitis, which do not always respond to estrogen by mouth, must have a supplemental estrogen vaginal cream. It is important to teach the patient to rub the estrogen cream on the outside, particularly around the posterior fourchette and just into the introitus. It is important to instruct the patient to start the estrogen vaginal cream just above the anus and rub it carefully into the perineum, particularly the posterior fourchette. This increases the amount of vulvar and vaginal tissues, and usually stops the itching and discomfort that occurs with intercourse.

In the past couple of years, alendronate therapy has been shown to restore bone mass, but, when discontinued, the loss of bone mass continues. In the elderly, alendronate therapy is often associated with gastrointestinal symptoms, particularly esophagitis. Ideally, the alendronate must be taken first thing in the morning on an empty stomach with a glass of tap water. Carbonated water and fruit juices must be avoided at this time. Following the ingestion of alendronate and one glass of tap water, the patient is instructed not to eat or drink anything for half an hour, and the patient must not lie down during this time.

Recently, designer estrogens (SERMs) have been introduced. These agents behave like estrogen in some tissues, but block its action in others. The drug raloxifene has demonstrated ability for maintaining bone density in postmenopausal women. Reports indicate that it provides protection against endometrial cancer and breast cancer. Like estrogen replacement therapy, it increases the incidence of blood clots in veins. The media publicity has been great for the recent designer estrogens, but more data must be accumulated before they are prescribed for every patient.

## OSTEOPOROSIS

Although the subject is covered in detail in another part of this book (Chapter 14), it is important to review it briefly in this chapter. Many women visiting their family practitioner or the obstetrician/gynecologist, especially those in the postmenopausal years, inquire about osteoporosis. Osteoporosis has been called the silent disease. Technically this is because it usually produces absolutely no symptoms until a fracture occurs. In reality, osteoporosis is not a disease per se, but rather the end result of severe or prolonged bone loss. Osteoporosis is a painful, disfiguring and debilitating process. It is a women's issue. Osteoporosis cannot be cured, but with alendronate bone mass can be restored. However, it can be prevented and the symptomatology relieved. A great number of women visiting their gynecologist for backache after they have been thoroughly evaluated by an orthopedic doctor may be found to have osteoporosis. Usual X-ray studies cannot identify osteoporosis until it is far advanced. When it shows up on the usual radiographs, there is about a 30% bone mass loss. However, by use of single photon absorptiometry or dual photon absorptiometry, a diagnosis can be made at an early stage and the patient treated for symptoms, and hopefully the progress of the osteoporosis stopped. In an overall evaluation, osteoporosis is really a pediatric disease. Therefore, prevention should start in early childhood, including a well-balanced diet, structured exercise and, above all, prohibition of smoking and drinking.

The patient who is predisposed to developing osteoporosis is a postmenopausal woman who is slender in weight, with very fair skin and small bone structure. There are other contributing factors that may predispose the patient to osteoporosis, namely a family history of the disease, Asian background, nulligravida, lack of physical activity, poor diet, calcium deficiency, vitamin D deficiency, smoking, alcohol, change in estrogen balance, and change in calcium metabolism. Therapy for established disease includes calcium supplements, at least 1500 mg, vitamin D 400 IU, estrogens, androgens, fluoride, and calcitonin. Alendronate has recently been introduced and has the ability, when calcium supplements and vitamin D are given, to restore bone mass. Treatment should be carried out under strict control conditions. It can be stated that osteoporosis cannot be cured, but, with alendronate, bone mass can be restored, but can only be maintained if alendronate is given continuously. However, the patient can be made more comfortable by treatment, and it may be possible to prevent osteoporosis from progressing. Structured exercise and a well-balanced diet are particularly important in dealing with osteoporosis. The new designer estrogens have been effective in preventing and treating osteoporosis and, although the reports are suggestive, they are not conclusive.

## CARDIOVASCULAR DISEASE

There is a relationship between the loss of ovarian function and the development of heart disease. Approximately 450 000 American women die of heart attacks each year. Studies have shown the relationship between ovarian function, coronary atherosclerosis, and mortality. Up until the menopause, women have fewer coronary heart disease problems than men, but, within the first 10 years after the menopause, women who have not been given estrogen replacement have a rate as high as, or higher than that for men, whereas women who have been taking estrogen have a much lower rate of coronary heart disease. Therefore, the use of appropriate doses of estrogen may offer postmenopausal women protection against coronary heart disease. The protective effect of low doses of estrogen is mediated through a decrease in the low-density lipoproteins (LDLs), and an increase in the high-density lipoproteins (HDLs). If the dosage of estrogen is too high, hypertension may be produced, but this is very seldom seen in women taking appropriate doses of estrogen. In addition, it should be added that estrogen replacement therapy has been associated with an increased incidence of stroke, embolism or thrombophlebitis, and patients should be counseled accordingly.[4] Women receiving estrogen replacement therapy must be warned about the danger of smoking while taking estrogens.

Probably the most important indication for long-term hormonal therapy is the prevention of cardiovascular disease. This causes 10 times more death than breast cancer in the postmenopausal population. Estrogen therapy reverses the negative lipoprotein changes that usually occur after the menopause. Among women who have an intact uterus, a progestational agent should be added to the estrogen as part of the hormone replacement therapy. By the use of medroxyprogesterone acetate in small doses, such as 5 or 2.5 mg, the beneficial effect of estrogen on the lipid profile is not adversely affected. The role of the designer estrogen remains to be determined as far as the value in preventing cardiovascular disease is concerned.

There is increasing evidence in the literature that estrogen replacement therapy returns sex hormones to the premenopausal level, and it has been proposed as one method for reducing cardiovascular disease. In postmenopausal women treated with estrogen replacement therapy, it is anticipated that there will be a 50% decrease in all-cause mortality, compared to women who did not receive estrogen replacement therapy. On further examining the analysis of the data, it is evident that the largest effect on mortality was in decreasing ischemic heart disease. Although not every woman is a candidate for estrogen replacement therapy, if this treatment is prescribed judiciously and with full knowledge of its clinical effects, it can both offer patients lower mortality for cardiovascular disease and enhance quality of life. Recently it has been shown that estrogen therapy can slow aging of the brain and, if the patient has been taking estrogen replacement therapy for five or more years, it decreases the incidence of Alzheimer's disease by 60%. The effect of designer estrogens on the brain is to be determined.

## SEXUALITY

With better nutrition, more cholesterol in the diet, more rest and better health, women are maintaining an interest in sexual function well into their postmenopausal years. Continued sexual outlets and functioning are the most important factors in maintaining sexual interest and capacity in the menopausal woman. If for any reason a woman is sexually inactive for some years in the postmenopausal period, there may be difficulty with re-institution of sexual function.

Women generally experience little serious loss of sexual capacity because of age alone. Those changes that do occur are mainly in the shape, flexibility and lubrication of the vagina. These can be traced directly to lowered levels of the hormone estrogen during and after the menopause. Women who have severe problems can be treated successfully with estrogen replacement therapy and are then able to carry on an active sex life.

As stated above, while Kinsey reported that the sexual activity of unmarried women remains relatively constant until age 55, the activity of unmarried men declines progressively from adolescence.[1] Among married couples also, the frequency of sexual intercourse appears to decline in a similar fashion with aging. Kinsey concluded from these observations that, in women, age has no effect on sexual activity until very late in life, and suggested that subsequent reduction in sexual activity may be due primarily to diminution in the sexuality of the male partner.

Alterations in sexual response associated with aging are a result of generalized decrease in tone, strength and elasticity of tissues and lengthening of response time. In older women it may take 3–5 min for vaginal lubrication to occur, whereas in the young woman it takes only 15–20 s. At the same level of arousal, the older woman will have a smaller volume of lubrication. Again, provided that she is in good health and especially if there has been continuing of sexual function, lubrication for intercourse will be adequate. Use of commonly available lubricants may be helpful. Currently, Upsher-Smith Laboratories, Inc. has introduced Lubrin®, a vaginal lubricating insert which is unscented, colorless and convenient, as well as Replens®, which provides long-lasting lubrication for sexual intercourse. Some women find that Astro-Glide® serves as an adequate lubrication.

Sexual dysfunction may be lifelong, in the sense that the woman has brought the condition into her marriage or other relationships, or it may have been acquired after a period of successful functioning. The dysfunction may affect both partners, or it may be situational in the sense that it is present in only one partner, usually the male. Many instances of sexual incompatibility are based on insufficient foreplay or preparation by the partner. Although the blame may be assigned to the partner, the failure is that of the woman herself, for she should assume responsibility for her own sexual pleasure, and be able to communicate effectively her needs to her partner. If her partner rejects the explicit request, the problem may be of general marital dysfunction and not strictly sexual.

The menopausal woman complaining of sexual inadequacy is often told by her physician that loss of sexual function is to be expected with the change of life, and there is nothing to be done about it. Although sexual behavior is the sum total of the individual make-up, including chromosomal sex, gender identification, gonadal adequacy, childhood rearing, environmental influences, a possible hypothalamic sensitization, and hormone factors, there is a definite role for hormone therapy in modifying sexual responsiveness. A combination of estrogen and androgen is often beneficial. Conjugated estrogen or its equivalent in a dose of 0.625 mg, or 5 mg of methyltestosterone, is recommended. In some women, methyltestosterone, 10 mg three times a day for 2 weeks, will often increase the libido and fantasy level, and, if the patient indulges in intercourse, the desires will continue without needing any further stimulation from hormonal therapy. Androgens are not important for the physiological sexual response, but they are critical for the cognitive aspects of a woman's sexual functioning, such as desire. In women for whom intercourse is difficult because of shrinkage secondary to estrogen withdrawal, hormonal cream is often beneficial. This should be applied locally on the outside, around the inside lip of the small labia, up around the clitoris, and particularly around the posterior fourchette. It is important not only to apply the estrogen cream, but also to rub it into the tissue. The treatment should be carried out two to three times a week until the tissue has undergone a period of rejuvenation. The treatment should then be continued at less frequent intervals. A quarter of an applicator of estrogenic cream inserted into the vagina every 2–3 weeks usually keeps the upper part of the vagina healthy.

Masters and Johnson have shown that all four stages of the response cycle (excitement, plateau, orgasm, and resolution) are somewhat diminished with increased age.[3] In the excitement phase, breasts are less engorged and the sexual flush may be absent. The clitoris enlarges normally, but there is no noticeable change in the labia majora. Vaginal lubrication is reduced. Vaginal ballooning occurs later in the plateau phase and is often less marked. Orgasms continue to occur, but their duration is shorter, and muscular contraction may also be less intense. Uterine spasms may render some orgasms painful. The resolution phase is rapid in elderly women and occasionally, because of urethral trauma, is accompanied by a desire to void. Decrease in the strength of vaginal contractions occurring with orgasm is another change that occurs in elderly women. This effect is recordable and documented. However, older women may report no diminution in the experience of pleasure or release gratification. Viagra® (sildenafil citrate) is receiving a great deal of media attention at present, and other female stimulants are also actively under investigation.

## MAJOR GYNECOLOGICAL SURGICAL PROCEDURES IN THE AGED

Advances in preoperative, operative and post-operative management have considerably reduced the hazards of surgery for the postmenopausal patient. Older women are increasingly requesting surgery for gynecological problems in order to improve the quality of their lives.

A number of published studies have demonstrated that there is very little increase in the morbidity or mortality or length of stay in hospitals for patients undergoing major and minor gynecological surgery when compared with the younger age group, provided that due respect is paid to the patient's general condition. Most procedures can be performed with regional or local anesthesia, with minimal discomfort to the patient, if general anesthesia is contraindicated. The majority of operative procedures are for the definitive treatment of genital prolapse and the diagnosis of the cause of postmenopausal bleeding, followed by surgery for uterine and vulvar lesions. Patients who are 90 years and older can undergo successful major surgery. The problem is that, in the post-

anesthesia stage, the patient may appear to be confused, and stroke and pulmonary emboli must be ruled out.

As the postmenopausal population increases and women no longer accept age alone as a barrier to active life, more elective surgery will be demanded by patients and performed by gynecological surgeons. Disorders of the female genital organs are certainly not among the major causes of death. Yet they give rise to important illnesses producing discomfort and disability and, therefore, warrant treatment. Most of the gynecological complaints of elderly women are related to genital prolapse. These conditions cause daily discomfort and anxiety. Contrary to the practice in younger patients, most of the operations in the elderly are carried out by the vaginal route. Vaginal hysterectomy is the procedure most often chosen to correct uterine prolapse. However, in rare situations, either the Manchester or LeFort operations may be employed.

Medical advancements in diagnosis and treatment, and the better understanding of physiological and pathophysiological processes in the elderly now justify the performance of major operations in this group. Reports from numerous authors have shown that age alone does not contraindicate surgical intervention if due regard is paid to the patient's general condition. Better anesthesia and antibiotic therapy have resulted in greater security in the postoperative course. It is important for the physician to bear in mind that sexual activity in some women continues into very old age. Therefore, vaginal surgery should be performed with this in mind.

The duration of operation should be kept as short as possible, because the prolonged lithotomy position invites more complications than does prolonged anesthesia. Many postmenopausal patients develop hallucinations and disorientation following the anesthesia. This gives rise to the question of whether the patient has thrown an embolism or has had a cerebral accident. Unfortunately, these patients must be subjected to the usual evaluation for these conditions.

Contraindications to surgical intervention should not include chronological age. The role for peri-operative low-molecular weight heparin is presently being investigated. Cancer patients who have abdominal surgery are at very high risk of venous thrombo-embolism, and should receive an additive means of prophylaxis in addition to sequential compression boots. This may be started on postoperative day one and continued while patients are in the hospital at least for the present time. The full extent of the duration of prophylaxis is being investigated as well as the dosing regimen for a preoperative schedule.[5]

## NUTRITION AND AGING

The elderly need a healthy, balanced diet. Preventative medicine is now taking center stage, and nutrition is the important part of this lifestyle. The keystone of this diet recommends at least five servings of fresh fruit and also five fresh vegetables per day. This is usually a fairly heavy diet for the elderly and it is difficult for them to absorb and take in this much food. However, preparations such as cooking, baking and roasting often destroy important micronutrients for patient nutrition. Therefore, it is important to make plans (phyto) for a well-balanced diet that is tolerable and can be managed by the patient.

A new process has been able to maintain the micronutrients by first using a standard method to get rid of water and excess sugar. Beyond this, the vegetables, fruits and berries, each treated separately, are made into a mash and then, by low temperature desiccation, a powder is formed which is put into capsules. The process is safely scrutinized at every step to make sure there are no pesticides or other contaminants. After one month of using these capsules, it has been shown in the blood plasma levels that the antioxidants are greatly increased. It is now a whole food product, but does not take the place of fresh fruits and fresh vegetables, however it contains all the nutrients that are found in fresh fruits and fresh vegetables.

- The fruits made up by this method are called an orchard blend. It is made up of apples, oranges, pineapples, cranberries, peaches, cherries, and papaya.
- The garden blend is made up of carrots, spinach, broccoli, kale, cabbage, parsley, beets, and tomatoes.
- The grains are barley, and oats.
- The vineyard powder is made up of blueberries, blackberries, bilberries, raspberries, cranberries, elderberries, blackcurrants, redcurrants, and Concord groups.

These are made up from fresh fruits and vegetables and are constituted by the same process which maintains their micronutrients and a very high level of effective antioxidants. If two capsules are taken three times a day with eight ounces (approximately 250 ml), then perhaps all the nutritional protection that the body needs is supplied. Some patients complain that it seems to produce a great deal of gas, but this can usually be controlled very successfully by Beano.

Richard Boronow, MD, in a personal communication, provided an easy method to explain a free radical and a suggestion of how to manage them.

$$H_2O - water (H^+ H^+ O^{--})$$
$$\overset{.}{O}H - hydroxyl\ radical$$

A perfect control would be oxidation as controlled by the antioxidant system. Oxidative byproducts of normal metabolism cause extensive damage to DNA, protein and lipids. This damage is the same as that produced by radiation, and is a major contributor to aging and degenerative diseases of aging such as cancer, cardiovascular disease, immune system decline, brain dysfunction, and cataracts.

NSA (National Safety Associates) is a company that conceived of the idea, resulting in a balanced food supplement called Juice Plus +. They do not advertise and we have no interests to disclose in the product, but the product thus far has been subjected to the most intensive research of any vitamin or food supplement. The food supplement or more information can be obtained by calling the toll-free number +1-866-862-5448.

Sugar and water are removed by a standard method and then by mashing the fresh fruits and vegetables, desiccation under low temperature produces a powder that is put in the capsules. The product is carefully scanned for pesticides and other contaminants. The test subjects showed significant increases in blood plasma levels of antioxidants after only 28 days on Juice Plus +. This is a whole food product that does not take the place of fresh fruits and fresh vegetables. As more and more preventative and protective agents are explored in the field of metabolism, this method will receive a great deal of attention.

## SUMMARY

Aging is a process that is continuous from conception to death. Aged is a term used to identify persons generally according to some established arbitrary chronological decision. In this conceptual system of the unitary man, aging is a developmental process. Moreover, aging is a continuously creative process directed towards a growing diversity of field pattern and organization. It is not a running down. The aged need less sleep and the pattern frequency of sleep/wakefulness is more diverse. Aging is not a disease. New lifestyles are being promulgated by the postmenopausal patient. It is obvious that the postmenopausal patients represent a significant part of the population and that they add stability through their maturity and wisdom.

The word menopause means a final cessation of menstruation. This gives the grossly erroneous idea that yesterday all was well, tomorrow has changed; it also implies that a hysterectomy causes the menopause. Menopause occurs if the ovaries are removed or cease to function. Climacteric, meaning the period of change, is a better word because it expresses the all-important concept of a time-scale, but is not in common use.

The quality of life for the postmenopausal woman can be significantly improved by active investigation and treatment of gynecological disorders, such as postmenopausal osteoporosis, and consideration of the best method of administering hormones and rehabilitation plans when illness strikes. Whereas patients were once considered elderly at age 60 years, this has now been advanced to a retirement age of 70 years. Many women in their 80s are living a very active lifestyle. With the improvements in technology, food, rest, leisure time, and a variety of methods of physiotherapy, patients are staying younger much longer than previously. Surgical intervention should never be excluded simply on the basis of chronological age.

Sexuality in postmenopausal life is a healthy sign and free discussion should be had with the patient so that she understands that it is all part of her life. The Victorian age is over. Many menopausal and postmenopausal patients have adopted a new lifestyle which parallels the freedom of younger patients.

Most women want and are able to lead an active, satisfying sex life. With age, women do not ordinarily lose their physical capacity for orgasm, nor men their capacity for erection and ejaculation. There is, however, a gradual slowing of response, especially in men, which is a process currently considered a part of normal aging, but perhaps eventually treatable or even reversible. In the postmenopausal patient, sex often improves because of several factors. One is that her husband has reached a stable level in business and the children have grown up, so a couple have more time together. In addition, ovarian androgen secretion increases for a period of time after the menopause. In patients who have been studied, it has been found that a relatively higher testosterone/estrogen ratio in women after the ovaries have undergone follicular depletion may contribute to increased libido and fantasy.

The incidence of illness and disability increases with age. Although they can affect sexuality in later life, even the most serious diseases rarely warrant stopping sexual activity. Public acceptance of sexuality in later life is gradually increasing. Physicians can expect that the day will come when special aspects of sexuality in the postmenopausal patient are generally understood, and when diagnosis and treatment of sexual problems is refined to a greater degree. It is obvious that the postmenopausal patient has developed a new lifestyle that is much more liberal than previously.

Osteoporosis is not a disease per se, but rather is the end result of severe or prolonged bone loss. Osteoporosis cannot be cured, but it can be prevented. Recently, alendronate has been approved by the Food and Drug Administration (FDA), and can restore bone loss, but must be continued otherwise the bone mass will decrease. Estrogen replacement therapy is a vital factor in osteoporosis therapy, as well as an important factor in treating other symptoms of the menopause. Articles have finally appeared which indicate that estrogen therapy does not cause breast cancer. One risk factor relates to stimulating the development of endometrial carcinoma, but with the addition of progesterone this risk is negated. Furthermore, with progesterone therapy, the endometrium is protected against development of a malignant process. It is the height of professional responsibility to provide estrogen when it is needed, and to withhold it when it is contraindicated or not needed.

The problem of the menopause and the management of gynecological problems during this period has taken on added significance in the past three decades. Women are living longer and can anticipate spending approximately one-third of their lives in the postmenopausal period. It is important, therefore, for physicians to be prepared to handle the problems that arise during this time.

# REFERENCES

1.  Kinsey AC et al. Sexual Behavior in the Human Female. Philadelphia: W.B. Saunders; Bloomington, IN: Indiana University Press, 1953/1998.
2.  Anderson GL et al. Effects of conjugated equine estrogen in postmenopausal women with hysterectomy: the Women's Health Initiative randomized controlled trial. JAMA. 2004 Apr 14; 291(14): 1701–12.
3.  Kolodny R, Johnson VE, Masters WH. Masters and Johnson on Sex and Human Loving.
4.  Martino M, Eskin BA. Estrogen and the postmenopausal heart. Female Patient 1999; 24: 19–28.
5.  Martino MA, Borges E, Williamson E et al. Pulmonary embolism after major abdominal surgery in gynecologic oncology. Obstet Gynecol 2006; 107: 666–71.

# FURTHER READING

Andrews W. What's new in preventing and treating osteoporosis? Postgrad Med 1998; 104: 89.

Avioli L, ed. The Osteoporosis Syndrome. New York: Grune and Straton, 1983.

Barber HRK. Ovarian Carcinoma. Etiology, Diagnosis and Treatment. New York: Masson Publishing, 1981.

Barber HRK, Sommers SC, eds. Carcinoma of the endometrium. Etiology.

Diagnosis and Treatment. New York: Masson Publishing, 1981.

Block G, Patterson B, Subar A. Fruit, vegetables and cancer prevention: a review of the epidemiologic evidence. Nutr Cancer 1992; 18: 1–29.

Brown ADG. Postmenopausal urinary problems. Clin Obstet Gynecol 1977; 4: 181.

American Cancer Society. Cancer Facts and Figures – 1999. Washington DC: American Cancer Society.

Coutifaris B, Chryssicopoulos A, Botsis D. Primary carcinoma of the fallopian tube. Int Surg 1980; 65: 83.

DeLancey JO. Anatomy and biomechanics of genital prolapse. Clin Obstet Gynecol 1993; 36: 897.

de Ple S, West CE, Muhilal et al. Lancet 1995; 346: 75–81.

Frederick EJ Jr. Vulvar Disease. Philadelphia: WB Saunders, 1976.

Giovannucci E, Ascherio A, Rimm EB, Stampfer MJ, Colditz GA, Willett WC. Intake of carotenoids and retinol in relation to risk of prostate cancer. J Nat Cancer Inst 1995; 87: 1767–76.

Gruis MG, Wagner NN. Sexuality during the climacteric. Postgrad Med 1979; 65: 197.

Hennekens CH, Buring JE, Manson JE et al. Lack of effect of long-term supplementation with beta carotene on the incident of malignant and cardiovascular disease. N Engl J Med 1996; 334: 1145–9.

Heung AW, Comstock GW, Abbey H, Polk F. Retinol, carotenoids and toccophenol and risk of prostate cancer. J Natl Cancer Inst 1990; 82: 941–6.

Ho CT, Rosen RT, eds. Food phytochemicals for cancer prevention in fruits and vegetables. Washington, DC: American Chemical Society, 1994: 258–71.

Hoffman RH, Gardner HL. Vulvar dystrophies. Clin Obstet Gynecol 1978; 21: 1801.

Huffman JW. Gynecologic disorders in the geriatric patient. Geriatr Gynecol Postgrad Med 1982; 71: 38.

Huffman JW. The diagnosis and treatment of gynecologic disorders in elderly patients. Compr Ther 1983; 9: 54.

Jordan HL. Hormonal dynamics associated with the menopause. Clin Obstet Gynecol 1976; 19: 775.

Kaplan HS. The Illustrated Manual of Sex Therapy. New York: Quadrangle/New York Times, 1975.

Macozzi MS, Brown ED, Edwards BK. Plasma carotenoid response to chronic intake of selected foods and beta carotene supplements in men. Am J Clin Nutr 1992: 55: 1120–5.

Marshall VF, Marchetti KE. The correction of stress incontinence by simple vesicourethral suspension. Surg Gynecol Obstet 1949; 88: 509.

Masters WH. The sexual response cycle of the human female: vaginal lubrication. Ann NY Acad Sci 1959; 83: 301.

McKeithen WS. Major gynecologic surgery in the elderly female. Am J Obstet Gynecol 1975; 59: 63.

Munoz KA, Krebs-Smith SM, Ballard-Barbash R, Cleveland LE. Food intake of US children and adolescents compared with recommendations. Pediatrics 1997; 100: 323–9.

Plotnick GD, Corretti MC, Vogel RA, Hesslink R Jr, Wise JA. Effect of supplemental phytonutrients on impairment of the flour-mediated brachial artery vasoactivity after a single high-fat meal. Am Coll of Cardiology 2003; 41: 1743.

Reid RL. Effects of the menstrual cycle on medical disorders. Arch Intern Med 1998; 158: 1405–12.

Romoff A (with Yalof I). Estrogen, How and Why It Can Save Your life. New York: Golden Books, 1999.

Sagar PM, Pemberton JH. Dysfunction of the posterior pelvic floor and disorders of defecation. J Pelvic Surg 1993; 1: 92.

Te Linde RW. Prolapse of the uterus and allied conditions. Am J Obstet Gynecol 1966; 94: 444.

Wall LL. The muscles of the pelvic floor. Clin Obstet Gynecol 1993; 36: 910.

Yanik R, Ries LD, Yates JW. Ovarian cancer in the elderly: an analysis of surveillance, epidemiology and end results program data. Am J Obstet Gynecol 1980; 154: 639–47.

# Chapter 14

# Osteoporosis

Brian M Berger

## INTRODUCTION

Osteoporosis is a skeletal disorder characterized by low bone mass and an increased susceptibility to fracture. The past two decades have seen an increase in our understanding of the epidemiology of fractures at the three most frequent sites (the hip, wrist, and vertebral body). These new insights have led to the delineation of preventive strategies against these fractures for both the general population and those individuals at highest risk. A new definition of osteoporosis moves this disorder from a disease of fractures to a disease of fracture risks. The goal of osteoporosis therapy is to prevent the morbidity and mortality that arise from the disease. This can be best accomplished by vigorous screening programs and public awareness of the magnitude of the disease.

## PREVALENCE

The incidence of osteoporosis varies from country to country and among different races. In many countries, hip fractures occupy 20% of hospital beds. In England and Wales, the cost of osteoporosis has been estimated at £500 million every year.[1] Osteoporosis affects an enormous number of people, and its prevalence will increase as the population ages. It is estimated that between 13% and 18% of postmenopausal white women in the US (4–6 million) have osteoporosis, and an additional 30–50% (13–17 million) have low bone density at the hip. Health care expenditures attributable to osteoporotic fractures in 1995 were estimated at $US13.8 billion, of which $US10.3 billion (75.1%) was for the treatment of white women, $US2.5 billion (18.4%) for white men, $US0.7 billion (5.3%)

for non-white women and $US0.2 billion (1.3%) for non-white men.[2]

The most common fractures are those of the proximal femur (hip), vertebrae (spine), and distal forearm (wrist), but because osteoporosis is a systemic disease causing bone loss throughout the skeleton, almost all fractures in older adults are due in part to low bone density. Unfortunately, this is a silent epidemic which may present with pain or fractures, or cause damage in an insidious manner until the presentation is far more severe.

Hip fracture can result in up to 10–25% mortality within one year. Additionally, up to 25% of hip fracture patients may require long-term nursing-home care, and only one-third fully regain their prefracture level of independence. One year after hip fracture, 40% of patients are still unable to walk independently, 60% have difficulty with at least one essential activity of daily living, and 80% are restricted in other activities, such as driving and grocery shopping. Moreover, 27% of these patients enter a nursing home for the first time.[3] After adjusting for other factors associated with mortality, women with fractures of the hip or pelvis have a 2.4-fold increase in mortality. Although some of these deaths are undoubtedly the result of chronic conditions that contribute to the hip or pelvic fracture, up to 20% are directly due to the fracture itself.[4]

Vertebral fractures also cause significant complications including back pain, height loss and kyphosis. Morbidity and mortality arising from vertebral fracture are less secure than those of the hip and radius.[5] Reasons relate to the uncertain definition of vertebral fracture and its variable clinical expression, and hence its incidence is not known.[3] Using radiological criteria, 50% or more of vertebral fractures may be asymptomatic.

Although the true incidence of vertebral fracture is unknown, there is evidence that it increases exponentially with age in much the same way as for hip fracture. Between the ages of 60 and 90 years, the apparent incidence rises approximately 20-fold in women, compared to a 50-fold increase in risk of hip fracture.[6] Postural and height changes associated with kyphosis may limit activity, including bending and reaching, and their cosmetic effects may erode self-esteem, although there does not appear to be any correlation between kyphosis and back pain.[7] Multiple thoracic fractures may result in restrictive lung disease, and lumbar fractures may alter abdominal anatomy, leading to constipation, abdominal pain, distention, reduced appetite, and premature satiety.

## THE PHYSIOLOGY OF BONE

Bone undergoes perpetual remodeling of units aptly named bone remodeling units. These units are continuously changing throughout life, in a balance between bone resorption and formation. The two bone types involved in bone remodeling are cortical and trabecular bone. Cortical bone constitutes 80% of total bone, while trabecular bone makes up the remainder. Trabecular bone is the predominant bone type in the spinal column, and is less dense, consisting of a honeycomb structure of marrow and fat. Age-related trabecular bone loss is characterized not simply by a global loss of bone, but also by cortical porosity and loss of trabecular connections.

The two main cell types involved are the osteoblasts and osteoclasts, with osteocytes and lining cells performing a supportive role. Osteoblasts are prominent in bone surfaces when bone growth or remodeling is taking place. They secrete collagen to form a non-mineralized matrix which consists of a seam or border of osteoid. The osteoid matures over a period of 1–2 weeks, and lays down a matrix of hydroxyapatite. Among the proteins involved in this process are osteocalcin and alkaline phosphatase, which serve as markers of bone formation (Table 14.2).

Osteoclasts are multinucleated giant cells found at the surface of cells undergoing bone resorption. They form pits or lacunae known as the lacunae of Howship. Osteoclasts are responsive to parathyroid hormone (PTH), and are inhibited by calci-

tonin. They contain lysosomal enzymes which resorb collagen, and markers of collagen resorption such as urinary hydroxyproline and pyridinoline cross-links are used to measure osteoclastic activity.

Parathyroid hormone plays a vital role in the homeostasis of calcium within the bloodstream. A decrease in calcium causes an increase in PTH secretion by the parathyroid glands. This stimulates the production of 1,25–vitamin D in the kidneys which, in turn, increases the calcium absorption from the intestines. Parathyroid hormone-related protein (PTHrP), a genetically and structurally distinct hormone which displays similar binding and activation profiles to PTH, has greatly facilitated the effort to establish a structure–biological function relationship by allowing for direct comparisons.[8]

Extracellular or plasma calcium ion concentration is held constant at 5 mg/dl through the combined actions of PTH, vitamin D and calcitonin on their target organs, kidney, and bone. The thresholds of renal tubular calcium reabsorption and bone resorption and formation are both set at 5 mg/dl. The set point of PTH secretion is also fixed at 5 mg/dl plasma calcium ion. Therefore, the sensing system (parathyroid cell) and the effectors, kidney and bone, are all set to maintain plasma calcium at 5 mg/dl, perhaps through membrane-bound calcium sensor proteins. The effectiveness of this system depends upon the presence of bone remodeling, which allows a swift shift of plasma calcium from and to bone in response to PTH and calcitonin, respectively. In this regard, directing hematopoiesis to bone marrow that provides bone resorbing osteoclasts is critical. It is likely that this shift of hematopoiesis occurred through evolution at the transition from aquatic to terrestrial life, and this event is directed by expression of homing molecule in bone marrow stromal cells.

The recent cloning of receptors for calcitonin and PTH/PTHrP has enabled very rapid progress in understanding the molecular and cell biology of these receptors. In particular, much has been learned about the tissue distribution of these receptors, as well as their mode of interaction with ligands, signal transduction and regulation of expression.[9] A second calcium-regulating hormone (calcitonin) is released by hypercalcemia, and lowers plasma calcium by inhibiting osteolysis. Specifically, it lowers serum calcium by decreasing bone resorption and tubular calcium reabsorption. It is a straight-chain peptide with

32 amino acids and a seven-membered disulfide ring at the N-terminal. It is produced by C cells which arise from the neural crest, and is considered a neuropeptide hormone. It is produced in the thyroid of mammals and the ultimobranchial glands of lower vertebrates.[10] An analgesic action, possibly mediated via beta-endorphins, is also evident. Parenteral calcitonin has been shown to stabilize and increase indices of cortical and trabecular bone mass and total body calcium, when administered to patients with established osteoporosis. The routine use of this route of administration has been limited by poor patient compliance and tolerability. An intranasal preparation of calcitonin has provided a more convenient means of administration.[11] The form most widely used in therapy is salmon calcitonin because of its tremendous potency, compared to human calcitonin.[12]

## RISK FACTORS

Vertebral bone strength is determined by several factors: cortical thickness, bone size, trabecular bone density, and microarchitecture. All these factors change with age as a result of the two dynamic processes: remodeling and modeling. When the changes become pronounced, osteoporotic fractures occur.

Aspects of bone quality to be considered are bone architecture, matrix, mineralization and fatigue damage. The trabecular network becomes progressively disconnected and weaker with age. Death of old osteocytes leads to hypermineralization and brittleness of bone. The stability of bone collagen declines with age, and unremodeled bone accumulates fatigue damage. The lower bone fragility rates in males than in females may be due to a combination of the larger male skeleton, greater cortical bone density after age 60 years, and greater bone turnover which would replace fatigue-damaged bone.

### Endowment of skeletal mass

The amount of skeletal mass acquired during adolescence is one of the most important determinants for the risk of postmenopausal and involutional osteoporosis In both sexes, a large variance in bone mineral density (BMD) and content (BMC) is observed among healthy individuals at the beginning of the third decade. In females,

bone mass accumulation occurs predominantly from age 11 to 14 years, and is drastically reduced by 16 years of age in both the lumbar spine and femoral neck.[13,14] A sharp reduction occurs between the second and fourth years after menarche.[15] Although more than 60% of peak bone mineral mass is gained during puberty (mostly at the expense of an increase in bone size while volumetric bone density slightly changes), familial resemblance for most bone traits is already present between daughters and their mothers before puberty.[16] These results indicate that genetic susceptibility to osteoporosis may already be detectable in early childhood. Up to 5% of trabecular bone and 1.5% of total bone will be lost per year after the menopause.

Physical activity has been related to enhanced bone mass and improved physical functioning and, thus, may reduce the risk for osteoporotic fracture. In one study, higher levels of leisure time, sport activity and household chores, and fewer hours of sitting daily were associated with a significantly reduced relative risk for hip fracture, but not wrist or vertebral fracture after adjustment for age, dietary factors, falls at baseline, and functional and health status.[17] Very active women (fourth and fifth quintiles) had a statistically significant 36% reduction in hip fractures (relative risk, 0.64; 95% confidence interval (CI), 0.45–0.891), compared with the least active women (lowest quintile).[17] Other studies have arrived at similar conclusions.[8,19]

### Low serum hormone levels

Women with undetectable serum estradiol concentrations (<5 pg/ml) have a relative risk of 2.5 for subsequent hip fracture and subsequent vertebral fracture, compared to women with detectable serum estradiol concentrations.[20] Women with both undetectable serum estradiol concentrations and serum sex hormone-binding globulin concentrations of 1 µg/dl or more have a relative risk of 6.9 for hip fracture and 7.9 for vertebral fracture.[20]

### Glucocorticoid use

Glucocorticoids cause bone loss by altering the bone remodeling sequence: bone resorption by osteoclasts is increased, and bone formation by osteoblasts is decreased. Serum levels of osteocalcin are decreased with glucocorticoid therapy, further evidence of decreased osteoblast function.

Glucocorticoids decrease calcium absorption by the gastrointestinal tract, and increase renal calcium excretion. Several recent studies suggest that low-dose glucocorticoid therapy is not associated with bone loss.[21,22]

## Thyroid function

Hyperthyroidism and use of thyroid hormone to suppress thyroid-stimulating hormone (TSH) because of thyroid cancer, goiters, or nodules seem to have an adverse effect on bone, especially in postmenopausal women; the largest effect is on cortical bone.[23] Although some studies have found that thyroid hormone replacement seems to have a minimal negative clinical effect on bone,[24] there is no consistent evidence that low TSH, a sensitive biochemical marker of excess thyroid hormone, is associated with low BMD or accelerated bone loss in older ambulatory women.[25]

## Smoking

The use of tobacco products is detrimental to the skeleton as well as to overall health. The Framingham Study found that current estrogen use appeared to be protective against bone fractures (adjusted odds ratio, AOR, 0.38; 95% CI, 0.12–1.21; $P = 0.10$).[26] Among current smokers, however, estrogen use did not protect against fracture (AOR for current use, 1.26; 95% CI, 0.29–5.45), whereas estrogen was protective in non-smokers (AOR for current or past use, 0.37; 95% CI, 0.19–0.75; $P = 0.005$). Therefore, smoking may negate the protective skeletal effects of estrogen replacement therapy.[26] Smokers are at increased risk of hip fracture, and their risk rises with greater cigarette consumption. Risk declines among former smokers, but the benefit is not observed until 10 years after cessation.[27]

## MONITORING BONE STATUS

### Measuring bone density

Bone mineral density (BMD) measurement (Table 14.1) can be used to establish or confirm a diagnosis of osteoporosis, predict future fracture risk, and monitor changes in BMD due to medical conditions or therapy. BMD has a continuous, graded, inverse relationship to the risk of fracture: the lower the BMD, the greater the risk.

**Table 14.1** Radiological measurement of bone mineral density (BMD)

| Type | Bone type assessed |
| --- | --- |
| Dual energy X-ray absorptiometry (DEXA) | Trabecular, cortical, whole body |
| Single-energy X-ray absorptiometry (SXA) | Cortical |
| Radiographic absorptiometry (RA) | Trabecular |
| Quantitative computed tomography (QCT) | Trabecular, cortical |
| Ultrasound densitometry | Cortical? |

Measurements of BMD at any skeletal site have value in predicting fracture risk. There is a variety of densitometers in clinical use that provide reliable assessment of fracture risk. BMD is expressed as a relationship to two norms: the expected BMD for the patient's age and sex (Z-score), or for young normal adults of the same sex (T-score). The difference between the patient's score and the norm is expressed as a standard deviation (SD) above or below the mean.

### Dual-energy X-ray absorptiometry

Dual-energy X-ray absorptiometry (DEXA) is the best method of measuring bone density and, thus, the best available indicator of osteoporotic fracture risk. DEXA can be used to measure bone mineral density in the spine, hip or wrist – the most common sites for osteoporotic fractures. Radiation hazard is small with patient-effective doses of the order of a few microsieverts.[28] In vivo measurement precision of the order of 1% is achievable for posteroanterior (PA) scans of the lumbar spine. Lateral scans can achieve measurement precision of the order of 4%.[29] Recent technological developments using X-ray fan beams and multi-element detector arrays on C-arm devices have resulted in faster scan times, higher resolution images, and an ability to perform PA and lateral scanning without the need to reposition the patient. Accuracy of DEXA is dependent upon specific instrumentation and data reduction algorithms, but results generally correlate well with ashed bone measurements.[30]

While total-body scans may be precise and offer the advantage of total-body composition determination, BMD values derived from total-body scans cannot currently replace direct measurements.

Site-specific measurements are required to assess regional osteopenia. Bone mineral density should be measured only to assist in making a clinical management choice. Measurement of the lumbar spine and femoral neck is standard, but a different site or a single measurement is recommended in specific cases. Unless accelerated bone loss is suspected, DEXA should be repeated every 2–4 years for patients receiving ovarian hormone therapy, and 1–2 years for patients undergoing biphosphonate therapy. Measurements and reporting of results must provide actual measurement and its relation to peak bone mass.

## Single-energy X-ray absorptiometry

These techniques measure bone density in the forearm, finger and sometimes the heel. Single-energy X-ray absorptiometry (SXA) is a device which incorporates an X-ray tube as a photon source. SXA delivers a radiation exposure of 1.68 mrem, with image quality and spatial resolution comparable to DEXA.[31,32]

## Radiographic absorptiometry

Radiographic absorptiometry (RA) is a technique that is based on a standard radiograph or computer-generated radiograph of the hand with a metal wedge in the same field. RA is used for bone mass measurement from radiographs of peripheral sites, most commonly the hand or heel. Recently developed new computer-assisted methods have improved RA precision, thus providing a simple and inexpensive technique for screening of bone mineral status of large populations.[33]

## Quantitative computed tomography

Quantitative computed tomography (QCT) measures trabecular and cortical bone density at several sites in the body, but is most commonly used to measure trabecular bone density in the spine. It may be used as an alternative to DEXA for vertebral measurements.[34]

## Ultrasound densitometry

Ultrasound assesses bone in the heel, tibia, patella or other peripheral sites where the bones are relatively superficial. Changes in the calcaneal ultrasound parameters in response to treatment of osteoporosis are not a reflection of mineral changes occurring in the lumbar spine and femoral neck in a given individual, and, in this regard, calcaneal ultrasonometry is not a substitute for direct-site DEXA measurement of the lumbar spine and femur, but may be useful in a clinical setting when DEXA access is poor.[35]

## Serum and urinary measurements of bone turnover

The non-invasive assessment of bone turnover (Table 14.2) has received increasing attention over the past few years because of the need for sensitive markers in the clinical investigation of osteoporosis. Markers of bone formation include serum total and bone-specific alkaline phosphatase, serum osteocalcin and serum type I collagen extension peptides. Assessment of bone resorption can be achieved with measurement of urinary hydroxyproline, urinary excretion of the pyridinium cross-links (Pyr and D-Pyr) and plasma tartarate resistant acid phosphatase (TRAP) activity.[36] The immunoassay of human osteocalcin recognizing the intact molecule and its major proteolytic fragment, and that of bone alkaline phosphatase, are currently the most sensitive markers to assess bone formation.[37] For bone resorption, the total urinary excretion of pyridinoline cross-links measured by high pressure liquid chromatography has shown its superiority over all other markers for the clinical assessment of osteoporosis.[38] The recent development of immunoassays recognizing either the free pyridinoline cross-links or pyridinoline crosslinked type I collagen peptides in urine and serum should allow a broad use of this sensitive resorption marker. Programs combining bone mass measurement and assessment of bone turnover in women at the time of the menopause have been developed in an attempt to improve the assessment of the risk for osteoporosis.[39]

## TREATMENT (TABLE 14.3)

### Calcium

A lifelong intake of adequate calcium is necessary for the acquisition of peak bone mass and maintenance of bone health. The skeleton contains 99% of the body's calcium stores; when the exogenous supply is inadequate, calcium is extracted from the skeleton to maintain serum calcium at a constant level.

**Table 14.2** Biochemical measurement of bone mineral turnover

| Marker | Source | Marker Type |
|---|---|---|
| Bone-specific alkaline phosphatase | Serum | Formation |
| Osteocalcin | Serum | Formation |
| Type I collagen extension peptides | Serum | Formation |
| Hydroxyproline | Urine | Formation |
| Pyridinium cross-links (Pyr and D-Pyr) | Urine | Resorption |
| Deoxypyridinoline | Urine | Resorption |
| Pyridinoline | Urine | Resorption |

**Table 14.3** Treatments used for prevention of bone loss

- Estrogens
- Alendronate
- Calcitonin
- Raloxifene
- Zoledronic acid
- Tibolone
- Calcium
- Vitamin D
- Exercise
- Parathyroid hormone (teriparatide)

The recent cloning of an extracellular calcium ($Ca^{2+}$)-sensing receptor (CaR) from the parathyroid gland and the kidney has provided novel insights into the mechanisms that underlie the direct actions of $Ca^{2+}$ on various cells. The receptor is a member of the superfamily of G protein-coupled receptors, activating phospholipase C (PLC), and probably also inhibiting adenylate cyclase in target tissues. In the parathyroid gland it is a key mediator of the inhibition by high $Ca^{2+}$ of PTH secretion and, perhaps, *PTH* gene expression and parathyroid cellular proliferation. It also appears to represent the major mechanism through which $Ca^{2+}$ stimulates the secretion of calcitonin from the thyroidal C cells. In the kidney, the CaR directly inhibits tubular reabsorption of calcium and magnesium in the thick ascending limb, and may be responsible for the long-recognized, but poorly understood, inhibition of urinary-concentrating ability by hypercalcemia.[9]

Controlled clinical trials have demonstrated that the combination of supplemental calcium and vitamin D reduces the risk of fracture of the spine, hip and other sites. This positive effect on BMD has been demonstrated, even in a group of women of early postmenopausal age, with a fairly good initial calcium and vitamin D status.[40]

After peak bone mass in women is attained, the benefits of increased dietary calcium or supplemental calcium are uncertain. Some investigators have found that premenopausal women in the fifth decade lose about 1% of spinal trabecular mineral yearly, in spite of a normal serum estradiol level and ample calcium intake.[41] However, calcium supplementation in postmenopausal or oophorectomized women who had been undergoing unopposed estrogen therapy for at least 2 years, and whose serum calcium level was suppressed to below the normal range, potentiated the effect of estrogen.[42]

Long-term administration of calcium supplements to elderly women may partially reverse age-related increases in serum PTH level and bone resorption and decrease bone loss. However, the effects on bone loss are weaker than those reported for estrogen, biphosphonates, or calcitonin therapy, indicating that calcium supplements alone cannot substitute for these in treating established osteoporosis.[43]

Nonetheless, because of their safety, high tolerance and low expense, increasing daily calcium is a cost-effective way to help reduce fracture risk.

### Vitamin D

Vitamin D plays a major role in calcium absorption and bone health. Chief dietary sources of vitamin D include vitamin D-fortified milk (400 IU per litre) and cereals (50 IU per serving), egg yolks, salt-water fish and liver. Some calcium supplements and most multivitamin tablets also contain vitamin D. Low-dose vitamin D supplementation has been shown to have only a minor effect in the prevention of osteoporosis in non-osteoporotic, early postmenopausal women, and does not give any benefit additional to that of hormone replacement therapy (HRT) alone.[44] Supplementation with 400 IU vitamin $D_3$ daily in elderly women has been found to decrease PTH secretion slightly and increase bone mineral density at the femoral neck, but no changes in the biochemical markers of bone turnover were seen.[45] An intake of 400–800 IU of vitamin D per day is recommended for those at risk of deficiency, such as elderly, chronically ill, housebound, or institutionalized individuals.[46]

## EXERCISE

In postmenopausal women with low bone density, bone loss can be slowed or prevented by exercise plus calcium supplementation or estrogen–progesterone replacement (Table 14.3). Some studies have found that exercise plus estrogen is more effective than estrogen alone.[47] The amount and type of exercise needed to prevent bone loss is largely unknown. One study found that short-term (7 months') exercise with intensity above the anaerobic threshold is safe and effective in preventing postmenopausal bone loss.[48] A recent meta-analysis of studies on bone loss and the effects of exercise found that the exercise-training programs prevented or reversed almost 1% of bone loss per year in both the lumbar spine and femoral neck for both pre- and postmenopausal women.[49] Another meta-analysis showed a significant effect of physical activity on the bone mineral density at the L2–4 level of the lumbar column in studies published after 1991 (effect sizes (ES) = 0.8745, $P < 0.05$). No effect could be seen, however, on forearm and femoral bone mass.[50] These meta-analyses suggest that exercise programs in a population of postmenopausal women over 50 years of age are effective for preventing spinal bone mineral density loss at the L2–4 level. Further studies are needed to evaluate the effects on the forearm and femoral bone/hip.

### Hormone replacement therapy

Estrogen with or without progesterone replacement therapy is the most studied and proven therapy for the prevention of bone loss in estrogen-deficient women. The results of the Postmenopausal Estrogen/Progestin Intervention (PEPI) trial showed significant differences in patients on active treatment, and are worth reviewing.[51] Treatments were: placebo; conjugated equine estrogens (CEEs), 0.625 mg/day; CEEs, 0.625 mg/day plus medroxyprogesterone acetate (MPA), 10 mg/day for 12 days per month; CEEs, 0.625 mg/day plus MPA, 2.5 mg/day daily; or

CEEs, 0.625 mg/day plus micronized progesterone 200 mg/day for 12 days per month. Over a time course of 36 months, participants assigned to the placebo group lost an average of 1.8% of spine BMD, and 1.7% of hip BMD by the 36-month visit, while those assigned to active regimens gained BMD at both sites, ranging from 3.5% to 5.0% mean total increases in spinal BMD and a mean total increase of 1.7% of BMD in the hip. Women assigned to CEEs plus continuous MPA had significantly greater increases in spinal BMD (increase of 5%) than those assigned to the other three active regimens (average increase, 3.8%). Findings were similar among those adhering to assigned therapy, although, among adherent participants, there were no significant differences in BMD changes among the four active treatment groups.[51] Many other studies have confirmed these results.

In another multicenter study on 9704 ambulatory non-black women 65 years of age or older, current estrogen use was associated with a decrease in the risk for wrist fractures (relative risk, RR 0.39; 95% CI, 0.24–0.64) and for all nonspinal fractures (RR, 0.66; 95% CI, 0.54–0.80), when compared with no estrogen use.[52] Results in this study were similar for women using unopposed estrogen or estrogen plus progestin.[52] The potential benefits may be influenced by genotypes of the vitamin D receptor and estrogen receptor. In a study examining BMD, differential gains in women of varying receptor status, vitamin D receptor and estrogen receptor loci varied from approximately 1.0% (for the total body BMC changes in combined placebo and HRT groups) to approximately 18.7% (for the spine BMD changes in the HRT group).[53] These results suggest that individual genotypes are important factors in determining changes in bone mass in the elderly with and without HRT, and thus may need to be considered with respect to the treatment to preserve bone mass in elderly Caucasian women.

Another study examined the effect of various doses on BMD, and found that esterified estrogens at doses from 0.3 to 1.25 mg/day, administered unopposed by progestin, produce a continuum of positive changes on bone and lipids.[54] Plasma estradiol concentrations increased with esterified estrogens dose and were related to positive bone mineral densities. The 0.3 mg dose resulted in positive bone and lipid changes without inducing endometrial hyperplasia.[54] These benefits appear to be evident in women receiving transdermal estrogen replacement as well.[55]

An intriguing study of 65 pairs of twins who were discordant for HRT use showed that among current users of estrogen, BMD was consistently and significantly higher than in non-users at both the lumbar spine and femoral neck.[56] Past users of HRT did not, however, show the same benefits. The clinical implications of these findings are that HRT needs to be used continuously to influence BMD, and that alternative treatments need to be considered in those who discontinue HRT.

## Alendronate

Alendronate is a member of the biphosphonate group of drugs along with etidronate, clodronate, pamidronate, tiludronate and residronate. The biphosphonates bind to bone mineral where they inhibit bone resorption. Well-conducted controlled clinical trials utilizing alendronate sodium indicate that treatment reduces the incidence of fracture at the spine, hip and wrist in patients with osteoporosis. In a large study of 447 women who had recently experienced the menopause, alendronate at 5, 10 and 20 mg/day increased BMD from baseline at the lumbar spine, femoral neck and trochanter by 1–4% and in the total body by 0.3–1.0%.[57] In a study undertaken to determine the response to alendronate therapy in women with postmenopausal osteoporosis who were non-responders to intermittent cyclical etidronate therapy, 25 women with postmenopausal osteoporosis (mean ± SD, 65.1 ± 1.9 years of age), previously treated with intermittent cyclical etidronate with no increase of spine BMD, were then changed to alendronate 10 mg/day, which they received for 1.3 ± 0.1 years.[58] After treatment with alendronate, BMD increased significantly at the lumbar spine (4.4 ± 0.7% annualized, $P < 0.0001$) and at all hip sites. Bone markers also changed significantly after alendronate treatment: urine deoxypyridinoline fell from 6.8 ± 0.8 to 5.5 ± 0.6 µmol/mol creatinine ($P < 0.0001$) and serum bone-specific alkaline phosphatase rose from 4.6 ± 0.5 to 11.9 ± 1.0 ng/ml ($P < 0.0001$). This study suggests that alendronate causes more complete suppression of bone resorption and less inhibition (or stimulation) of bone formation.

In a three-year study of alendronate therapy at three different dosages, BMD continued to increase over the entire three-year study duration in the alendronate-treated groups and, compared with the other dosage groups (5 mg and 20 mg), 10 mg alendronate produced the largest gains in BMD during the third year.[59]

A more recent study looking at a 10-year experience with alendronate in 994 postmenopausal women treated with 10 mg of alendronate daily showed mean increases in bone mineral density of 13.7% at the lumbar spine (95% CI, 12.0–15.5%), 10.3% at the trochanter (95% CI, 8.1 to 12.4 percent), 5.4% at the femoral neck (95% CI, 3.5–7.4%), and 6.7% at the total proximal femur (95% CI, 4.4–9.1%) as compared with baseline values; smaller gains occurred in the group given 5 mg daily.[60]

Alendronate therapy is associated with gastrointestinal side-effects. It must therefore be taken on an empty stomach, first thing in the morning, with a large glass of water, at least 30 min before eating or drinking. Patients should remain upright during this interval. The 5 mg dose has been approved by the Food and Drug Administration (FDA) for prevention of osteoporosis, and the 10 mg dose has been approved for treatment. A rare reported complication of alendronate (probably <1%) is esophageal ulceration.

## Calcitonin

Salmon calcitonin, a hormone that inhibits bone resorption, is FDA approved for the treatment of osteoporosis. It is delivered as a single daily intranasal spray that provides 200 IU of the drug.

Epidemiological, retrospective and prospective studies provide a convergent network of evidence that calcitonin administration in osteoporosis contributes to reduce significantly the frequency of subsequent fractures, both in the spine, and in the hip. In a randomized controlled study, the rate of patients with new fractures was reduced significantly in the women treated with salcatonin, to about one-third of that in the non-calcitonin-treated women (RR, 0.23; 95% CI, 0.07–0.77).[61] Nasal calcitonin also possesses a potent analgesic effect, and decreases the number of concomitant analgesic medications.[62]

## Raloxifene

Raloxifene hydrochloride is a selective estrogen receptor modulator (SERM) with estrogen agonist effects on bone and lipid metabolism, and estrogen antagonist effects on reproductive tissues, including the breast. Tissue selectivity of raloxifene may be achieved through several mechanisms: the ligand structure, interaction of the ligand with different estrogen receptor subtypes in various tissues, and intracellular events after ligand binding. Raloxifene, a non-steroidal benzothiophene, cannot be used to treat menopausal symptoms, and it has no beneficial effects on hot flushes or vaginal symptoms. In contrast to estrogen, raloxifene does not induce histopathological evidence of endometrial stimulation in healthy postmenopausal women.[63] In addition, raloxifene lowers serum concentrations of total and low-density lipoprotein cholesterol, and lowers serum lipoprotein(a) levels.[64,65] It also has a favorable, dose-related effect on plasma homocysteine levels in postmenopausal women.[66]

The Multiple Outcomes of Raloxifene Evaluation (MORE), a multicenter, randomized, double-blind trial, in which women taking raloxifene or placebo were followed up for a median of 40 months, showed that raloxifene decreased the risk of estrogen receptor-positive breast cancer by 90% (RR, 0.10; 95% CI, 0.04–0.24), but not estrogen receptor-negative invasive breast cancer (RR, 0.88; 95% CI, 0.26–3.0). Raloxifene increased the risk of venous thromboembolic disease (RR, 3.1; 95% CI, 1.5–6.2), but did not increase the risk of endometrial cancer (RR, 0.8; 95% CI, 0.2–2.7).[67]

## Tibolone

Tibolone, a synthetic steroid with estrogenic, androgenic and progestogenic properties, relieves climacteric symptoms, and prevents post-menopausal bone loss. Although no studies on fracture risk have been performed, tibolone appears to be at least as efficacious as other forms of HRT with regard to climacteric symptoms. In a randomized controlled trial, tibolone increased bone mass in the spine and prevented bone loss in the forearm in late postmenopausal women, as determined by densitometry and several biochemical parameters of bone turnover. This occurred at two doses (1.25 and 2.5 mg/day), indicating that even lower doses may be efficacious.[68] In a second randomized controlled trial, tibolone induced a significant increase in trabecular (lumbar spine) and cortical (femoral neck) bone mass in postmenopausal osteoporotic women, compared to placebo.[69] Administration of tibolone in association with gonadotropin-releasing hormone analog (GnRH-a) reduced vasomotor symptoms and prevented bone loss, without compromising the therapeutic efficacy of GnRH-a alone.[70]

## Anabolic agents

Probably the most important development in recent years in anti-osteoporosis therapy was the recent release of teriparatide. This agent is given subcutaneously, on a once-daily basis. When supported with adequate calcium and vitamin D, teriparatide produces increases in bone mass of 10% to 15% per year.[71] More importantly it reduces risk of all vertebral fractures by two-thirds, and of severe and multiple vertebral fractures by approximately 85%. It also reduces non-vertebral fracture rates by approximately 50%. When given in combination with estrogen, teriparatide has increased spine bone density by 30%, and hip bone density by 12% at two years. In contrast to the antiresorptive drugs, teriparatide acts by directly stimulating osteoblastic bone formation at both trabecular and cortical sites.

Because the agent is so new, there is virtually no practice experience to describe; it is likely that the use of teriparatide will be concentrated initially in patients with severe osteoporosis, with a treatment duration of probably 18 to 24 months, and with a transition to an antiresorptive agent at the end of that time. In clinical trials the drug has been well tolerated, producing only mild transient hypercalcemia, a moderate increase in urine calcium, and an unexplained mild increase in serum uric acid–all without symptoms.[72]

## Zoledronic acid

Zoledronic acid is a very potent intravenous bisphosphonate that takes minutes to administer and is also approved for the treatment of hypercalcemia of malignancy. Reid et al. reported the results of a one-year randomized, placebo-controlled trial of zoledronic acid in post-menopausal women with low bone mineral density.[73] As compared with placebo, zoledronic acid given every three months, every six months, or as a single dose increased bone density at the spine and hip and suppressed markers of bone turnover. All treatment regimens had similar effects, which were also similar to those reported with the oral bisphosphonates in current use. The suggestion that an intravenous dose of zoledronic acid once a year, or even less often, might effectively treat postmenopausal osteoporosis is encouraging. More studies are clearly needed to determine whether the risk of fractures is actually reduced, and to determine whether long-term use of this medication is safe.

## CONCLUSION

In the 50-year modern history of osteoporosis, advances in therapy and monitoring have given the clinician an enormous armamentarium with which to battle osteoporosis. The challenge for the next 50 years is to reduce bone fracture risk by maintaining and restoring the constituents of BMD. This must be achieved while concomitantly maintaining quality of life and reducing the symptoms of estrogen excess and/or deprivation. Advances in the selective estrogen receptor modulators (SERM), and recent release of an anabolic agent, promise to revolutionize the future management of osteoporosis. These innovations will allow clinicians to provide effective prevention of bone fracture morbidity and mortality, while minimizing some of the undesirable side-effects of earlier-generation medications.

## REFERENCES

1. Cummings SR, Kelsey JL, Nevitt MC, O'Dowd KJ. Epidemiology of osteoporosis and osteoporotic fractures. Epidemiol Rev 1985; 7: 178–208.
2. Ray NF, Chan JK, Thamer M, Melton LJ. Medical expenditures for the treatment of osteoporotic fractures in the United States in 1995; report from the National Osteoporosis Foundation. J Bone Miner Res 1997; 12: 24–35.
3. Cooper C. The crippling consequences of fractures and their impact on quality of life. Am J Med 1997; 103: 12S–17S.
4. Browner WS, Pressman AR, Nevitt MC, Cummings SR. Mortality following fractures in older women. The study of osteoporotic fractures. Arch Intern Med 1996; 156: 1521–6.
5. Nevitt MC, Ettinger B, Black DM et al. The association of radiographically detected vertebral fractures with back pain and function: a prospective study. Ann Intern Med 1998; 128: 793–800.
6. Kanis JA, McCloskey EV. Epidemiology of vertebral osteoporosis. Bone 1992; 13 (Suppl 12): S1–10.
7. Ettinger B, Black DM, Palermo L, Nevitt MC, Melnikoff S, Cummings SR. Kyphosis in older women and its relation to back pain, disability and osteopenia: the study of osteoporotic fractures. Osteoporos Int 1994; 4: 55–60.
8. Mierke DF, Pellegrini M. Parathyroid hormone and parathyroid hormone-related protein: model systems for the development of an osteoporosis therapy. Curr Pharm Des 1999; 5: 21–36.
9. Brown EM, Hebert SC. The First Annual Bayard D. Catherwood Memorial Lecture. Ca$^{2+}$-receptor-mediated regulation of parathyroid and renal function. Am J Med Sci 1996; 312: 99–109.
10. Copp DH. Calcitonin: discovery, development, and clinical application. Clin Invest Med 1994; 17: 268–77.
11. Reginster JY. Calcitonins: newer routes of delivery. Osteoporos Int 1993; 3 (Suppl 2): S3–7.
12. Gennari C, Agnusdei D, Camporeale A. Long-term treatment with calcitonin in osteoporosis. Horm Metab Res 1993; 25: 484–5.
13. Theintz G, Buchs B, Rizzoli R et al. Longitudinal monitoring of bone mass accumulation in healthy adolescents: evidence for a marked reduction after 16 years of age at the levels of lumbar spine and femoral neck in female subjects. J Clin Endocrinol Metab 1992; 75: 1060–5.
14. Kroger H, Kotaniemi A, Kroger L, Alhava E. Development of bone mass and bone density of the spine and femoral neck – a prospective study of 65 children and adolescents. Bone Miner 1993; 23: 171–82.
15. Bonjour JP, Theintz G, Buchs B, Slosman D, Rizzoli R. Critical years and stages of puberty for spinal and femoral bone mass accumulation during adolescence. J Clin Endocrinol Metab 1991; 73: 555–63.
16. Ferrari S, Rizzoli R, Slosman D, Bonjour JP. Familial resemblance for bone mineral mass is expressed before puberty. J Clin Endocrinol Metab 1998; 83: 358–61.
17. Gregg EW, Cauley JA, Seeley DG, Ensrud KE, Bauer DC. Physical activity and osteoporotic fracture risk in older women. Study of Osteoporotic Fractures Research Group. Ann Intern Med 1998; 129: 81–8.
18. Kannus P. Preventing osteoporosis, falls, and fractures among elderly people. Promotion of lifelong physical activity is essential [Editorial]. BMJ 1999; 318: 205–6.
19. Whooley MA, Kip KE, Cauley JA, Ensrud KE, Nevitt MC, Browner WS. Depression, falls, and risk of fracture in older women. Study of Osteoporotic Fractures Research Group. Arch Intern Med 1999; 159: 484–90.
20. Cummings SR, Browner WS, Bauer D et al. Endogenous hormones and the risk of hip and vertebral fractures among older women. Study of Osteoporotic Fractures Research Group. N Engl J Med 1998; 339: 733–8.
21. Reid IR. Glucocorticoid effects on bone [Editorial]. J Clin Endocrinol Metab 1998; 83: 1860–2.
22. Baylink DJ. Glucocorticoid-induced osteoporosis [Editorial]. N Engl J Med 1983; 309: 306–8.
23. Greenspan SL, Greenspan FS. The effect of thyroid hormone on skeletal integrity. Ann Intern Med 1999; 130: 750–8.
24. Affinito P, Sorrentino C, Farace MJ et al. Effects of thyroxine therapy on bone metabolism in postmenopausal women with hypothyroidism. Acta Obstet Gynecol Scand 1996; 75: 843–8.
25. Bauer DC, Nevitt MC, Ettinger B, Stone K. Low thyrotropin levels are not associated with bone loss in older women: a prospective study. J Clin Endocrinol Metab 1997; 82: 2931–6.
26. Kiel DP, Baron JA, Anderson JJ, Hannan MT, Felson DT. Smoking eliminates the protective effect of oral estrogens on the risk for hip fracture among women. Ann Intern Med 1992; 116: 716–21.
27. Cornuz J, Feskanich D, Willett WC, Colditz GA. Smoking, smoking cessation, and risk of hip fracture in women. Am J Med 1999; 106: 311–14.
28. Huda W, Morin RL. Patient doses in bone mineral densitometry. Br J Radiol 1996; 69: 422–5.
29. Seto H, Kageyama M, Nomura K, Kakishita M, Tonami S. Precision of total-body and regional bone mineral measurement by dual-energy X-ray absorptiometry. Radiat Med 1991; 9: 110–13.
30. Tothill P, Avenell A. Errors in dual-energy X-ray absorptiometry of the lumbar spine owing to fat distribution

and soft tissue thickness during weight change. Br J Radiol 1994; 67: 71–5.

31. Borg J, Mollgaard A, Riis BJ. Single X-ray absorptiometry: performance characteristics and comparison with single photon absorptiometry. Osteoporos Int 1995; 5: 377–81.

32. Kelly TL, Crane G, Baran DT. Single X-ray absorptiometry of the forearm: precision, correlation, and reference data. Calcif Tissue Int 1994; 54: 212–18.

33. Rossini M, Viapiana O, Adami S. Instrumental diagnosis of osteoporosis. Aging (Milano) 1998; 10: 240–8.

34. Guglielmi G. Quantitative computed tomography (QCT) and dual X-ray absorptiometry (DXA) in the diagnosis of osteoporosis. Eur J Radiol 1995; 20: 185–7.

35. Rosenthall L, Caminis J, Tenehouse A. Calcaneal ultrasonometry: response to treatment in comparison with dual x-ray absorptiometry measurements of the lumbar spine and femur. Calcif Tissue Int 1999; 64: 200–4.

36. Christenson RH. Biochemical markers of bone metabolism: an overview. Clin Biochem 1997; 30: 573–93.

37. Adachi JD. The correlation of bone mineral density and biochemical markers to fracture risk. Calcif Tissue Int 1996; 59 (Suppl 1): 16–19.

38. Garnero P, Delmas PD. New developments in biochemical markers for osteoporosis. Calcif Tissue Int 1996; 59: 2–9.

39. Miura H, Yamamoto I, Yuu I et al. Estimation of bone mineral density and bone loss by means of bone metabolic markers in postmenopausal women. Endocr J 1995; 42: 797–802.

40. Baeksgaard L, Andersen KP, Hyldstrup L. Calcium and vitamin D supplementation increases spinal BMD in healthy, postmenopausal women. Osteoporos Int 1998; 8: 255–60.

41. Citron JT, Ettinger B, Genant HK. Spinal bone mineral loss in estrogen-replete, calcium-replete premenopausal women. Osteoporos Int 1995; 5: 228–33.

42. Mizunuma H, Okano H, Soda M et al. Calcium supplements increase bone mineral density in women with low serum calcium levels during long-term estrogen therapy. Endocr J 1996; 43: 411–15.

43. Riggs BL, O'Fallon WM, Muhs J, O'Connor MK, Kumar R, Melton LJ. Long-term effects of calcium supplementation on serum parathyroid hormone level, bone turnover, and bone loss in elderly women. J Bone Miner Res 1998; 13: 168–74.

44. Komulainen M, Tuppurainen MT, Kroger H et al. Vitamin D and HRT: no benefit additional to that of HRT alone in prevention of bone loss in early postmenopausal women. A 2.5-year randomized placebo-controlled study. Osteoporos Int 1997; 7: 126–32.

45. Ooms ME, Roos JC, Bezemer PD, van der Vijgh WJ, Bouter LM, Lips P. Prevention of bone loss by vitamin D supplementation in elderly women: a randomized double-blind trial. J Clin Endocrinol Metab 1995; 80: 1052–8.

46. Ringe JD. Vitamin D deficiency and osteopathies. Osteoporos Int 1998; 8 (Suppl 2): S35–9.

47. Prince RL, Smith M, Dick IM et al. Prevention of postmenopausal osteoporosis. A comparative study of exercise, calcium supplementation, and hormone-replacement therapy. N Engl J Med 1991; 325: 1189–95.

48. Hatori M, Hasegawa A, Adachi H et al. The effects of walking at the anaerobic threshold level on vertebral bone loss in postmenopausal women. Calcif Tissue Int 1993; 52: 411–14.

49. Wolff I, van Croonenberg JJ, Kemper HC, Kostense PJ, Twisk JW. The effect of exercise training programs on bone mass: a meta-analysis of published controlled trials in pre-and postmenopausal women. Osteoporos Int 1999; 9: 1–12.

50. Berard A, Bravo G, Gauthier P. Meta-analysis of the effectiveness of physical activity for the prevention of bone loss in postmenopausal women. Osteoporos Int 1997; 7: 331–7.

51. Anonymous. Effects of hormone therapy on bone mineral density: results from the postmenopausal estrogen/progestin interventions (PEPI) trial. The Writing Group for the PEPI. J Am Med Assoc 1996; 276: 1389–96.

52. Cauley JA, Seeley DG, Ensrud K, Ettinger B, Black D, Cummings SR. Estrogen replacement therapy and fractures in older women. Study of Osteoporotic Fractures Research Group. Ann Intern Med 1995; 122: 9–16.

53. Deng HW, Li J, Li JL et al. Change of bone mass in postmenopausal Caucasian women with and without hormone replacement therapy is associated with vitamin D receptor and estrogen receptor genotypes. Hum Genet 1998; 103: 576–85.

54. Genant HK, Lucas J, Weiss S et al. Low-dose esterified estrogen therapy: effects on bone, plasma estradiol concentrations, endometrium, and lipid levels. Estratab/Osteoporosis Study Group. Arch Intern Med 1997; 157: 2609–15.

55. Stevenson JC, Cust MP, Gangar KF, Hillard TC, Lees B, Whitehead MI. Effects of transdermal versus oral hormone replacement therapy on bone density in spine and proximal femur in postmenopausal women. Lancet 1990; 336: 265–9.

56. George GH, MacGregor AJ, Spector TD. Influence of current and past hormone replacement therapy on bone mineral density: a study of discordant postmenopausal twins. Osteoporos Int 1999; 9: 158–62.

57. McClung M, Clemmesen B, Daifotis A et al. Alendronate prevents postmenopausal bone loss in women without osteoporosis. A double-blind, randomized, controlled trial. Alendronate Osteoporosis Prevention Study Group. Ann Intern Med 1998; 128: 253–61.

58. Watts NB, Becker P. Alendronate increases spine and hip bone mineral density in women with postmenopausal osteoporosis who failed to respond to intermittent cyclical etidronate. Bone 1999; 24: 65–8.

59. Devogelaer JP, Broll H, Correa-Rotter R et al. Oral alendronate induces progressive increases in bone mass of the spine, hip, and total body over 3 years in postmenopausal women with osteoporosis [Erratum Bone 1996; 19: 78]. Bone 1996; 18: 141–50.

60. Bone HG, Hosking D, Devogelaer J-P et al. Ten years' experience with alendronate for osteoporosis in postmenopausal women. N Engl J Med 2004; 350: 1189–99.

61. Overgaard K, Hansen MA, Jensen SB, Christiansen C. Effect of salcatonin given intranasally on bone mass and fracture rates in established osteoporosis a dose–response study. BMJ 1992; 305: 556–61.

62. Franceschini R, Cataldi A, Cianciosi P et al. Calcitonin and beta-endorphin secretion. Biomed Pharmacother 1993; 47: 305–9.

63. Boss SM, Huster WJ, Neild JA, Glant MD, Eisenhut CC, Draper MW. Effects of raloxifene hydrochloride on the endometrium of postmenopausal women. Am J Obstet Gynecol 1997; 177: 1458–64.

64. Mijatovic V, van der Mooren MJ, Kenemans P, de Valk-de RG, Netelenbos C. Raloxifene lowers serum lipoprotein(a) in healthy postmenopausal women: a randomized, double-blind, placebo-controlled comparison with conjugated equine estrogens. Menopause 1999; 6: 134–7.

65. Delmas PD, Bjarnason NH, Mitlak BH et al. Effects of raloxifene on bone mineral density, serum cholesterol concentrations, and uterine endometrium in postmenopausal women. N Engl J Med 1997; 337: 1641–7.

66. Mijatovic V, Netelenbos C, van der Mooren MJ, de Valk-de RG, Jakobs C, Kenemans P. Randomized, double-blind, placebo-controlled study of the effects of raloxifene and conjugated equine estrogen on plasma homocysteine levels in healthy postmenopausal women. Fertil Steril 1998; 70: 1085–9.

67. Cummings SR, Eckert S, Krueger KA et al. The effect of raloxifene on risk of breast cancer in postmenopausal women: results from the MORE randomized trial. Multiple Outcomes of Raloxifene Evaluation. J Am Med Assoc 1999; 281: 2189–97.

68. Bjarnason NH, Bjarnason K, Haarbo J, Rosenquist C, Christiansen C. Tibolone: prevention of bone loss in late postmenopausal women [see Comments]. J Clin Endocrinol Metab 1996; 81: 2419–22.

69. Bjarnason NH, Bjarnason K, Hassager C, Christiansen C. The response in spinal bone mass to tibolone treatment is related to bone turnover in elderly women. Bone 1997; 20: 151–5.

70. Palomba S, Affinito P, Tommaselli GA, Nappi C. A clinical trial of the effects of tibolone administered with gonadotropin-releasing hormone analogues for the treatment of uterine leiomyomata. Fertil Steril 1998; 70: 111–18.

71. Hodsman AB, Hanley DA, Ettinger MP et al. Efficacy and safety of human parathyroid hormone-(1–84) in increasing bone mineral density in postmenopausal osteoporosis. J Clin Endocrinol Metab 2003; 88: 5212–20.

72. Neer RM, Arnaud CD, Zanchetta JR et al. Effect of parathyroid hormone (1–34) on fractures and bone mineral density in postmenopausal women with osteoporosis. N Engl J Med 2001; 344: 1434–41.

73. Reid IR, Brown JP, Burckhardt P et al. Intravenous zoledronic acid in postmenopausal women with low bone mineral density. N Engl J Med 2002; 346: 653–61.

# Chapter 15

# Cognition in the menopause

Karen L Dahlman and Kim P Kelly

## INTRODUCTION

As the proportion of the population over age 50 increases, the field of geropsychology in general has expanded rapidly. Issues related to the menopause have become the focus of much attention as well, with much of this work focused on hormone replacement therapy (HRT) and its effects on cognition, mood, vasomotor symptoms, and sexuality of peri- and postmenopausal women. The changes in our basic understanding about cognition in the menopause have been significant over the past few years, and these changes highlight the importance of evidence-based medical care for women.[1] While menopause management has always been challenging for physicians, the state of the art has never before shifted as dramatically as it has very recently. With the abrupt discontinuation after only four of the planned seven years of a major longitudinal study, the Women's Health Initiative (WHI),[2] current wisdom has settled in unexpected and sometimes surprising ways. This chapter will frame what we now know about cognition in the menopause, in terms of how the normal aging process affects women in this stage of life; in addition, we will discuss the major abnormal conditions that must be understood when treating menopausal patients: mild cognitive impairment, dementia, and depression.

## NORMAL AGING AND COGNITION

A key issue in the assessment of aging patients is the need to discriminate between normal age-related intellectual changes and those changes that are clinically significant. Although many cognitive functions decline as a part of the normal aging process,[3–5] the extent and pattern of the decline varies according to both the individual and the type of function being examined. Aspects of cognitive functioning that deal with well-rehearsed, overlearned activities change very little across the lifespan. Crystallized cognitive abilities such as knowledge and expertise in certain areas may even continue to increase into old age.[3,6] Other cognitive functions, including speeded tasks, processing of unfamiliar information, complex problem-solving, delayed recall, mental flexibility, perceptual manipulation tasks, and sensory and sensorimotor abilities, do tend to decline as individuals age.[3,6,7] Considerable individual differences exist in terms of aging, and these differences often are first noticed by women in the perimenopause. Despite the subjective complaints that often exist about cognitive changes experienced as part of the menopausal transition, there is no clear evidence that the perimenopause is associated with significant cognitive decline.[8] Cognitive functioning falls on a spectrum ranging from impaired to normal to successful at any given point in the aging process. Using the example of normative standards from the Wechsler Memory Scale,[4] it is clear that those individuals who performed at the highest levels (e.g. 99th percentile) in their youth on a variety of cognitive domains tend to decline relatively less throughout their lifespan. Individuals who performed at lower levels (e.g. 2nd percentile) when younger exhibit not only a marked decline as they age, but the decline seen in lower functioning individuals is more dramatic than that of individuals in the upper percentile ranges. The individuals at the top of the distribution consistently outperform those at the lower levels by a progressively greater extent as they become older.

Whalley and colleagues explain this phenomenon with the construct of cognitive reserve, which they define as 'the hypothesized capacity of the mature adult brain to sustain the effects of disease or injury sufficient to cause clinical dementia'.[9] Generally individuals with a high level of cognitive reserve are highly educated, have high premorbid intelligence levels, are or were engaged in mentally stimulating occupations, and have a more active lifestyle.[9-11] These are thought to be protective factors against the risk of developing a degenerative dementia, such as Alzheimer's disease.[12,13] One recent study, based on data from the large longitudinal study of the School Sisters of Notre Dame religious congregation, found that nuns who had strong linguistic abilities early in life (i.e. high idea density) were less at risk for developing cognitive impairment later in life (e.g. 60 years later). Additionally, the study showed that low idea density early in life was significantly correlated with greater concentrations of neurofibrillary lesions, but not of plaques, on postmortem neuropathological examination.[14] These findings support the notion that cognitive reserve is positively correlated with preserved cognitive functioning later in life.

It is critical in the assessment of aging individuals to take into account the relative nature of observed cognitive deficits; relative, that is, to the patient's own previous levels of functioning. Current functioning, in terms of engagement in life, as well as the presence/absence of disease and cognitive normalcy, must be viewed against the individual's overall level of previous functioning.

## COGNITIVE FUNCTION AND ESTROGEN

In general, the role of the menopause in cognitive changes is complex. There are estrogen receptors in the brain, and estrogen has a vasodilatory effect that could impact blood supply to the brain; estrogen also appears to be involved in the maintenance of the cholinergic neurotransmitter system, which mediates memory and attentional functioning. Despite this, there is little evidence that estrogen has beneficial effects on cognition in women, either in studies of women in different stages of the natural reproductive cycle,[15] or in studies focusing on hormone replacement or estrogen replacement therapy in healthy postmenopausal women.[16-18] Lifelong estrogen exposure is typically difficult to measure in observational studies.

This is because there is wide variability in the length and level of estrogen replacement treatment received by individual women; studies that distinguish simply between ever-users and never-users are limited because the length and level of treatment are too variable across individual study participants to be compared for effectiveness. One major observational study, the PATH Through Life Study found no significant effect of lifelong estrogen exposure on cognitive performance.[15] It remains to be determined whether factors such as older age (>69 years), type of menopause, and type of treatment, including dosage and duration of treatment, could impact memory function to a clinically relevant extent. Although in the last two decades evidence from several studies provided evidence that estrogen may have some protective effect on memory, a number of recent longitudinal and cross-sectional studies, including those from the WHI Memory Study, have failed to confirm these data.[2] Thus current thinking is that hormone therapy should not be initiated in the late postmenopause with the goal of improving memory, preventing cognitive decline, reducing risk of developing dementia, or improving symptoms of pre-existing Alzheimer's disease. Rather, the critical window hypothesis suggests that effects of early hormone therapy may differ from those of hormone therapy initiated in the late postmenopause.[19-22] Specifically, there appears to be a difference between studies that find a protective effect and those that do not, such that, in the former studies, treatment with estrogen began at the time of menopause, while in the latter studies, estrogen was introduced for the first time many years after the onset of menopause. Evidence from these studies, both in humans and animals, argues that there is a window of opportunity for the protection of memory in women, when estrogen is administered at the time of onset of menopause or soon after ovariectomy.

## MILD COGNITIVE IMPAIRMENT (MCI)

Mild cognitive impairment (MCI) refers to impairments that are objectively observable but not prominent in more than one cognitive area, and are not severe enough to affect activities of daily living.[6,23] MCI generally refers to an intermediary stage occurring between normal cognition and mild dementia.[24,25] Amnestic MCI, generally considered a prodromal phase phase of Alzheimer's disease (AD), refers to a syndrome in which memory complaints are the prominent symptoms, with preserved general cognitive functioning in other areas as well as activities of daily functioning. Approximately 10 to 15% of those with an amnestic MCI diagnosis will progress to AD per year. In comparison, only 1 to 2% of those aging normally will develop AD.[24,25] Non-amnestic forms of MCI also exist, and individuals with non-amnestic MCI generally exhibit mild impairments in a single non-memory domain (e.g. language, executive functioning). Data from the WHI suggests that estrogen plus progestin therapy did not prevent MCI in these women. Currently these data suggests that HRT risk may outweigh the benefit of treatment for women over 65 years of age.[26]

## CLINICAL EVALUATION OF THE MENOPAUSAL WOMAN WITH COGNITIVE COMPLAINTS

In addition to a thorough medical history, including a review of any diseases, psychiatric or medical, and known neurological disorders, history of head trauma, alcohol or other substance abuse, as well as exposure to toxins should be reviewed. Because these and other contributing factors (e.g. human immunodeficiency virus (HIV), diabetes, urinary tract infection) may affect cognitive functioning, a careful interview should document any illness or infection, past or present. Medication history is also an important part of the initial evaluation because drug-induced cognitive changes are among the most easily reversible. All medications, including over-the-counter (OTC) formulas, could have an effect on cognition, especially in combination. When performing a physical examination on a menopausal or postmenopausal woman, a brief neurological evaluation, designed to identify lesions, vascular illness, or infection, is advisable. Illnesses, such as urinary tract infection or medication toxicity, are assessed in order to rule out or address delirium. The physical examination needs to incorporate a check for signs of contusions that may indicate either accidental injuries or domestic abuse of the patient. Keeping an eye out for such signs is particularly important, given studies showing that between 25% and 37% of patients seen in primary care settings have experienced intimate partner violence (IPV) at some point in their lifetime and between 2% and 12%

have experienced IPV during the past year,[27–29] and that patients who suffer from domestic abuse tend to seek treatment in primary care, not mental health, settings.[30] These patients will often present with other difficulties in addition to their physical complaints, including psychological and emotional distress, suicidality, and substance abuse.[27–29] Recent research indicates that approximately 1.5 million older American adults are affected by elder mistreatment such as abuse, neglect, and abandonment by family members, caregivers, and friends,[31] and these individuals, if they report the abuse, are more likely to present for treatment at an emergency room than to their primary physician or a mental health counselor.[32]

A family history of dementia and other conditions (such as Huntington's disease and schizophrenia) should be established, as the genetic component of these illnesses is significant.[33–37] It is important, for example, when evaluating patients who present with psychotic symptoms (i.e. delusions and hallucinations), to weigh family and personal history of schizophrenia in making a decision about the primary disorder in the clinical picture.

The history taking should include a review of educational level, career, physical activity, and hobbies, along with socioeconomic, ethnic, and cultural background. These factors are important to assess because they potentially impact the overall level of cognitive functioning, and serve as a basis to assist in establishing the patient's estimated premorbid level of functioning.[3] When assessing cognitive decline, the patient's performance on formal cognitive testing should be compared not only to established norms, but also to the patient's own level of premorbid functioning.

The evaluation should take into account the possibility of either minimization or exaggeration of symptoms. Information on major life events and social supports, and especially recent changes, are necessary because of their possible contribution to the individual's performance on tests of cognitive functioning. The frequency of changes in living situations, support systems, and resources among elderly patients is common. The impact on a woman's adjustment vis-a-vis changes in family structure as children move out of the home and begin independent lives may be profound; changes for the worse in the marital relationship may be formidable as well. Research indicates that stress and social and environmental factors may be associated with an exacerbation in severity of symptoms during the menopause.[38]

## DEPRESSION

Depression is twice as prevalent among women relative to men, and one small study recently demonstrated that risk of a depressive episode was 14 times greater in the two years around the final menstrual period in a woman's life than in the premenopausal years.[39] The Study of Women's Health Across the Nation (SWAN), a large longitudinal study emphasizing active recruitment of minorities, suggests that there is increased psychological distress in the perimenopausal period.[40] Variables including race, education, marital status, and level of social support were all shown to mediate level of distress. Because the perimenopause is generally viewed as a vulnerable time for new-onset depression, there is a clear need to assess this carefully. The assessment of depression in patients presenting with cognitive impairment involves some level of sophistication in order to parse out the relative contributions of affective, neurological, or other medical illness. This is critical because of treatment selection issues; if cognitive impairment is attributed to incipient dementia, a treatable affective disorder may be overlooked. Rabheru notes that major depressive disorder often goes undetected and untreated, particularly in older patients.[41] Assessment of psychotropic medications used by the patient throughout the course of the psychiatric illness needs to be ascertained, as certain medications (e.g. anticholinergic medication) are associated with cognitive impairments in the elderly.[42]

If the patient's cognitive dysfunction can be attributed with some degree of certainty to depression, the clinician has strong reasons to pursue vigorous antidepressant treatment. The failure to treat a primary depression is potentially disastrous for a patient, especially given the fairly good response of depressed patients in general to various treatments.[43–45] However, if the patient's cognitive impairment is due to a primary memory disorder, then aggressive treatment of depressive symptoms may not substantially improve the quality of the patient's life. Complicating the picture is the fact that depression is often a comorbid illness with dementia and MCI.[46] Overall, the issue is one of careful assessment of the clinical picture.

The differential diagnosis of behavioral and cognitive disorders in aging patients is made more complicated by depression, which can produce symptoms that mimic those of early dementia, as well as MCI.[47] This is understandable given evidence from neuroimaging studies showing that patients with late-onset depression have enlarged ventricles, sulcal widening, and decreased brain density, particularly in the frontal lobes, hippocampus, and caudate nucleus.[48–50] Estimates of the incidence of depression in the elderly indicate that an estimated 15% of Americans over the age of 65 years experience clinically significant depressive symptoms,[51] and it may be the most common emotional problem among elderly patients.[52,53] Depressive symptoms are often precipitated by a traumatic loss, or by an event such as retirement or poor health. In cases such as these, the depression is reactive, and fits better with the diagnosis of adjustment disorder with depressed mood than with major depressive disorder. While a chronic physical illness greatly increases the likelihood of depression in an older patient, making the diagnosis of depression in a physically sick patient is often complicated by iatrogenic factors. Depressive symptoms may arise either from an illness itself, or from medication used to treat it.[48,54,55] Also, the somatic symptoms of depression, such as fatigue or weight loss, may actually be caused by a physical illness rather than by a depressive episode, making it especially difficult to tease apart the etiology.[54]

Assessment of depression in the perimenopausal patient usually begins with clinical interview of the patient, and, ideally, this is supplemented by corroborative information from a family member. The assessment must focus on objective symptoms of depression, including mood, behavior, anxiety, and vegetative symptoms such as sleep disturbance, anhedonia, anergia, and loss of appetite, as well as the subjective experiences outlined by the individual. The diagnosis of perimenopause-related depression is made in the same way as that for depression at any other time in the lifespan; however, with the perimenopausal woman, the depression must occur in the context of endocrine evidence of the perimenopause.

Menopause-related depression is defined by the onset of depression (major or minor) in association with changes in an individual's menstrual cycle and evidence of endocrine changes (e.g. elevations of plasma follicle-stimulating hormone (FSH) levels). Vasomotor or other physiological symptoms associated with menopause may lead to affective changes, rather then the menopause status itself. Persistent hot flashes may disturb sleep patterns, which can result in fatigue, diminished ability to concentrate, and irritability; these symptoms may disrupt daily functioning.

Major and/or less significant depression may occur in the perimenopause. Women may also present with a mixed anxiety–depressive disorder. The affective symptoms are often described as having a gradual onset and sometimes as occurring during hot flashes.[56] It is the relative prominence of the mood and behavioral symptoms compared to the somatic complaints that leads to the diagnosis of a depressive syndrome. One reliable scale frequently used to measure depression is the Beck Depression Inventory-II, in which the patient checks 21 four-choice statements presented on a single page, for the choice or choices most appropriate. The statements refer to the following areas: sadness, pessimism/discouragement, sense of failure, dissatisfaction, guilt, expectation of punishment, self-dislike, self-blame, suicidality, tearfulness, irritability, social withdrawal, indecisiveness, unattractiveness, work difficulty, sleep disruption, fatigue, appetite loss, weight loss, somatization, and diminished libido.[57]

## Prevalence of depression in the perimenopause

It remains controversial whether postmenopausal women are more vulnerable to the development of depression. Some investigators have concluded that there is little evidence suggesting women in perimenopause are at increased risk for developing depression.[58–61] More recently, however, epidemiological studies and clinic-based surveys have reported that as many as 10% of women participating in longitudinal community-based studies have been observed to have perimenopause-related changes in mood.[62,63] Other reports indicate that both perimenopausal and postmenopausal women have higher prevalence of depressive symptoms than do premenopausal women, and that perimenopausal women are more symptomatic than postmenopausal women.[64–67]

Ladd and colleagues note that between 15% and 30% of women experience depressive symptomatology during perimenopause, and, compared to those without hot flashes, women experiencing hot flashes are four times more likely to experience depression.[43] Improvement in mood, attention, concentration, and libido in postmenopausal women without clinical depression has been observed with estrogen replacement therapy,[68] as has improvement in perimenopausal women with some depressive symptoms.[61,69,70] Because of the number of women entering the menopause at any

given point in time, it is important to understand the nature of the relationship between affective disorders and the perimenopause. Weissman suggests a peak in the onset of depressive illness during the perimenopausal years (age 45–50 years).[71] Other writers suggest that the etiology of major depressive illness occurring in the context of menopause may be related to changes in reproductive hormones that occur at that time.[72] Rather than the direct effects of these hormones, or the absolute levels of the hormones, it may be the rate of change of hormone levels or their indirect effects on neurotransmitter, neuroendocrine, or circadian systems that lead to mood alteration.[38,73–76] Another explanation is that psychosocial factors such as perceived social support, employment state and marital status are related to the occurrence of depression.[38,73,77] In addition to the etiology of depression in perimenopausal women being fundamentally different than in other patient groups, both the nature of the depression itself and response to treatment may be unique as well.[56]

## Effects of hormone replacement therapy on menopausal depression

Now that evidence exists that HRT is not indicated to prevent cognitive changes in the menopause, what can we say about the use of HRT for treatment of depression associated with the menopause? HRT most commonly consists of estrogen and progesterone administered in a cyclical manner. A number of different estrogen preparations with and without progesterone have been studied in both mood and cognitive disorders. Unfortunately negative mood symptoms may be associated with cyclical estrogen and progesterone administration, particularly after the introduction of progesterone in the treatment cycle. These effects seem to be dose related, increasing with the progesterone dose.[78,79] Estrogen acts as a serotoninergic and cholinergic agonist, but also selectively increases norephinephrine (noradrenaline) in the brain. Administration of estrogen has been shown to decrease dopamine type 2 receptors, and possibly other dopamine receptor subtypes.[74] It has mixed actions on endorphins. It has been suggested that decreases in postmenopausal serotonergic and noradrenergic functioning are associated with declining levels in estrogen. It is unclear if HRT decreases the vulnerability caused by this hypofunctioning. Studies have suggested that monoamine oxidase (MAO) activity is decreased by estrogen administration in depressed postmenopausal women.[80]

Some studies suggest that estrogen augmentation to antidepressant medication may benefit women with menopausal depressions,[75,81,82] though the addition of estrogen supplements to tricyclic antidepressants (TCAs) may induce rapid mood cycling or other undesirable side-effects in some patients.[83,84] Estrogen as a monotherapy does not seem to have impressive antidepressant properties, but may be useful for mood stabilization.[85]

A number of studies have offered evidence about the effectiveness of low-dose, short-term estrogen replacement therapy (ERT) plus antidepressant (selective serotonin reuptake inhibitor (SSRI)) treatment in the treatment of climacteric disorders, hot flashes and depressive symptoms.[86,87] Because periods of hormonal fluctuations are associated with exacerbation of existing psychiatric disorders, especially the incidence of premenstrual dysphoria and depressive symptoms during the peri-menopause, it has been speculated that steroids such as estrogens, progestogens, testosterone, and dehydroepiandrosterone (DHEA) exert a significant modulating effect on brain functioning, which is likely to be mediated across neurotransmitter systems.[18] It stands to reason that when these hormones are dramatically altered, interference with mood and behavior will result. Quite a bit of data suggest that hormonal supplements, such as raloxifene and continuous combined estrogen plus progestin, may provide relief from depressive symptoms during the menopause.[88] Another study found that the combination of 2 mg estradiol valerate and 2 mg dienogest was an effective treatment option for women with mild to moderate depression during the postmenopausal period,[89] while Schiff et al reported an improvement in depressive symptoms among postmenopausal women over 60 years of age as the result of treatment with transdermal estradiol.[90]

HRT also seems to buffer the association between naturally occurring low cholesterol levels and increased depressive symptoms in post-menopausal women. In one study, increased levels of depression have been found to be associated with lower levels of cholesterol and low-density lipoprotein (LDL)-C among healthy, postmenopausal women who were not receiving HRT. The interaction of depression and HRT explained about 17% of the variance in LDL-C and 16% of the variance in total cholesterol, respectively, following adjustment for the influences of age, body mass index, and the main effects of HRT and depressive symptoms.[91] This suggests that postmenopausal women with naturally lower levels of cholesterol have increased depressive symptoms; this relationship is only apparent among women not receiving HRT. The combination of low-dose estrogen with SSRI (fluvoxamine) was also found to be effective at relieving symptoms of depression and hot flashes, in a study of oophorectomized women with these complaints; these data suggest that the combination of low-dose estrogen combined with SSRI is more effective than low-dose estrogen alone.[83]

## HRT AND COGNITION IN POSTMENOPAUSAL WOMEN: WHAT IS THE LAST WORD?

### Cognitive changes in the menopause

It has long been suspected that estrogen deficiency may be a cause of memory loss in postmenopausal women. If true, men should have less memory loss with age than women. However, one large-scale study found weak or absent sex differences in cognitive decline with aging.[92] These findings, known as the Rancho Bernardo Study, do not support the idea that estrogen deficiency is associated with a decline in cognitive functioning among postmenopausal women. Recent work confirms that transition through the menopause is not accompanied by decline in working memory and perceptual speed.[93] There are quite a few studies that demonstrate a clear improvement on verbal recall tasks, but no changes in visual recall tasks,[94–96] while others show no effects of estrogen treatment on memory.[68,97] A review of the literature by Rice et al concludes that the epidemiological evidence for an association between estrogen and cognitive function among postmenopausal women remains controversial.[98] Overall, the evidence for a positive relationship comes primarily from randomized clinical trials, which suggest an acute effect on specific verbal memory tasks as well as some tasks that incorporate concept formation and reasoning.

While estrogen in a therapeutic dosage was shown to alter brain activation patterns in post-menopausal women during the performance of certain memory tasks, no significant performance differences were found.[99] Some writers have pointed out that the equivocal data on estrogen effects on cognition in menopausal women may be due to the artifacts of group membership. In at least one large-scale, community-based study, ever-users had significantly higher levels of education, and presumably, IQ, than never-users.[94] Other factors that may contribute to explaining inconsistencies in the data produced by these studies include concomitant medication use, different types of estrogen preparations, and a disparity in psychometric tests used as dependent variables. In summary, although there was some encouraging early evidence from observational studies for the beneficial use of estrogen on cognitive function, especially verbal memory, that evidence is outweighed by the results from the WHI work.

Little consistent benefit of HRT on cognition in healthy postmenopausal women has been demonstrated in recent years. A randomized, placebo-controlled study of a transdermal estrogen preparation composed of 17β-estradiol found that, although little overall beneficial effect of estrogen was found, the number of years since menopause was significantly related to change in executive functioning, such that more recently postmenopausal women demonstrated greater positive change than older women. Body mass index, thought to be a gross estimate of circulating estrogen, was significantly positively related to change in attentional and psychomotor ability regardless of treatment group.[100] These findings suggest that reproductive events and levels of endogenous estrogen play a part in determining clinical response to HRT. In a substudy utilizing a subgroup of participants from the Women's Memory Study (WMS), a large-scale longitudinal observational study of never- and ever-users of HRT, there was no significant difference between the two groups on any cognitive outcome measures.[101] Likewise, another observational study, despite corrections for age and educational levels, failed to confirm benefit any significant benefit of HRT to cognitive functioning in postmenopausal women.[102] Another study sought to determine whether reduction of homocysteine is a mechanism by which estrogen may enhance cognitive functioning on postmenopausal women; results failed to support such an interaction.[103]

## Rationale for HRT treatment of postmenopausal women with dementia

The rationale for estrogen treatment for AD is based on preclinical, epidemiological, and preliminary treatment studies. Evidence from these stud-ies indicates that estrogen receptors are present in the nucleus basilus of Meynert,[104] and in the hippocampus and hypothalamus.[105] A decline in choline acetyl transferase activity in the frontal cortex and hippocampus can be prevented by the administration of estrogen.[106,107] Estrogen has been shown to mediate the neuronal sprouting response to injury and survival. It also potentiates neurite outgrowth, dendritic spine and synapse formation.[108,109] The changes seen in the estrus cycle are also seen in the hippocampus, an area well known to be associated with memory and learning. Here, the rise in progesterone is associated with involution of neuronal elements in the CA1 region, a phenomenon which is also reversed by estrogen use.[110]

A mechanism whereby estrogen affects cognition in AD is still not well understood. There are several possibilities: Hagino's work with rats demonstrated that early aging females exhibited a decrease in hippocampal function that was restored with supplemental estradiol administration.[111] Arai et al suggested that estrogen may play a role in the reparative neuronal response to injury.[112] Arimatsu demonstrated that estrogen enhanced the survival of amygdala neurons in culture.[109] Goldman's work revealed an increase in cerebral blood flow to the frontal cortex, the hippocampus, the basal ganglia, and the cerebellum with administration of estrogen to rats, a finding that was more robust in female than in male rats.[113]

The area of the central nervous system responsive to estrogen possesses estrogen receptors, and these areas, including the basal forebrain nuclei and cholinergic neurons, are the ones predominantly affected in AD.[114] These cholinergic neurons with estrogen receptors also have receptors for nerve growth factor whose expression is modulated by the hormone. Estrogen also affects norepinephrine (noradrenaline) and other neurotransmitter systems. Beta-endorphin neurons are lost in the face of chronic estradiol exposure. Female patients with AD have been reported to have lower serum estrone sulfate levels than non-senile females.[104]

Estrogen may affect the progression of AD via its effects on the metabolism of amyloid precursor protein (APP).[115] In the cell culture, physiological concentration of 17β-estradiol increases the secretory metabolism of the soluble fragment of APP without increasing the intracellular levels of APP. Hence, the deposition of beta amyloid and plaque formation may be reduced. Estrogen reduces plasma levels of apolipoprotein E.[116,117] Plaque formation may also be reduced by the modification of the inflammatory response by estrogen, via its effects on interleukin 6, a cytokine postulated to participate in plaque formation.[118,119] Estrogen has also been found to have anti-oxidant properties, via its action on free radicals.[120,121] Estrogen prevents platelet aggregation by influencing the production of prostacyclin which opposes thromboxane. It is thought to do this via cyclo-oxygenase 2 and phospholipase stimulation. Prostaglandins are thought to be possible mediators of histopathological damage in AD; they inhibit nitric oxide (NO) production and decrease NO synthetase mRNA, whereas estrogen increases NO production by upgrading NO synthetase.[122] This influence is also seen in vessel walls; estrogen may exert antihypertensive effects in premenopausal women; other studies have revealed that it increases both cerebral blood flow and cerebral glucose utilization.[123]

HRT has been shown to blunt stress-induced cortisol levels; it is known that cortisol levels are elevated in AD.[124] Stress has detrimental effects on memory and may lead to neuronal damage in the hippocampus. After the menopause, aromatization of androgens provides most estrogen. In addition, recent evidence suggests that prior HRT use may be associated with reduced risk of AD, although current HRT use has no clear benefit unless use has exceeded 10 years.[125] For example, four years of treatment with HRT did not result in improved cognitive function in postmenopausal women with coronary disease.[126] In an interesting study of brain-injured women, low levels of estradiol therapy seemed to exert a protective effect by slowing the progression of the injury and diminishing the effect of cell death through suppression of apoptic cell death pathways and enhancing expression of genes that optimize cell survival.[127]

Despite findings from the WHI that for women aged 65 years or older, HRT had an adverse effect on cognition, which was greater among older women with lower cognitive ability at initiation of treatment,[128,129] reviews of the results of the WHI suggest that long-term postmenopausal hormone therapy should not be precluded, and that the primary prevention of Alzheimer's disease through HRT may still be a possibility.[130–132] This seems to be true especially for younger women in their 50s, who are closer to the menopausal transition.[133] A meta-analysis suggests that, overall, this is highly unlikely; and that data from a large randomized trial indicate that HRT does not decrease dementia risk despite the evidence from observational studies.[134] Among postmenopausal women aged 65 years or older, estrogen plus progestin did not improve cognitive function when compared with placebo in the WHI Memory Study; in fact, a small increased risk of clinically significant cognitive decline was documented in this group,[135] as was higher risk of ischemic stroke in these generally healthy women.[136]

## HRT and risk of Alzheimer's disease

Early studies of estrogen therapy effects on cognitive function yielded results suggesting that improvements were found in language comprehension, naming and arithmetic; for example, Ditkoff et al and Fillit et al reported improvements in cognition with estradiol treatment in postmenopausal women with AD.[68,137] This was later confirmed by a placebo-controlled double-blind trial by Honjo et al.[138] Ohkura's group also showed increases in cerebral blood flow.[139] Paganini-Hill and Henderson performed a case-controlled study nested within a large prospective cohort of women in a retirement community in southern California.[140] The results showed that ever-users of HRT had a 30% decreased risk of developing AD compared with never-users, with a positive relationship between dosage and duration. The Puget Sound HMO organization found a similar magnitude in risk reduction for development of AD.[141] Results from another large sample longitudinal study of elderly women in New York City indicate that 12.5% of women reported taking estrogen after the menopause.[142] Among this group, the age of AD onset was significantly later, with a reduced relative risk of 5.8% adjusted for education, ethnic origin and apolipoprotein E genotype compared with those not taking estrogen. Results also confirmed the results of other investigators that use greater than one year in duration was associated with a greater reduction in risk. Barrett-Conner and Kritz-Silverstein did not find an association between the use of estrogen and impaired cognitive function in late life.[96]

In Ohkura's study of seven patients with mild to moderate dementia of the Alzheimer's type, who received long-term low-dose HRT over a period of 5–45 months, four of the seven showed improvements on a brief cognitive rating scale and on a dementia rating scale over pretreatment levels during HRT; these results decreased when HRT was stopped.[143] Schneider et al examined at the effects of HRT on response to tacrine in patients with AD.[144] Results indicated that women on HRT performed better on measures of cognition and overall functioning than those not on HRT. The authors suggested that the improvements may have been related to the increase in choline acetyltransferase activity in the hippocampus.

It is clear that the findings discussed above, drawn from observational studies, point in a different direction than do the data from randomized controlled trials. How can this be explained? Meta-analyses of observational trials suggest that there is a protective effect of HRT against the development of AD; however, as discussed above, differences in length of time on HRT and differences in dosages used by participants in observational studies, as well as differences in participant characteristics, limit the ability to draw conclusions from observational studies alone about the benefits of HRT over time. Specifically, women on HRT tend to be better educated, with higher socioeconomic status and better access to medical care than those not treated with HRT.[145] In contrast to observational studies, randomized controlled trials have failed to confirm any significant benefit on the cognitive functioning of patients who have already developed AD.[146]

# REFERENCES

1. Richardson MK. Commentary: what's the deal with menopause management? Postgrad Med 2005; 118: 21–6.
2. Rossouw JE, Anderson GL, Prentice RL et al. Writing Group for the Women's Health Initiative Investigators. Risks and benefits of estrogen plus progestin in healthy postmenopausal women: principal results from the Women's Health Initiative randomized controlled trial. JAMA 2002; 288: 321–33.
3. Anstey KJ, Low LF. Normal cognitive changes in aging. Aust Fam Physician 2004; 33: 783–7.
4. Wechsler D. Wechsler Memory Scale – III Administration and Scoring Manual. San Antonio, TX: The Psychological Corporation, 1997.
5. Wechsler D. Wechsler Adult Intelligence Scale – III Administration and Scoring Manual. San Antonio, TX: The Psychological Corporation, 1997.
6. Lindeboom J, Weinstein H. Neuropsychology of cognitive ageing, minimal cognitive impairment, Alzheimer's disease, and vascular cognitive impairment. Eur J Pharmacol 2004; 490: 83–6.
7. Harvey PD, Dahlman KL. Neuropsychological assessment of dementia. In: Chalev A, ed. Neuropsychological Assessment of Neuropsychiatric Disorders. Washington: American Psychiatric Press, 1999.
8. Fuh JL, Wang SJ, Lee SJ, Lu SR, Juang KD. A longitudinal study of cognition change during early menopausal transition in a rural community. Maturitas 2006; 53: 447–53.
9. Whalley LJ, Deary IJ, Appleton CL, Starr JM. Cognitive reserve and the neurobiology of cognitive aging. Ageing Res Rev 2004; 3: 369–82.
10. Fratiglioni L, Paillard-Borg S, Winblad B. An active and socially integrated lifestyle in late life might protect against dementia. Lancet Neurol 2004; 3: 343–53.
11. Newson RS, Kemps EB. General lifestyle activities as a predictor of current cognition and cognitive change in older adults: A cross-sectional and longitudinal examination. J Gerontol 2005; 60: 113–20.
12. Scarmeas N, Stern Y. Cognitive reserve and lifestyle. J Clin Exp Neuropsychol 2003; 25: 625–33.
13. Scarmeas N, Stern Y. Cognitive reserve: Implications for diagnosis and prevention of Alzheimer's disease. Curr Neurol Neurosci Rep 2004; 4: 374–80.
14. Riley KP, Snowdon DA, Desrosiers MF, Markesbery WR. Early life linguistic ability, late life cognitive function, and neuropathology: Findings from the Nun Study. Neurobiol Aging 2005; 26: 341–47.
15. Low LF, Anstey KJ, Jorm AF, Rodgers B, Christensen H. Reproductive period and cognitive function in a representative sample of naturally postmenopausal women aged 60–64 years. Climacteric 2005; 8: 380–9.
16. Hogervorst E, Yaffe K, Richards M et al. Hormone replacement therapy for cognitive function in postmenopausal women. Cochrane Database Syst Rev 2002; 3: CD003122.
17. Morse CA, Rice K. Memory after menopause: preliminary considerations of hormone influence on cognitive functioning. Arch Women Ment Health 2005; 8: 155–62.
18. Low LF, Anstey KJ, Jorm AF, Christensen H, Rodgers B. Hormone replacement therapy and cognition in an Australian representative sample aged 60–64 years. Maturitas, 2006; 54: 84–94.
19. Sherwin BB. Estrogen and cognitive aging in women. Neuroscience, 2006; 138: 1021–6.
20. Henderson VW. Menopause and disorders of the central nervous system. Minerva Ginecol 2005; 57: 579–925.
21. Gibbs RB, Gabor R. Estrogen and cognition: applying preclinical findings to clinical perspectives. J Neurosci Res 2003; 74: 637–43.
22. Hammond CB. The Women's Health Initiative Study: perspectives and implications for clinical practice. Rev Endocr Metab Disord 2005; 6: 93–9.
23. Maruff P, Collie A, Darby D, Weaver-Cargin J, Masters C, Currie J. Subtle memory decline over 12 months in mild cognitive impairment. Dement Geriatr Cogn Disord 2004; 18: 342–8.
24. Grundman M, Petersen RC, Ferris SH et al. Alzheimer's Disease Cooperative Study. Mild cognitive impairment can be distinguished from Alzheimer disease and normal aging for clinical trials. Arch Neurol 2004; 61: 59–66.
25. Petersen RC, Doody R, Kurz A et al. Current concepts in mild cognitive impairment. Arch Neurol 2001; 58: 1985–92.
26. Shumaker SA, Legault C, Rapp SR et al. Estrogen plus progestin and the incidence of dementia and mild cognitive impairment in postmenopausal women: The Women's Health Initiative Memory Study: a randomized controlled Trial. JAMA 2003; 289: 2651–62.
27. Jaffee KD, Epling JW, Grant W, Ghandour RM, Callendar E. Physician-identified barriers to intimate partner violence screening. J Womens Health 2005; 14: 713–20.

28. Kramer A, Lorenzon D, Mueller G. Prevalence of intimate partner violence and health implications for women using emergency departments and primary care clinics. Womens Health Iss 2004; 14: 19–29.

29. Richardson J, Coid J, Petruckevitch A, Chung WS, Moorey S, Feder G. Identifying domestic violence: cross sectional study in primary care. BMJ 2002; 324: 1–6.

30. Samson AY, Benson S, Beck A, Price D, Nimmer C. Post traumatic stress disorder in primary care. J Fam Pract 1999; 48: 222–7.

31. Fulmer T, Guadagno L, Bolton MM. Elder mistreatment in women. J Obstet Gynecol Neonatal Nurs 2004; 33: 657–63.

32. Kleinschmidt KC. Elder abuse: a review. Ann Emerg Med 1997; 30: 463–72.

33. Bachman DL, Wolf, PA, Linn RT et al. Incidence of dementia and probable Alzheimer's disease in a general population: The Framingham Study. Neurology 1993; 43: 515–19.

34. Bierer LM, Silverman JM, Mohs RC et al. Morbid risk to first degree relatives of neuropathologically confirmed cases of Alzheimer's disease. Dementia 1992; 3: 134–9.

35. Goldberg TE, Ragland JD, Torrey EF et al. Neuro-psychological assessment of monozygotic twins discordant for schizophrenia. Arch Gen Psychiatry 1990; 47: 1066.

36. Mayeux R, Ottman R, Tang MX et al. Genetic susceptibility and head injury as risk factors for Alzheimer's disease among community dwelling elderly persons and their first degree relatives. Ann Neurol 1993; 33: 494–501.

37. Schellenberg GD, Bird TD, Wijsman EM et al. Genetic linkage evidence for a familial Alzheimer's disease locus on chromosome 14. Science 1992; 258: 668–71.

38. O'Connell E. Mood, energy, cognition, and physical complaints: A mind/body approach to symptom management during the climacteric. J Obstet Gynecol Neonatal Nurs 2005; 34: 274–9.

39. Schmidt PJ, Haq NA, Rubinow DR. A longitudinal evaluation of the relationship between reproductive status and mood in perimenopausal women. Am J Psychiatry 2004; 161: 2238–44.

40. Bromberger JT, Meyer PM, Kravitz HM et al. Psychologic distress and natural menopause: a multiethnic community study. Am J Public Health 2001; 91: 1435–42.

41. Rabheru K. Special issues in the management of depression in older patients. Can J Psychiatry 2004; 49: 41S–50S.

42. Drimer T, Shahal B, Barak Y. Effects of discontinuation of long-term anticholinergic treatment in elderly and schizophrenic patients. Int Clin Psychopharmacol 2004; 19: 27–9.

43. Ladd CO, Newport DJ, Ragan KA, Loughhead A, Stowe ZN. Venlafaxine in the treatment of depressive and vasomotor symptoms in women with perimenopausal depression. Depress Anxiety 2005; 22: 94–7.

44. Nickel MK, Nickel C, Lahmann C et al. Changes in instrumental activities of daily living disability after treatment of depressive symptoms in elderly women with chronic musculoskeletal pain: a double-blind, placebo-controlled trial. Aging Clin Exp Res 2005; 17: 293–6.

45. Thase ME, Entsuah R, Cantillon M, Kornstein SG. Relative antidepressant efficacy of venlafaxine and SSRIs: sex-age interactions. J Womens Health 2005; 14: 609–16.

46. Modrego PJ, Ferrandez, J. Depression in patients with mild cognitive impairment increases the risk of developing dementia of the Alzheimer type: a prospective cohort study. Arch Neurol 2004; 61: 1290–3.

47. Lopez OL, Jagust WJ, Dulberg C et al. Risk factors for mild cognitive impairment in the Cardiovascular Health Study Cognition Study: part 2. Arch Neurol 2003; 60: 1394–9.

48. Alexopoulos GS, Schultz SK, Lebowitz BD. Late-life depression: a model for medical classification in geriatric depression. Biol Psychiatry 2005; 58: 283–9.

49. Schweitzer I, Tuckwell V, Ames D, O'Brien J. Structural neuroimaging studies in late-life depression: A review. World J Biol Psychiatry 2001; 2: 83–8.

50. Schweitzer I, Tuckwell V, O'Brien J, Ames D. Is late onset depression a prodrome to dementia? Int J Geriatr Psychiatry 2002; 17: 997–1005.

51. Harman JS, Edlund MJ, Fortney JC, Kallas H. The influence of comorbid chronic medical conditions on the adequacy of depression care for older Americans. J Am Geriatr Soc 2005; 53: 2178–83.

52. Mayall E, Oathamshaw S, Lovell K, Pusey H. Development and piloting of a multidisciplinary training course for detecting and managing depression in the older person. J Psychiatr Ment Health Nurs 2004; 11: 165–71.

53. Hassinger M, Smith G, LaRue A. Assessing depression in older adults. In: Hunt T, Lindley CJ, eds. Testing older Adults: A Reference Guide for Geropsychological Assessments. Austin, TX: Pro-Ed, 1989.

54. Drayer RA, Mulsant BH, Lenze EJ et al. Somatic symptoms of depression in elderly patients with medical comorbidities. Int J Geriatr Psychiatry 2005; 20: 973–82.

55. Meeks S, Murrel SA, Mehl RC. Longitudinal relationships between depressive symptoms and health in normal older and middle-aged adults. Psychol Aging 2000; 15: 100–9.

56. Schmidt PJ, Roca CA, Rubinow DR. Clinical evaluation in studies of perimenopausal women: Position paper. Psychopharmacol Bull 1998; 34: 309–11.

57. Beck AT, Steer RA. Beck Depression Inventory Manual. San Antonio, TX: Psychological Corporation, 1993.

58. Avis NE, Brambilla D, McKinaly SM et al. A longitudinal analysis of the association bwtewen menpause and depression: Results from the Massachusetts Women's Health Study. Ann Epidemiol 1994; 4: 214–20.

59. Kaufert PA, Gilbert P, Tate R. The Manitoba Project: a re-examination of the link between menopause and depression. Maturitas 1992; 14: 143–55.

60. McKinlay JB, McKinlay SM, Brambilla D. The relative contributions of endocrine changes and social circumstances to depression in mid-aged women. J Health Soc Behav 1987; 28: 345–63.

61. Schmidt PJ. Depression, the perimenopause, and estrogen therapy. Ann NY Acad Sci 2005; 1052: 27–40.

62. Hunter M. The South-East England longitudinal study of the climacteric and postmenopause. Mauritas 1992; 14: 117–26.

63. Matthews KA. Myths and realities of the menopause. Psychosom Med 1992; 54: 1–9.

64. Dennerstein L, Smith AMA, Morse C et al. Menopausal symptoms in Australian women. Med J Aust 1993; 159: 232–6.

65. Freeman EW, Sammel MD, Liu L et al. Hormones and menopausal status as predictors of depression in women in transition to menopause. Arch Gen Psychiatry 2004; 61: 62–70.

66. Hay AG, Bancroft J, Johnstone EC. Affective symptoms in women attending a menopause clinic. Br J Psychiatry 1994; 164: 513–16.

67. Stewart DE, Boydell K, Derzko C, Marshall V. Psychologic distress during the menopausal years in women attending a menopause clinic. Int J Psychiatry Med 1992; 22: 213–20.

68. Ditkoff EC, Crary WG, Cristo M, Lobo RA. Estrogen improves psychological function in asymptomatic postmenopausal women. Obstet Gynecol 1991; 78: 991–5.

69. Schmidt PJ, Nieman L, Danaceau, MA et al. Estrogen replacement therapy in perimenopause-related depression: a preliminary report. Am J Obstet Gynecol 2000; 183: 414–20.

70. Soares CD, Almeida OP, Joffe H et al. Efficacy or estradiol for the treatment of depressive disorders in perimenopausal women: a double-blind, randomized, placebo-controlled trial. Arch Gen Psychiatry 2001; 58: 529–34.

71. Weissman MW. Epidemiology of Major Depression in Women. Women and the Controversies in Hormonal Replacement Therapy. Presented at the American Psychiatric Association Meeting, New York, 4 May 1996.

72. Haynes P, Parry BL. Mood disorders and the reproductive cycle: affective disorders during the menopause and premenstrual dysphoric disorder. Psychopharmacol Bull 1998; 34: 313–18.

73. Cohen LS, Soares CN, Joffe H. Diagnosis and management of mood disorders during the menopausal transition. Am J Med 2005; 118: 935–75.

74. Halbreich U. Role of estrogen in postmenopausal depression. Neurology 1997; 48 (Suppl 7): S16–9.

75. Schneider LS, Small GW, Hamilton SH, Bystritsky A, Nemeroff CB, Meyers BS, and the Fluoxetine Collaborative Study Group. Estrogen replacement and response to fluoxetine in a multicenter geriatric depression trial. Am J Geriatr Psychiatry 1997; 5: 97–106.

76. Soares CD, Cohen LS. The perimenopause, depressive disorders, and hormonal variability. Sao Paulo Med J/Rev Paul Med 2001; 119: 78–83.

77. Maartens LWF, Knottnerus JA, Pop VJ. Menopausal transition and increased depressive symptomatology. Maturitas 2002; 42: 195–200.

78. Magos AL, Collins WP, Studd JW. Management of the premenstrual syndrome by subcutaneous implants of estradiol. J Psychosom Obstet Gynaecol 1984; 3: 93–9.

79. Magos AL, Brewster E, Singh R, O'Dowd T, Brincat M, Studd JW. The effects of norethisterone in postmenopausal women on estrogen replacement therapy: a model for the premenstrual syndrome. Br J Obstet Gynaecol 1986; 93: 1290–6.

80. Holsboer F, Benkert O, Demisch L. Changes in MAO activity during estrogen treatment of females with endogenous depression. Mod Probl Pharmacopsychiatry 1983; 19: 321–6.

81. Stahl SM. Role of Hormone Therapies for Refractory Depression. Presented at the American Psychiatric Association Annual Meeting, New York, 4 May 1996.

82. Klaiber EL, Broverman DM, Vogel W, Kobayashi Y. Estrogen therapy for severe persistent depressions in women. Arch Gen Psychiatry 1979; 36: 550–4.

83. Oppenheim, G. A case of rapid mood cycling with estrogen: Implications for therapy. J Clin Psychiatry 1984; 45: 34–5.

84. Shapira B, Oppenheim G, Zohar J, Segal M, Malach D, Belmaker R. Lack of efficacy of estrogen supplementation to imipramine in resistant female depressives. Biol Psychiatry 1985; 20: 570–83.

85. Stahl SM: Augmentation of antidepressants by estrogen. Psychopharmacol Bull 1998; 34: 319–21.

86. Nagata H, Nozaki M, Nakano H. Short-term combinational therapy of low-dose estrogen with selective serotonin re-uptake inhibitor (fluvoxamine) for oophorectomized women with hot flashes and depressive tendencies. J Obstet Gynaecol Res 2005; 31: 107–14.

87. Morgan ML, Cook IA, Rapkin AJ, Leuchter AF. Estrogen augmentation of antidepressants in perimenopausal depression: a pilot study. J Clin Psychiatry 2005: 66: 774–80.

88. Carranza-Lira S, MacGregor-Gooch AL, Sarachaga-Osterwalder M. Mood modifications with raloxifene and continuous combined estrogen plus progestin hormone therapy. Int J Fertil Womens Med 2004; 49: 120–2.

89. Rudolph I, Palombo-Kinne E, Kirsch B, Mellinger U, Breitbarth H, Graser T. Influence of a continuous combined HRT (2 mg estradiol valerate and 2 mg dienogest) on postmenopausal depression. Climacteric 2004; 7: 301–11.

90. Schiff R, Bulpitt CJ, Wesnes KA, Rajkumar C. Short term transdermal estradiol therapy, cognition and depressive symptoms in healthy older women. A randomized placebo controlled pilot cross-over study. Psychoneuroendocrinology 2005; 30: 309–15.

91. Brown RA, Giggey PP, Dennis KE, Waldstein SR. Depression and lipoprotein lipids in healthy, postmenopausal women: the moderating effects of hormone replacement therapy. J Psychosom Res 2004; 56: 171–6.

92. Barrett-Connor E, Kritz-Silverstein D. Gender differences in cognitive function with age: The Rancho Bernardo Study. J Am Geriatr Soc 1999; 47: 159–64.

93. Meyer PM, Powell LH, Wilson RS et al. A population-based longitudinal study of cognitive functioning in the menopausal transition. Neurology 2003; 61: 801–6.

94. Jacobs DM, Tang MX, Stern Y et al. Cognitive function in nondemented older women who took estrogen after menopause. Neurology 1998; 50: 368–73.

95. Philips S, Sherwin BB. Effects of estrogen on memory function in surgically menopausal women. Psychoneuroendocrinology 1992; 17: 485–95.

96. Sherwin BB, Philips S. Estrogen and cognitive functioning in surgically menopausal women. Ann NY Acad Sci 1990; 592: 474–5.

97. Barrett-Connor E, Kritz-Silverstein D. Estrogen replacement therapy and cognitive function in older women. JAMA 1993; 269: 2637–41.

98. Rice MM, Graves AB, McCurry SM, Larson EB. Estrogen replacement therapy and cognitive function in postmenopausal women without dementia. Am J Med 1997; 103 (3A): 26S–35S.

99. Shaywitz SE, Shaywitz BA, Pugh KR et al. Effect of estrogen on brain activation patterns in postmenopausal women during working memory tasks. JAMA 1999; 281: 1197–202.

100. Dunkin J, Rasgon N, Wagner-Steh K, David S, Altschuler L, Rapkin A. Reproductive events modify the effects of estrogen replacement therapy on cognition in healthy postmenopausal women. Psychoneuroendocrinology 2005; 30: 284–96.

101. Buckwalter JG, Crooks VC, Robins SB, Petitti DB. Hormone use and cognitive performance in women of advanced age. J Am Geriatr Soc 2004; 52: 182–6.

102. Mitchell JL, Cruickshanks KJ, Klein BE, Palta M, Nondahl DM. Postmenopausal hormone therapy and its association with cognitive impairment. Arch Intern Med 2003; 163: 2485–90.

103. Whitmer RA, Haan MN, Miller JW, Yaffe K. Hormone replacement therapy and cognitive performance: the role of homocysteine. J Gerontol 2003; 58A: 324–30.

104. Luine V, McEwen BS. Sex differences in cholinergic enzymes of diagonal band nuclei in the rat preoptic area. Neuroendocrinology 1983; 36: 475–82.

105. Gould E, Wooley C, Franfurt M, McEwen BS. Gonadal steroids regulate pyramidal cells in dendritic spine density in hippocampal adulthood. J Neurosci 1990; 10: 1286–91.

106. Singh M, Meyer EM, Huang FS et al. Ovariectomy reduces CHAT activity and NGF MRNA levels in the frontal cortex and hippocampus of the female Sprague-Dawley rat. Abstr Soc Neurosci 1993; 19: 1254.

107. Singh M, Meyer EM, Simpkins JW. The effect of ovariectomy and estradiol replacement on brain derived neurotrophic factor messenger ribonucleic acid expression in cortical and hippocampal brain regions of female Sprague-Dawley rats. Endocrinology 1995; 136: 2320–4.

108. Simpkins JW, Meharvan S, Bishop J. The potential role for estrogen replacement therapy in the treatment of the cognitive decline and neurodegeneration associated with Alzheimer's disease. Neurobiol Aging 1994; 15: 195–7.

109. Arimatsu Y, Hatanaka H. Estrogen treatment enhances survival of cultured amygdala neurons in a defined medium. Dev Brain Res 1986; 26: 151–9.

110. Woolley CS, McEwen BS. Estradiol mediates fluctuation in hippocampal synapse density during the estrous cycle in the adult rat. J Neurosci 1992; 12: 2549–54.

111. Hagino N. Aged limbic system: interactions of estrogen with catecholaminergic and peptidergic synaptic transmissions. Biomed Res 1982: 85–108.

112. Arai Y, Matsumoto A, Nishizuka M. Synaptogenic action of estrogen on the hypothalamic arcuate nucleus (ARCN) of the developing rat brain and of the deafferented adult brain in female rats. In: Dorner G, Kawakami M (eds). Hormones and Brain Development, North Holland, Amsterdam: Elsevier: 43–8, 1978.

113. Goldman H, Skelley EB, Sandman CA et al. Hormones and regional blood flow. Pharmacol Biochem Behav 1976; 5 (Suppl 1): 165–9.

114. Toran-Allerand CD, Miranda RC, Betham WDL et al. Estrogen receptors co-localize with low-affinity nerve growth factor receptors in cholinergic neurons of the basal forebrain. Proc Natl Acad Sci USA 1992; 89: 4668–72.

115. Jaffe AB, Toran-Allerand CD, Greengard P, Gandy SE. Estrogen regulates metabolism of Alzheimer amyloid beta precursor protein. J Biochem 1994; 269: 13065–8.

116. Honjo H, Tanaka K, Kashiwagi T et al. Senile dementia – Alzheimer's type and estrogen. Horm Metab Res 1995; 27: 204–7.

117. Applebaum-Bowden D, McClean P, Steinmetz A et al. Lipoprotein, apolipoprotein, and lipolytic enzyme changes following estrogen administration in post menopausal women. J Lipid Res 1989; 30: 1895–906.

118. Bauer J, Ganter U, Strauss S et al. The participation of interleukin-6 in pathogenesis of Alzheimer's disease. Res Immunol 1992; 43: 650–7.

119. Ershler WB. Interleukin-6: a cytokine for gerontologists. J Am Geriatr Soc 1993; 41: 176–81.

120. Niki E, Nakano M. Estrogens as antioxidants. Meth Enzymol 1990; 186: 330–3.

121. Mooradian AD. Antioxidant properties of steriods. J Steriod Biochem Mol Biol 1993; 45: 509–11.

122. Gambassi G, Landi F, Bernabei R. Oestrogen and Alzheimer's disease [letter]. Lancet 1996; 348: 1029.

123. Belfort MA, Saade GR, Snabes M et al. Hormonal status affects the reactivity of the cerebral vasculature. Am J Obstet Gynecol 1995; 172: 1273–8.

124. Peskind ER, Wilkinson CW, Petrie EC, Schellenberg GD, Raskind MA. Increased CSF cortisol in AD is a function of APOE genotype. Neurology 2001; 56: 1094–8.

125. Zandi PP, Carlson MC, Plassman BL et al. Hormone replacement therapy and incidence of Alzheimer disease in older women. JAMA 2002; 288: 2123–9.

126. Grady D, Yaffe K, Kristof M, Lin F, Richards C, and Barrett-Connor E. Effect of postmenopausal hormone therapy on cognitive function: the Heart and estrogen/progestin replacement study. Am J Med 2002; 113: 543–8.

127. Wise PM, Dubal DB, Rau SW, Brown CM, Suzuki S. Are estrogens protective or risk factors in brain injury and neurodegeneration? Reevaluation after the Women's Health Initiative. Endocr Rev 2005; 26: 308–12.

128. Espeland MA, Rapp SR, Shukaker SA et al. Conjugated equine estrogens and global cognitive function in postmenopausal women: Women's Heath Initiative Memory Study. JAMA 2004; 291: 2959–68.

129. Shumaker SA, Legault C, Kuller L et al. Conjugated equine estrogens and incidence of probable dementia and mild cognitive impairment in postmenopausal women: Women's Health Initiative Memory Study. JAMA 2004; 291: 2947–58.

130. Speroff, L. Clinical appraisal of the Women's Health Initiative. J Obstet Gynaecol Res 2005; 31: 80–93.

131. Craig MC, Maki PM, Murphy DGM. The Women's Health Initiative Memory Study: findings and implications for treatment. Lancet Neurol 2005; 4: 190–4.

132. Asthana S. Estrogen and cognition: a true relationship? J Am Geriatr Soc 2004; 52: 316–18.

133. Schneider LS. Estrogen and dementia: Insights from the Women's Health Initiative Memory Study. JAMA 2004; 291: 3005–7.

134. The American College of Obstetricians and Gynecologists Women's Health Care Physicians. Cognition and dementia. Obstet Gynecol 2004; 10(4 Suppl): 25S–40S.

135. Rapp SR, Espeland MA, Shumaker SA et al. Effect of estrogen plus progestin on global cognitive function in postmenopausal women. The Women's Health

Initiative Memory Study: a randomized controlled trial. JAMA 2003; 28: 2663–72.

136. Wassertheil-Smoller S, Hendrix SL, Limacher M et al. Effect of estrogen plus progestin on stroke in post-menopausal women: The Women's Health Initiative: a randomized trial. JAMA 2003; 289: 2673–84.

137. Fillit H, Weinraub H, Cholst L et al. Observations in a preliminary open trial of estradiol therapy for senile dementia-Alzheimer's type. Psychoneuroendo-crinology 1986; 11: 337–45.

138. Honjo H, Ogino Y, Tanaka K et al. An effect of conju-gated estrogen to cognitive impairment in women with senile dementia – Alzheimer's type: a placebo controlled double blind study. J Menopause Soc 1993; 167–71.

139. Ohkura T, Isse K, Akazawa K, Hamamoto M et al. Evaluation of estrogen treatment in female patients with dementia of the Alzheimer's type. Endocr J 1994; 41: 361–71.

140. Paganini-Hill A, Henderson VW. Estrogen replace-ment therapy and risk of Alzheimer's disease. Arch Intern Med 1996; 156: 2213–17.

141. Brenner D, Kukull WA, Stergachis A et al. Postmenopausal estrogen replacement therapy and the risk of Alzheimer's disease: a population-based case-controlled study. Am J Epidemiol 1994; 140: 262–7.

142. Tang MX, Jacobs D, Stern Y, Marder K et al. Effects of estrogen during menopause on risk and age of onset of Alzheimer's disease. Lancet 1996; 348: 429–32.

143. Ohkura T, Isse K, Akazawa K, Hamamoto M et al. Long term estrogen replacement therapy in female patients with dementia of the Alzheimer's type: 7 case reports. Dementia 1995; 6: 99–107.

144. Schneider LS, Farlow MR, Henderson VW, Pogoda JM. Effects of estrogen replacement therapy on response to tacrine in patients with Alzheimer's disease. Neurology 1996; 46: 1580–4.

145. Marder K, Sano M. Estrogen to treat Alzheimer's dis-ease: too little, too late? So what's a woman to do? Neurology 2000; 2035–7.

146. Maki P. HRT and cognitive decline. Best Pract Res Clin Endocrinol Metab 2003; 17: 105–22.

# Chapter 16

# Gynecological oncology in the menopause

Martin A Martino and Hugh RK Barber

## INTRODUCTION

Menopause is a product of reproductive aging. Aging is one of the facts of life, it occurs both day and night. How women deal with aging during the menopause will prepare them medically, intellectually, and spiritually for 'the geripause.' Geripause was first described by Eskin to be the time in a woman's life after the menopause from the ages 65 years and above.[1] With the average female life expectancy steadily on the rise, nearly half of a women's life will include the menopausal/geripausal years. For these reasons, it is important to review some of the major malignancies that these females present with as well as to describe the recent approaches to managing women during this important time. In this chapter, we will describe some of the most common gynecological malignancies such as breast cancer, ovarian cancer, uterine cancer, and vulvar/vaginal cancer. Further, we will describe the recent advances in minimally invasive surgery and its potential role in gynecological oncology. Finally, we will conclude with an insight into the direction that cancer-related care is heading, from translational research, to the clinical setting and unique approaches to the management of gynecologic malignancies in the 21st century with techniques such as gene expression profiling.

## WHAT IS CANCER?

Cancer is, by definition, the unrestricted growth of cells.[2] The understanding of this growth cycle expanded when p53 was named in 1993 by the journal Science as the 'molecule of the year'.[3] TP53 is a tumor suppressor gene which interacts in a complex mechanism with other genes and proteins. For simplicity, p53 functions as the 'brakes' on the cell cycle. These brakes are released through genetic alterations or mutations. The 'gas' on the cell cycle is provided through proto-oncogenes, cytokines, and growth factors that signal a cell to continue to divide. While the balance between proto-oncogenes and tumor suppressor genes is believed to be involved in the regulation of the cell cycle and growth, there is much more to learn about the specific molecular characteristics of each tumor.

## SCREENING FOR GYNECOLOGICAL CANCERS IN THE MENOPAUSE

Aging is a risk factor for many malignancies. The roles of the physician and nurse clinicians are to not only manage presenting problems such as a pelvic mass or postmenopausal bleeding, but to offer comprehensive care individualized to each patient. Often, patients are unsure as to the time of their last screening mammography or colonoscopy. They may remember their last Pap smear, but that might be years ago, since they might have heard that a Pap smear after a hysterectomy is not necessary. Unfortunately, patients are hearing the message 'you may not need a Pap smear', and equating this with ceasing routine gynecological annual care. Let's be clear about this, there remain unquestionably many health benefits that are important to wellness care that are provided at the time of the annual exam.

## Breast mammography

The first and foremost benefit is that the patient maintains communication with their physician so that general cancer screening may be performed. The American Cancer Society recommends women over the age of 40 years to have annual mammography performed to screen for breast cancer.[4] Females who are in their 20s and 30s should do self-breast examinations monthly and have a clinical breast examination (CBE) as part of a periodic (regular) health examination by a health professional at least every three years. After age 40 years, women should have a breast examination by a health professional every year.

## Colon cancer screening

The American Cancer Society recommends that patients over the age of 50 years are encouraged to consider screening with a colonoscopy every 10 years, unless hereditary non-polyposis colorectal cancer (HNPCC) or familiar polyposis coli are prevalent in a patient's family history, in which case these patients should undergo closer screening and examination.[4] Further, they recommend annual fecal occult blood testing with a flexible sigmoidoscopy at least every five years. Future screening tests are under development, to determine the most cost-effective method to screen for a large population.

## Cervical cancer screening

The Pap smear has been responsible for dramatically lowering the cause-specific mortality from cervical cancer. Unfortunately, many patients presenting with cervical cancer do not report a recent cervical smear within the past year. The early identification of disease with increased surveillance by colposcopy are important components in the management of cervical dysplasia. The human papillomavirus (HPV) vaccine in women appears to have great promise and the Food and Drugs Administration (FDA) may approve a vaccine for use to attempt to decrease the overall incidence of cervical cancer. Further, the National Institutes of Health (NIH) have recently granted 10 million dollars to researchers at the H Lee Moffitt Cancer Center to study the role of the HPV vaccine in men.

## Ovarian cancer screening

Seventy-five per cent of women with ovarian cancer present at an advanced stage with an unfortunate 5-year survival between 30% and 40%. There is presently no reliable screening test to evaluate either the urine or the serum for ovarian cancer. CA-125 remains useful in the management of disease after diagnosis, but it is not a screening test for ovarian cancer. The combination of CA-125, ultrasound, and pelvic examination have also been evaluated, however, the benefits of this remain to be unclear in the literature. In 1998, lysophosphatidic acid (LPA) was reported in the Journal of the American Medical Association by Xu et al as a potential serum biomarker for early detection of ovarian cancer.[5] In 2004, Sutphen et al, at the Moffitt Cancer Center evaluated 117 patients with pre-operative serum levels in a controlled setting.[6] The combination of 16:0-LPA and 20:4-LPA yielded the best discrimination between preoperative case samples and control samples, with 93.1% correct classification, 91.1% sensitivity, and 96.3% specificity. Research with LPA and other serum biomarkers including serum proteonomics may produce a suitable test, but this is still investigational.

The future for prevention and early detection appears to involve nanotechnology, where the NIH have recently made large commitments to develop core centers to focus on this new field. The NIH intend researchers to combine engineering, mathematics, physics, chemistry, and biology, and integrate these disciplines with medicine to find a potential new biomarker. In conclusion, there is presently no commercially available screening test for ovarian cancer and we for the present time we continue to recommend an annual physical examination to attempt to identify any new pelvic masses or signs on physical examination.

## Uterine cancer screening

Uterine cancer is the most common gynecological malignancy in females, with over 36 000 cases being diagnosed in 2004 in the US. The most common clinical presenting sign is postmenopausal vaginal bleeding. Since over 95% of uterine cancers are in women over the age of 40 years, it is imperative for the physician to perform an endometrial sampling to rule out endometrial cancer, as this is often the earliest sign of disease. Recent investigations and attempts have been made to evaluate the usefulness of transvaginal ultrasound in identifying early disease, however, the studies are still not clearly in favor of this screening mechanism. There have been no randomized studies performed looking at screening uterine cancer, and there do not appear to be any being planned. Further, the American Cancer Society does not recommend any methods of annual screening for uterine cancer. Even in women on tamoxifen, ultrasound is not recommended to screen for the possibility of malignancy in this high-risk group. The best present methods are to use the known risk factors such as obesity, nulliparity, diabetes mellitus, and unopposed estrogen exposure. When these risk factors are present, the most beneficial thing physicians can do is to directly ask their patients whether they have had any irregular bleeding, and, if so, then proceed to sampling. Often simply asking the correct questions will lead to the right diagnosis. In the future, perhaps molecular markers may be identified through microarray help to identify a panel of genes which may predict the development of uterine cancer. One such gene we are aware of is *HNPCC*. Studies indicate that patients with this genetic predisposition have at least a 10-fold increased risk of uterine cancer by age 70 years. In this select population, yearly endometrial sampling is recommended, and perhaps hysterectomy for prophylactic measures.

## Vulvar/vaginal cancer screening

Vulvar and vaginal cancer is predominantly a disease which presents itself in geripausal years. Often times, diagnostic delay both due to the physician and the patient lead to an invasive malignancy. Primary treatment of early-stage disease involves surgical management with evaluation of lymph nodes in the groin and/or pelvis, to determine the appropriate stage of disease. While there are no reliable screening tests available, routine gynecological care on an annual basis may often allow patients and physicians to identify early lesions that warrant further evaluation. Annual examinations are necessary for physicians to identify these lesions even after a hysterectomy

might have been done, and this is perhaps the best screening method we presently have available.

# GYNECOLOGICAL CANCERS

## The ovary

Ovarian cancer is the leading cause of death from gynecological cancer. It is one of the most challenging issues in gynecological oncology. Often it is not possible to make an early diagnosis, as evidenced by the fact that 60–70% of patients are already in stages III and IV when they present for initial examination and treatment. The overall survival rate for the truly invasive epithelial ovarian cancers is seldom better than 25% 5-year survival, though with optimal debulking surgery and platinum-based chemotherapy this appears to be closer to 40%. Ovarian tumors have a complex classification, but may be considered under the headings of gonadal–stromal, germ cell, mixed, common epithelial ovarian cancer, and metastatic tumors. The greatest number of cases of common epithelial ovarian cancer occur between the ages of 50 and 70 years, with a peak incidence of occurrence at about age 77 years. It is obvious that the ovary becomes too old to function, but never becomes too old to form a cancer.

While it has been stated that there are no early symptoms of ovarian cancer, reports in the literature contradict this statement. A great number of women with ovarian cancer have vague abdominal complaints for a long time before the diagnosis is made. Many of these women have had a thorough work-up, including barium enema and gastrointestinal series, computed tomography (CT) scan or magnetic resonance imaging (MRI), but a serious attempt at a pelvic or rectal examination has not been carried out. It is important, therefore, to rule out ovarian cancer in any woman over 40 years, particularly one who is nulliparous, or has a history of involuntary sterility or multiple spontaneous abortions, and who presents with vague abdominal symptoms. This is accomplished by careful attention to physical examination, and possibly a transvaginal ultrasound. If a pelvic mass is identified on examination, or the ultrasound has evidence of a complex adnexal mass, then referral to a gynecological oncologist is the proper management for these patients. The routine use of tumor markers to pre-emptively screen patients is not that helpful prior to a diagnosis, and often creates additional anxiety for the patient. Understanding the role of CA-125 and its use is important for the practicing physician. This is a useful adjunct post-diagnosis to follow patients on treatment, and for clinical studies, but its utility as a screening tool has clearly not been proven.

Any woman who is postmenopausal and presents with a palpable ovary that is abnormal in size must have a careful work-up, and, if on repeat examination findings are confirmed, surgical exploration should be carried out without delay. This ovarian finding has been designated the postmenopausal palpable ovary syndrome. This syndrome does not refer to the small cysts that are found on ultrasound examination, and may be a normal finding in women as old as 80 years of age. In these patients, the risk of surgical mortality has been described to be as high as 10%, so judicious use of this means to make a diagnosis is necessary, since the risk factors are very high. These cysts often represent the last follicle left in the ovary, followed by connective tissue surrounding the cavity giving a small coin-like lesion.

Of the gonadal–stromal tumors, the granulosa theca cell tumor is the most important. These tumors occur at any age, but may become manifest during the climacteric with the average age at 52 years. About 65% occur in the postmenopausal period. Probably as a result of their frequent hormone production, numerous associated conditions are found along with these tumors, and include such entities as endometrial carcinoma, leiomyomas, breast carcinoma, and mammary dysplasia. Approximately 25% of these tumors are functioning, and about 25% are malignant. The bilaterality rate is about 5%. The Sertoli–Leydig cell tumor is associated with masculinization when it functions, but only about 25% do so. They have a malignancy rate of about 25% and about 5% are bilateral. When the gonadal–stromal tumors appear in the menopausal and postmenopausal years, the proper treatment involves a surgical staging, with a total hysterectomy, bilateral salpingoooophorectomy, cytological washing, and omentectomy as deemed in the best interest of the patients. The benefit of lymphadenectomy is left to the discretion of the gynecological oncologist.

The germ cell tumors usually occur in the childbearing years, and most commonly occur from birth to age 20 years. They are seldom seen in the postmenopausal period, but, when they are diag-nosed at this time, referral to a gynecological oncologist for treatment options are recommended. The Gynecologic Oncology Group (GOG) has performed several studies evaluating the role of triple agent chemotherapy, and at present bleomycin, etoposide, and platinum is recommended.[7] The ovary is unique in that not only does it give rise to a great number of primary tumors and malignancies, but it is also itself a recipient of metastases from a variety of organs. Since breast and colon cancers are among the leading killers of women from cancer and have a propensity for metastasizing to the ovary, it is important to do a very thorough evaluation in any patient suspected of having ovarian cancer. Although all metastatic tumors to the ovary are referred to as Krükenberg, this is not strictly correct. The Krükenberg tumor is usually a metastatic tumor that involves both ovaries, giving them a kidney-shaped appearance, and, on microscopic examination, has a characteristic signet ring cell dispersed with an inactively responsive connective tissue. The usual primary is somewhere along the gastrointestinal tract, most often the stomach, particularly the pyloric end.

The treatment for common epithelial ovarian cancer is surgical removal of the uterus, tubes, ovary, omentum, and appendix, and possible lymph node sampling. The surgery should be aggressive without creating inordinate morbidity and mortality. For the common epithelial ovarian cancer, the adjuvant treatment of choice is a combination of anticancer chemotherapy, and the drugs most often employed are Carboplatin (platinum) and Taxol® (paclitaxel). With GOG 158, Carboplatin and Taxol became the standard frontline therapy in treatment.[8]

In January, 2006, the National Cancer Institute issued a clinical alert to co-incide with the publication of GOG 172 which recommended Intraperitoneal Therapy as a preferred treatment for Optimally debulked stage 3C patients. This study identified a 16 month improvement in survival when compared to 24 hour taxol with cisplatin. A debate continue as to whether or not to evaluate 3 hour taxol and Carboplatin with the preferred treatment arm of GOG 172(IP chemotherapy consisting of Day 1 IV taxol, Day 2 IP Cisplatin, Day 8 IP Taxol every 3 weeks.[9]

In addition to this study, the GOG has recently completed accrual of GOG 182 which evaluates five arms in a doublet regimen, and these results are being evaluated to determine if our firstline treatment will change. (www.gog.org) In the second line, options are generally based on whether the patient is considered platinum-resistant or -sensitive. In the platinum-resistant patient, there appears to be equivalency between doxil and topotecan, and thus the use depends on the side-effects and the patient/physician preference. However, with the platinum-sensitive group, controversy remains as to whether retreatment with a platinum/taxane is better than either single agent platinum, doxil, or other regimens. Doxil and topotecan have recently been evaluated by Gordon et al, and reports indicate that in the platinum-sensitive patient, doxil may have a greater benefit compared to topotecan, but this is still being evaluated.[10]

## The Fallopian tube

Primary adenocarcinoma of the Fallopian tube accounts for less than 1% of the malignant neoplasms of the female genital tract. However, the true incidence is difficult to assess as, in many cases, the primary site of origin of the neoplasm cannot be determined. Some cases of ovarian and endometrial cancer spread to the Fallopian tube. Although the reverse is also true, lesions of ambiguous origin are not usually assigned to the tube, in view of the greater frequency of ovarian and uterine carcinoma.

Fallopian tube adenocarcinoma usually occurs in postmenopausal patients between the ages of 45 and 55 years. Approximately 60% of patients are infertile, which may be the result of the pre-existing inflammation. The tumors are usually asymptomatic until they infiltrate locally or metastasize. The patient may then present with a triad of pain, serosanguinous or watery vaginal discharge, or frank bleeding. Any adnexal mass in postmenopausal patients should suggest the possibility of ovarian or tubal carcinoma. The spread is similar to that found with the common epithelial ovarian cancer and the same treatment is employed for carcinoma of the tube as is employed for carcinoma of the ovary.

## The uterus

The uterus undergoes retrogressive changes and becomes small and atrophic. Leiomyomas tend to atrophy, although they may still present problems. There are many causes for postmenopausal genital bleeding, but endometrial carcinoma must be ruled out when it occurs in this age group.

Bleeding may be a result of estrogen therapy, a collection of bloody fluid in the endometrial cavity bursting through an occluded cervix, an estrogen-producing ovarian tumor, a lesion of the vagina or vulva, or coital, instrumental or digital trauma. Whatever the presumed cause, it is mandatory that such procedures as are necessary be performed to exclude endometrial cancer or other genital cancer. Endometrial biopsies and lavages are often ill-suited for study in the endometrium of the postmenopausal patient. The use of ultrasound to measure the thickness of the endometrium may help in making the diagnosis. If there is any question, the patient should be hospitalized in an ambulatory setting and, under anesthesia, have a careful pelvic examination and a dilation and curettage. Carcinoma of the endometrium ranks as the fifth most common cause of death in women in whom cancer develops and who are 75 years of age or older. Diabetes mellitus, obesity, certain ovarian tumors and hypertension are among the risk factors for uterine cancer. Any treatment with estrogens, anticoagulants or a number of other medications, as well as the possibility of blood dyscrasias, should always be included in the differential diagnosis. In patients who are unable to distinguish bleeding from the urethra, vagina or anal canal, it may be necessary to perform cystoscopy and sigmoidoscopy, in addition to investigating the reproductive tract.

The management of endometrial cancer has evolved from using preoperative radiation followed by hysterectomy to doing surgery as an initial procedure, and then making a decision about the type and extent of external radiation. The Society of Gynecologic Oncology recommends that any patient with a diagnosis of uterine cancer be managed by a gynecological oncologist, due to the increased complexities of management scenarios. Recently, GOG 99 and the PORTEC studies were released which defined the rates of recurrence matched with risk factors such as age, grade, and stage.[11,12] There is no question that brachytherapy has reduced the number of vaginal vault recurrences. Thus, patients with carcinoma of the endometrium may be given brachytherapy, however the decision for pelvic radiation in the management of early uterine cancer is left to the decision between the patient, the radiation oncologist, and the gynecological oncologist. The use of postoperative chemotherapy or radiation for the treatment of intermediate risk Stage IC uterine cancers are still being evaluated.

The advent of laparoscopy and its application to gynecological oncology are discussed elsewhere in this chapter. However, the role in management of uterine cancers via the laparoscope have been directly addressed by the GOG in the GOGLAP2 study which is now complete, and results are pending. This was a phase III study of over 2500 patients with patients randomized to either a laparotomy with hysterectomy, bilateral salpingoophorectomy (BSO) and lymph node dissection (LND) or a laparoscopic approach with a laparoscopic assisted hysterectomy, BSO and LND.

## The cervix

The histology of the cervix is quite different from that of the corpus with regard to its epithelium, glands, and stroma. The epithelium is of two varieties, the stratified squamous, and the glandular–columnar. The stratified squamous epithelium lines the pars vaginalis or portio, and it has inconspicuous subepithelial papillae and no cornification. This epithelium extends to the external os with some variation of demarcation line. The glandular–columnar epithelium is tall, non-ciliated, and picket-fence in appearance, and within the endocervical canal. Nuclei are deeply stained and basal, and the cytoplasm, which is rich in mucins, stains faintly basophilic or is neutral and unstained. The transition zone, of vital importance clinically with respect to carcinoma of the cervix, may be gradual or abrupt. In the postmenopausal patient, the squamocolumnar junction is found higher in the endocervical canal than is generally seen in the premenopausal patient.

The cervix presents an atrophic picture similar to the vulva and the vagina in the postmenopausal patient. The cervix shrinks to become flush with the vaginal vault and presents as a relatively avascular fibrous nodule; the cervical canal may become stenosed. Vaginal bleeding is a signal for further evaluation of the patient. Bleeding may occur as a result of atrophic vaginitis, with or without infection, or benign polyps of the cervix, but cervical cancer can and does occur in the elderly population, and cervical smears, colposcopic examination, biopsies, and possibly fractional curettage are indicated if the lesion is present on the cervix, or cervical smear shows abnormal cytological findings.

Cervical erosion, ulcer, and ectropion are three conditions that become increasingly important with aging. In erosion of the acquired type, there is a loss of superficial layers of the epithelium by a local destructive influence which may be unclear etiologically. It may be the result of pH change, or bacterial toxicity, or a combination of the two.

The basal cuboidal cells have been exposed. A congenital form of erosion may also be a pathogenetic factor. Cervical ectropion is manifested by an inflamed and edematous endocervical mucosa, which hangs out of the endocervical canal and is easily visible. True cervical ulcers present gross and histological findings as with any ulcer. There is complete loss of epithelium, revealing a base of more or less active granulation tissue, with an increasingly fibrous base with time.

Non-specific cervicitis is extremely common and often afflicts almost every multiparous female. A variety of organisms have been implicated. The non-specific cervicitis most commonly results from child-bearing, instrumentation, pH change, contaminating coitus, estrogen depletion, cervical eversion and others. Chlamydia is starting to be found in the menopausal and postmenopausal patient, as well as in the young patient. This is also true of HPV. Occasionally, herpes simplex type 2 may cause a lesion on the cervix. The increasing incidence of chlamydia, HPV and herpes simplex virus 2 being found in the vagina and on the cervix of the menopausal and postmenopausal woman may represent a change in lifestyle today.

Whereas carcinoma in situ of the cervix occurs premenopausally, the average age being 38 years, the invasive phase of this disease affects women with a peak occurrence in the 40–49 year range, after which the rate remains constant with advancing age. However, in the past few years, it has been found that the incidence of carcinoma in situ of the cervix appears to be increasing in the postmenopausal period. Again, this may be the result of a change in lifestyle.

Invasive cancer of the cervix is encountered less often in the postmenopausal patient than in the younger patient. Elderly patients should be examined for cervical carcinoma just as they were premenopausally. In patients under 70 years, with a stage IB or IIA carcinoma, radical hysterectomy and pelvic node dissection is usually chosen unless there is a medical contraindication.

However, in stages IIB, III and IV, chemotherapy and radiation therapy are the treatment of choice.

## The vulva

The vulvar and vaginal tissues of most women who are several years postmenopausal, and who are not on estrogen replacement therapy are more or less atrophic. The vulva presents an atrophic appearance, and there is loss of subcutaneous fat and hair. The labia tend to blend into the surrounding skin. The shrinkage, loss of elasticity and dryness of vaginal mucosa are due to estrogen withdrawal. Puckering of the vulvar tissue with atrophy of the introitus, even in multiparous women, may make penile intromission exquisitely painful, and deflection of the penis anteriorly by a rigid perineum may create pressure on the urethral meatus causing urethritis, local inflammation, and dysuria. Loss of, or graying of, pubic hair is often psychologically traumatic to these women. An attempt must be made to assure them that it is a normal process and has no pathological significance.

Many vulvar diseases are similar in different age groups. In the postmenopausal and geripausal patient, there are increases in the incidence of diabetic vulvitis, hypotrophic dystrophy, and lichen sclerosus. Patients with these lesions often present with burning, pruritus or difficulty in coitus. Intertrigo is frequently seen in obese, postmenopausal patients who have difficultly in bathing and cleansing their perineums and vulvae. As a consequence, the skin covering their perineums, genital crura folds, labia majora, and thighs is constantly moistened by preparations, and soiled by urine. Those with intertrigo usually complain of perineal itching and burning. Inspection shows the area to be superficially denuded, shiny, hyperemic and moist; a scanty, malodorous discharge may cover the affected areas. Treatment is best effected by good hygiene, clearing up any infection with a bactericidal cream, or fungi with an antimycotic cream. After the area has been cleared of any irritation and infection, the patient may protect herself by using cornstarch in the area.

Senile angiomata are small, usually multiple, up to 3 mm in diameter, red, elevated papules that bleed freely when scrubbed or scratched. They are quite innocent, but the bleeding caused when they are traumatized frightens patients. This usually occurs after a hot bath when the area is vigorously rubbed with a bath towel. Angiomata and telangiectasias are not excised unless the patient is unduly alarmed or disturbed by their presence. They can then be treated by laser therapy.

Sebaceous cysts of the vulva form small, rarely 1 cm diameter, yellowish-gray nodules in the skin covering the labia. The foul-smelling, purulent material extruded when a sebaceous cyst becomes infected and ruptured, as is often the case, or the discovery of a small lump in the vulva, may be quite disturbing to the patient. Very large sebaceous cysts that become repeatedly infected should be removed. Clitoral phimosis may cause an inspissated smegma to collect beneath the prepuce, producing discomfort. The area is usually very red and resembles balanitis in men. Persistence of the inflamed area is treated surgically by making an incision over the top of the prepuce, and removing the inspissated smegma.

The urethral caruncle is a small, reddened, sensitive, fleshy outgrowth at the urethral meatus. Most represent an ectropion of the urethra or infections at the urethral meatus. Occasionally there are vascular anomalies, or benign or malignant neoplasms, which may also cause caruncle formation. The vast majority of caruncles are benign, but any persistent lesion which becomes progressively larger must be biopsied and treated according to the findings. The caruncles may occur at any age, but postmenopausal women are most commonly affected.

The vulvar dystrophies are a group of conditions characterized by disordered growth, sometimes disordered maturation, of the vulvar squamous epithelium. Their etiology is unknown, although recently an association between vulvar dystrophy and achlorhydria has been demonstrated, and a papillomavirus has been identified in some cases. A rationalized and simplified classification and nomenclature of vulvar dystrophies has been established. It includes lichen sclerosus, hypertrophic dystrophy, and mixed dystrophy.

Dystrophic lesions appear as white patches in the epithelium known as leukoplakia. In addition, the mucocutaneous tissue becomes dry, shriveled and brittle, a condition clinically known as kraurosis vulvae. These are clinical terms, similar to dystrophy, used to describe the gross appearance of the lesion. They do not indicate specific pathological disease entities. Leukoplakia can be caused by a wide variety of abnormalities other than dystrophy. The diagnosis of specific conditions depends largely on careful histological evaluation.

White lesions of the vulva were once treated as a group. They were considered premalignant. The white appearance of the lesion is due to the keratin, a deep pigmentation and relative avascularity. All three of these mechanisms are present in the vulvar dystrophies. It is now recognized that white lesions of the vulva are not premalignant or malignant. Much of the confusion in the past resulted from the fact that there was no uniform terminology.

The skin of the vulva consists of two parts: dermis and epidermis, which interact and, therefore, modify each other. Each group does not necessarily respond to the same nutritional or other conditioning patterns. Estrogen lack has little effect on vulvar epidermis. However, it has a considerable effect on the dermis, reversing fibrosis and shrinking of the introitus and loss of fat from the labia majora. The vulva is not part of the integument. Embryologically, from the mons pubis to the anus, it is an organ. Its lymphatic drainage and blood supply are its own, and not merged with those of the surrounding skin, although they are related in varying degrees to the connecting vaginal mucosa.

Relief may be obtained by using the following method: place a folded paper tissue in the freezing part of the refrigerator and coat it with plain yogurt; it can be applied to the vulva and will give relief without causing an ice burn. It has no direct therapeutic value. Based on clinical and histological characteristics, the vulvar dystrophies may be subdivided into three groups: lichen sclerosus, hyperplastic and mixed. In the latter two groups, it may occur with or without atypia.

### Lichen sclerosus

Lichen sclerosus is the most common of the three groups of white lesions. It usually occurs in postmenopausal patients, but it can affect persons of all ages, including children. Clinical examination reveals the skin of the vulva to be thin, atrophic, parchment-like, dry, and white or yellow. The final diagnosis should be made on histological examination.

Lichen sclerosus is best treated with testosterone applications, which result in some epithelial activation, perhaps by blocking chalone receptor sites or by simply activating the growth potential and increasing the blood supply to the epithelium. Current reports indicate that testos-

terone is metabolized in much larger quantities in skin from lichen sclerotic patients than in normal vulvar skin. Although not always successful, testosterone ointment can be applied freely for 2–3 weeks, then once or twice a week, or more frequently if the pruritus returns, and finally is needed to promote patient comfort. Testosterone propionate ointment has its greatest benefit when there is burning rather than itching. Judicious use of corticosteroid ointment may help to reduce the disturbing edema of the prepuce and clitoris, but if it is continued for any length of time it may be dangerous because the thin skin is then easily ulcerated. Testosterone propionate 2% is made up in white petrolatum in 60 g units.

### Hyperplastic dystrophy

Hyperplastic dystrophy is also called hyperplastic vulvitis, neurodermatitis, and leukokeratosis. The resulting clinical picture is one of thickening and lightening of the vulva and adjacent skin. Unlike lichen sclerosus, the perineal and perianal areas are seldom affected. Pruritus is almost always present and, owing to the uncontrollable urge to scratch, changes occur in the primary lesion.

Since these patients present with marked itching, therapy must be directed towards controlling this symptom. It is important to teach the patient proper hygiene. Any soap with detergent should be excluded. For example, Ivory® soap is very alkaline and dries the area, and aggravates the itching and burning. The patient should be instructed to use baby soap or Neutrogena®. The tense, nervous patient, particularly one whose focus is on the vulvar itching, should be treated with a mild tranquilizer for a short period of time. Atarax® (hydropyzine hydrochloride) is used widely among dermatologists as an adjuvant treatment for itching. Topical corticosteroids provide the backbone for treatment. They should be applied twice a day. Although the itching is controlled rather rapidly, it takes about 6–8 weeks before any visible change is seen in the gross lesion. Patients who do not respond to the corticosteroids should have cream made up of eurax and corticosteroids, consisting of 30% eurax and 70% corticosteroids, and should be made up in 60 g lots. The cream should be applied twice daily until the itching is controlled. The patient can then resume using topical corticosteroids and switch to the eurax and corticosteroid combination only when the itching is bad. Burning is best treated with testosterone propionate 2% in white petrolatum. Progesterone in oil 400 mg in 4 oz aquaphor has been successfully used in most cases of dystrophy that were unresponsive or unsuited to testosterone.

## Mixed dystrophy

Approximately 15% of all cases of vulvar dystrophy show a mixed pattern. Both lichen sclerosus and hyperplastic dystrophy can be found on the same vulva, and constitute the condition known as mixed dystrophy. In studying these lesions, some areas show the gross and microscopic features of lichen sclerosus, while others show the features of hyperplastic dystrophy. A wrinkled, parchment-like appearance usually signifies an area of lichen sclerosus, and heaped-up white plaque is usually associated with a hyperplasia. It is important to take multiple biopsy specimens from these lesions. In a differential diagnosis, lichen sclerosus with hyperkeratotic plaques, superimposed fungal infections and carcinoma in situ must be considered.

The management is similar to that of other dystrophies. Attention should be given to soap, underclothes and personal hygiene. Pantyhose seem to aggravate the problem. The vulva should be treated with corticosteroids and, when the hyperplastic areas disappear, it may be necessary to treat the lichen sclerosus with 2% testosterone propionate in petrolatum base. The corticosteroids and testosterone preparations may have to be alternated. In order to control the itching in some resistant cases, it may be necessary to give alcohol injections, but this is very infrequent. Laser therapy has been employed in some of these patients, but there are not enough data to determine its value accurately.

## Vitiligo

Vitiligo may occur in the vulva. It is usually associated with a generalized condition of the skin. It may occur early in life and is seen more often in the female than in the male. Hyperkeratosis presents clinically as elevated, thickened patches of white skin or mucosa. Chronic inflammatory lesions may become hypertrophic because of the irritation from scratching. Senile atrophy occurs in elderly women. It is usually accompanied by shrinkage and by very dry, thin tissue, often with multiple telangiectasias present.

## Carcinoma in situ

Carcinoma in situ of the vulva is perhaps the most puzzling dystrophy, and the one which the physi-

cian relates to carcinoma of the cervix, to which it bears a superficial relationship. The possibility exists that carcinoma in situ is a sexually transmitted disease, at least in an associated or triggering role. Carcinoma in situ of the vulva may be either unifocal or multifocal, two-thirds being multifocal. Whether this represents exposure to persistent carcinogens on the one hand, or a single stimulus on the other, is unclear. It is important to rule out microinvasion or frank invasion in any vulvar lesion.

The treatment of in situ lesions may be observation, removal or destruction. However, it is important to make certain of the diagnosis by using a biopsy technique to document the histology. Although the treatment of carcinoma in situ has gone through many phases from simple vulvectomy, skinning procedures or applications of 5-fluorouracil, the use of laser surgery is now playing an increasingly important role in the management of these lesions.

In addition to in situ carcinomas, there is at least a 20%, probably greater, association of the vulvae with malignancies in other organs that are perhaps quite unrelated. The cervix is the most common site, but the breast and gut are also common.

## Paget's disease

Paget's disease is not truly a dystrophy; however, as it is a hyperplastic change within the epithelium and is confined by the basement membrane, it is considered in the in situ category. Pruritus is predominant as a symptom, and soreness comes much later. It should not be confused with fungal infestation which causes soreness and redness of the vulva. The typical picture is a velvety red background with white patches scattered throughout the area. It is important that a biopsy be taken that is deep enough to encompass the epidermis and dermis, so that a sweat gland or Bartholin's gland cancer is not missed. Having made an accurate diagnosis of carcinoma in situ, the patient with Paget's disease can be treated as any other in situ patient, with wide local excision. The biopsy must be carried down through the dermis so that the invasive cancer is not missed. The breasts must be carefully evaluated as there may be a concomitant breast lesion.

Primary malignant disease of the vulva represents about 5–10% of female cancers. The most common lesion is epidermoid cancer, which may be invasive or intraepithelial, and is primarily seen in women aged well over age 60 years.

Epithelial dysplasia coexists with about 50% of invasive cancers, and is considered by many oncologists to be a premalignant vulvar disease. A second primary malignancy affecting the cervix, breast or uterus is found in about 50% of patients, often in association with a primary vulvar neoplasm. It is obvious that these patients should have careful evaluation with biopsy. Treatment of invasive cancer of the vulva is primarily surgical, with radical or modified radical excisional vulvectomy and inguinal node dissection. Sentinel lymph node biopsy is still under clinical investigation and being evaluated by the GOG. The decision about excision of the deep nodes is usually left to the responsible surgeon. Radiotherapy is reserved to treat the deep nodes in the pelvis.

## The vagina

The reduction of estrogen support for the vaginal tissues is responsible for most of the common symptoms associated with vaginal disorders. The vaginal epithelium is thin and relatively avascular and inelastic; rugae disappear and the epithelium presents a dry, glazed appearance. These conditions cause no discomfort for many patients, but those who are sexually active may complain of dyspareunia, even if they had no coital distress when they were younger.

The most common symptoms suggestive of vaginal disease are leukorrhea, frequency and urgency of urination, dyspareunia, itching, and bleeding. In this age group, 80% of the patients studied cytologically are estrogen deficient. Older patients who complain of these symptoms may have no findings other than those associated with atrophic vaginitis. In the absence of a proven pathogen, the most common treatment for atrophic vaginitis is topical estrogen cream. This should be carried out for at least one month. The patient should be instructed to insert about one-quarter of an applicator of estrogen cream into the vagina every third or fourth night, for approximately 2 months. Inserting a full applicator of cream usually results in some of the cream running out. Having been mixed with vaginal secretion, it may cause a marked irritation around the vulva.

Trichomonas vaginalis and occasionally candida may be superimposed upon some atrophic vaginitis. The diagnosis should be made and, in addition to treating the atrophic vaginitis, trichomonas infestation should be treated with metronidazole for 10 days by mouth, or by metronidazole gel vaginally for 5 days, and the candida infestation treated with topical antifungal agent for approximately the same time. Postmenopausal patients are often helped by douching once a week with a half-cup of vinegar in approximately a liter of lukewarm water. This substitutes for the acidity of the normal vagina.

Women who have been treated for carcinoma in situ of the cervix by hysterectomy should have routine Pap smears, because the transformation zone has been found to extend to the vagina in 5% of normal women. Occasionally, in situ lesions will be identified in the vagina. These lesions should be biopsied and then treated. Treatment with 5-fluorouracil, laser surgery and surgical excision are usually the methods chosen. Having treated the patient, a structured regimen for Pap smears must be instituted.

Primary vaginal carcinoma is uncommon, accounting for less than 1% of cancers of the female reproductive tract. It is usually epidermoid, presenting as an ulcer high in the posterior vaginal fornix. Any persistent lesion of the vagina must be biopsied, and the decision then made about its management. In this age group, radiation therapy is usually the method of treatment chosen.

## The breast

Carcinoma of the breast is the second leading cause of death from cancer among women. There are approximately 215 900 new cases and 40 100 women are anticipated to die of the disease in 2004 in the US according the American Cancer Society. One woman in eight will develop a carcinoma of the breast by age 70 years. Although breast cancer is covered in another chapter in this book (see Chapter 19), it is important that attention be directed towards reducing breast cancer mortality. The principles that should be followed are:

1. breast examinations are an integral part routine gynecological examination for all patients
2. patients must receive instructions in the proper technique of lifelong periodic breast self-examination
3. proper ambulatory surgical facilities for performing breast biopsies must be developed
4. the final diagnosis of pathology rests on careful histological examination of a biopsy specimen (biopsy is recommended for all true, solid, three-dimensional masses)
5. research, both basic and clinical, and etiology, diagnosis, and treatment of breast lesions are

to be encouraged. Innovative screening programs for high-risk patients must be included in this effort. Residency training programs in obstetrics and gynecology must include specific instructions in early detection techniques of breast carcinoma, including biopsy examination. The American Cancer Society has monographs on the step-like fashion for breast examination by the physician, as well as monographs for the patient to learn breast self-examination (see www.cancer.org).

6. research should continue to be directed to evaluate designer estrogens (selective estrogen receptor modulators or SERMs) and their role in the prevention and treatment for the patient who has survived breast cancer

7. tamoxifen, the first known SERM has extended millions of lives by acting as an anti-estrogen in breast cancer. It is suggested, but not conclusive, that it may prevent breast cancer. Newer SERMs are being compared to tamoxifen such as raloxifen in the STAR Trial as this is nearing completion.

### The implications of the breast and ovarian cancer gene, BRCA

While 90% of cancers are due to sporadic genetic alterations at specific loci, at least 10% are due to a hereditary alteration passed on between family members until it is phenotypically expressed. Recently, Pal et al from the Moffitt Cancer Center have reported on the outcome of the Tampa Bay Ovarian Cancer Study, which was a prospective trial to determine the underlying incidence of BRCA in patients newly diagnosed with ovarian cancer.[13] There were over 15% of our patients carried a mutation in BRCA, with the majority of mutations presenting in BRCA1. Interestingly, family history was only positive in 70% of these patients, and hence not a very specific screening question to select whom to test. In light of these findings, and with the recent advances in minimally invasive surgery for prophylaxis, we believe it is important to refer all newly diagnosed patients to genetic counseling for consideration of testing. If there were not other options for management in the positive patient, then this may not be all that useful. However, the data are impressive that prophylactic surgery lowers the overall incidence for the development of breast and ovarian cancer.

The hereditary breast and ovarian cancer syndrome (HBOCS) may now be detected by examining serum for genetic alterations in the BRCA1 or BRCA2 gene. Patients with a BRCA1 mutation have a lifetime risk of up to 84% for the development of breast cancer, and up to a 40% risk for the development of ovarian cancer. Patients with a BRCA2 mutation have up to a 60% lifetime risk of developing breast cancer, and up to a 20% risk of developing ovarian cancer. With these increased lifetime risks, patients who have a family history of ovarian cancer or personal history of breast cancer are encouraged to see genetics counselors. After an evaluation, options now exist that may significantly lower their future risk of developing malignancy.

The options for patients who are BRCA-positive are best made after a detailed discussion regarding the present evidence published in the literature, and the subsequent rates of malignancy balanced with the complications of prophylactic procedures. Options include close observation with or without imaging, or prophylactic risk-reducing surgery. In the end, the final decision is left up to the patient and her family.

### Breast surgery

Large prospective trials have been performed to determine the effect of the strategy of risk-reducing surgery. The PROSE trial was reported in 2004.[14] In the study, Rebbeck et al reported on their study of 483 patients who were BRCA-postitve, to determine the outcome of risk-reducing surgery. Cases were patients who underwent prophylactic mastectomy ($n = 105$), and they were followed up over six years. During this time, only two cases of breast cancer were diagnosed. In matched controls, there were 184/378 patients who were diagnosed with breast cancer over a similar six-year period. This important study answers several questions. First, it comfirms that the lifetime risk of a BRCA patient developing breast cancer is indeed very high, as nearly 50% of these observation patients developed breast cancer over just six years. Second, it confirms that a risk-reducing strategy may reduce the risk of breast cancer by over 90%.

### Minimally invasive surgery and bilateral salpingo-oophorectomy (BSO)

Advances in molecular oncology and the development of cancer control and prevention centers within NCI Cancer Centers have resulted in growing numbers of women participating in genetic testing protocols. Recently, Kauff et al reported on the first prospective clinical trial in women with *BRCA1* and *BRCA2* genetic alterations.[15] This study identified that there was a significant benefit from prophylactic BSO in high-risk patients. In this prospective study involving 170 female patients, the estimated 5-year cancer-free estimates were 96% for the group ($n = 98$) choosing prophylactic BSO, and 69% for the group ($n = 72$) choosing intensive surveillance ($P = 0.006$). There were also three additional cases of early epithelial ovarian cancers diagnosed at the time of prophylactic surgery.

While prophylactic BSO may be considered an effective risk-reducing procedure, the benefit of adding hysterectomy to this procedure has been controversial. Reasons for this are unclear, however recent reports have identified *BRCA*-positive patients also may develop Fallopian tube carcinoma. Controversy remains as to what extent these patients may benefit from completing the intent of the risk-reducing procedure.

Powell et al asked an interesting study question: what is the detection rate of cancer in their 67 patients who underwent a risk-reducing BSO (RRSO) for mutations in *BRCA*?[16] Interestingly, their study stressed the importance of pathologists performing multiple serial sections on both the ovaries and Fallopian tubes. They identified 7/67 cases of early malignancy, but more concerning was that 4/7 had malignancy in the Fallopian tube. With this report identifying 10–17% of incidental pelvic malignancies at the time of RRSO, and with the majority of these cancers identified in the Fallopian tube, can one justify performing a complete risk-reducing surgery in a high-risk patient by doing only a BSO, and not including the remainder of the Fallopian tube that is within the uterine cornual region? Recently, Agoff et al reported that with a change to their pathological evaluation, two additional cases of BRCA-positive Fallopian tube carcinoma were identified.[17] This remains a controversial issue that is still being debated and evaluated.

With the advances that have occurred over the past decade in laparoscopy and minimally invasive surgery, once a patient elects to undergo surgery for risk reduction, her options may include either a BSO only or a BSO with a completion hysterectomy. Ultimately, the final decision rests with the patient after she understands the genetic basis for this recommendation, and in consultation with her physician.

## CONCLUSION

Scientists and physicians have come to learn more about cancer cell growth, apoptosis and the thought that each human cell is uniquely destined by its preset genetic composition. This understanding has been accelerated with the cloning of the human genome, and the modernization of molecular biology. The science of cancer is emerging into gene expression analysis, proteomics, and immunotherapy with monoclonal antibodies. Early identification, prevention, and treatment delivery systems are being creating on a daily basis. With the potential application of nanotechnology into this exciting field of research, hopefully oncologists will be much more successful in accurately detecting early disease, and develop newer treatment agents to improve survival. With each step, we are one step closer to finding a cure to cancer.

## REFERENCES

1. Eskin B, Troen B. The Geripause: Medical Management During the Late Menopause. London: Parthenon Publishing Group, 2003.
2. National Cancer Institute: www.cancer.gov/dictionary (accessed 3 April 2006).
3. Culotta E, Koshland DR Jr. p53 sweeps through cancer research. Science 1993; 262: 1958–61.
4. American Cancer Society. www.cancer.org (accessed 3 April 2006).
5. Xu Y, Shen Z, Wiper DW et al. Lysophosphatidic acid as a potential biomarker for ovarian and other gynecologic cancers. JAMA 1998; 280: 719–23.
6. Sutphen R, Xu J, Wilbanks GW et al. Lysophospholipids are potential biomarkers of ovarian cancer. Cancer Epidemiol Biomarkers Prev 2004; 13: 1185–91.
7. Hoskins WJ, Young RC, Markman M et al (eds). Hoskins' Principles and Practice of Gynecologic Oncology, 4th edn. Baltimore: Lippincott, Williams and Wilkins, 2005.
8. Bookman M, Greer BE, Ozols RF. Optimal therapy of advanced ovarian cancer: carboplatin and paclitaxel vs. cisplatin and paclitaxel (GOG 1 58) and an update on GOG0 182–ICON5. Int J Gynecol Cancer 2003; 13: 735–40.
9. Armstrong DK, Bundy B, Wenzel L et al. Intraperitoneal cisplatin and paclitaxel in ovarian cancer. N Engl J Med 2006; 354: 34–43.
10. Gordon AN, Tonda M, Sun S et al. Long-term survival advantage for women treated with pegylated liposomal doxorubicin compared with topotecan in a phase 3 randomized study of recurrent and refractory epithelial ovarian cancer. Gynecol Oncol 2004; 95: 1–8.

11. GOG 99. Keys HM, Roberts JA, Brunetto VL et al. A phase III trial of surgery with or without adjunctive external pelvic radiation therapy in intermediate risk endometrial adenocarcinoma: a Gynecologic Oncology Group study. Gynecol Oncol 2004; 92: 744–51.

12. PORTEC Study Group. Survival after relapse in patients with endometrial cancer: results from a randomized trial. Gynecol Oncol 2003; 89: 201–9.

13. Pal T, Permuth-Wey J, Betts JA et al. BRCA1 and BRCA2 mutations account for a large proportion of ovarian carcinoma cases. Cancer 2005; 104: 2807–16.

14. Rebbeck TR, Friebel T, Lynch HT et al. Bilateral prophylactic mastectomy reduces breast cancer risk in *BRCA1* and *BRCA2* mutation carriers: the PROSE Study Group. J Clin Oncol 2004; 22: 1055–62.

15. Kauff ND, Satagopan JM, Robosn ME et al. Risk-reducing salpingo-oophorectomy in women with a *BRCA1* or *BRCA2* mutation. N Engl J Med 2002; 346: 1609–15.

16. Powell CB, Kenley E, Chen LM et al. Risk-reducing salpingo-oophorectomy in *BRCA* mutation carriers: role of serial sectioning in the detection of occult malignancy. J Clin Oncol 2005; 23: 127–32.

17. Agoff SN, Garcia RL, Goff B et al. Unexpected gynecologic neoplasms in patients with proven or suspected *BRCA-1* or *-2* mutations: implications for gross examination, cytology, and clinical follow-up. Am J Surg Pathol 2002; 26: 171–8.

# Chapter 17

# Urological problems

Nina S Davis

## INTRODUCTION

Age truly has become a negligible consideration in the treatment of urological disease, as increased life expectancy, improved general health, and enhanced safety of anesthesia have allowed us to offer the full range of medical and surgical therapies to our patients. Further, increased understanding of the normal anatomy and physiology of the pelvis and urogenital system, as well as pathological disturbances of their structure and function has resulted in the introduction of new classes of drugs as well as novel, minimally invasive techniques for the treatment of all types of voiding disorders. These developments have significantly expanded our therapeutic armamentarium, making the treatment of our menopausal patients more effective and, thereby, more gratifying.

In spite of significant medical advancements, however, there still remains a significant gap in the knowledge and understanding of urological problems, particularly voiding disorders, and their potential therapies among practitioners and patients alike. Patients are told or continue to believe that such problems as incontinence and overactive bladder are 'normal' concomitants of aging and are, therefore, to be tolerated. Others may be relegated to diapers or chronic catheterization because it is assumed that no better options are available for treating their voiding dysfunction. Fears of surgery and its complications may prevent patients from seeking specialty consultation, or they and their physicians may assume that they are too infirm or too old to be treated. Though many urological problems affecting aging women may not be life-threatening, they dramatically impact quality of life. Menopausal women, who have nothing more wrong with them than severe

urgency and frequency, may become invalids because they are worried about bathroom access, are afraid of public accidents, or have been embarrassed by such episodes in the past. Although complete resolution of some urological disorders with appropriate therapy may not always be possible, incremental improvements in symptoms or function can often reverse the negative psychological and physical effects of such chronic problems, restoring patients' independence and sense of wellbeing.

There is still much progress to be made in understanding the physiological correlates of lower urinary tract dysfunction in aging women, but it is hoped that the material contained herein will permit physicians to educate themselves and their patients about established and emerging therapies. By increasing patients' understanding of available treatments and facilitating access to specialty care, physicians will be able to dramatically and positively impact their patients' quality of life and, by extension, their overall health. As George William Curtis so aptly commented, 'Age is a matter of feeling, not of years.'

## NORMAL ANATOMY AND PHYSIOLOGY OF THE BLADDER AND URETHRA

The bladder is an organ that lies in the true pelvis and functions as a urinary reservoir. Its wall is comprised of interdigitating fascicles of smooth muscle arranged in a random fashion, collectively known as the detrusor muscle. The triangular portion of the bladder base where the ureteral orifices are situated is the trigone. Here, the smooth muscle takes on a more complex architecture with a longitudinal muscle layer overlying the detrusor and taking on a circular configuration to encompass the intramural portion of the ureters, and to contribute to the valvular mechanism of the distal ureters. The bladder is lined by transitional epithelium (urothelium) which is covered by a glycosaminoglycan (GAG) layer. The exact role of the GAG layer remains controversial. It may have a role in preventing bacterial adherence and urothelial damage by large macromolecules; however, its ability to serve as a plasma–urine barrier has been questioned.[1]

A woman's urethra is approximately 4 cm in length. It begins at the bladder neck and courses along the distal third of the anterior vaginal wall to the urethral meatus. It is lined by transitional epithelium that gradually converts to non-keratinized stratified squamous epithelium distally. Passive coaptation of the urethral wall is maintained by a subepithelial layer of of spongy vascular tissue, an important component of the female continence mechanism.[2] The mucosal and submucosal layers are both estrogen sensitive. In men, there are distinct sphincteric entities that effect continence; however, maintenance of female continence is more complex and dependent upon both intrinsic urethral musculature and pelvic floor support. The entire length of the wall of the female urethra consists of a thick, longitudinal smooth muscle layer surrounded by a thinner circular layer. The distal two-thirds of the urethra is enveloped by striated muscle which is designated the external urinary sphincter (EUS) or rhabdosphincter. Its fibers become attenuated posteriorly, inserting into the vaginal wall to form the compressor urethrae, which contracts to close the urethra against the anterior vaginal wall.[3] Just proximal to the vaginal vestibule, the urethrovaginal sphincter is formed as striated muscle encompasses the urethra and vagina. Contraction of this sphincter and the bulbospongiosis muscle produces tightening of the urogenital hiatus. Continence, as well as prevention of prolapse, is also dependent on the integrity of the pelvic floor musculature and fasciae, as well as the ligamentous attachments of the pelvic viscera.[4–6]

Understanding the innervation of the bladder and urethra is the key to effective pharmacological manipulation of their function. They are served by both autonomic and somatic nerves. Parasympathetic fibers from S2–S4 travel via the pelvic nerve to the pelvic plexus and stimulate muscarinic receptors in the bladder wall via the release of acetylcholine, producing contraction of the detrusor. Sympathetic fibers from T1–L2 course through the hypogastric plexus, and reach the urethra via the hypogastric nerve, increasing alpha-adrenergic tone and outlet resistance. Indeed, measurements taken during hypogastric nerve stimulation in male cats demonstrate augmentation of urethral pressure in the region of the EUS, suggesting that adrenergic receptors play a role in EUS function.[7] This finding has been extrapolated to human females as well, and has been reinforced by the efficacy of alpha-blockade in diminishing EUS overactivity in women with functional voiding disorders. Another site of sympathetic innervation is the bladder body where scattered beta-adrenergic receptors facilitate relaxation of the detrusor during filling. Somatic nerves derived from the S2–S4 supply the EUS via the pudendal nerve. Voluntary contraction of the sphincter is mediated by acetylcholine.

The normal micturition cycle consists of a filling/storage phase, and an emptying or elimination phase which are modulated by the pontine motor nucleus of the central nervous system, but which require co-ordination at all levels of the brain and spinal cord, and signal implementation via peripheral autonomic and somatic nerves. During the storage phase, the bladder accommodates increasing volumes of urine, while the detrusor pressure remains lower than urethral resting pressure. This distensibility or compliance is facilitated by the viscoelastic properties of the bladder wall, by central suppression of reflex contractions by cortical centers, and by sympathetic detrusor relaxation. Urethral tone remains high due to alpha-adrenergic stimulation of the EUS. Normal voiding is then initiated by voluntary relaxation of the striated sphincter, followed by relaxation of the bladder neck and proximal urethra. Finally, parasympathetically mediated contraction of the detrusor results in expulsion of the bladder contents. Normal micturition is therefore a highly complex, co-ordinated event, and the disruption of any part of the process can result in significant dysfunction.

## PATHOPHYSIOLOGY OF THE AGING BLADDER

Age-associated disorders of the bladder and urethra result from intrinsic and extrinsic changes that alter the composition, relations, and function of the urogenital structures. The decline in estrogen levels that is the sine qua non of the menopause is similarly responsible for alterations in the structure and function of the genitourinary tract. There is decreased cellularity, thinning, and increased friability of the vaginal and urethral tissues, as well as a decrease in tissue elasticity. The vagina atrophies and shortens, causing the urethral meatus to recede along the anterior vaginal wall.[8–10] Atrophy also contributes to pelvic floor prolapse. Vaginal secretions decrease in volume and lose the acidity that protects against cystitis and vaginitis.

Estrogen receptors populate the urethra and bladder, particularly the trigone, so hypoestrogenism negatively impacts urethral closure mechanisms, predisposing to incontinence. A number of animal studies have suggested that hormone withdrawal can affect receptor density and sensitivity in the bladder and urethra. Restoration of normal estrogen levels reverses these effects, increasing the number and responsiveness of muscarinic and adrenergic receptors. However, although several investigators have attempted to demonstrate that estrogen deficiency causes detrusor instability in menopausal women, and replacement therapy ameliorates it, the data remain equivocal and the issue controversial. It has also been postulated that diminished estrogen levels may provoke a global decrease in responsiveness to nerve stimulation.[11] This correlates with the observed decrease in smooth muscle tone with aging.

On a microscopic level, histological and ultrastructural studies have identified distinct degenerative changes in aging smooth and striated muscle that may predispose to vesicourethral dysfunction, even though these abnormalities may be present in individuals without apparent genitourinary pathology. Fibrosis is the most common degenerative change associated with the aging bladder. Although previously attributed to outlet obstruction, it has been demonstrated in the bladder walls of normal elderly women.[12] One explanation may be the recent observation that atherosclerosis produces ischemia of the bladder wall and subsequent fibrotic change.[13]

In order to better understand the functional correlates of observed age-related structural changes, a number of investigators have performed histological comparisons of tissues from normal and symptomatic patients. Levy and Wight focused on the bladder submucosa, as it constitutes 25% of the thickness of the bladder wall.[14] Optical and electron microscopic examination of bladder biopsies revealed progressive separation and disorganization of the collagen fascicles, which was most pronounced in association with bladder outlet obstruction. In the case of urgency alone, collagen could barely be detected. In an elegant and detailed series of papers correlating urodynamic findings with ultratsructural data from detrusor biopsies, Elbadawi and colleagues identified histological patterns that consistently correlated with given clinical entities.[15–18] They described a 'dense band' pattern of degeneration in the normal aging bladder. Associated degeneration of muscle cells and axons were linked to impaired contractility. A 'dysjunction pattern' correlated with detrusor instability, and 'myohypertrophy' was characteristic of obstruction. Combinations of these patterns correlated with parallel symptom complexes. More recently, ultrastructural studies of the hypotonic bladder demonstrated high numbers of disrupted cells.[19] Investigators have also examined changes in the EUS with aging.[20] Accelerated apoptosis, programmed cell death, appears to be responsible for muscle cell loss. This is postulated to induce stress incontinence in the elderly.

## URINARY INCONTINENCE

When one thinks of urological problems in the menopausal woman and beyond, one invariably thinks of urinary incontinence, a non-specific term for a constellation of voiding disorders that are highly prevalent and often become increasingly complex as patients age, owing to the cumulative effects of childbirth, lifestyle, hormonal changes, gravity, aging, pelvic surgeries, and diseases unique to older adults such as diabetes, stroke, and parkinsonism. All of these directly affect the constitutional integrity of the urethrovesical unit or its relations with the pelvic floor, leading to diverse complaints ranging from inability to maintain urinary control, to inability to effectively empty with urination.

It is estimated that 13 million Americans suffer from urinary incontinence, and women are 2–4 times as likely as men to experience incontinence.[21] Although prevalence data vary, and some feel that incontinence is underreported due to a large number of women who do not seek help for this problem, it is generally believed that the prevalence of all types of incontinence ranges from 40% to 50%. In one study of women 60 years and older, mixed incontinence was most prevalent (55.3%), followed by stress incontinence (26.7%), urge incontinence (9.1%), and other forms of incontinence (8.9%).[22] When a broader population is considered as in the Norwegian EPINCONT study,[23] 50% of participants reported stress incontinence, 36% reported mixed incontinence, and 11% reported urge incontinence. It should be noted that the prevalence of urge incontinence increased with age, such that mixed incontinence occurred in up to 48% of women aged 60–90 years. Hence, available data suggest that in postmenopausal women, urge incontinence, either alone or in combination with stress incontinence, is most prevalent.

## Classification of incontinence

Over the years, incontinence disorders have been subject to a number of classification systems in an effort to standardize diagnostic categories and to guide therapeutic decision-making. Most have proved cumbersome, complex, and confusing, and have, therefore, been abandoned. In general, it is now customary to use descriptive nomenclature to classify the subtypes of incontinence regardless of etiology. Conceptually, the definitions are related to the dual aspects of vesicourethral function, storage and elimination. Recently, the International Continence Society (ICS) updated its standardized terminology to make it compatible with the International Classification of Diseases and the World Health Organization (WHO) International Classification of Functioning, Disability and Health.[24,25] Further, the ICS used observational descriptions based on urodynamic data as the foundation for the definitions, so as to facilitate communication between investigators and allow valid comparisons of study results.

Problems related to urinary storage include *stress urinary incontinence*, newly defined as involuntary leakage on effort or exertion, or on sneezing or coughing; *urge urinary incontinence*, involuntary leakage accompanied by or immediately preceded by urgency; *mixed urinary incontinence*, involuntary leakage associated with urgency and also with exertion, effort, sneezing, or coughing; and *continuous urinary incontinence*, continuous leakage. The latter was previously referred to as total incontinence, and generally referred to the leakage resulting from genitourinary fistulae. The ICS has designated other types of incontinence as situational, for instance, incontinence during sexual intercourse. However, no reference is made to what is generally referred to as *spontaneous incontinence* or insensate leakage. This is a type of voiding dysfunction that is fre-

quently manifested by older postmenopausal women, and is poorly researched and poorly understood. In this author's experience, it generally presents in women who have had multiple pelvic surgeries, and can be quite severe. Urodynamic correlates have not been defined. It is presumed to be neuropathic in origin, but does not respond to conventional therapy for neurogenic bladder. It does, however, respond to sacral neuromodulation (see p. xx).

In terms of impaired elimination or voiding symptoms, slow stream refers to a perception of reduced urine flow; *intermittency* describes staccato flow; *hesitancy* refers to difficulty initiating micturition resulting in a delay in the onset of voiding after the individual feels ready to pass urine; and *straining* describes the muscular effort to initiate, maintain, or improve the urinary stream. *Urinary retention* in ICS terminology is a condition rather than a symptom, and may be acute or chronic. It is defined in anatomical terms by a painful palpable or percussible bladder, without the ability to pass urine in the acute situation, and non-painful bladder distention after voiding in the chronic situation. The latter may be associated with incontinence. The ICS rejects the term *overflow incontinence* because of its imprecision.

Although the ICS has attempted to provide a comprehensive vocabulary for the diagnosis, evaluation, and treatment of voiding disorders, in complex situations, it is sometimes necessary to revert to older, yet generally understood, terminology. For instance, a unique subset of geriatric patients present with detrusor instability (involuntary detrusor contractions) in conjunction with impaired bladder contractility (acronym DHIC) such that the patients exhibit both incomplete emptying, and incontinence between voids.[26] This type of voiding dysfunction is particularly prominent in patients with Parkinson's disease. DHIC may mimic many other pathological voiding states, so urodynamic testing is particularly beneficial in establishing the diagnosis. The implications for treatment are also significant, since antimuscarinics may produce urinary retention, and surgery for presumed stress incontinence may result in the worsening of both the retention and the incontinence, due to the introduction of a component of urethral obstruction.

Particularly in view of the potential complexity of voiding disorders in the older postmenopausal patient, it is necessary to obtain a detailed history, thorough abdominal and pelvic examinations, and judicious testing to establish the exact nature of the patient's dysfunction and to identify the relevant pathology. Such careful assessment permits more appropriate and precise therapeutic intervention.

### Evaluation of the incontinent patient

As with any voiding dysfunction, the historical context is critical to establishing etiology. Therefore, determining time of onset (inciting event), duration, character, course, and prior treatments and their efficacy will provide valuable clues as to the nature of the patient's problem. Specifics of patients' voiding habits must be elucidated including daytime frequency, nocturia, number and types of pads used, and effects on lifestyle. Resnick has outlined factors that must be considered when evaluating incontinence in the geriatric population and has systematized them into a mnemonic – DIAPPERS (delirium, infection, atrophy, pharmaceuticals, psychological, excessive urine output, restricted mobility, and stool impaction).[27] It is also helpful to assess the risk factors for the development of urinary incontinence. These include vaginal delivery, age, estrogen deficiency, back problems, neurological disorders, constipation, and obesity. In particular, vaginal delivery may cause muscle, nerve, and connective tissue damage that may not be manifest until many years after the insult.[28] Prolonged second-stage labor, episiotomy, and instrumentation all can produce significant pelvic floor injury. Conditions commonly associated with chronic increases in intra-abdominal pressure correlate with incontinence as well. Besides constipation and obesity, these include coughing from smoking or asthma, and occupational or recreational heavy lifting. Detrusor instability and resultant irritative symptoms such as frequency, urgency, nocturia, and urge incontinence are characteristic of the autonomic neuropathy that occurs in patients with diabetes mellitus. Obtaining details of pelvic surgeries, especially prior incontinence procedures, is critical, as they may produce urethral scarring leading to intrinsic sphincter deficiency (ISD), urethral obstruction, or fistulae. Physicians should review all medications and herbal remedies with particular attention to systemic or local hormonal therapy or medications with anticholinergic effects that may impair urination.

The consensus is that a bladder diary is the single most important tool in the evaluation of voiding dysfunction. Ideally, the patient provides a three- to seven-day log that details daily fluid intake, number and volume of voids, and number of incontinence episodes in each 24-hour period. Each incontinence episode should be accompanied by a notation regarding associated activity or the presence of urge. It is also helpful to know the types of fluid the patient drinks. The data provided in the diary will help elucidate the pattern of incontinence and will direct behavioral interventions such as fluid restriction.

Although it is important to perform a complete physical assessment of the incontinent patient, the key components of the physical examination are the abdominal and pelvic examinations. The abdomen should be inspected for scars and distention, and the bladder should be percussed. Palpation will reveal focal areas of tenderness, masses, and hernias. If there is any question of incomplete emptying, either a sonographic bladder scan should be performed, or the patient should be sterilely catheterized for residual urine (post-void residual). As the patient moves down the table into the lithotomy position, observe for leakage, a sign of stress incontinence due to ISD. On initial inspection of the vulva and perineum, lesions should be sought, the degree of atrophy should be assessed, and the length and integrity of the perineal body should be noted. Often a caruncle, an erythematous, polypoid mass associated with estrogen difficiency, is visible at the urethral meatus. Anocutaneous and bulbocavernosus reflexes are tested to determine the integrity of the S2–S4 spinal segments. A speculum examination is then used to evaluate the vagina and cervix, if present, as well as the adequacy of pelvic floor support. After inspection of the vagina and cervix for lesions or discharge, the patient is asked to bear down, so that the degree of pelvic organ prolapse (POP) can be determined. A number of systems are available for the grading of POP.[29–31] The examiner must also try to determine the nature of the prolapse, whether it represents a cystocele, enterocele, rectocele, or a combination of these. This is abetted by the 'half-speculum examination' which allows separate manipulation of the anterior and posterior vaginal walls. Bimanual examination then permits not only evaluation of the bladder, uterus and adnexa, but also palpation of the pelvic floor musculature to evaluate symmetry, strength, and tone. Pelvic masses or areas of tenderness may also be detected. The urethra should be a supple, non tender structure, but palpation will, on occasion, reveal a cyst or diverticulum, or the gritty firmness of urethral carcinoma. When compression of the urethra produces purulent drainage, an infected diverticulum is usually present, though these are unusual in post-menopausal women. A cough test can be used to demonstrate urethral hypermobility and stress incontinence. Some practitioners prefer a Q-tip test to assess hypermobility. A fixed urethra usually indicates ISD. The presence of a vaginal discharge should prompt a wet-prep microscopic examination and/or culture as appropriate.

A urinalysis should always be included as part of the evaluation of the incontinent patient. Frequently, an occult infection is detected, and treatment of this alone may significantly improve or eradicate the incontinence. The presence of microscopic blood in the urine should alert the examiner to the possibility of a genitourinary neoplasm. In the absence of a positive urine culture, hematuria should not be attributed to infection. Any suspicion of malignancy should prompt submission of a urine cytology and initiation of a formal workup. Hematuria and urinary tract infection are discussed in more detail later in this chapter.

*Urodynamic testing in the evaluation of urinary incontinence*

Urodynamics, as used in this context, refers to sophisticated clinical studies of vesicourethral anatomy and function that are used to help elucidate the nature of complex voiding disorders. Although there is no consensus as to the indications for urodynamic testing, most would agree that it is not necessary for the assessment of patients with straightforward stress or urge incontinence. However, urodynamic evaluation should be considered in those patients who have voiding dysfunction after multiple pelvic surgeries, who have failed empiric medical therapy for urge incontinence, whose anti-incontinence procedure was unsuccessful or exacerbated their lower urinary tract symptoms, or who are suspected of having a neuropathic component to their voiding disorder. Further, many practitioners insist on urodynamics before proceeding with any pelvic floor reconstructive surgery, as the information obtained can be invaluable in counseling patients regarding risks, outcomes, and prognosis.

To perform urodynamics, an intraurethral catheter is sterilely placed for the measurement of intravesical pressure, and a balloon catheter is inserted into the rectum or vagina to measure intra-abdominal pressure. Detrusor pressure is therefore a subtracted pressure, intravesical pressure minus the intra-abdominal pressure. The primary components of urodynamic testing include:

- *uroflowmetry*: measures the pattern and rate of urinary flow. To have a valid study, the patient must void at least 150 ml. In normal micturition, the flow curve exhibits a steep upslope to a peak followed by a more gradual downslope. It should take no longer than 23 s to discharge a bladder volume of 400 ml.[32] In women, maximal flow is not affected by age, and ranges from 15 to 36 ml/s. A common uroflow abnormality is the 'stutter-step' intermittency characteristic of abdominal straining in the context of an atonic bladder (Valsalva voiding), or external urethral sphincter (EUS) spasticity interrupting urinary flow. Therefore diminished voiding velocities may indicate obstruction or a weak bladder.
- *cystometry* is a test of bladder storage. It assesses capacity and compliance. It also offers an indirect means of evaluating bladder sensation. To perform this study, the bladder is filled at a steady rate with fluid, and several parameters are measured including filling pressure, sensation, capacity, compliance, the presence of involuntary (uninhibited) detrusor contractions, and the ability to suppress voiding. A normal bladder should maintain low pressures throughout the storage phase. In general, filling pressures should not exceed 5–10 cmH$_2$O, and the capacity should generally range from 400 ml to 600 ml. Sustained filling pressures >40 cmH$_2$O produce renal damage via the transmission of pressure to the upper tracts.[33]
- *voiding pressure–flow studies* (micturition studies) reproduce the emptying phase of the micturition cycle, thereby establishing the presence of detrusor contractility and quantifying it as voiding pressure. These studies, which may be performed in the supine, sitting, or standing positions, are useful for detecting bladder outlet obstruction or abnormal voiding patterns. After her bladder is filled to capacity, the patient is asked to void to completion. The flow rate and pattern, as well as the voiding pressures, are noted. A post-void residual volume should be measured. Generally, voiding pressures should be less than 60 cmH$_2$O, particularly in women: their voiding pressures tend to be quite low because of the diminished outlet resistance

conferred by their short urethras. Failure to relax the EUS during voiding, however, results in the characteristic pattern of a reduced flow rate accompanied by a high voiding pressure. In elderly women it is more common to see a reduced flow rate and a low voiding pressure, with or without an elevated post-void residual, findings consistent with a decompensated or flaccid (atonic) bladder. The pressure–flow study, therefore, expands and corroborates the findings on initial uroflowmetry.

- *electromyography* (EMG) is performed as an adjunct to cystometry and pressure–flow testing as it allows simultaneous assessment of EUS function. It is a critical component of neurophysiological testing. Patch electrodes are placed perianally to detect pelvic floor activity. Normally, the sphincter exhibits increasing tone as the bladder fills, or when patients attempt to suppress an IDC or stress leakage. Conversely, EMG activity should be negligible during voiding. When detrusor-external sphincter dyssynergia is present, there is an inappropriate increase in EMG activity during voiding, resulting in elevated voiding pressures and reduced urinary velocity. This may occur in conjunction with neurological diseases such as multiple sclerosis or functional voiding disorders.

- *leak-point pressure testing* generally refers to the measurement of abdominal or Valsalva leak-point pressure (VLPP), defined as the degree of straining required to elicit urinary leakage. It is a test of urethral competence, as it determines the pressure at which urethral resistance is overcome. This study is used to distinguish stress incontinence due to ISD from that due to urethral hypermobility. Classically, VLPPs less than 60 cmH$_2$O are indicative of ISD, while those exceeding 90 cmH$_2$O signal urethral hypermobility.[34] A mixed situation exists when pressures lie between 60 and 90 cmH$_2$O, and clinical correlation usually allows identification of the predominant cause of the patient's incontinence.

- *videourodynamics* refers to measurement of urodynamic parameters with simultaneous fluoroscopic visualization of the bladder and urethra. Contrast is used for bladder filling instead of the usual irrigant. The advantages of this method include more precise correlation of measurements to vesicourethral function, identification of artifactual measure-

ments, and enhanced definition of the patient's anatomy. Videourodynamics are therefore particularly valuable in sorting out complicated voiding complaints. Recently, Nitti and colleagues found that the diagnosis and etiology of subtle outlet obstruction in women could be most accurately established using videourodynamic pressure–flow studies.[35]

A number of studies have been performed using urodynamics to characterize detrusor dysfunction in the aging bladder. It is generally agreed that bladder capacity and flow rates are universally diminished and that post-void residuals are higher.[36,37] Detrusor sensory function is thought to be impaired as well.[38] Changes in urethral function with aging are much more difficult to measure, and findings are contradictory in many instances. However, one large study demonstrated lower urethral pressure and decreased sphincteric function with age.[39] It is not clear to what extent age-related changes in vesicourethral function contribute to the pathogenesis of incontinence and other voiding disorders in postmenopausal women.

Besides videourodynamics, cystoscopy is another means of assessing vesicourethral anatomy, but is rarely indicated in the evaluation of incontinence. It should be considered in cases of sterile hematuria or pyuria, bladder pain, recent onset of irritative voiding symptoms, or suspected genitourinary pathology.

### Treatment of urinary incontinence in the postmenopausal patient

The available therapies for urinary incontinence may be organized into three broad categories: behavioral therapy/physiotherapy, pharmacological agents, and surgical interventions. These are not mutually exclusive, and combined modalities may be the most effective treatment for a given individual. It is clear that a detailed understanding of a patient's particular voiding complaints as well as a basic knowledge of the pathophysiological principles underlying her disorder are necessary to optimize therapy and ensure a successful outcome.

#### Behavioral interventions and pelvic floor physiotherapy

Behavioral modification begins with a careful review of the voiding diary. Excessive fluid intake is a common finding in incontinent patients and can easily be adjusted downward to provide more manageable urinary volumes.[40] Further, significant intake of caffeinated beverages, especially at night, can produce symptoms of overactive bladder (OAB), including frequency, urgency, and nocturia. Substitution of water or decaffeinated drinks, avoidance of caffeine before bed, and fluid restriction after dinner can decrease daytime and night-time urinary frequency.

For patients taking diuretics and suffering from nocturia, changing the dosing to late afternoon will produce a diuresis before bedtime, thereby decreasing night-time polyuria and resultant nocturia or nocturnal enuresis. If getting to the toilet is problematic, providing a commode or otherwise improving access to bathroom facilities will promote continence.

Chronic constipation and fecal impaction are endemic in the postmenopausal population, and can both produce and exacerbate incontinence. Aggressive treatment with a high-fiber diet, increased water intake, increased activity, and judicious use of stool softeners and laxatives can normalize bowel function. It is also important to establish healthy long-term habits for maintaining regularity.

'Bladder training' refers to regulating bladder function through the use of timed voiding and urge suppression. Generally, the patient is directed to void on a schedule, usually every 1.5 to 2 h, so that her bladder will not reach the critical volume that triggers incontinence. Then, using Kegels or other maneuvers to 'distract the bladder' and reduce urgency, the patient gradually acquires the ability to hold her urine for increasingly longer periods. Bladder training may be used for the treatment of both stress and urge incontinence.

Pelvic floor physiotherapy encompasses the use of such varied modalities as physical therapy, biofeedback, electrical stimulation, vaginal weights, massage, scar release, and breathing techniques to strengthen and balance the pelvic floor. Although Kegel exercises have long been advocated for the enhancement of pelvic floor support, they are often performed incorrectly. A properly designed and supervised regimen that is individualized to the patient can dramatically improve or cure incontinence. These techniques are also very effective in the treatment of functional voiding disorders and pelvic pain syndromes. Many patients choose pelvic floor physiotherapy because the 'holistic' nature of the treatment is more appealing than medication or surgery. It is essential to refer patients to qualified personnel, usually nurse practitioners in continence centers or physical therapists in established rehabilitation facilities. Studies show that frequent monitoring of patients' progress and offering positive reinforcement reduce attrition and enhance performance.[41]

*Pharmacological therapy of urinary incontinence*

Although drug therapy has traditionally been employed in the treatment of milder forms of *genuine stress incontinence* (GSUI), there is no Food and Drug Administration (FDA)-approved agent currently available in the US for this indication. Previously, phenylpropanolamine, an alpha-agonist, and various antihistamine decongestants were often tried as initial therapy for GSUI. However, phenylpropanolamine was recently withdrawn from the market, and most practitioners have lost their enthusiasm for this class of agents. Imipramine, which has been used extensively for the treatment of bedwetting in children, is a central inhibitor of norepinephrine (NE, noradrenaline) and serotonin (5-HT). Its peripheral anticholinergic and alpha-agonist properties have prompted its use in GSUI, as it acts on both the detrusor (relaxation) and the urethra (increased tone).

It is also used to treat *nocturia* and *nocturnal enuresis* in adults, even though there are no studies demonstrating efficacy for these problems. Recent advances in our understanding of the neurophysiology of the lower urinary tract, however, suggest that there may also be CNS-based mechanisms of action for imipramine and other drugs that provide a rationale for their use in GSUI. One drug that holds particular promise is duloxetine, a selective serotonin reuptake inhibitor (SSRI) whose effects on 5-HT and NE reuptake in the brain are potent and balanced.[42] It is currently FDA-approved for the treatment of major depression and diabetic neuropathy, but in trials has been effective in the treatment of GSUI. Interestingly, a recent international study demonstrated that combined treatment of GSUI with duloxetine and pelvic floor muscle training was more effective than either modality alone, though both exhibited efficacy in the trial.[43]

Whereas medication is not a mainstay of the treatment of GSUI, medical management is considered firstline therapy for the treatment of *urge incontinence*, *mixed incontinence*, and other micturition disorders that are thought to result from detrusor overactivity. Indeed, the prevalence of such disorders prompted the International Continence Society to define a syndrome, known as OAB or *overactive bladder*, consisting of urinary urgency with or without urge incontinence, and usually associated with urinary frequency and nocturia.[24,25] OAB is further classified as 'wet' when the patient is incontinent, and 'dry' when the symptom complex does not include urge incontinence. Again, because of increased focus on the neurophysiology of micturition, it is now understood that implicating the detrusor alone in the production of urge-related symptoms is too simplistic, and explains why current therapies that largely affect detrusor (motor) function are not consistently beneficial. We now appreciate that the interplay of detrusor, central and peripheral nerves, growth factors and substances such as prostaglandin determines bladder behavior. In the future, this growing body of knowledge will give rise to whole new classes of pharmaceuticals.

In the meantime, physicians still rely on anticholinergic/antimuscarinic agents for the treatment of OAB symptoms and urge incontinence. Currently approved medications and their dosages are listed in Table 17.1. All of the drugs in this class produce significant dry mouth and constipation in many patients, side-effects that are shared by a number of medications commonly administered to the elderly. The additive side-effects may produce significant disability. To make matters worse, some anticholinergics are associated with major cognitive impairment in older patients, another potentially serious complication of therapy. For this reason, it is important to consider both receptor selectivity and the ability to cross the blood–brain barrier when prescribing these agents.[44]

It is now known that there are five muscarinic receptor subtypes, designated M1–M5, that mediate cholinergic function. In the bladder, the M3 receptors are principally responsible for detrusor contractility,[45] whereas M1 receptors predominate in the cerebral cortex. A new class of antimuscarinics specific for M3 inhibition diminish detrusor contractility while avoiding significant CNS side-effects. Two such agents have recently been approved in the US – solifenacin and darifenacin. Theoretically, their M3 specificity confers greater potency in the bladder, but the presence of M3 receptors in salivary glands and bowel means that dry mouth and constipation remain significant side-effects. Finally, although these drugs consti-

tute a new class of anticholinergics, they really do not represent a major therapeutic advancement, as they still largely modulate the efferent side of detrusor function.

### Surgical treatment of urinary incontinence

Surgical intervention constitutes definitive treatment for significant stress urinary incontinence (GSUI), with or without associated pelvic organ prolapse. Except in cases of severe, refractory detrusor overactivity, surgery is not considered conventional therapy for urge incontinence (see p. xx). Procedures for GSUI may be performed via the transabdominal or transvaginal routes, and fall into the following categories: retropubic suspensions, pubovaginal (bladder neck) slings, midurethral slings, and periurethral injections with bulking agents. The dual objectives of all anti-incontinence procedures are

1.  re-establishing urethral support and stabilizing/restoring the normal anatomical relationship of the bladder and urethra
2.  creating urethral coaptation or and/or compression, thereby increasing urethral resistance. There are myriad approaches to achieving these goals.

The classic retropubic procedure is the Burch culposuspension which involves placing suspension sutures on either side of the bladder neck and bringing them up to Cooper's ligament. This produces both high rates of success and durable cures. Complications are the same as for all anti-incontinence procedures: urinary retention, generally transient; de novo detrusor overactivity; and prolapse. The other retropubic operation is the Marshall–Marchetti–Krantz procedure, which is similar to the Burch culposuspension, except that the sutures are placed in the periurethral fascia and brought up to the periosteum of the symphysis pubis. It has largely fallen into disfavor because of the associated risk of osteitis pubis and the tendency of the procedure to cause urethral obstruction and secondary voiding dysfunction.

Many pelvic floor surgeons preferentially perform their procedures through the vagina, as pain is significantly diminished and recuperative time is reduced. Further, a vaginal approach allows concomitant repair of any pelvic floor defects. The standard of care for all transvaginal approaches is to place a suburethral sling to restore urethral support. Slings are placed at either the bladder neck or the midurethra. The current trend is to perform

**Table 17.1**   Pharmacological agents employed in the treatment of overactive bladder

| Classification/name | Dosage | Comments |
|---|---|---|
| **Antimuscarinic quarternary amines** | | Minimal transmission across blood–brain barrier; advocated for elderly patients; adult use uncommon |
| Trospium chloride | 20 mg bid | |
| Propantheline bromide | 15–30 mg qid | |
| Non-specific antimuscarinics | | |
| Oxybutynin | | Also has muscle relaxant and local anesthetic effects; patch avoids first-pass phenomenon |
| IR | 5 mg bid–qid | |
| ER | 5–30 mg qd | |
| TDS | 2×/week | |
| Tolterodine | | |
| IR | 2 mg bid–qid | |
| LA | 4 mg qd | |
| Hyoscyamine | | May be used as adjunctive therapy with other anticholinergics |
| SL | 0.125 mg q4h | |
| ER | 0.375 mg bid | |
| **M3 inhibitors** | | |
| Darifenacin | 7.5–15 mg qd | |
| Solifenacin | 10–20 mg qd | Long (50 h) half-life |
| **Tricyclic antidepressant** | | |
| Imipramine | 25–50 mg bid | Anticholinergic + alpha-agonist effects |

OAB, overactive bladder; qid, four times a day; bid, two times a day; qd, once daily; 2×/week, twice per week; q4h, every four hours; IR, immediate release; ER, extended release; TDS, transdermal system; LA, long-acting; SL, sublingual.

minimally invasive synthetic slings on an outpatient basis. The differences between the various slings center on the material used for the sling, the approach for sling placement, the location of the sling, and the technique used for securing the sling. Bladder neck slings are suspended either by tying them over the recti suprapubically, by attaching them to the posterior aspect of the pubis via bone anchors, or by using serrated mesh extensions to hold the sling within the supporting tissue. The trochars or needles that carry the slings may be directed from vagina to suprapubic region, or vice versa. Sling materials range from the patient's own fascia (rectus or fascia lata) to xenografts such as pigskin and bovine pericardium, to polygalactan mesh. It has been shown that a larger weave promotes tissue ingrowth to better incorporate the sling into the patient's own tissue. Traditional slings have been placed at the bladder neck, but midurethral placement is in vogue based on Delancey's 'hammock theory'.[5] Finally, variations on the transobturator sling are gaining momentum among both urologists and gynecologists. Early results are excellent, and this approach has several advantages. Two small incisions are made in the genital creases opposite the clitoris, and a small midurethral opening is made in the vaginal wall, with dissection only to the level of the lateral pelvic fascia. A special carrier needle is then brought through the vulvar incisions and obturator foramen, then out through the vagina. Various types of sling material are then attached to the needle and brought into position. The transobturator approach is thought to reproduce the course of the urethropelvic ligament, does not violate the endopelvic fascia, and completely avoids entering the pelvis, a distinct advantage in a patient with multiple prior abdominal or pelvic surgeries.

For the patient with GSUI who is a poor surgical risk, is surgically averse, or is not very active, periurethral bulking agents offer an effective, minimally invasive alternative. The procedure can be performed in the office under local anesthesia. The agent is injected submucosally via cystoscopy to produce mucosal coaptation. Continence is usually immediate, and lasts for variable periods, usually 6–24 months; however, more than one session may be needed initially to get the patient dry. Since the procedure is rapid and minimally morbid, the need for repeat sessions does not pose a hardship to most patients. Risks include infection, transient retention, and minor hematuria. Administering a 3-day course of antibiotics usually prevents perioperative infection.

### Nocturia and nocturnal enuresis

Nocturia or nocturnal frequency is a complex voiding dysfunction which is multifactorial in etiology. It is equally prevalent in women and men, and increases with advancing age. Contributing factors include diminished bladder capacity, decreased renal concentrating ability, increased secretion of atrial natriuretic peptide, diminished activity of the renin-angiotensin-aldosterone system, and loss of circadian secretion of antidiuretic hormone.[46] The latter is the basis for treatment with DDAVP, a synthetic analog of arginine vasopressin. It is available as a tablet or spray. Dosages should not exceed 40 µg/day. It is essential that the patient be monitored closely upon initiating therapy, as profound hyponatremia can rapidly develop. Electrolytes must be checked early and often. The use of behavioral modification and imipramine for the treatment of nocturia have already been mentioned. In general, anticholinergics are not very effective for this disorder.

Bedwetting or nocturnal enuresis is a poorly understood, and extremely distressing disorder. It is also difficult to treat. Any intervention that diminishes night-time urinary volume can be beneficial. Pharmacotherapy is identical to that for nocturia. Sacral neuromodulation may also be helpful when nocturnal enuresis occurs as part of an urgency-frequency syndrome (see p. 201).

### Urinary retention

Urinary retention ranges from incomplete emptying to the inability to void at all. The incidence increases with age, and it is not unusual for a patient to be unaware of the problem, as bladder sensation is often impaired. Secondary signs of retention include a weak urinary stream, straining to void, frequency, urge, overflow, or spontaneous incontinence. It is particularly common in diabetes and may be heralded by asymptomatic bacteriuria. Other causes include cerebrovascular accident (CVA), lower spinal cord tumors, disk disease below T12, and pernicious anemia. Iatrogenic retention occurs when patients are administered medications with anticholinergic properties. In a woman with retention, it is most important to rule out urethral carcinoma. Hematuria will be present, and a mass will be palpable on physical examination.

The treatment of urinary retention is governed by etiology and patient preference. When retention is relatively minor (residuals 150–200 ml) and no infection is present, no intervention is needed. Medications should be adjusted as necessary to minimize anticholinergic effects. Unfortunately, there are no medications that reliably facilitate bladder emptying. The cholinergic agent, bethanecol chloride, is available, but its efficacy is compromised by its inability to stimulate a coordinated detrusor contraction. Neuropathic lesions may need to be treated with clean intermittent catheterization by the patient or her caretaker, or suprapubic cystostomy. More complex forms of diversion are rarely necessary. In cases of benign urethral obstruction such as seen with connective tissue disorders, periodic urethral dilation may be sufficient to preserve normal lower urinary tract function. Severe prolapse can kink the urethra. Pessaries or manual reduction to permit voiding are temporary maneuvers until definitive repair can be accomplished.

### Refractory voiding dysfunction

In the past, when patients remained incontinent or continued to retain urine in spite of our best efforts, we could only offer them some form of urinary catheterization or diversion. Those in retention who lacked the capability or caretaker to perform clean intermittent catheterization were forced into chronic catheterization, a suprapubic cystostomy always being preferred over a urethral Foley. Incontinent patients could also be treated with some form of catheterization, but often residual detrusor instability prevented dryness, even with concomitant muscarinic blockade. Therefore, more complex solutions involving bladder augmentations using bowel or urinary conduits offered the only reliable means of eliminating incontinence.

Happily, this situation has changed with the advent of two new minimally invasive therapies, both of which were made possible by advancements in the understanding of the neurophysiology of the lower genitourinary tract.

Patients who have non-obstructive incontinence due to detrusor overactivity, spontaneous leakage, or an idiopathic etiology or who have detrusor–external sphincter dyssynergia may benefit from injection of botulinum toxin, type A (BTX-A).[47] Known primarily for its use in cosmetic enhancement, this neurotoxin is seeing increasing off-label use in the treatment of urological disorders. Between 100 and 300 units are diluted in sterile saline then injected submucosally into the bladder wall to reduce detrusor overactivity, and into the striated muscle of the external urinary sphincter to diminish outlet resistance. Maximal effect is noted 7–30 days after injection.[48] Adverse effects are uncommon with an overall incidence of 2–5%. These include generalized lethargy from systemic absorption, rapidly resolving retention in the case of detrusor injection, and stress incontinence after sphincter injection. Rarely, patients develop antibodies to BTX-A, rendering subsequent injections ineffective. Unfortunately, as has been observed with cosmetic use, the effects generally last only six to nine months. Some reports indicate that repeated injection may, in some cases, produce more durable results.[47]

Sacral nerve stimulation (SNS) or sacral neuromodulation is a more permanent therapeutic modality which is FDA-approved in the US and employed throughout Europe and Asia for the treatment of intractable urgency-frequency or urge incontinence, as well as urinary retention.[49,50] The technique involves placement of a quadripolar lead into the S3 foramen under fluoroscopic guidance, with subsequent connection of the lead to a pulse generator (IPG) that is implanted beneath the skin. This is generally performed as a two-stage procedure, the first stage being conducted under local anesthesia with sedation, so that the patient is responsive and can guide lead placement. The lead is connected to an external stimulator that is worn for a variable period, generally 1–2 weeks. If the patient experiences at least 50% improvement in voiding function during the test phase as indicated by a voiding diary, she continues to stage 2, implantation of the IPG, usually in the upper, outer quadrant of one of the buttocks. External programming is done via a magnetic device that communicates with the IPG through the skin. Results are often dramatic, with immediate normalization of voiding function. Urinary retention tends to respond more slowly and less completely than detrusor overactivity.[51]

Morbidity for both stages of the procedure is quite low, with pain at the IPG site and infection being most common.[52,53] Lead migration and equipment problems follow in frequency, and generally require surgical revision. Reported revision rates range from 20% to 30%. Explantation is usually performed for lack of response during test stimulation, loss of response after IPG placement, or for infection. In one contemporary series, the stage I and stage II explantation rates were 28% and 12%, respectively.[52] In spite of the relatively frequent need for re-operation to either obtain or optimize response to SNS, the minimally invasive and relatively brief nature of these outpatient procedures makes them very appealing to patients. Fortunately, no serious complications or long-term sequelae have been noted. It should be emphasized that there is no evidence that age and, by extension, duration of disability, affect the outcome of SNS. The major consideration with regard to age is the patient's ability to communicate and to manage programming of the device. Even in cases of severe and longstanding urinary incontinence or retention, near-resolution of symptoms can be achieved regardless of patient age. With this remarkable technology, one can indeed teach an old bladder new tricks!

## URINARY TRACT INFECTION

Nearly half of all women will experience a urinary tract infection (UTI) in their lifetime, and advanced age is known to be an independent risk factor for UTI. UTI accounts for 25% of all infections in the non-institutionalized elderly, while catheter-associated UTI is the most common nosocomial infection.[54] Other established risk factors for UTI include diabetes mellitus, urinary retention, neurogenic bladder, immunocompromise, sexual activity, and prior history of UTI.[55] Hypoestrogenism has also been implicated as a contributing factor to UTI in the postmenopausal woman because of its association with urogenital atrophy as well as alterations in vaginal pH and normal vaginal flora. The benefit of systemic hormone replacement in the prevention of UTI remains controversial, while the salutary prophylactic effect of local estrogen therapy is generally accepted.[56–58] Options available for topical estrogen delivery are presented earlier in the text.

Patients with UTI present with various constellations of symptoms, which may include frequency, urgency, dysuria, urge incontinence, suprapubic pressure or pain, flank pain, fever, or lethargy. Physical examination will often reveal suprapubic tenderness and fullness. The urethra and bladder base may also be tender to palpation. Costovertebral tenderness is an unusual finding, and is generally associated with pyelonephritis. A midstream clean-catch urine specimen should be sent for culture. Occasionally, catheterization may be necessary to obtain a specimen when there is concern regarding vaginal contamination. Preliminary dipstick reading of the urine as well as microscopic examination of a centrifuged specimen can help with establishing the presence of a UTI and determining empirical therapy. The presence of leukocyte esterase alone on dipstick is not specific for infection, as it will frequently read positive with even minor vaginal contamination or non-specific inflammation of the bladder or urethra. However, when a positive nitrite reading is obtained, this usually means that a gram-negative organism is present, and one would expect to see rods on microscopic examination. If there is no nitrite present on dipstick, cocci may be seen under the microscope, and treatment can be tailored accordingly. Occasionally, because of a dilution effect in urines with low specific gravities, bacteria will not be seen on microscopic urine examination, but will grow out in culture.

Except in cases of sporadic, uncomplicated UTI, the presence of infection should be established by a positive culture containing $10^5$ colony-forming units (cfu)/ml of a pathogenic organism, although in a symptomatic, immunocompromised patient, a pure culture demonstrating a lesser quantity of bacteria or fungus mandates treatment. Regardless of whether the UTI is uncomplicated or complicated, nosocomial, or community-acquired, the most common uropathogen is *E. coli*.

In patients with uncomplicated UTIs, usual pathogens include *Staphylococcus saprophyticus*, Klebsiella species, Proteus species, and enterococci. In institutionalized patients, and those with complicated infections, more virulent gram-negative organisms such as *Pseudomonas aeruginosa* and Morganella, Citrobacter, and Acinetobacter species and gram-positive bacteria such as *S. aureus* and *S. epidermidis* produce significant morbidity. Candida species constitute another class of opportunistic organisms that can cause severe illness in older, compromised patients. In postmenopausal women, the native lactobacilli found in the vagina are often replaced by gram-negative bacteria, thus providing a reservoir of potential pathogens, and contributing to the high incidence of asymptomatic bacteriuria in this population.

Asymptomatic bacteriuria refers to the condition whereby the urine culture of an asymptomatic individual grows out $>10^5$ cfu of a single uropathogen. Although the exact incidence is unknown, it is common in the geriatric population, and highest among the institutionalized elderly. Many physicians are confused by the lack of connection between symptoms and evidence of infection, and are uncertain regarding indications for treatment. Although this is often termed an 'infection', the majority of the time, no treatment is indicated. Numerous studies have shown that if patients are given appropriate antibiotics, the urine will clear temporarily, but most will recolonize, frequently with a more virulent or resistant strain of the same organism. Further, the presence of asymptomatic bacteria is not an independent predictor of either morbidity or mortality in the elderly.[59] Screening for asymptomatic bacteriuria is therefore not advocated, even in such high-risk patients as those with diabetes.[60–62] Treatment of asymptomatic bacteriuria should be reserved solely for immunocompromised patients such as those undergoing chemotherapy for cancer, for patients growing Proteus because this organism predisposes to urinary stone formation, and for patients undergoing surgical procedures, particularly those involving implantation of artificial joints or manipulation of the urinary tract.

Another dilemma relating to the geriatric population is the management of bacterial colonization and infection in patients with chronic indwelling catheters. It is generally agreed that those who are symptom-free should be treated similarly to patients with asymptomatic bacteriuria. For symptomatic individuals, the choice of antibiotic(s) should be based on the results of culture and sensitivity testing. A catheter change should be performed after initiation of therapy. The duration of treatment will depend on the organism, the extent of involvement of the urinary tract, and on the patient's response to therapy. For the patient with recurrent symptomatic infections, prophylactic daily antibiotics should be considered after completion of the full-dose regimen.

In summary, UTI remains a common problem in postmenopausal women, even those that are healthy. However, judicious use of topical estrogen, antibiotics, and prophylactic regimens can minimize morbidity. Therapeutic guidelines are the same as for uncomplicated and complicated infections in younger patients. That is, for uncomplicated UTI, 3 days of an appropriate antibiotic is usually sufficient, while, for complicated UTI, 7–14 days of coverage is advocated. In cases of bacteremia and sepsis, longer courses of antibiotics may be appropriate. Current US and international guidelines for the treatment of UTI have been summarized in a recent publication.[63] Prophylactic antibiotics should be considered in those with recurrent symptomatic infections, those who are immunocompromised, or those who are at risk for serious sequelae of UTI. For patients with recurrent UTIs without underlying pathology, a six-month course of a daily, low-level antibiotic will allow restoration of the patient's natural defense mechanisms. Indefinite prophylaxis may be indicated in patients whose impaired health puts them at high risk for significant morbidity from UTI. It should be emphasized that, whenever possible, predisposing factors for UTI should be addressed to minimize the risk of developing symptomatic infection. Holistic remedies such as taking cranberry extracts in various forms (juice, tablets), and maintaining healthy lactobacillus colonization of the vagina via the ingestion of yogurt with live cultures, acidophilus tablets, or acidophilus powder remain popular, and are largely supported by scientific data.[64–66]

## HEMATURIA

Hematuria, either gross (visible) or microscopic, is one of the most common reasons for urological referral as it is often a harbinger of genitourinary pathology. Even a single episode of gross hematuria is reason for concern and demands investigation. However, until recently, what constituted significant microscopic hematuria was cause for debate. The controversy was settled when the American Urological Association appointed a Best Practice Policy Panel consisting of representatives from urology, nephrology, and family practice who were charged with establishing guidelines for the detection and evaluation of microscopic hematuria. The consensus recommendation defined clinically significant microscopic hematuria as 'three or more red blood cells per high-power field on microscopic evaluation of the urinary sediment, from two or three properly collected urinalysis specimens'.[67–69] Nevertheless, if the patient is a smoker or is otherwise at risk for genitourinary malignancy, any degree of microhematuria should be considered significant and should be investigated. This is particularly applicable in older individuals as it has been shown that the incidence of malignancy in patients over 50 years is 7.5% overall, and 34.5% in those with gross blood in their urine.[70]

The standard work-up of hematuria consists of either an intravenous pyelogram (IVP) or a helical computed tomographic (CT) urogram for imaging of the kidneys and upper tracts followed by cystourethrography for direct inspection of the bladder. For patients with painful hematuria or a history of urolithiasis, a CT scan without contrast may be substituted, but the most complete information is obtained by obtaining a CT scan of the abdomen and pelvis without and with contrast (unenhanced followed by enhanced CT). The unenhanced imaging study will demonstrate urinary tract stones regardless of composition as well as gross anatomical features of the urinary tract, while subsequent contrast administration will provide details of anatomy and function. Tumors are best seen with the use of intravenous contrast. For those patients with an elevated creatinine or a contrast allergy precluding performing an IVP or CT urogram, a renal ultrasound followed by cystourethrography with bilateral retrograde pyelography is considered equivalent.

The most common etiologies of hematuria in women aged 40–60 years are acute UTI, stones, and bladder cancer. In those 60 years of age or older, bladder cancer and UTI are most frequent. Although rare, urethral carcinoma should always be considered in the differential diagnosis of microhematuria in the mature woman, because it is most prevalent in this age group and is often not detected until it is advanced. It is often associated with a mass or urethral thickening and obstructive voiding/retention as well. Renal cell carcinoma, particularly in smokers, must also be considered.

Postmenopausal hematuria may also be caused by non-malignant entities. Caruncles are polypoid lesions of the urethral meatus that may bleed or, less frequently, produce discomfort. Intervention is rarely indicated, but if the caruncle is friable with active bleeding or bothersome to the patient, excision is easily accomplished under local anesthesia in the office. Other inflammatory disorders may affect the bladder and mimic cancer. Chronic cystitis, which resembles carcinoma in situ of the bladder, may not have an apparent microbial source. Only biopsy can distinguish carcinoma in situ from inflammation. Tuberculosis can affect any portion of the genitourinary system causing pyuria and hematuria. In the diabetic patient or one who abuses non-steroidal anti-inflammatory drugs, IVP may demonstrate calyceal blunting, characteristic of papillary necrosis. During the acute phase of the disorder, sloughed papillae may appear as polypoid intrarenal or ureteral masses that mimic tumors. Patients may actually suffer renal colic from transient obstruction related to the passage of a sloughed papilla. They often report gross hematuria and passage of tissue fragments in their urine in association with the flank pain.

Painful hematuria, gross or microscopic, is most commonly associated with renal or ureteral calculi. Irritative voiding symptoms may indicate the presence of a stone in the distal ureter, heralding the imminent passage of the calculus.

Finally, conditions unique to the postmenopausal woman may produce microhematuria. Women taking combined hormone replacement therapy (HRT) can experience occult or overt bleeding per vagina. Contamination of the urine with vaginal secretions then results in the detection of blood on dipstick or formal urinalysis. Conversely, in women who are not being treated with local or systemic HRT, atrophy alone, because of the associated tissue fragility, may produce microhematuria.

## REFERENCES

1.  Chancellor MB, Yoshimura N. Physiology and pharmacology of the bladder and urethra. In: Walsh PC, Retik AB, Vaughan ED, Wein AJ, eds Campbell's Urology, 8th edn. Philadelphia: WB Saunders, 2002: 831–86.
2.  Raz S, Caine M, Ziegler M. The vascular component in the production of intraurethral pressure. J Urol 1972; 108: 93–6.
3.  Delancey JOL. Structural aspects of urethrovesical function in the female. Neurourol Urodyn 1988; 7: 509–20.
4.  Delancey JOL. Pubovesical ligaments: a separate structure from the urethral supports ('pubourethral ligaments'). Neurourol Urodyn 1989; 8: 53–62.
5.  Delancey JOL. Structural support of the urethra as it relates to stress urinary incontinence: the hammock hypothesis. Am J Obstet Gynecol 1994; 170: 1713–20.
6.  Mostwin JL. Current concepts of female pelvic anatomy and physiology. Urol Clin North Am 1991; 18: 175–95.
7.  Kakizaki H, Koyanagi T, Kato M. Sympathetic innervation of the male feline urethral rhabdosphincter. Neurosci Lett 1991; 129: 165–7.
8.  Greendale GA, Lee NP, Arriola ER. The menopause. Lancet 1999; 353: 571–80.
9.  Brown ADG. Postmenopausal urinary problems. Clin Obstet Gynecol 1977; 4: 181–206.
10. Ouslander JG. Aging and the lower urinary tract. Am J Med Sci 1997; 314: 214–8.
11. Longhurst PA, Kauer J, Leggett RE et al. The influence of ovariectomy and estradiol replacement on urinary bladder function in rats. J Urol 1992; 148: 915–19.
12. Holm NR, Horn T, Hald T. Detrusor in aging and obstruction. Scand J Urol Nephrol 1995; 29: 45–9.
13. Azadzoi KM, Tarcan T, Siroky MB et al. Atherosclerosis-induced chronic ischemia causes bladder fibrosis and non-compliance in the rabbit. J Urol 1999; 161: 1626–35.
14. Levy BJ, Wight TN. Structural changes in the aging submucosa: new morphologic criteria for the evaluation of the unstable human bladder. J Urol 1990; 144: 1044–55.
15. Elbadawi A, Yalla SV, Resnick NM. Structural basis of geriatric voiding dysfunction. I. Methods of a prospective ultrastructural/urodynamic study and an overview of the findings. J Urol 1993; 150: 1650–6.
16. Elbadawi A, Yalla SV, Resnick NM. Structural basis of geriatric voiding dysfunction. II. Aging detrusor: normal versus impaired contractility. J Urol 1993; 150: 1657–67.
17. Elbadawi A, Yalla SV, Resnick NM. Structural basis of geriatric voiding dysfunction. III. Detrusor overactivity. J Urol 1993; 150: 1668–80.
18. Elbadawi A, Yalla Sv, Resnick NM. Structural basis of geriatric voiding dysfunction. IV. Bladder outlet obstruction. J Urol 1993; 150: 1681–95.
19. Brierly RD, Hindley RG, McLarty E et al. A prospective controlled quantitative study of ultrastructural changes in the underactive detrusor. J Urol 2003; 169: 1374–8.
20. Strasser H, Tiefenthaler M, Steinlechner M et al. Apoptosis of rhabdosphincter cells: the main cause of urinary incontinence with advancing age? J Urol 1999; 161 (Suppl): 254.
21. Nihira MA, Henderson N. Epidemiology of urinary incontinence in women. Curr Womens Health Rep 2003; 3: 340–7.
22. Diokno AL, Brock BM, Brown MB et al. Prevalence of urinary incontinence and other urologic symptoms in the non-institutionalized elderly. J Urol 1986; 136: 1022–8.
23. Hannestad YS, Rortveit G, Sandvik H et al. A community-based epidemiologic survey of female urinary incontinence. The Norwegian EPINCONT Study. J Clin Epidemiol 2000; 53: 1150–7.
24. Abrams P, Cardozo L, Fall M et al. The standardisation of terminology in lower urinary tract function: report from the standardisation sub-committee of the International Continence Society. Neurourol Urodyn 2002; 21: 167–78.

25. Abrams P, Cardozo L, Fall M et al. The standardisation of terminology in lower urinary tract function: report from the standardisation sub-committee of the International Continence Society. Urology 2003; 61: 37–49.

26. Resnick NM, Yalla SV. Detrusor hyperactivity with impaired contractile function: an unrecognized but common cause of incontinence in elderly patients. JAMA 1987; 257: 3076–81.

27. Resnick NM. Geriatric incontinence. Urol Clin North Am 1996; 23: 55–74.

28. Baessler K, Schuessler B. Childbirth-induced trauma to the urethral continence mechanism: review and recommendations. Urology 2003; 62 (Suppl 4a): 39–44.

29. Bump RC, Mattiason A, Bo K et al. The standardization of terminology of female pelvic organ prolapse and pelvic floor dysfunction. Am J Obstet Gynecol 1996; 175: 10–17.

30. Kobashi K, Leach GE. Pelvic prolapse. J Urol 2000; 164; 1879–90.

31. Harrison BP, Cespedes RD. Pelvic organ prolapse. Emerg Med Clin North Am 2001; 19: 781–97.

32. Boone TR, Kim YH. Uroflowmetry. In: Nitti VW, ed. Practical Urodynamics. Philadelphia: WB Saunders, 1998: 28–34.

33. McGuire EJ, Woodside JR, Borden TA. Prognostic value of urodynamic testing on myelodysplastic children. J Urol 1981: 126: 205–9.

34. McGuire EJ, Fitzpatrick CC, Wan J et al. Clinical assessment of urethral sphincter function. J Urol 1993; 150: 1452–4.

35. Nitti VW, Tu LM, Gitlin J. Diagnosing bladder outlet obstruction in women. J Urol 1999; 161: 1535–40.

36. Brocklehurst JC, Dillane JB. Studies of the female bladder in old age. I. Cystometrograms in non-incontinent women. Gerontol Clin 1966; 8: 285–305.

37. Madersbacher S, Pycha A, Schatzel et al. The aging lower urinary tract: a comparative urodynamic study of men and women. Urology 1998; 51: 206–12.

38. Wagg AS, Lieu PIC, Ding YY et al. A urodynamic analysis of age-associated changes in urethral function in women with lower urinary tract symptoms. J Urol 1984; 156: 1984–90.

39. Collas DM, Malone-Lee JG. Age-associated changes in detrusor sensory function in women with lower urinary tract symptoms. Int Urogynecol J 1996; 7: 24–9.

40. Davila GW, Guerette N. Current treatment options for female urinary incontinence – a review. Int J Fertil 2004; 49: 102–112.

41. Bo K, Hagen RR, Kvarstein B et al. Pelvic floor muscle exercises for the treatment of female stress urinary incontinence. III. Effect of two different degrees of pelvic floor muscle exercises. Neurourol Urodyn 1990; 9: 489–502.

42. Nitti VW. Duloxetine: a new pharmacologic therapy for stress urinary incontinence. Rev Urol 1004; 6 (Suppl 3): S48–S55.

43. Ghoneim GM, Vanleeuwen JS, Elser DM et al. A randomized controlled trial of duloxetine alone, pelvic floor muscle training alone, combined treatment and no active treatment in women with stress urinary incontinence. J Urol 2005; 173: 1647–53.

44. Kay GG, Granville LJ. Antimuscarinic agents: implications and concerns in the management of overactive bladder in the elderly. Clin Ther 2005; 27: 127–38.

45. Hashim H, Abrams P. Drug treatment of overactive bladder. Efficacy, cost and quality-of-life considerations. Drugs 2004; 64: 1643–56.

46. Lose G, Alling-Moller L, Jennum P. Nocturia in women. Am J Obstet Gyn 2001; 185: 514–21.

47. Chancellor MB, Smith CP. Emerging role of botulinum toxin in the management of voiding dysfunction. J Urol 2004; 171, 2128–37.

48. Smith CP, Nishiguchi J, O'Leary M et al. Single-institution experience in 110 patients with botulinum toxin A injection into bladder or urethra. Urology 2005; 65: 37–41.

49. Chancellor MB, Chartier-Kastler EJ. Principles of sacral nerve stimulation (SNS) for the treatment of bladder and urethral sphincter dysfunction. Nueromodulation 2000; 3: 15–26.

50. Leng WW, Chancellor MB. How sacral nerve stimulation neuromodulation works. Urol Clin North Am 2005: 32: 11–18.

51. Jones U, Fowler CJ, Grunewald V. Efficacy of sacral nerve stimulation for urinary retention: results up to 18 months after implantation. In: Jones U, Grunewald V, eds. New Perspectives in Sacral Nerve Stimulation. London: Martin Dunitz, 2002: 150–8.

52. Hijaz A, Vasavada S. Complications and troubleshooting of sacral neuromodulation therapy. Urol Clin North Am 2005; 32: 65–9.

53. Jones U, Van den Hombergh U. Complications of sacral nerve stimulation. In Jones U, Grunewald, eds. New Perspectives in Sacral Nerve Stimulation. London: Martin Dunitz, 2002: 183–96.

54. Foxman B. Epidemiology of urinary tract infections: incidence, morbidity and economic costs. Am J Med 2002; 113 (Suppl 1A): 5S–13S.

55. Hu KK, Boyko, Scholes D et al. Risk factors for urinary tract infection in postmenopausal women. Arch Int Med 2004; 164: 989–93.

56. Raz R, Stamm WE. A controlled trial of intravaginal estriol in postmenopausal women with recurrent urinary tract infections. N Engl J Med 1993; 329: 753–6.

57. Stern JA, Hsieh YC, Schaeffer AJ. Residual urine in an elderly female population: novel implications for oral estrogen replacement and impact on recurrent UTI. J Urol 2004; 171: 768–70.

58. Rozenberg S, Pastijn A, Gevers R et al. Estrogen therapy in older patients with recurrent urinary tract infections: a review. Int J Fertil Womens Med 2004; 49: 71–4.

59. Abrutyn E, Mossey J, Berlin JA et al. Does asymptomatic bacteriuria predict mortality and does antimicrobial treatment reduce mortality in elderly ambulatory women. Ann Int Med 1994; 120: 827–33.

60. Hardy GK, Zhanel GG, Nicolle LE et al. Antimicrobial treatment in diabetic women with asymptomatic bacteriuria. N Engl J Med 2002; 347: 1576–83.

61. Nicolle LE. Urinary tract infection in geriatric and institutionalized patients. Curr Opin Urol 2002; 12: 51–5.

62. Nicolle LE. Asymptomatic bacteriuria: when to screen and when to treat. Infect Dis Clin North Am 2003; 17: 367–94.

63. Nickel JC. Management of urinary tract infections: historical perspectives and current strategies: Part 2 – modern management. J Urol 2005; 173: 27–32.

64. Jepson RG, Mihaljevic L, Craig J. Cranberries for preventing urinary tract infections. Cochrane Database Syst Rev 2004; (2): CD 001321.

65. Raz R, Chazen B, Dan M. Cranberry juice and urinary tract infection. Clin Infect Dis 2004; 38: 1413–19.
66. Fernandez MF, Boris S, Barbes C. Probiotic properties of human lactobacilli strains to be used in the gastro-intestinal tract. J Appl Microbiol 2003; 94: 449–55.
67. Grossfeld GD, Litwin MS, Wolf JS et al. Evaluation of asymptomatic microscopic hematuria in adults: the American Urological Association best practice policy – Part I: definition, detection, prevalence, and etiology. Urology 2001; 57: 599–603.
68. Grossfeld GD, Litwin MS, Wolf JS et al. Evaluation of asymptomatic microscopic hematuria in adults: the American Urological Association best practice policy – Part II: Patient evaluation, cytology, voided markers, imaging, cystoscopy, nephrology evaluation, and follow-up. Urology 2001; 57: 604–10.
69. Grossfeld GD, Wolf JS, Litwin MS et al. Asymptomatic microscopic hematuria in adults: summary of the AUA best practice policy recommendations. Am Fam Phys 2001; 63: 1145–54.
70. Sultana SR, Goodman CM, Byrne DJ et al. Microscopic haematuria: urological investigation using a standard protocol. Br J Urol 1996; 78: 691–6.

# Chapter 18

# The menopause and cardiovascular disease

William P Castelli

## INTRODUCTION

The number one cause of death in women is a disease related to atherosclerosis such as coronary heart disease, stroke, peripheral vascular disease, or other manifestations of vascular disease. Almost twice as many women die from these diseases as from all the cancers put together. In the vital statistics of the US it amounted to 45% of deaths in women.[1] As important as the death rates are, the morbidity from vascular diseases is even greater considering that prior to age 65 years, only about 15% of women die when they develop coronary heart disease; 85% of these women live. Over the age of 65 years, the death rate is 20–25%, but 75% live. Almost half of the people who live have a lower quality of life; many lose their jobs.

Over 75% of the women destined to develop cardiovascular disease could be identified years in advance of their clinical manifestations, if their physicians were willing to measure a few simple things on their bodies. These things have come to be known as the risk factors and deal with those well-known items such as cholesterol, blood pressure, smoking, blood sugar, weight, and many other variables that are described in this chapter.

Women, more recently, have been involved in trials to lower the risk factor numbers, and the studies have led to clinical strategies to prevent cardiovascular disease in women and offer better treatments for those who have developed the disease. Those health professionals involved with the care of women after the menopause need to recognize the importance of assessing these women for diseases other than just those associated with the reproductive status of women.

## RATES OF CARDIOVASCULAR DISEASE

Prior to the menopause only about eight women in the Framingham study developed coronary heart disease.[2] These women can be found in any town in the world. They have familial hypercholesterolemia, familial combined hyperlipoproteinemia, hypertriglyceridemia or diabetes, and smoke at the same time. Once women pass through the menopause it takes them about 10 years to catch up to the same rates of coronary heart disease as occur in men, as indicated in Figure 18.1. The lifetime risk of cardiovascular diseases is another way of looking at these rates in the Framingham study. The lifetime risk of women starting at age 40 years, for coronary disease is 31.7% (95% confidence interval (CI), 29.2 to 34.2), which when added to the risk of cerebrovascular diseases (9%) and other vascular disease (7%) adds up to 47% of the women developing cardiovascular disease over their lifetime compared to 54% percent of men.[3]

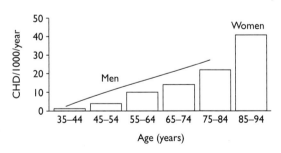

**Figure 18.1**  Annual coronary heart disease (CHD) rate for men and women. (Reproduced from the Framingham Heart Study, courtesy of the National Heart, Lung and Blood Institute, Boston University School of Medicine.)

## BLOOD LIPIDS

### Total cholesterol

One of the first lipids to be looked at in the Framingham Heart study was total cholesterol. As Figure 18.2 shows, at any age, the higher the total cholesterol level, the higher the subsequent rate of coronary heart disease. Note that older women do not tolerate cholesterol better than do younger women. The absolute rate of coronary heart disease in a 70-year-old women is double that of 50-year-old women at the same level of cholesterol, everything else being equal.

As shown in Figure 18.3, the total cholesterol level is not sufficient by itself to identify 90% of the women at risk. The bell-shaped curve for all the cholesterols of the men and women of the

Framingham Heart study who stayed free of coronary heart disease in the first 26 years of the study overlapped the bell-shaped curve, with the men and women who develop coronary heart disease when the total cholesterols are between 150 and 300 mg/dl.

We understand three kinds of risk in medicine: relative, absolute, and attributable risk. Relative risk shows that the people with a total cholesterol level of 300 mg/dl have five times the rate of disease as people with 150 mg/dl. Absolute risk shows that for people with a cholesterol level of 300 mg/dl higher, 90/100 are likely to develop coronary heart disease. It is generally agreed that people with such high cholesterol levels should be treated at any age, because the chance of treating someone who does not need it, is low. Attributable risk is more complex. There are several attributa-

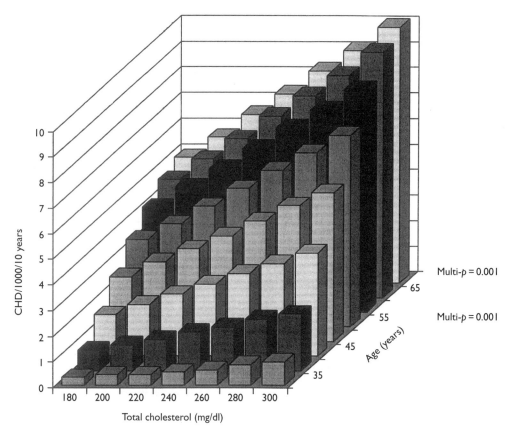

**Figure 18.2**  Coronary heart disease (CHD) and total cholesterol in low-risk women. Multi-$P$ = 0.001. (Trend adjusted on multivariate analysis for systolic blood pressure, cigarettes, diabetes and LVH.) (Reproduced from the Framingham Heart Study, National Heart, Lung and Blood Institute, Boston University School of Medicine: Anderson et al. Circulation 1991; 83: 357–63,[4] and Kannel WB, Wolf PA, Garrison RJ, Framingham Study Section 34, 30 year follow-up. NIH publication No 87-2703.[5])

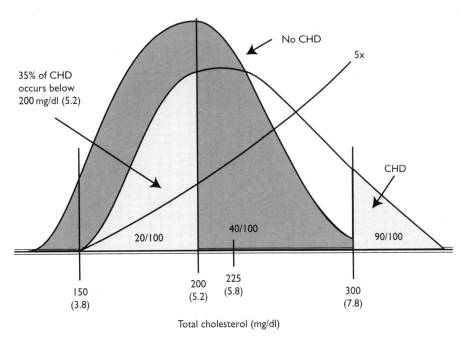

No CHD

5x

35% of CHD
occurs below
200 mg/dl (5.2)

CHD

20/100

40/100

90/100

150
(3.8)

200
(5.2)

225
(5.8)

300
(7.8)

Total cholesterol (mg/dl)

**Figure 18.3**
Relative, absolute,
population-
attributable risk
fraction. CHD,
coronary heart
disease. (Reproduced
from the Framingham
Heart Study, the
National Heart, Lung
and Blood Institute,
Boston University
School of Medicine:
Castelli. Can J Cardiol
1988; 4 (Suppl A):
5A–10A,[6] with
permission from the
publisher.)

ble risks, but that illustrated in Figure 18.3 is the population-attributable risk fraction. This is the fraction of heart attacks that one would attribute to a particular level of cholesterol. For example, twice as many women with a cholesterol level between 150 and 200 mg/dl all their lives are likely to develop coronary disease as those with a cholesterol level of 300 mg/dl or higher. The National Cholesterol Education Program (NCEP) considered a cholesterol level under 200 mg/dl as desirable. Why should this be so, when twice as many women and men develop coronary disease at this level than over 300 mg/dl? It is largely because the NCEP program ignored attributable risk. They understood absolute risk and therefore, the rate at cholesterol levels between 150 and 200 mg/dl being 20/100, was lower than the rate of 90/100 for people with cholesterol over 300 mg/dl. The reason that there are more heart attacks at 20/100 than 90/100 is that the incidence at 20/100 relates to 45% of the population, whereas the incidence of 90/100 relates to just 3% of the population. If we eliminate all the heart attacks occurring at a cholesterol at 300 mg/dl, the rate of coronary disease will fall by 10–15%. Eventually we have to find a way to prevent the 35% of the heart attacks that occurred at cholesterol levels between 150 and 200 mg/dl. The worse cholesterol level in this regard is around 225 mg/dl, because more coronary disease occurs at that level of cholesterol than any other, and the

rate is 40/100. How does one find just the 20, 40, and 90 out of hundred at these different levels of cholesterol so that one does not treat people who do not need it? This is when one must look at the other kinds of cholesterol found in the blood, of which there are 20 known to date. One other point: if the total cholesterol level is under 150 mg/dl, then the person is like the billions of people living on this earth who cannot develop atherosclerotic diseases. These people live in the poorest sections of Asia, Africa and Latin America. Unfortunately, they are now adopting many of the Western dietary practices, for example fast food.

### High-density lipoprotein cholesterol

Of the 20 different kinds of cholesterol particles, the one that needs to be looked at first is the high-density lipoprotein (HDL) cholesterol. There are five sizes of HDL cholesterol particles. Figure 18.4 shows the level of the total cholesterol stratified by the HDL cholesterol level in men and women in the Framingham Heart Study. It can be seen that the higher the HDL level, the lower is the rate of coronary heart disease. The first row of this figure indicates that the high-risk people with a total cholesterol level under 200 mg/dl have a low HDL level, and this is true of all the other levels of cholesterol, but the higher the total cholesterol level, the higher the level of HDL cholesterol needed for protection. Rather than memorizing a different HDL level for each total cholesterol level, a simple ratio was sufficient: the total cholesterol divided by the HDL cholesterol. This is the best lipid predictor in the Framingham study,[8] the Lipid Research Clinic Trial, the Physicians' Health Study,[10] the Harvard Nurses Study,[11] the Scandinavian, Simvastin Survivors' (4S) study,[12] the AirForce/Texas Coronary Atherosclerosis Prevention Study (AFCAPS/TexCaps) study,[13] indeed any study that took the time to measure it.[6] Figure 18.5 shows the ratio of total cholesterol/HDL cholesterol in women. There is another way to think about risk: normal, average, and ideal (Dawber TR, personal communication). For too many years the guideline writers called average normal. You do not want to be like the average American, it would be better to be like average Chinese who cannot develop this disease in those small communities of China where individuals have a total cholesterol around 127 mg/dl. We need to think about a more ideal level; for now we would choose a total / HDL ratio of less than 4 for primary prevention and a ratio of under 3 if we want to shrink the deposits in people who have vascular disease, diabetes or a Framingham Risk Calulator score of 20% or higher.

## Low-density lipoprotein cholesterol

Figure 18.6 shows that the higher the level of low density lipoprotein (LDL) as measured by the $S_f$ 0–20 (Svedborg ultracentrifuge measures) lipoproteins, the higher the rate of coronary heart disease. The NCEP guidelines used to evaluate the lipid numbers currently call for an LDL under 160 mg/dl for people without other risk factors or disease. Those with two or more other risk factors but no vascular disease should have an LDL cholesterol level under 130 mg/dl, however a new option was introduced after the Anglo-Scandinavian Cardiac Outcomes Trial (ASCOT) showed that people with two or more other risk factors do better with an LDL under 100 mg/dl.[14] Those with vascular disease, diabetes, or a high Framingham Risk Calculator Score should have an LDL cholesterol under 70 mg/dl as recently shown in the Prove-it Study.[15] The other risk factors defined in the guidelines are a family history of vascular disease before the age of 55 years, hypertension, cigarette smoking, and an HDL cholesterol level under 35 mg/dl. However, a level of 160 mg/dl seems inappropriate because the average level of LDL cholesterol level of someone who

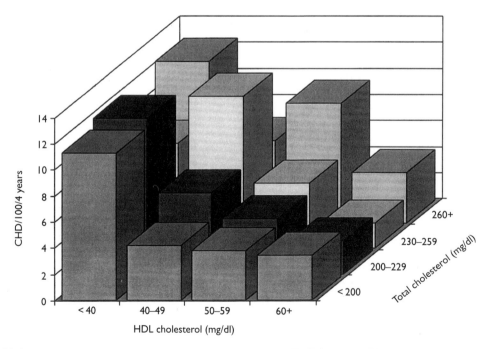

**Figure 18.4** Coronary heart disease (CHD) and total and high-density lipoprotein (HDL) cholesterol on men and women aged 50–60+ years. (Reproduced from the Framingham Heart Study, National Heart, Lung and Blood Institute, Boston University School of Medicine: Castelli et al. JAMA 1986; 256: 2835–8,[6] with permission from the publisher.)

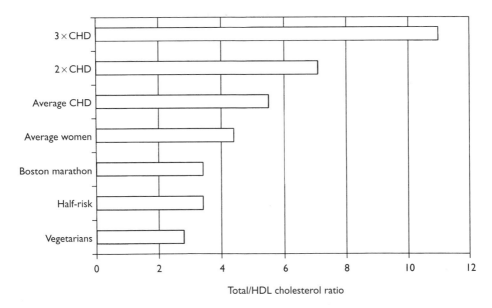

**Figure 18.5**   Total cholesterol/high-density lipoprotein (HDL) cholesterol ratio in women. (Reproduced from the Framingham Heart Study, the National Heart, Lung and Blood Institute, Boston University School of Medicine: Castelli. Can J Cardiol 1988; 4 (Suppl A): 5A–10A,[6] with permission from the publisher.)

dies of coronary heart disease in the US is under 150 mg/dl. The targets for the average person should be a lot lower than that. Two new studies have helped to change these guidelines. ASCOT, in people with marked hypertension, but largely free of cardiovascular disease, who had their LDL cholesterols lowered from 131 mg/dl to 90 mg/dl, on just 10 mg of atorvastatin (Lipitor), ran a 36% lower rate of the prime coronary endpoints in just 3.3 years.[14] The Prove-it study in subjects with coronary heart disease ran a significantly lower heart disease rate in people taken to an LDL of 62 mg/dl on atorvastatin, than people taken to 95 mg/dl on pravastatin in 6 months.[15] Even though there were not enough women in either of these two studies, the current consensus is that these goals should be used for women as well.

### The seven LDLs

There are seven LDL cholesterols, and the smaller the LDL particle's size, the higher the heart attack rate.[16] A recent study in Quebec showed that people with the small dense LDL ran three-times the heart attack rates of people with the large LDL, who, because of their higher levels of LDL, were running twice the heart attack rate of the control group.[17] As the triglycerides rise, as shown in Figure 18.7, the size of the LDL particles falls and

the level of the HDL cholesterols falls. When the triglycerides exceed 100 mg/dl, these changes in size are accelerated, and when people get to an LDL of 150 mg/dl they have mostly the smaller sizes of LDL.[18]

### Triglycerides

As Figure 18.6 shows, the higher the triglyceride level in women, the higher the heart attack rate.[6] There are four major classes of triglyceride: two are not atherogenic; one type is the chylomicrons, appearing in blood shortly after a high-fat meal, and the other type is the large very low-density lipoproteins that come out of the liver after a vegetarian diet, the intake of estrogen, alcohol, or a resin, The two that are atherogenic are the chylomicron remnants and the small, dense very low-density lipoproteins. The chylomicron remnants are derived from the chylomicrons after they have had some of their triglyceride fat removed by the action of lipoprotein lipases, and the small dense low-density lipoproteins come out of the liver, after diets high in saturated fat and cholesterol. Chylomicrons and chylomicron remnants have been poorly studied because of the necessity for a prolonged fast prior to measuring blood lipids. The large and very small low-density lipoproteins constitute the bulk of the triglyceride in fasting

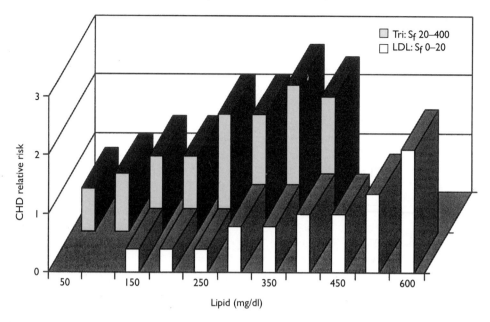

**Figure 18.6** Coronary heart disease (CHD) relative risk and low-density lipoprotein (LDL), and triglycerides (Tri) in women. (Reproduced from the Framingham Heart Study, the National Heart, Lung and Blood Institute, Boston University School of Medicine: Castelli. Can J Cardiol 1988; 4 (Suppl A): 5A–10A,[6] with permission from the publisher.)

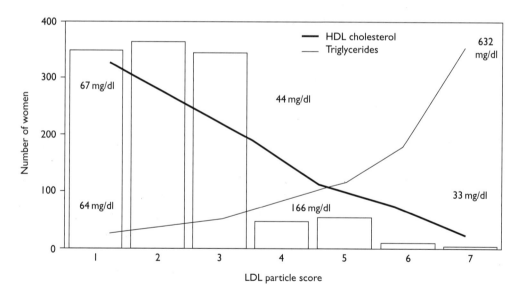

**Figure 18.7** Low-density lipoprotein (LDL) particle size. (Reproduced from the Framingham Heart Study, National Heart, Lung and Blood Institute, Lipid Metabolism Laboratory, USDA: Tufts University: Campos. Arterioscl Thromb 1992; 12: 1410–19,[18] with permission from the publisher.)

blood, with 70% being in the small dense low-density lipoproteins.[19]

However, similar to total cholesterol and LDL cholesterol, triglyceride risk is better ascertained if the HDL cholesterol is known. As Figure 18.8 shows, it is particularly the women with high triglyceride and low HDL levels who incur the highest rates of coronary heart disease, and these women have also been found to have other problems. Reaven showed they have increased insulin resistance and hypertension, and called this combination Syndrome X,[20] Kaplan emphasizes the work of Jean Vaque, the French physician who drew attention to the dangers of central obesity.[21] Others[22,23] have shown studies enforcing the evidence on hypertension, insulin resistance and dislipidemia. As triglyceride levels rise above 80 to 90 mg/dl there is a shift in the size of LDLs from larger to smaller ones that are more atherogenic. From Figure 18.8, we are not happy if a woman has a triglyceride of 100 mg/dl when her HDL is under 50 mg/dl; we consider that already to be too high a risk. The newest term to describe this syndrome is the metabolic syndrome (Figure 18.9).[24] In addition to the high triglycerides and low HDL and central obesity, women with this syndrome have higher levels of the clotting factors such as fibrinogen and plasminogen activator inhibitor-1 (PAI-1).[25] They also have higher uric acid levels, which have been associated with higher risk, and usually hypertension and pre-diabetes. The reason the guidelines have been less stringent with regard to triglycerides is that it has only been recently shown that they are an independent risk factor; however, triglycerides are a lot worse in women than in men.[26]

The most practical way to identify women with a dangerous triglyceride concentration is to find those with a triglyceride of 100 mg/dl and an HDL under 50 mg/dl, as shown in Figure 18.8. They have a significantly higher heart attack rate, and are largely ignored in medicine because their total cholesterols can frequently be under 200 mg/dl, and their LDL cholesterols are frequently under 130 mg/dl; in addition, unfortunately, they have the very atherogenic small dense very low-density lipoproteins (β-VLDL).

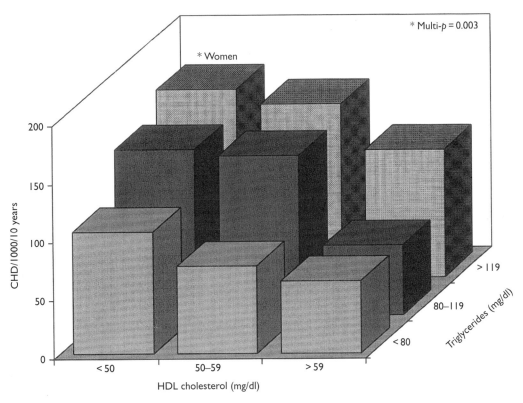

**Figure 18.8** Coronary heart disease (CHD), and high-density lipoprotein (HDL) cholesterol, and triglycerides in women. *, multi-P − 0.003. (Reproduced from the Framingham Heart Study, the National Heart, Lung and Blood Institute, Boston University School of Medicine: Castelli. Can J Cardiol 1988; 4 (Suppl A): 5A–10A,[6] with permission from the publisher.)

When waist/hip exceeds 0.8
>    Glucose   5.5 mmol/l (100 mg/dl)
>    Insulin resistance
>        insulin > 25 mU/l
>        C peptide > 1.3 nmol/l
>    BP over 120/80
>    Triglycerides   1.7 mmol/l (150 mg/dl)
>        small dense β VLDL
>    HDL cholesterol   1.17 mmol/l (45 mg/dl)
>    LDL
>        small dense pattern β
>    Uric acid 0.4 mmol/l (7)
>    Plasminogen activator inhibitor-1 (PAI-1)
>    Microalbuminuria, increased Na/Li
>    exchange

**Figure 18.9**   Metabolic syndrome.[20–24]

## Genetic disorders of lipids

About 5% of post menopausal women who have a very high risk of vascular disease associated with their inherited tendency have high levels of LDL cholesterol, triglycerides or both. These are generally traits that have run in their families, and many will have a family history of premature vascular disease occurring before the age of 60 years. Table 18.1 gives the cutoff points proposed by Schaefer and Levy to identify the women at any age who are most likely to have a genetic tendency to develop high cardiovascular disease rates due to their lipids.[27] Those with LDL cholesterol levels at or above that listed for their age are a type IIA hypolipoproteinemic. Those with a triglyceride level at or above that cited for their age are type IV hyperlipoproteinemic.[27] Those who equal or exceed both numbers for their age are combined type IIB hyperliproteinemic.[20] In addition to treating these women more aggressively, it is important to measure the lipid levels of all their children. The type IIAs are generally autosomal dominant genetic disorders, and half of their children will inherit this disorder.

## Lipoprotein(a)

A newly recognized risk factor is lipoprotein(a). It is a combination of an LDL particle with a small 'a' protein which blocks the conversion of plasminogen to plasmin, which dissolves fibrin on the

**Table 18.1**   Cutoff points for familial lipid disorders.

| Age (years) | Men LDL-II | Men Triglycerides-IV | Women LDL-II | Women Triglycerides-IV |
|---|---|---|---|---|
| 0–4 | | 84 | | 96 |
| 5–9 | 117 | 85 | 125 | 90 |
| 10–14 | 122 | 102 | 126 | 114 |
| 15–19 | 123 | 120 | 126 | 107 |
| 20–24 | 138 | 165 | 136 | 112 |
| 25–29 | 157 | 199 | 141 | 116 |
| 30–34 | 166 | 213 | 142 | 123 |
| 35–39 | 176 | 251 | 161 | 137 |
| 40–44 | 173 | 248 | 164 | 155 |
| 45–49 | 186 | 253 | 173 | 171 |
| 50–54 | 185 | 250 | 192 | 186 |
| 55–59 | 191 | 235 | 204 | 204 |
| 60–64 | 188 | 235 | 201 | 202 |
| 65–69 | 199 | 208 | 208 | 204 |
| 70+ | 182 | 212 | 189 | 204 |

LDL, low-density lipoprotein. Reproduced from Schaefer EJ and Levy RI. N Engl J Med 1985; 312: 1300–10,[27] with permission from the publisher.

endothelial cells. We live in this 'drizzle' of platelets clumping and unclumping, and fibrinogen being converted to fibin all day long. When the fibin hits the endothelial cells it stimulates the cells to send tissue type plasminogen activator and urokinase to activate plasminogen to convert to plasmin, which will dissolve the fibrin. Figure 18.10 shows the first evidence in women that lipoprotein(a) is associated with increased risk of coronary heart disease.[28] The difficulty with lipoprotein(a) is therapy. Primarily estrogen and high doses of crystalline niacin have been able to lower the lipoprotin(a) under 30 mg/dl, which would be the safer level to achieve. If this is not possible it is possible to take away the risk of lipoprotein(a) by getting the LDL level under 80 mg/dl, and the triglycerides to levels under 90 mg/dl.

## Lipids and the menopause

When women pass through the menopause, there is a significant rise in LDL cholesterol, and a fall in HDL cholesterol. Triglycerides continue to rise. The total cholesterol/HDL ratio and the apolipoprotein B/A ratio rise significantly, as indicated in Table 18.2.[29]

## ESTROGEN AND THE MENOPAUSE

One of the most important events said to happen during the menopause is the fall in estrogen. Estrogen is anti-atherogenic. The best data come from the work of Clarkson and colleagues in the cynamolgus macaques.[30] These monkeys have 98% of the human genome; they have the same male–female difference in HDL. When they are fed an atherogenic diet, the male total cholesterol/HDL ratio was increased to almost 12. In control females with their higher HDL, the ratio increases to eight; they develop appreciable atherosclerosis but not as much as the males. If the females are given a second-generation progestin which raises LDL and lowers HDL such as norgestrel, the ratio is increased to 12, but if it is given in the form of a birth control pill with a higher dose of estrogen, the atherosclerosis is

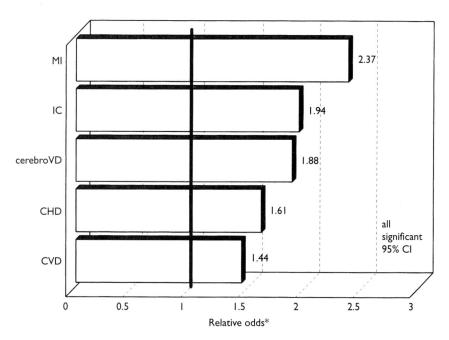

**Figure 18.10** Sinking pre-β lipoprotein(a) in women. *Relative odds adjusted for age, body mass index, systolic blood pressure, cigarette use, high-density lipoprotein, low-density lipoprotein, glucose, left ventricular hypertrophy on electrocardiogram. MI, myocardial infarction; IC, intermittent claudication; CerebroVD, cerebrovascular disease; CHD, coronary heart disease; CVD, cardiovascular disease; CI, confidence interval. (Reproduced from the Framingham Heart Study, the National Heart, Lung and Blood Institute, Boston University School of Medicine: Bostom et al. Circulation 1994; 90: 1688–95,[28] with permission from the publisher.)

**Table 18.2**   Lipid changes with the menopause

|  | Premenopausal | Postmenopausal | P value |
|---|---|---|---|
| Total cholesterol | 208 | 227 | 0.08 |
| LDL cholesterol | 134 | 156 | 0.03 |
| Triglycerides | 87 | 98 | 0.30 |
| HDL cholesterol | 56 | 51 | 0.10 |
| Total/HDL ratio | 3.71 | 4.45 | 0.02 |
| Apo A-1/Apo B | 2.41 | 1.86 | 0.04 |

LDL, low-density lipoprotein; HDL, high-density lipoprotein; Apo, apolipoprotein. Reproduced from Campos H et al. J Clin Endocrinol Metab 1988; 67: 30–5,[29] with permission from the publisher.

greatly diminished. With a second-generation progestin such as levonorgestrel without the estrogen, a high total cholesterol and HDL ratio, and increased atherosclerosis result.[30] The same is probably true in human females. In the Harvard Nurses Study, in nurses who took the first-generation birth control pills, which caused thrombosis-related deaths, nonetheless it recorded a 20% lower rate of coronary heart disease if they survived to the menopause.[31]

The use of estrogen is a double-edged sword. At any dose it is anti-atherogenic, as long as we are talking about true human ethinyl estradiol and not conjugated estrogens from the urine of pregnant mares. But as the dose rises, the blood starts to clot and this will, at higher doses, lead to coronary heart disease and stroke as it did in the postmenopausal women in Framingham who were taking 2.5 and 3.5 mg of conjugated estrogens.[32] In the Harvard Nurses Study, postmenopausal women taking estrogen at a dose above 1.25 mg more than doubled their rate of coronary disease.[31] Also men given estrogen in the Coronary Drug Project, at a dose of 2.5 mg conjugated estrogens, died at a significantly higher rate of coronary disease, and this arm of the study was stopped prematurely.[33] The birth control pill is one of the few medicines in use for which a dose–response curve was never determined. The dose fell in the history of the birth control pills from 150 µg ethinyl estradiol down eventually to 20 µg, but lower doses have never been fully tested. Recently, lower doses have been looked at in the field of hormone replacement therapy (HRT), 5 and 10 µg ethinyl estradiol with norethindrone provide the same osteoporosis prevention as do higher doses.[34]

While some epidemiological studies showed that women taking HRT incur about a 50% lower heart attack rate than those not taking it, these are not random trials, and the benefits could have been explained by the healthy cohort effect, namely that the women who self-select to take estrogen are richer and smarter than the women who do not, and do all kinds of other things to improve their risk, and that is why they incur such a low heart attack rate.[35] The first random trial of giving HRT was the Heart Estrogen/Progestin Replacement Study (HERS); while not in women free of disease, it showed only a small fall in vascular events after several years, and even suggested that there was a higher rate of coronary death in the first year, which was probably a statistical artifact due to the very low rate of coronary disease in the first year of the control group compared to years 2, 3, 4, and 5.[36] The only women in the HERS study who benefited from taking estrogen therapy were women who had an elevated lipoprotein(a). Less than 10% of the women on the estrogen had their LDLs taken under 100 mg/dl, let alone under 70 mg/dl. Estrogen therapy is not a substitute for aggressive control of the risk factors.

The Woman's Health Initiative has now provided us with the best evidence concerning the use of conjugated estrogen and medroxyprogesterone use after the menopause (Table 18.3).[37,38] Whether use of lower doses, less than 625 mg Premarin, or a different progestin or even use of progesterone itself, or even human estrogen would do better will await future trials.

One of the disconcerting findings in the Woman's Health Initiative was the increase in breast cancer. Given the data from the China study,[39] and from comparisons of women from Japan, Hawaii, and San Francisco,[40] where it appears that societies with higher plant protein diets protect women from breast cancer, whether giving them estrogen would increase their breast cancer, is unknown. Establishing enough evidence to study this would be quite difficult at this time in history.

As far as the clotting goes, with estrogen, besides considering a much lower dose, one wonders what would happen if women with a tendency to clot were excluded from estrogen therapy. Table 18.4 summarizes some of the new risk factors for thrombosis which, added to the old ones like fibrinogen or high factor VII, might provide a way to identify candidates who should not take estrogen.[41]

**Table 18.3** The Women's Health Initiative[36,37]

**Compared to placebo, estrogen and progestin resulted in:**
- increased risk of heart attack
- increased risk of stroke
- increased risk of blood clots
- increased risk of breast cancer
- fewer fractures
- increased risk of dementia
- reduced risk of colorectal cancer
- no protection against mild cognitive impairment

**Compared to placebo, estrogen alone resulted in:**
- no difference for heart attack
- increased risk of stroke
- increased risk of blood clots
- uncertain risk of breast cancer
- fewer fractures
- increased risk of dementia, statistically significant only in women over 65 years
- no difference in colorectal cancer
- no protection against mild cognitive impairment

## HYPERTENSION

It is only in those societies that eat a high-salt diet that the blood pressure rises with age. American women live in a society that eats 20 times the amount of salt they need, and the blood pressure rises with age such that shortly after women pass through the menopause over half will have a blood pressure at 140/90 mmHg or above. Of

**Table 18.4** Percentage prevalence of risk factors for thrombosis

| Risk factors | General population | Patients with thrombosis |
|---|---|---|
| Protein C deficiency | 0.2–0.4 | 3 |
| Protein S deficiency | Not known | 1–2 |
| Factor V Leiden | 5 | 20 |
| Prothrombin 20210A | 2 | 6 |
| Homocysteine >18 μmol/l | 5 | 10 |
| High factor VIII (>1500 IU/l) | 11 | 25 |
| Antithrombin deficiency | 0.02 | 1 |

Reproduced from Rosendaal. Lancet 1999; 353: 1167–73,[41] with permission from the publisher.

course this is not any longer the definition of hypertension; ideal blood pressure is under 120/80 mmHg.

As diastolic or systolic pressures rise in women, cardiovascular risk, particularly of stroke and heart attack, rise as shown in Figure 18.11. Of the two measures, systolic pressure is a better predictor than diastolic. Isolated systolic hypertension is also very dangerous. The elderly do not tolerate high blood pressure, which is the opposite of what was said for decades in medicine. Figure 18.12 shows elderly women with isolated systolic hypertension: the higher the value the worse the prognosis, and the older the woman the higher the risk.[5] Table 18.5 indicates that half of the coronary disease in women occurs at levels of blood pressure 120–139 mmHg for the systolic and 80–89 mmHg for the diastolic pressures. The latest joint National Commission on hypertension recommendations have tried to address at least half of this risk by setting a new cutoff point at 135/85 mmHg (Table 18.6).[42] However, the Hope study in Canada treating people with systolic pressures in the 130s (mmHg) with an angiotensin-converting enzyme (ACE) inhibitor showed a reduction in heart attacks, strokes, and the onset of diabetes.[43] Two studies treating people with systolic pressures in the 120s (mmHg), the old Study of Left Ventricular Dysfunction (SOLVD) study,[44] and now the new Camelot study with a calcium channel blocker amlodipine,[45] lowered the cardiovascular events by taking blood pressures below 120/80 mmHg.

## CIGARETTE SMOKING

In 1948, when the first women entered the Framingham study, of the 35% who said they smoked, virtually none inhaled. Of the major cancers beyond skin cancer, breast cancer was number one in incidence, and lung cancer was last. Women learned how to inhale in the 1950s, and by the 1960s they were paying the price for inhaling. The incidence of vascular disease and especially of lung cancer rose, and, in 1987, lung cancer overtook breast cancer and became the number one cancer cause of death in women for the first time in the history of the US, as it has been since time immemorial in men. Figure 18.13 is taken from the work of Rosenberg and her colleagues, and shows that the risk of myocardial infarction is dose related, rising from a relative risk of 2 for 1–14 cigarettes per day, to 7.2 for 35 or more.[46] Quitting

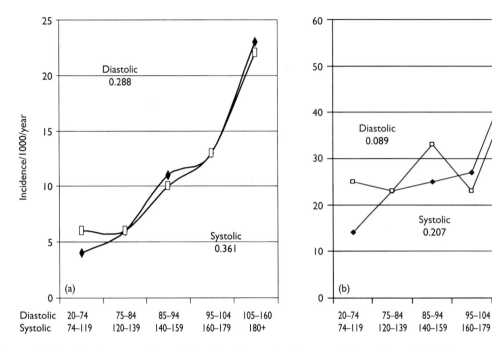

**Figure 18.11** Blood pressure (in mmHg) and cardiovascular disease in (a) women aged 35–64 years, and (b) women aged 65–94 years. (Reproduced from the Framingham Heart Study, the National Heart, Lung and Blood Institute, Boston University School of Medicine: Kannel et al. NIH publication No. 87–2703, 1987,[5] with permission from the publisher.)

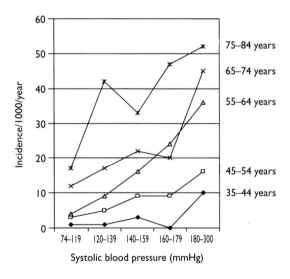

**Figure 18.12** Blood pressure and cardiovascular disease. (Reproduced from the Framingham Heart Study, the National Heart, Lung and Blood Institute, Boston University School of Medicine: Kannel et al. NIH publication No. 87–2703, 1987,[5] with permission from the publisher.)

returns the risk to that of non-smokers within three years in this study, but the benefit of quitting may be much quicker. It depends on how people define the quitter. In the Framingham study, where the smoker had to quit for the entire year to be called a quit smoker, the risk fell back within one year. Women apparently have more difficulty than men in giving up smoking.[47] Women also tend to smoke low yield cigarettes, perhaps believing them to be safer, but the evidence shows that these cigarettes are not safer, and lead to just as

**Table 18.5** Twelve-year coronary heart disease incidence according to blood pressure category in women[54]

| Blood pressure category | Person years | Events (%) | Relative odds |
|---|---|---|---|
| Normal | 20719 | 29 | 1 |
| High normal | 6043 | 16 | 1.31 (0.86–1.99) |
| Hypertension Stage I | 7242 | 32 | 1.78 (1.19–2.51) |
| Hypertension Stages II–IV | 4000 | 23 | 2.12 (1.42–3.17) |
| Total | 37995 | n = 227 | |

| Table 18.6   Joint National Commission on Hypertension VII: blood pressures | | |
|---|---|---|
| | Systolic pressure (mmHg) | Diastolic pressure (mmHg) |
| Normal | <120 | <80 |
| Prehypertension | 120–139 | 80–89 |
| Hypertension Stage I | 140–159 | 90–99 |
| Hypertension Stage II | ≥160 | ≥100 |

Reproduced from Chobanian et al. JAMA 2003; 289: 2560–72, with permission from the publisher.

much coronary heart disease as the old-fashioned higher tar and nicotine cigarettes.[48]

## BLOOD GLUCOSE

The higher the blood sugar, starting at levels even within the normal range, the higher the rate of cardiovascular diseases in the Framingham study. Figure 18.14 shows hemoglobin A1c levels and prospective risk in the study.[49] When glucose rises in the blood it combines with many of the noble proteins in the body. When it combines with proteins in the eye it becomes the number one cause of blindness; when it combines with the noble proteins in the kidney it is the number one cause of renal dialysis; when it combines with the noble

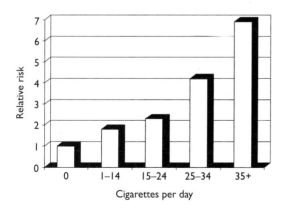

**Figure 18.13**   Myocardial infarction in women and cigarette smoking. (Reproduced from Rosenberg et al. N Engl Med 1990; 322: 214–17,[46] with permission from the publisher.)

proteins in the nerves it becomes the number one cause of neuropathy. Note that a big jump occurs when the hemoglobin $A_{1c}$ level hits 5.5 mg/dl and above. This dose is equivalent to a fasting blood sugar level of 110 mg/dl, but it is preferable to have the blood sugar level under 100 mg/dl. Diabetes is not diagnosed until the subject's blood sugar reaches 126 mg/dl. Do not wait for that to happen, start treating their sugars when they rise over 100 mg/dl.

The majority of diabetes in the US is related to obesity, and getting rid of central obesity would eliminate 80–90% of the diabetes. Female diabetics develop cardiovascular disease at the same rate as men their age. Most diabetics die of cardiovascular disease, and they should be treated as though they already have vascular diseases. Thus, in the new guidelines for cholesterol, they need to have their LDL cholesterol levels lowered to under 70 mg/dl; their triglyceride levels should be under 90 mg/dl, and their TC/HDL ratio below 3.

## WEIGHT

Weight gain from age 25 in the Framingham study is a very dangerous risk factor. As people gain weight, their atherogenic lipids rise, and the protective lipid HDL falls. Blood pressure, blood sugar, uric acid, left ventricular size, and insulin resistance all rise. Figure 18.15 shows that the incidence of cardiovascular disease, coronary disease, congestive heart failure, stroke, and sudden death all demonstrate an upward trend. On multivariate analysis, obesity is an independent risk factor for these endpoints.[50] The US is perhaps the fattest country in the world, with food consumption approaching 40% of the food eaten on this earth: not bad for just 7% of the people who live on this planet!

## EXERCISE

As Blair and his colleagues at the Cooper Clinic in Dallas showed, the women of America who exercise the most, die at the slowest rate. These women also go on to develop heart attacks at the slowest rate (Fig. 18.16), and incur a lowered cancer rate.[51] The low rates in this eight year study in 3120 women could be achieved with a 30 minute per day program.[51] The trade-off of exercise for calories seems unfair. Walking a mile burns off 100 calories – an American candy bar is

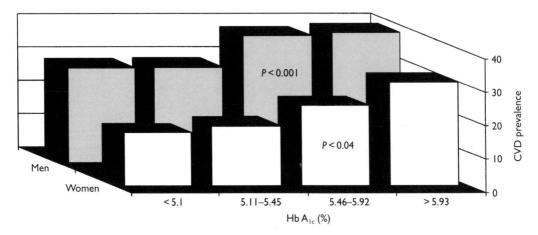

**Figure 18.14** Hemoglobin (Hb) A$_{1c}$ and cardiovascular disease (CVD). (Reproduced from the Framingham Heart Study, the National Heart, Lung and Blood Institute, Boston University School of Medicine: Singer et al. Diabetes 1992; 41: 202–8,[49] with permission from the publisher.)

2.5 miles, the Big Mac is 5.9 miles, the Burger King 'Whopper' is 8.6 miles. Of course some of these fast food places are not to be outdone, they are introducing the mega burger. It will have four hamburger patties: as Jay Leno the late-night comedian commented, one burger for each chamber of your heart. It takes about 35 miles to work off 1 lb of weight.

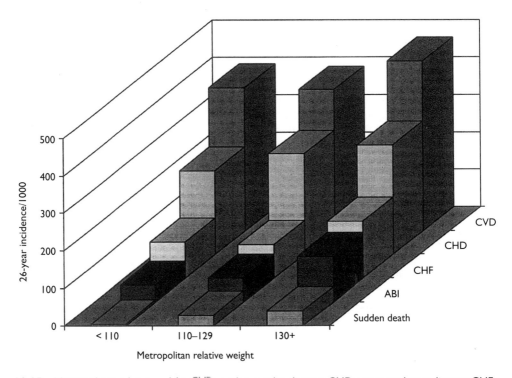

**Figure 10.15** Metropolitan relative weight. CVD, cardiovascular disease; CHD, coronary heart disease; CHF, congestive heart failure; ABI, atherothrombotic brain infarction. (Reproduced from the Framingham Heart Study, courtesy of the National Heart, Lung and Blood Institute, Boston University School of Medicine.[50])

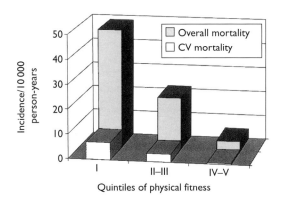

**Figure 18.16**   Cardiovascular (CV) and overall mortality (Cooper Clinic Women). Quintiles of Physical Fitness. (Reproduced from Blair et al. JAMA 1989; 262: 2395–401,[45] with permission from the publisher.[51])

## HOMOCYSTEINE

Homocysteine is an amino acid in the blood which is either excreted in the urine or converted back to methionine. Hyperhomocysteinemia is a recessive trait; children must inherit one gene from each parent to develop hyperhomocysteinemia, with values up usually above 100 mmol/l, and they develop atherosclerotic disease as teenagers, and occasionally even younger. The have homocysteinuria. Apart from these children, until fairly recently it was not thought that homocysteine played a role in medicine. Some 40% of the men and women of the Framingham study have elevated homocysteine, with values over 9 mmol/l, where they begin to pay the price. The upper five percentile is at 15 mmol/l or higher, but, as Figure 18.17 shows, much lower values, over 11 mmol/l, lead to significant stenosis in the carotid arteries as seen using ultrasound. These lesions lead to increased stroke, heart attack, and death, in the Framingham Original and Offspring cohorts. An ideal level would appear to be under 9 mmol/l.[52]

The blood of people with elevated homocysteine levels contains very low levels of folic acid and vitamin B$_6$. It was imagined at one point that the cure for most Americans would be 1 mg folic acid per day. For many people this is too little. Then, the recommendation was one B 100 capsule-with a hundred units of all the various B vitamins and 400 IU folic acid. More recently it has been learned that somewhere between 25% and 50% of the people in America cannot convert folic acid to

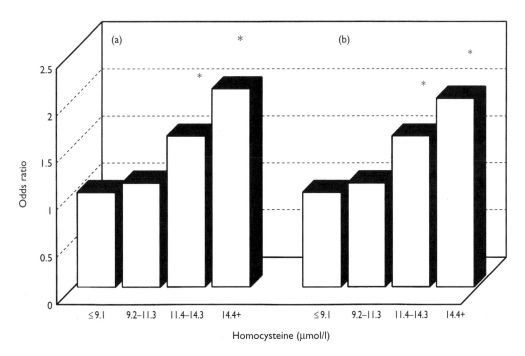

**Figure 18.17**   Homocysteine and carotid artery stenosis (a) adjusted for age and sex; (b) adjusted for sex, age, total cholesterol/high-density lipoprotein, cigarette use, and systolic blood pressure. *Significant 95% confidence interval. (Reproduced from Selhub et al. N Engl J Med 1995; 332: 286–91,[52] with permission from the publisher.)

methyl folate, and these people will need to take methyl folate to lower their homocysteine. Of the numerous trials which have lowered homocysteine to control the risk of cardiovascular diseases, so far only one of them, the Swiss study, has shown a benefit. This study is the only one to have lowered the homocysteine below 9 mmol/l.[53]

## ELECTROCARDIOGRAPHIC AND ECHOCARDIOGRAPHIC FINDINGS

First-degree atrioventricular block, atrial premature beats, and most isolated, less than one per hour premature ventricular beats, particularly late cycle, on an electrocardiogram that was otherwise normal, did not carry any increased risk. As Table 18.7 indicates, non-specific ST-T, left ventriclar hypertrophy, atrial fibrillation, and right and left bundle branch blocks all carry a statistically significant increased rate of coronary heart disease. Increased left ventricular mass on an echocardiogram is an independent risk factor for coronary heart disease.[54] Using older criteria, the prevalence of mitral valve prolapse was markedly overstated, using new criteria, it affects about 2–3% of women.

## STRESS

The women of the Framingham study who were bossy, pressed for time, driven to excel or to be the best, quick eaters, dissatisfied with their work but unable to take vacations, incurred twice the heart attack rate of their easy-going contemporaries. The only categorical job classification that was bad was a clerical-secretarial worker, married to a blue collar worker, working for an insensitive boss,

**Table 18.7** Coronary heart disease and electrocardiogram abnormalities in women: Framingham Heart Study, National Heart, Lung and Blood Institute, Boston University School of Medicine[54]

| Abnormality | Relative odds |
| --- | --- |
| Non-specific ST-T wave | 1.92 |
| Left ventricular hypertrophy | 3.22 |
| Atrial fibrillation | 2.70 |
| Right bundle branch block | 3.10 |
| Left bundle branch block | 4.20 |
| + ST segment/ recovery loop | 4.70 |

with three children. Of course these data were collected for a generation of women who mostly did not work outside the home. It remains for a futures study to decide what happens to the home-maker with lots of children, who also has a full-time demanding job – the career women of today.

## OTHER RISK-FACTORS

In past reports it was said that the rise of lipid levels during pregnancy was not a risk factor, but the number of pregnancies is emerging as a modest risk factor. No increase in risk was found for coffee consumption, hours of sleep, marital status, or area of residence. Fibrinogen, low and very high hematocrit, high pulse rate, low pulse variability, high white blood cell count, C reactive protein, especially the high-sensitivity C reactive protein, serum amyloid antigen, and positive family history, increase the rate of cardiovascular disease. As many as 240 risk factors have been described for cardiovascular diseases. It remains to be seen if specific therapies for each of them will lower risk, to decide where they will fit in a good preventive approach to this disease. This chapter has tried to focus on the major risk factors for which successful interventions exist.

## MULTIPLE RISK FACTORS

As Figure 18.18 shows, adding one risk factor to another increases the risk of vascular disease. In other renditions of multiple risk, the rate can vary as much as 70-fold from the lowest to the highest risk. Using a multiple risk factor approach, anyone could go into any town in the world and measure a few simple things on people's bodies, and identify over 75% of the people in that town destined to develop coronary heart disease or cardiovascular disease. Better than that, they could lower these risk factors and prevent the vast majority of vascular disease anywhere in the world. This also indicates that about 25% of the risk factors are still unknown. It remains the work of future generations to solve the rest of the puzzle.

Online, easily downloaded, from the National Institutes of Health, at http://hp2010.nhlbihin.net/atpiii/calculator.asp?usertype=pub, one can have the Framingham Risk Calculator up and running on a computer. All patients, at their first assessment have to have this run on their major

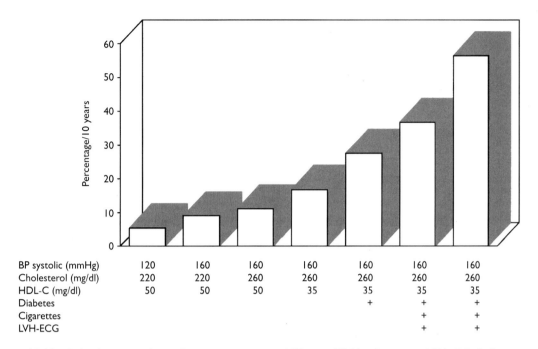

| BP systolic (mmHg) | 120 | 160 | 160 | 160 | 160 | 160 | 160 |
| Cholesterol (mg/dl) | 220 | 220 | 260 | 260 | 260 | 260 | 260 |
| HDL-C (mg/dl) | 50 | 50 | 50 | 35 | 35 | 35 | 35 |
| Diabetes | | | | | + | + | + |
| Cigarettes | | | | | | + | + |
| LVH-ECG | | | | | | + | + |

**Figure 18.18**  Risk of coronary heart disease in women aged 55 years. BP, blood pressure; HDL-C, high-density lipoprotein cholesterol; LVH-ECG, left ventricular hypertrophy on electrocardiogram. (Reproduced from the Framingham Heart Study, the National Heart, Lung and Blood Institute, Boston University School of Medicine: Wilson. Am J Hypertens 1994; 7: 75–125,[54] with permission from the publisher.)

risk factors to especially identify the people where the risk is 20% or greater. These people have a coronary heart disease equivalent risk, and in the new Adult Treatment Panel (ATP) III version the National Cholesterol Education Guidelines need to have their LDLs lowered to under 70 mg/dl, and as someday they will tell you, their triglycerides under 90 mg/dl and their total cholesterol/HDL ratios under 3!

## KNOW YOUR NUMBERS!

Life is a game of numbers. The gift of the people of the Framingham study was to teach us what the numbers mean. We started with half the men and women in the town in 1948, they were all mostly healthy. We measured all these variables on them and examined them every two years to find out who went on to develop cardiovascular and other kinds of diseases. They taught us the numbers relating to people who develop vascular disease, and these numbers eventually in medicine became known as the risk factors. They also taught us the numbers relating to people who stayed free of car-

diovascular disease, and eventually a third set of numbers derived from the treatment of people with disease would lead to the shrinking of the cholesterol deposits in their arteries. From this original cohort we now have under study their offspring, and grandchildren, two full additional generations of Framingham people.

The numbers needed to sail through life in persons without disease include a total cholesterol under 150 mg/dl, a total to HDL ratio of under four, an LDL level under 100 mg/dl, and a triglyceride level under 100 mg/dl as well. Blood pressure has to be under 120/80 mmHg, and blood sugar under 100 mg/dl, hemoglobin $A_{1c}$ under 5.5%, no cigarettes or other inhaled smoke, individuals should have a very narrow waist, homocysteine under 9 mmol/l, lipoprotein(a) under 20 mg/dl, they should do 2 miles of walking per day, consume less than 10 g of saturated fat per day, and less than 200 mg of dietary cholesterol per day. Eliminate all the refined carbohydrate in your diet including white flour and sugar-containing items; substitute whole grains and vegetables; keep calories low as dictated by exercise performance.

To reverse the deposits in your arteries we want the LDL level now under 70 mg/dl and the triglycerides under 90 mg/dl, in a way then it would probably not matter what the total/HDL ratio is, even though we would like that under 3. The other numbers should be as above for primary prevention, except in diets where the saturated fat consumption must absolutely be under 10 g per day, and the total cholesterol eaten under 100 mg per day.

## TREATMENT

Taking all the diet trials to date, the better they lowered the cholesterol and saturated fat in the diet, the better they lowered cholesterol, and the better they lowered cholesterol, the better they lowered heart attack rate. Taking all the drug trials to date, the better they lowered the cholesterol the better they lowered the heart attack rate. Most focused on lowering the LDL, but there are even trials now showing benefit from lowering the triglycerides. Over 10 000 women have been taking part in cholesterol-lowering trials, and they actually do a better job than the men, with on average a 4% fall in coronary heart disease for a 1% fall in cholesterol. With today's powerful statin medications, of which there are currently six different types on the market, a few tablets of the strongest statins will take most high-risk women to their goal. Of course the best way to lower risk is to adhere to a better diet and exercise program, as this actually improves the fall in heart disease at a given level of cholesterol better than doing it with just drug therapy. To achieve triglyceride levels that are really low, it is frequently necessary to add niacin and usually a fibrate to the statins to achieve low triglyceride levels. In people with triglycerides over 100 mg/dl, it is essential to have them take fish oils, or other sources of omega-3 oils, such as from flax seed, to optimize the fall in triglycerides. Lowering triglycerides to under 100 mg/dl and, better, to under 90 mg/dl it is possible to change the size of the LDLs and HDL's, to less atherogenic and more protective attributes. One of the most recent findings in all of this is the use of fish oils containing omega-3 acids, which not only help to lower the triglycerides, but lower the sudden-death, and the heart attack rates, and dementia in people in the Framingham study.

By the late 1970s in the US, the Hypertension, Detection and Follow-up Program (HDFP) showed that lowering blood pressure in women improved their outcome.[55] This was followed in the early 1980s in the UK with the Medical Research Council (MRC) trial.[56] More recently the Systolic Hypertension in the Elderly Study SHEP), treating women with isolated systolic hypertension, lowered the stroke rate by 38%.[57]

Random allocation to exercise in the Cardiac Rehabilitation Trials lowered the death rate by 37% in the first year compared to people randomized to the couch.[58]

## CONCLUSION

Medical providers who take care of women should realize that these women will progress through the menopause and find themselves on an accelerated path to atherosclerotic diseases, the number one cause of death and major disability for women. A few simple tests, available virtually everywhere in the world will allow identification of the women destined to experience cardiovascular disease, years in advance of their clinical episodes. Better than that, lowering the cholesterol, blood pressure, blood sugar, cigarettes, weight, etc, could prevent these diseases from happening. Women will live longer, but the real benefit is when you understand they usually do not die when they have a heart attack or stroke. Currently 10% to 15% under the age of 65 years, and 20% to 25% over the age of 65 years die when they have a heart attack. Of the 75–90% of them who live, half will have damaged their pump, so they could live out the rest of their lives chronically ill, and, all of this could have been prevented.

## REFERENCES

1. Thom TJ, Kannel WB, Siberhsatz H, D'Agostino RB Sr. Incidence, prevalence and mortality of cardiovascular disease in the United States. In: Alexander RW, Schlant RC, Fuster V, eds. Hurst's The Heart, Arteries, and Veins, 9th edn. New York: McGraw-Hill, 1997: 3–17.
2. Gordon T, Kannel WB, Hortland MC, McNamara PM. Menopause and coronary heart disease. Ann Intern Med 1978: 89: 157–61.
3. Lloyd-Jones DM, Larson MG, Beiser A, Levy D. Lifetime risk of developing coronary heart disease. Lancet 1999; 353: 89–92.
4. Anderson KM, Wilson PWF, Odell PM et al. An updated coronary risk profile: a statement for health professionals. Circulation 1991; 83: 357–63.
5. Kannel WB, Wolf PA, and Garrison RJ. Some Risk Factors Related to the Annual Incidence of Cardiovascular Disease and Death Using Pooled Repeated Biennial

Measurements: Framingham Heart Study, 30 Year Follow Up. 1987 NIH Pubication No. 87-2703,

6. Castelli WP. Cholesterol and lipids in the risk of coronary artery disease. The Framingham Heart Study. Can J Cardiol 1988; 4 (Suppl A): 5A–10A.

7. Executive Summary of the Third Report of The National Cholesterol Education Program (NCEP) Expert Panel on Detection, Evaluation, and Treatment of High Blood Cholesterol in Adults (Adult Treatment Panel III). JAMA 2001; 285: 2486–497.

8. Castelli WP, Garrison RJ, Wilson PWF et al. Incidence of coronary heart disease and lipoprotein cholesterol levels. The Framingham Study. JAMA 1986; 256: 2835–8.

9. The Lipid Research Clinics Coronary Primary Prevention Trial results. 1. Reduction in incidence of coronary heart disease. JAMA 1984; 251: 351–64.

10. Stampfer MJ, Sacks FM, Salvini S, Willett WC, Hennekens CH. A prospective study of cholesterol, apolipoproteins, and the risk of myocardial infaction. N Engl J Med 1991 325: 373–81.

11. Shai I, Rimm EB, Hankinson SE et al. Multivariate assessment of lipid parameters as predictors of coronary heart disease among postmenopausal women: potential implications for clinical guidelines. Circulation 2004; 110: 2824–30.

12. Scandinavian Simvastatin Survival Study Group. Randomised trial of cholesterol lowering in 4444 patients with coronary heart disease: the Scandinavian Simvastatin Survival Study (4S). Lancet 1994; 344: 1383–9.

13. Downs JR, Clearfield M, Weis S et al. Primary prevention of acute coronary events with lovastatin in men and women with average cholesterol levels: results of AFCAPS/TexCAPS. Air Force/Texas Coronary Atherosclerosis Prevention Study. JAMA 1998; 279: 1615–22.

14. Sever PS, Dahlof B, Poulter NR et al. Prevention of coronary and stroke events with atorvastatin in hypertensive patients who have average or lower-than-average cholesterol concentrations in the Anglo-Scandanavian Cardiac Outcomes Trial-Lipid Lowering Arm (ASCOT-LLA): a multicentre randomised controlled trial. Lancet 2003; 361: 1149–58.

15. Cannon CP, Braunwald E, McCabe CH et al. Intensive versus moderate lipid lowering with statins after acute coronary syndromes. N Engl J Med 2004; 350: 1495–504.

16. Austin MA, Breslow JL, Hennekens CH et al. Low-density lipoprotein sublclass patterns and risk of myocardial infarction. JAMA 1988; 260: 1917–21.

17. Lamarche B, Tchernof A, Moorjani S et al. Small dense low-density lipoprotein particles as a predictor of the risk of ischemic heart disease in men: prospective results from the Quebec Cardiovascular Study. Circulation 1997; 95: 69–75.

18. Campos H. Low density lipoprotein particle size and coronary heart disease. Arterioscl Thromb 1992; 12: 1410–19.

19. Proapst M, Reardon M, Steiner G. Relative contribution of triglyceride-rich lipoprotein size and number to plasma triglyceride concentration. Arteriosclerosis 1985; 4: 381–90.

20. Reaven GM. Banting. Lecture 1988: Role of insulin resistance in human disease. Diabetes 1988; 37: 1585–607.

21. Kaplan NM. The deadly quartet and the insulin resistance syndrome: an historical overview. Hypertens Res 1996; 199 (Suppl 1): S9–11.

22. Williams RR, Hunt SC, Hopkins PN et al. Familial dyslipidemia hypertension: evidence from 58 Utah families for a syndrome pressent in approximately 12 percent of patients with the essential hypertension. JAMA 1988; 209: 3579–86.

23. De Franz RA, Ferransimi E. insulin resistance: a multifaceted syndrome responsible for an NIDDM, obesity, hypertension, dyslipidemia, and atherosclerotic cardiovascular disease. Diabetes Care 1991; 14: 173–94.

24. Grundy SM. Hypertriglyceridemia, atherogenic dyslipidemia and the metabolic syndrome. Am J Cardiol 1998; 81: 18–25B.

25. Juhan-Vague I, Collen D. On the role of coagulation and fibrinolysis in atherosclerosis. Ann Epidemiol 1992; 2: 427–38.

26. Hokanson JE, Austin MA. Plasma triglyceride level is a risk factor for cardiovascular disease independent of high-density lipoprotein cholesterol level: a meta-analysis of population based prospective studies. J Cardiovasc Risk 1996; 3: 213–19.

27. Schaefer EJ, Levy RI. Pathogenesis and management of lipoprotein disorders. N Engl J Med 1985; 312: 1300–10.

28. Bostom AG, Gagnon DR, Cupples LA et al. A prospective investigation of elevated lipoprotein(a) detected by electrophoresis and cardiovascular disease in women. The Framingham Heart Study. Circulation 1994; 90: 1688–95.

29. Campos H, McNamara JR, Wilson PWF, Ordovas JM, Schaefer EJ. Differences in low-density lipoprotein subfractions and apolipoproteins in pre-menopausal and post-menopausal women. J Clin Endocrinol Metab 1988; 67: 30–5.

30. Clarkson TB, Adams MR, Kaplan JR, Shively CA, Koritnik DR. From menarche to menopause: coronary artery atherosclerosis and protection in cynomolgus monkeys. Am J Obstet Gynecol 1989; 160: 1280–5.

31. Stampfer MJ, Willett WC, Colditz GA, Speizer FE, Hennekens CH. A prospective study of past use of oral contraceptive agents and risk of cardiovascular diseases. N Engl J Med 1991; 325: 756–62.

32. Wilson PF, Garrison RJ, Castelli WP. Post menopausal estrogen use, cigarette smoking and cardiovascular morbidity in women over 50. The Framingham Study. N Engl J Med 1985; 312: 1038–43.

33. Canner PL, Berge KG, Wenger NK et al. 15 year mortality in coronary Drug Project patients: long term benefit with niacin. J Am Coll Cardiol 1986; 8: 1245–55.

34. Speroff L, Rowan J, Symons J, Genant H, Wilborn W, For the CHART group. The comparative effect bone density, endometrium and lipids of continuous hormone as replacement therapy (CHART study). a randomized controlled trial. JAMA 1996; 276: 1397–408.

35. Grodstein F, Stampfer MJ, Colditz GA et al. Post menopausal hormone therapy and mortality. N Engl J Med 1997; 336: 1769–75.

36. Hulley S, Grady D, Bush T et al. Randomized trial of estrogen plus progestin for secondary prevention of coronary heart disease in postmenopausal women. JAMA 1998; 280: 605–13.

37. Writing Group for the Women's Health Intiative Investigators. Risk and benefits of estrogen plus progestin in healthy postmenopausal women: principal

results from the Women's Health Initiative Randomized Controlled Trial. JAMA 2002; 288: 321–33.

38. Shumaker SA, Legault C, Kuller L et al. Conjugated equine estrogen and incidence of probable dementia and mild cognitive impairment in postmenopausal women. JAMA 2004; 291: 2947–58.

39. Campbell TC. The China Study. Dallas: BenBella Books, 2005.

40. McPherson K, Steel CM, Dixon JM. Breast cancer – epidemiology, risk factors, and genetics. BMJ 2000; 321: 624–8.

41. Rosendaal FR. Venous thrombosis: A multicausal disease. Lancet 1999; 353: 1167–73.

42. Joint National Committee on Detection Evaluation and Treatment of High Blood Pressure. The seventh report of the Joint National Committee on Detection Evaluation and Treatment of High Blood Pressure (JNCV). Hypertension 2003; 42: 1206–52.

43. The Heart Outcomes Prevention Evaluation Study Investigators. Effects of an angiotensin-converting-enzyme inhibitor ramipril, on cardiovascular events in high-risk patients. N Engl J Med 2000; 342: 145–53.

44. The SOLVD Investigators. Effect of enalapril on survival in patients with reduced left ventricular ejection fractions and congestive heart failure. N Engl J Med 1991; 325: 293–302.

45. Nissen SE, Tuzen EM, Libby P et al. Effect of antihypertensive agents on cardiovascular events in patients with coronary disease and normal blood pressure: the Camelot Study: a randomized controlled trial. JAMA 2004; 292: 2217–25.

46. Rosenberg L, Palmer JR, Shapiro S. D. Decline in the risk of myocardial infarction among women who stops smoking. N Engl J Med 1990; 322: 214–17.

47. Fiore MC, Vovotny TE, Pierce JJP, Hatzianddreu EJ, Patel KM, Davis RM. Trends in cigarette smoking in the United States: the changing influence of gender and race. JAMA 1989; 261: 49–55.

48. Palmer JR, Rosenberg L, Shapiro S. 'Low-yield' cigarettes and the risk of non-fatal myocardial infarction in women. N Engl J Med 1989; 320: 1569–73.

49. Singer DE, Nathan DM, Anderson KM et al. Association of hemoglobin $A_{1c}$ with prevalent cardiovascular disease in the original cohort of the Framingham Heart Study. Diabetes 1992; 41: 202–8.

50. Hubert HB, Feinleib M, McNamara P, Castelli WP. obesity as an independent risk factor for cardiovascular disease; a 26 year follow-up of participants in the Framingham Heart Study. Circulation 1983; 67: 768–77.

51. Blair SN, Kohl HW III, Paffenbarger RS, Clark DG, Cooper RH, Gibbons LW, Physical fitness and all cause mortality. A prospective study of healthy men and women JAMA 1989; 262: 2395–401.

52. Selhub J, Jacques PF, Bostom AG et al. Association between plasma homocysteine and carotid stenosis. N Engl J Med 1995; 332: 286–91.

53. Schnyder G, Roffi M, Flammer Y et al. Effect of homocysteine-lowering therapy with folic acid, vitamin B12, and vitamin B6 on clinical outcome after percutaneous coronary intervention: the Swiss Heart Study: a randomized controlled trial. JAMA 2002; 288: 973–9.

54. Wilson PWF. Coronary heart disease prediction. Am J Hypertens 1994; 7: 75–125.

55. Hypertension Detection and Follow-up Program Cooperative Group. Five-year findings of the Hypertension Detection and Follow-up Program. I. Reduction in mortality of persons with high blood pressure including mild hypertension. JAMA 1979; 242: 2562–71.

56. Medical Research Council Working Party. MRC trial of treatment of mild hypertension: principal results. BMJ 1985; 291: 97–104.

57. SHEP Cooperative Research Group. Prevention of stroke by anti hypertensive drug treatment in older persons with isolated systolic hypertension: final results of the Systolic Hypertension in the Elderly Program (SHEP). JAMA 1991; 265: 3255–64.

58. O'Connor GT, Buring JE, Yusuf S et al. An overview of randomized trials of rehabilitation with exercise after myocardial infarction. Circulation 1989; 80: 234–44.

# Chapter 19

# The breast in the menopause

Ari D Brooks and Honesto Poblete

The menopause brings many changes to the female breast brought on by normal aging and the altered concentrations of estrogen and progesterone. The primary function of the breast is production and delivery of milk from the nursing mother to the infant child. Yet, few women would feel that this is the sole purpose of the breast. The breast is also integral to a woman's sense of appearance, emotional wellbeing, and sexual identity. This chapter will review the anatomy and development of the breast, and then discuss the diseases of the breast, with particular emphasis on cancer of the breast, which is of central importance to women in the menopause.

## ANATOMY

The female breasts are modified sweat glands which lie as paired structures on the anterior chest wall comprised of glandular, fibrous, and adipose tissue. Their appearance may vary greatly as influenced by age, genetics, ethnicity, parity, and stage of the menstrual cycle in premenopausal women. Clinically, each breast is divided into four quadrants: upper outer, upper inner, lower outer, and lower inner. Alternatively, regions of the breast may be described using the 'clock face' method. Any masses or structures described on or in the breast should be localized and described using either of these conventions.

Each breast lies directly over the thoracic musculature. Two-thirds of the breast lies over the pectoralis major and the deep pectoral fascia, and the remaining one-third over the serratus anterior and its fascia (Figure 19.1a). In addition, a small tapering segment of the breast may extend along the infero-lateral border of the pectoralis major towards the axilla, and is known as the axillary tail

of Spence. The deep fascial plane and the breast are separated by a potential space known as the retromammary space or bursa, which is invested with loose connective tissue, lymphatics, and small vessels. Anteriorly, the breast is firmly attached to the overlying dermis by fibrous condensations of connective tissue called the suspensory ligaments of Cooper. These ligaments fuse with the superficial fascia of the breast and intertwine between the glandular tissues, forming the interlobular fascia of the breast parenchyma (Figure 19.1b). These ligamentous attachments to the skin are responsible for the retraction of skin in the dimpled appearance in certain breast masses or conditions.[1]

The medially located areola has a thinned layer of overlying skin, and contains numerous small sebaceous glands that secrete an oily protective substance that guards the areola and nipple against drying and chafing in the nursing mother. The nipple is the central elevated segment of the areola, which is invested with nerves, elastic tissue and muscle fibers capable of erectile patterns in response to nursing or arousal. The nipple is perforated by 15–20 small, circumferentially arranged openings, which represent the terminal portions of the breast's functional subunits, the lobules. Each of these openings represents a lactiferous duct and the contributing lobules which secrete into the primary duct.

The glandular tissue of the breast comprises multiple functional units termed a lobule. The smallest subunit of a lobule is the terminal duct or acinus. Myoepithelial cells similar to smooth muscle are resident in the basement membrane, and aid in the secretion of produced milk into the tertiary and secondary ducts that terminate in the primary ducts, which have a dilatation prior to their opening at the nipple. Each primary duct is fed by multiple lobular subunits. This system serves to deliver and secrete the milk into the nursing child's mouth. During the menopause the glandular tissue of the breast gradually atrophies and becomes less evident. This may have significant impact when assessing breast masses or discharge in the menopausal breast.

The blood supply of the breast is abundant. Medially, the arterial blood supply of the breast is provided by branches of the internal mammary (internal thoracic) artery. Laterally, the lateral thoracic and thoracoacromial arteries (branches of the axillary artery) and posterior intercostal arteries supply the breast. Venous drainage of the breast is primarily via branches of the axillary vein, and less so the internal thoracic vein. The breast has a rich supply of lymphatic channels and draining nodes.[2] Knowledge of the lymphatic drainage of the breast is helpful in understanding the principals of surgical staging and treatment of breast cancer. For example, the 'peau d'orange' seen in some breast cancers is due to obstruction of these lymphatic channels by malignant cells. Overall, about 75% of the lymphatics drain into the nodal groups on the lateral aspect of the breast. The remaining medial portions drain into the parasternal or internal mammary nodes. The modern 'sen-tinel node' will almost invariably be harvested from the lowest axillary lymph nodes.[3]

## BREAST DEVELOPMENT

Early development of the female breast becomes evident at the onset of puberty. The breasts continue to develop throughout a woman's life, and may only reach full potential maturity at the end of the first full-term pregnancy.[4] The mammary glands develop initially as primordial cysts in the prepubertal girl. The first sign of a girl's entrance into puberty is the development of the breast bud or thelarche. There is increased fat deposition, elongation and development of ducts, and the initial appearance of lobular units. This development of the female breast is influenced by multiple hormonal influences. Estrogen, progesterone, thyroid hormones (tri-iodothyronine ($T_3$) and thyroxine ($T_4$)), adrenal hormones, pituitary hormones, and insulin, or insulin-like growth factor have all been shown to influence and mediate the development of the female breast. There also appear to be locally acting factors that act as paracrine mediators influencing the maturation of the breast. The amounts of each of the breasts' primary compo-

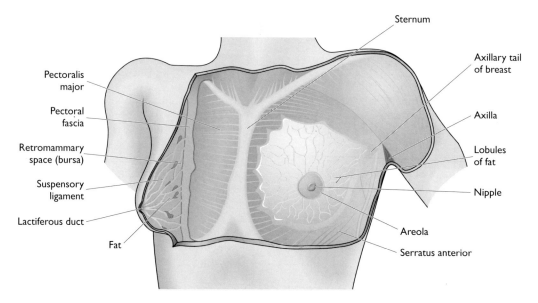

**Figure 19.1a** Superficial dissection of the pectoral region of the female. On the left side, observe the breast (skin removed) extending from the 2nd through the 6th ribs. Observe also the axillary tail extending into the axilla. The nonlactating breast consists primarily of fat. On the right side, observe the deep pectoral fascia covering the pectoralis major. Observe that the mammary gland lies in the subcutaneous connective tissue, or superficial fascia, between the skin and deep fascia. (Reproduced from Moore K and Dalley AF. Clinically Oriented Anatomy. Philadelphia, PA: Lippincott Williams & Wilkins, 2005.)

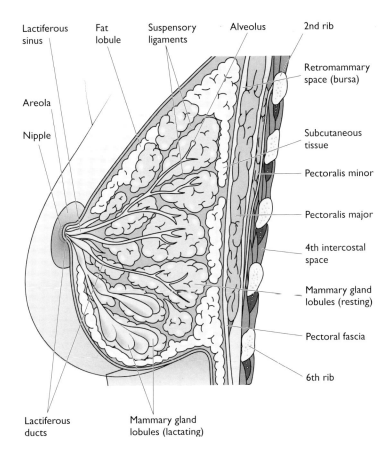

Lactiferous sinus

Fat lobule

Suspensory ligaments

Alveolus

2nd rib

Retromammary space (bursa)

Areola

Subcutaneous tissue

Nipple

Pectoralis minor

Pectoralis major

4th intercostal space

Mammary gland lobules (resting)

Pectoral fascia

6th rib

Lactiferous ducts

Mammary gland lobules (lactating)

**Figure 19.1b**  Sagittal section of the breast and anterior thoracic wall. The breast consists of glandular tissue and fibrous and adipose tissue between the lobes and lobules of glandular tissue, together with blood vessels, lymphatic vessels, and nerves. The superior two-thirds show schematically the suspensory ligaments and alveoli of the breast with resting mammary gland lobules. The inferior part shows lactating mammary gland lobules. (Reproduced from Moore K and Dalley AF. Clinically Oriented Anatomy. Philadelphia, PA: Lippincott Williams & Wilkins, 2005.)

nents: glandular, stromal, and adipose tissue will all vary dependent on a woman's developmental stage and parity, as well as an individual's genetic influences. These factors may also have a role in the appearance of symptoms or onset of disease in the mature and postmenopausal breast.

The cyclical variation of estrogen and progesterone concentrations in the premenstrual woman will have anatomical and physiological influences. During phases of estrogen elevation, the duct size increases by cellular hypertrophy. Progesterone elevations effect a cellular hyperplasia and increased production of prelactation secretions. Some breast symptomatology may be attributed to these effects. If the produced secretions are not readily reabsorbed, cystic accumulations and inflammation may result in breast pain, and fibrous reactions may result in fibrocystic nodules.

The glandular tissues or lobules of the breast may have distinct compositions depending on a woman's cyclical status, parity and menopausal stage. Type 1 lobules are the initial type seen in the developing breast, and formation occurs between one and two years after menarche. In the adult

these lobules are characterized as having 10–20 acini, termed alveolar buds. In contrast the type 2 and 3 lobules have more abundant alveolar buds, which are now termed ductules, and number about 50 to 80 respectively, and are seen more abundantly in premenstrual and parous women. A type 4 lobule describes an actively lactating lobule. The type of lobule present throughout a woman's life is dependent upon parity, and hormonal influences may have impact on subsequent susceptibility to tumorigenesis.[5]

## THE MENOPAUSE

The cyclical estrogen and progesterone elevations become attenuated in adulthood and gradually deteriorate over time. This deterioration becomes more rapid in the perimenopause and menopause, and the availability of estrogen and progesterone receptors decreases due to lack of stimulus. The physical changes of the breast include loss of subcutaneous fat and stroma. The lobular duct system atrophies and regresses. The supportive fibrous and elastic tissues degenerate, and the breast loses its firmness and results in an elongated and concave appearance. The skin overlying the breast also ages, though in a non-hormonal process. The skin thins and dries due to decreased cellular regeneration. The vascularity of the nipple–areola complex also decreases, and the pigmentation may lighten.

The glandular tissue of the female breast continues to change as well. The ducts become predominated by lobule type 1. In the nulliparous woman, the percentages go relatively unchanged. In the parous woman the change to a preponderance of type 1 lobule usually occurs late into the fifth decade of life. In all women, type 1 becomes the dominant lobule after the menopause.

The changing anatomy of the breast in menopause will affect the clinical approach and assessment of the breast. The decreased stromal and epithelial content allows for better palpation of new masses or lesions. The increased fat content allows for much clearer mammographic evaluation of the breast, with less stroma to confound the detection of signs of breast disease. In obese women this decline of functional tissue can be delayed for long periods owing to increased estrone concentrations from extra-ovarian androgen metabolism. These women's breasts may maintain a semifunctional state even more than a decade after menopause.[6] This persistence of functional tissue is also seen in women undergoing hormonal replacement therapy (HRT), with the reversal of atrophy and persistence of stromal and radiodense tissue. Radiologists and examining physicians should have a clear history regarding HRT when evaluating a woman's breast for disease.

## DISEASES OF THE BREAST IN THE MENOPAUSE

### Benign breast disease

Benign breast disease encompasses a group of often under-emphasized conditions encountered by thousands of women. Much emphasis is placed on the malignant dangers of the female breast, and the significant morbidity of benign disease may be overlooked. Both benign and malignant breast disease are often influenced by age and the hormonal milieu attendant to certain ages in a woman's lifetime. The most common complaints of female patients visiting a physician for breast disease in order of occurrence are pain, mass, or nipple discharge.[7,8] The most common benign breast disease diagnosed is fibrocystic changes. Ironically, this disease has no universally accepted definition much less a universal treatment strategy. Other benign breast conditions which may require medical evaluation and treatment include inflammation or infection and conditions resulting from trauma.

*Breast pain* or *mastalgia* may be classified as cyclic or non-cyclic, and can often be differentiated by their respective qualities as well. Cyclic breast pain is commonly bilateral and related to the menstrual cycle. Non-cyclic breast pain is often unilateral and not related to the menstrual cycle. For peri- and postmenopausal women the predominant complaint is clearly non-cyclic, even in the presence of hormonal therapy which is commonly prescribed in a non-varying regimen. Menopausal women with a new complaint of breast pain should receive a thorough history and physical examination to identify a specific cause. Other sources should be ruled out such as musculoskeletal or pneumonitic pain. A diagnostic mammogram is indicated if no physiological cause is clearly identified. If the mammogram is abnormal, the underlying lesion should be addressed. If normal, the patient should receive reassurance and education on breast physiology. She should be made aware that spontaneous remission occurs in 60–80% of women complaining of breast pain. Treatment should begin with analgesics and good documentation by the patient of the pain. The documentation should include parameters such as frequency, severity (using a scale), associated symptoms, and exacerbating factors. Proper documentation will aid the patient and physician in gauging the progress of disease and effectiveness of any treatments. If the pain is persistent the only Food and Drugs Administaration (FDA)-approved treatment specifically for mastalgia is danazol (Danocrine) in a dosage of 100–400 mg daily. Non-cyclic breast pain has a response rate of 75%. However, side-effects occur in up to 20% of patients, and include menstrual irregularity, acne, weight gain, and hirsutism. Treatment, therefore, should be reserved for those with mastalgia that is debilitating or significantly impacts their lifestyle. Alternative treatments have also been reported with inconsistent results. Evening primrose oil, a compound high in gamma-linolenic acid, has been reported to resolve mastalgia in up to 40% of patients, though subsequent studies have not repeated these results.[9] Avoidance of caffeine and supplementation of vitamin E have also been anecdotally reported to have beneficial effects on breast pain, but no reliable prospective studies have shown significant benefit for these treatment modalities. A novel approach that has been investigated in cyclic mastalgia is treatment with supraphysiological levels of iodine.[10] Significant reduction of breast pain was observed after 3 months of treatment with dosages of 3–6 mg/day of iodine. The role of this treatment in non-cyclic mastalgia requires further investigation. Surgical treatment has no evident benefit in the treatment of breast pain in the absence of an identifiable lesion.

*Nipple discharge* is most commonly a benign process. It is seen in 10–15% of benign breast disease and 2–3% of malignant breast disease, and it is rarely the presenting sign. Nipple discharge is a non-specific finding, and under aspiration 50–80% of women may yield secretions without known disease. Pathological discharges are often spontaneous, unilateral, bloody, and may be associated with a mass. Malignant causes of nipple discharge become increasingly more common with age.[11] Benign nipple discharge may appear clear, white, yellow, or dark green. A separately considered entity is galactorrhea or inappropriate lactation.

The type of discharge is often identified by careful history and physical examination. Reproduction of the discharge with gentle milking should be attempted, to identify involved ducts. The fluid should be tested for occult blood. Cytology is rarely helpful as negative results do not rule out malignancy. However, an occasional diagnosis of malignant or suspicious cells can be seen on evaluation of bloody nipple discharge. Work-up with mammography should be performed. The mammography may include a magnification view of the subareolar region, and may be helpful in identifying pathology. Galactography may provide useful information in specific patients, though its role is controversial and has been promoted in recent studies as an important diagnostic test in breast cancers presenting with nipple discharge.[12] A galactogram should visualize the specific duct that has exhibited discharge, however, a negative galactogram cannot reliably rule out a malignancy.

Newer modalities being employed to investigate suspicious nipple discharge are ductal lavage and ductoscopy. Ductal lavage provides increased cellular yield as compared to nipple aspiration.[13] Ductoscopy allows direct visualization of the intraductal architecture, and also provides improved sampling for cytology. These techniques may be useful in the investigation of suspicious nipple discharge, and may be most helpful in those at high risk for diagnosis of intraductal malignancy.[14,15]

If the work-up is negative then reassurance and education are the only treatments indicated. The physician should also emphasize that physiological discharge is promoted by manipulation of the areola and nipple. Stimulation of the nipple should be avoided, and this often resolves the discharge. Bloody or pathological nipple discharge usually requires biopsy for definitive diagnosis. The exceptions are pregnant women and those with a single, non-reproducible episode with no imaged abnormalities. Pathological nipple discharge will most often be caused by an intraductal papilloma.[16] Papillomas are attached to the wall of the subareolar duct by a stalk. They develop as lesions with an epithelial layer covering a fibrovascular stroma. The second most common cause of pathological nipple discharge is ductal ectasia. This condition involves the dilatation of the major ducts, usually in the subareolar region.[17] The discharge is classically dark green and thick like 'toothpaste', though it may be serous, bloody or purulent. Management of intraductal papilloma and ductal ectasia is simple excision. This may be segmental resection or more selective terminal duct excision. If a malignant cause has been identified, the most common causative lesion is ductal carcinoma in situ. The specific management will depend on the extent of the disease, and should be determined by the surgeon.

Galactorrhea is a cause of nipple discharge whose pathology is not intrinsic to the breast. Galactorrhea is defined as the non-puerperal discharge of milky fluid from both nipples (more than two years after the cessation of breast feeding). The work-up should focus on identifying the underlying endocrine disorder causing elevated prolactin levels or other promoters of lactation. Etiologies include hypothyroidism, pituitary adenomas, trauma, and various medications. Some patients may have a physiological galactorrhea as a diagnosis of exclusion, in these patients a negative work-up for endocrine disorder should be followed by reassurance.

*Benign breast masses* are a cause of considerable concern to many women of all ages. The anxiety over a palpable or radiologically detected mass negatively affects the sense of wellbeing for any patient. The most common benign breast disease usually associated with a 'palpable mass' is fibrocystic change or disease more recently termed fibrocystic condition. The term 'fibrocystic change' has come under considerable criticism as a distinct disease entity.[3,18] The term has been used to describe variant clinical presentations most commonly distinguished by palpable thickening or lumpiness of both breasts associated with breast pain and tenderness. The condition appears to be an exaggerated response by breast tissue to circulating hormones and growth factors. The condition is most common in premenopausal women, and often improves in the menopause as the hormonal signaling decreases in the maturing woman. However, fibrocystic disease is still seen in postmenopausal women, indicating that multiple factors and signals are probably responsible. There is often a cystic component as detected by ultrasound, which is seen as multiple small cysts. The cystic component becomes less prominent in women as they age, though when present it is often associated with HRT. The approach to a woman suspected of having fibrocystic disease should concentrate on her chief complaints and verification of detectable masses. If the primary complaint is breast pain, the management should include assessment and management of breast pain as described earlier. The presence of palpable or radiologically detectable masses will require further work-up. In the young female, observation may be the only initial management indicated. In the menopausal patient the suspicion of malignancy is significantly greater and the threshold for performing a diagnostic biopsy is lower. Techniques of biopsy are further detailed later in this chapter. The findings on biopsy aid in the classification of the fibrocystic disease. The histological characterization helps the patient and physician understand the nature of the change and any implications for future breast disease (Table 19.1). The biopsy findings can be classified by activity defined as non-proliferative, proliferative without atypia or atypical hyperplasia. This classification allows determination of malignant potential and stratifies patients for observation or preventive therapy.[2,19]

When assessing the breast for masses, identification of a dominant breast mass should be done if possible. Cysts may present to the physician as initially reported by the patient, as a palpable mass or as a finding on screening mammogram. A stepwise approach should be followed for the diagnosis and treatment of cystic breast masses (Figure 19.2). A palpable breast cyst or macrocyst is most commonly seen in premenstrual women. In the older, menopausal woman, a breast cyst is

| **Table 19.1** Fibrocystic diseases of the breast |
|---|
| *Non-proliferative lesions with no increased relative risk of future invasive breast cancer* |
| • Adenosis |
| • Apocrine metaplasia (papillary) |
| • Simple cysts, small or large |
| • Mild hyperplasia |
| • Duct ectasia |
| • Fibroadenoma |
| • Fibrosis |
| • Mastitis, inflammatory |
| • Periductal mastitis |
| • Squamous metaplasia |
| • Epithelial related calcifications |
| *Proliferative lesions without atypia with slightly increased relative risk (1.5 to 2)* |
| • Moderate or florid hyperplasia |
| • Intraductal papilloma |
| • Sclerosing adenosis, well developed |
| *Atypical hyperplasia with moderately increased relative risk (4 to 5)* |
| • Ductal |
| • Lobular |

an uncommon finding, and in half of these women a history of HRT is present. If the presentation is a macrocyst it is difficult on physical examination alone to differentiate between solid and cystic masses. Ultrasound is used to confirm the cystic nature of the mass. In an asymptomatic patient with a cyst that meets the criteria for a simple cyst, an ultrasound observation may be attempted. If the patient is symptomatic, or if the cyst appears 'complicated' or 'complex', aspiration should be attempted and may be ultrasound guided.[20] Fine needle aspiration of a simple cyst is usually conducted using a 20 or 22 gauge needle and an adequately sized syringe. If the aspirate is non-bloody no further management may be needed. Routine cytology is rarely helpful in these cases, and does not change the need for subsequent follow-up. Cytology is warranted in a grossly bloody aspirate or if a residual mass or cyst is present after aspiration. The patient should be reassessed in 4 to 6 weeks, and if the cyst has not recurred and remains asymptomatic no further management is indicated other than routine follow-up. If the cyst recurs, a biopsy may be indicated. A biopsy is recommended if the cyst recurs with complex features or if cytology is suspicious.[2]

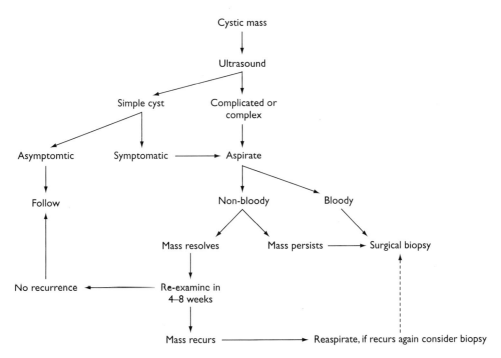

**Figure 19.2** Diagnosis and management of cystic breast masses.

Benign solid tumors of the breast often present with a dominant mass. The most common of these benign tumors is fibroadenoma. This tumor most often presents as a discrete palpable mass, though it may be multiple and bilateral. Fibroadenomas commonly enlarge in puberty and are most often seen in young women. The tumor may enlarge at times of increased estrogenic stimulation such as puberty, pregnancy, and in the older woman during HRT. Established fibroadenomas often regress during the menopause. Fibroadenomas usually present as a palpable mass in a young woman, and as a mammographic density in older women. Mammographic findings of macrocalcifications within a benign-appearing mass are characteristic of an involuted fibroadenoma. These masses do not develop after the later reproductive years, though they may only be discovered later during screening. Tumors are rubbery to firm, freely movable, and usually non-tender. Size may vary from less than 1 cm to large masses that can replace most of the breast. The classic radiographic appearance is of a large well-circumscribed, lobulated, 'popcorn' density. Calcification may also be clustered and be difficult to differentiate from more ominous tumors. The tumors arise from interlobular stroma, and grossly appear as rubbery, grayish-white masses. They may contain glandular or cystic spaces lined by epithelium. Management in a young female with a high likelihood of fibroadenoma may initially be observation, but in women over age 40 years, and certainly any women of menopausal age, a new solid breast mass should be suspected as malignant until proven benign. Malignant degeneration in fibroadenomas is a very rare event, but when seen is often associated with an increased cystic component. When planning management, diagnostic mammography or ultrasound should be obtained initially to better visualize the extent of the mass. A core biopsy may be obtained for diagnosis, though in the older patient excision of the mass is often the preferable approach. Other subtypes of fibroadenoma include the juvenile or giant fibroadenoma, almost exclusively seen in the young patient and unlikely to occur in the menopausal woman.

Phyllodes tumor is another tumor seen more commonly in older women as compared to the fibroadenoma, with the median age of diagnosis in the fifth decade of life. It usually presents as a palpable mass, but may be seen as a mammographic density. These tumors have also been referred to as 'cystosarcoma phyllodes', though they are predominantly benign and this term has fallen out of favor. Management is simple resection with wide margins. Axillary node dissection is not indicated because of the low incidence of spread. Rare high-grade lesions may recur, and when metastasis occurs it is spread hematogenously. Follow-up of patients should be similar to that of cancer patients for 2 to 3 years to provide reassurance and appropriate surveillance.

Other less common benign tumors that may occur in the breast include hamartomas, adenomas and lipoma. Hamartomas are firm, well circumscribed, and often appear as a well-defined density surrounded by a narrow zone of radiolucency or 'halo'.[21] Adenomas of the breast are well-defined, freely mobile masses, with no skin alterations and occasional tenderness. The subtypes of adenoma include lactating and tubular adenomas, and fibroadenolipomas. Excision of fibroadenomas is definitive management. Lipomas are most often found during the late reproductive years. Usually presenting as a soft, solitary mobile mass, they must be differentiated from the surrounding adipose tissue by identification of the delicate capsule. Angiolipomas are related tumors with distinctive vascularity on pathology. They may arise from resident lipomas that have suffered trauma.[22]

Traumatic injury to the breast often gives rise to a fatty necrosis, which may also be produced by radiation, previous surgery, infection, or radiation therapy. Often no history of trauma is recalled by the patient. Occurring most often in overweight women and those with large, pendulous breasts, it presents clinically as a small, hard irregular painless mass. Superficial lesions may have accompanying skin changes including thickening of the skin, dimpling, and retraction. The mammographic appearance can include spiculated masses, microcalcifications, and irregular architecture. The clinical impact is that these lesions closely mimic cancer in appearance. A confident diagnosis of fat necrosis can be made radiologically when the pathognomonic 'oil cyst', a well-circumscribed mass of mixed soft tissue and fat with a calcified rim is seen. In the absence of this finding, or without a clear association to trauma, biopsy is required.

*Mastitis* is a common disease of the breast which may present with edema and poorly defined 'masses'.[23] Less common in menopausal women, mastitis is commonly seen in pregnant or breast-feeding women. Antibiotic coverage commonly is directed against gram-positive infections, and a full course should be completed. If abscess formation requires incision and drainage, the procedure

should be done in an operative suite with adequate anesthesia lest an extensive debridement is required. Mondor's disease is a superficial phlebitis of the lateral chest wall with a painful thrombosed vein that is palpable as a fixed, fibrous cord. Incidence is most often associated with a previous breast biopsy. The appearance mimics cancer as the skin retracts laterally due to involvement of the lateral thoracic or thoracoepigastric vein, but once that has been ruled out reassurance, analgesics, and anti-inflammatory treatment is the indicated management. Antibiotics and anticoagulants have no established benefit.

Other systemic diseases which may present with breast masses or symptoms are rare. They include *cat scratch disease, granulomatous lesions* (tuberculosis and actinomycosis) and *diabetic mastopathy*.[24]

## BREAST CANCER

Breast cancer is the most common cancer among American women, and second only to lung cancer in cancer deaths among women. The American Cancer Society estimated that in 2005 nearly 213 000 new cases of invasive breast cancer would be diagnosed, along with more than 58 000 cases of non-invasive carcinoma.[25] In the same period about 42 000 women will die from breast cancer. The incidence over a woman's lifetime has increased from one in twenty in 1960, to one in eight today. Fortunately, the prognosis for those with breast cancer is has improved significantly. This improved prognosis is the result of improved detection and treatment resulting from concerted efforts of the healthcare establishment and support from government and private organizations. Health care workers must have a clear understanding of the enormous impact of this disease to individuals and society. The great majority of patients battling this disease are women in the menopause.

### Types of breast cancer

The great majority of breast cancers are adenocarcinomas, and the remaining types comprise only about 5% of all cases. Primary breast cancer is first determined to be non-invasive (in situ) or invasive carcinoma.

Non-invasive carcinomas include ductal carcinoma in situ (DCIS), lobular carcinoma in situ (LCIS), and Paget's disease. DCIS is the predominant form of carcinoma in situ and accounts for 15% to 30% of carcinomas found on screening, and nearly half of mammographically detected cancers. The morphology of DCIS has been divided into several subtypes including comedogenic, solid, cribriform, papillary, and micropapillary. Though DCIS may be made of a single cell type, most lesions will have a mixed cell type. DCIS may also have microinvasion defined as foci of tumor cells invading the stroma of less than 0.1 cm in diameter. These are most commonly seen in the comedogenic form. DCIS is thought to give rise to frankly invasive carcinoma and requires excision. Mastectomy is over 95% curative for DCIS. Breast-conserving therapy (BCT) is appropriate for DCIS with a slightly higher recurrence rate. Prognosis depends on grade, size and margins. Adjuvant therapy also plays a role in treatment of DCIS and will be discussed later in the chapter.

Paget's disease is a rare manifestation of breast carcinoma seen at the nipple, and may spread to the areola. The presentation is usually a unilateral erythematous, pruritic lesion with scaling or crust. The malignant Paget cells are extensions of an underlying DCIS within the ductal system onto the nipple. They do not cross the cell membrane but do disrupt the epithelium and allow extracellular fluid to exude onto the nipple surface. Nipple biopsy or cytology of the exudates detects Paget cells. Prognosis of the disease is primarily related to the extent of the underlying carcinoma.

LCIS is always non-palpable, often radiographically invisible, and is usually an incidental finding. LCIS represents only 1% to 6% of carcinomas. LCIS is bilateral in 20% to 40% when both breasts are biopsied, as compared to 10% to 20% of cases of DCIS. LCIS is also less common in older women, and up to 90% of the cases are diagnosed in premenopausal women. LCIS does not appear to give rise to invasive carcinoma but is considered a marker of invasive breast cancer risk. Patients followed over 24 years after finding LCIS showed a 35% chance of developing invasive carcinoma and up to a 12-fold increased risk of breast cancer.[26,27] Identification of LCIS on a biopsy identifies a high-risk individual. There is no need to re-excise to negative margins once the diagnosis is made, as this is not a directly pre-invasive condition.

Invasive carcinomas represent the majority of total breast cancers diagnosed. They often present as a firm, fixed, non-tender mass, and when palpable these tumors often already have axillary metastases. Larger tumors may be fixed to the chest wall, and involvement of the lymphatics causes lymphedema and thickening of the skin. This lymphedema along with retraction of the skin by tethering of the skin by Cooper's ligaments produces the orange peel or peau d'orange appearance. Retraction of the nipple may also occur in centrally located tumors. Inflammatory carcinoma refers to invasive carcinomas which present with extensive involvement of dermal lymphatics, resulting in enlarged, tender, erythematous breast. This diffuse infiltration indicates an aggressive pattern of growth and poor prognosis, though no specific histological type is necessarily associated.

Tumors may also over-express specific hormone receptors the most important include estrogen, progesterone and human epidermal growth factor receptor 2 (Her2/neu) receptors. Characterization of tumor receptors may direct selection of adjuvant therapy.

The most common type of invasive carcinoma is ductal carcinoma. This histological type represents approximately 80% of invasive breast cancers found. The second most common type is lobular carcinoma accounting for 10%, and the remaining types combine for the remaining 10%. Ductal carcinomas have varying amounts of DCIS accompanying the tumor. When large amounts of DCIS are present, wide margins are required upon excision to prevent recurrence.

Invasive lobular carcinoma often presents similarly to ductal carcinoma as a mammographic lesion or palpable mass. A significant number may present in a more diffuse pattern with only vague clinical or radiological irregularities. Lobular carcinoma has been reported to be more commonly bilateral, but these reports may have been biased by increased performance of bilateral surgery in these patients. The incidence of lobular carcinoma is noted to be increasing in older postmenopausal women, which may be associated with HRT.[28] The characteristic histological appearance of lobular carcinoma is the pattern of single infiltrating tumor cells aligned in 'indian file' though they may also present as loose clusters or sheets. Most lobular carcinomas are associated with a loss of a region on chromosome 16 (16q22.1) that contains genes responsible for cell adhesion. Similar to ductal carcinoma, these tumors often present along with a non-invasive carcinoma, and are often associated with varying amounts of LCIS. The pattern of metastasis differs distinctly from other forms of breast cancer. Metastases to the peritoneum, retroperitoneum, meninges (producing carcinomatous meningitis), gastrointestinal tract, ovaries and uterus are more common than in other types. Metastases to the lung and pleura are less likely. Prognosis is similar to ductal carcinoma when matched by grade.

Other less common types of breast carcinoma include medullary, mucinous or colloid, tubular, papillary, and metaplastic. These carcinomas are treated similarly to ductal carcinoma and generally have a more favorable prognosis, with tubular carcinoma having a particularly high rate of remission and cure.

Sarcomas of the breast include angiosarcoma, lymphangiosarcoma, rhabdomyosarcoma, liposarcoma, leiomysarcoma, chondrosarcoma, and osteosarcoma. These tumors are derived from the extrinsic tissues of the breast, and usually present as bulky palpable masses. Lymphatic spread is uncommon as these tumors exhibit hematogenous spread and often metastasize to the lung. Angiosarcomas are associated with prior radiation therapy.[29] Angiosarcoma is also seen as a long-term complication in a chronically edematous arm after ipsilateral mastectomy as Stewart–Treves syndrome. Management is wide excision with or without postoperative radiation therapy.

Other malignancies of the breast may arise from the skin, sweat glands, sebaceous gland, and hair shafts. These tumors are not inherent to the breast and will behave exactly as those types seen at other locations. Lymphomas may form primarily in the breast, or may be involved in a systemic lymphoma, and are usually the large cell type. Metastatic cancer to the breast is rare, and usually arises from a contralateral primary breast carcinoma. Other sources of metastatic cancer to the breast are melanoma and lung cancer.

## Risk factors for breast cancer

Other than sex, age is the most significant risk factor for acquiring breast cancer. Age is also the risk factor that will be common to nearly all peri- and postmenopausal women. Incidence increases rapidly during the reproductive years, then becomes more gradual over a women's lifetime.[30] The result is that risk for breast cancer at the age of 50 years (1 in 400) is more than ten-fold greater than at the age of 30 years (1 in 4200). The result of this increased risk is that about 50% of diagnosed breast cancer occurs in women aged 65 years and over.

Race is associated with increase in risk, with white women showing an increased incidence of breast cancer. However, breast cancers in young women are more often seen in African-American women.[31] Other ethnicities have significantly lower rates of breast cancer.

A woman's reproductive history can have significant impact on her risk for breast cancer. Early menarche and late menopause have both been associated with increased risk of breast cancer. For each two-year delay in menarche, a decrease in risk of 10% is seen. Women with onset of menopause after the age of 55 years have up to twice the risk of developing breast cancer. The mechanism is not fully understood, but many believe that these conditions increase a woman's exposure to estrogen, which may adversely affect her breast cancer susceptibility. Early or surgical menopause appears to have a somewhat protective effect. Other aspects of reproductive history that influence risk of breast cancer are age of first pregnancy and parity. Pregnancy before age 18 years is associated with a 50% decrease in risk compared to first pregnancy at greater than age 30 years. Overall, parity appears to have a protective effect for breast cancer. The protective effect of breast feeding has also been shown in large-scale studies. The longer a woman breast feeds throughout her life correlates directly with decreased incidence of breast cancer.[32] The lack of breast feeding, or short duration of feeding may make a major contribution to increased risk of breast cancer, and is most evident in developed countries.

History of benign breast disease may also have influence on breast cancer risk. A history of biopsy-proven proliferative breast disease such as hyperplasia increases a women's risk: from 1.5- to 2-fold for florid hyperplasia, 4- to 5-fold for atypical hyperplasia, and 8- to 10-fold for carcinoma in situ. The association of risk and non-proliferative or cystic forms of benign breast disease are not well established.

Lifestyle and environmental factors that influence breast cancer risk include alcohol intake, smoking, and ionizing radiation exposure. Alcohol intake has been linked to increased risk in the development of breast cancer.[33] Specifically, the study showed this link in postmenopausal women. Smokers have an increased clearance of estrogen. This hypoestrogenic effect was believed by some to have a protective effect against breast cancer. However, studies showed that cigarette smoking in those with previously identified risk factors for breast cancer revealed a 2.4-fold increased risk relative to non-smokers.[34] This risk increased to 5.8-fold when the patient had five or more first-degree relatives with breast or ovarian cancer. Previous radiation exposure conveys a highly increased risk. Relative risk ranges from 4.5 to 40, and risk is greatest for those women who underwent radiation therapy at 20 years of age or younger.

Fat intake has also been implicated as a risk factor, but studies have not yet shown a definite link to the development of breast cancer. However, an active lifestyle over one's lifetime does appear to be protective and most beneficial to menopausal women, and should be encouraged.[35]

A topic that has gained much attention in both medical literature and the media is genetic susceptibility to breast cancer. The great majority of breast cancer patients develop a sporadic cancer (absence of family history or identified genetic marker); however, a significant minority of cases may arise from women with genetic predispositions. A family history of breast cancer in a first-degree relative (sister, mother or daughter) can be identified in up to 30% of breast cancer patients. The factors that convey increased risk in women with strong family history of breast cancer are not completely understood, but specific gene mutations have been discovered that are responsible for a significant percentage, and inherited mutation in genes linked to the development of breast cancer may be detected in 5% to 10% of breast cancer patients. These mutations occur in *BRCA1* and *BRCA2*. They are both large genes located on chromosome 17q and 13q respectively, and both code for large proteins which probably have multiple functions. Among the functions suggested by experimental data include cellular DNA repair and maintenance of genomic integrity.[36] Patients should understand that only a minority of those with breast cancer will carry either of these mutations, and not all those who inherit a mutation in these genes will suffer breast cancer. Women who do have these gene mutations may have up to a 20-fold increased risk, and their likelihood of developing breast cancer has been estimated at 40% to 80%. Other cancers have been associated with these genes and *BRCA1* has been associated with increased rates of both ovarian and breast cancer. *BRCA2* has been associated with higher rates of breast cancer in men. The type of cancers seen also seems to be influenced by the mutation, and *BRCA1* mutation carriers have a higher percentage of medullary cancers. Widespread genetic testing for these mutations is not feasible currently, but those with strong family history should be referred for genetic counseling and possible testing for *BRCA1/2* mutations.

HRT is especially pertinent to the peri- and postmenopausal patient. HRT is an effective treatment against osteoporosis and symptoms of menopause, but much attention has been drawn to HRT's associated risk factors. The Women's Health Initiative trial which randomized over 10 000 women to receive estrogen plus progesterone treatment or placebo was discontinued because the observed increased incidence of breast cancer, cardiovascular events, and stroke exceeded predetermined limits for stopping the trial.[37] However, no increase in breast cancer was observed in women with hysterectomies receiving estrogen alone.[38] Subsequent studies have also shown that long-term use of combined estrogen–progesterone treatment appears to carry an increased risk of developing breast cancer. Short-term use carries an associated small reversible increased risk, and may be reasonable in the short-term treatment of menopausal symptoms. Estrogen-alone therapy probably does not increase breast cancer risk, though increased risk of ovarian cancer may still be present. The advised approach is to determine individualized therapy regimens appropriate to each patient.[39-41]

## Screening and diagnosis

In the past, diagnosis and management of breast cancer often began with a palpable mass followed by biopsy and subsequent mastectomy, with few alternatives or opportunities for preemptive management. Over the past 15 years the approach to breast cancer screening, diagnosis and management has changed dramatically, with advances such as routine screening, ultrasound, sentinel node biopsy, and emergence of alternative imaging modalities such as positron emission tomography (PET) scan and magnetic resonance imaging (MRI).

Breast self-examination is a low-cost screening tool that may be recommended monthly for all women aged 40 years and older. The exam consists of five steps taught to the patient (breastcancer.org):

1. stand facing a mirror with shoulders straight and hands at hips. The patient should look for usual size shape and color. The patient should note signs of swelling, redness, dimpling, or nipple inversion
2. the patient should then raise arms and observe for the same changes

3.  while at the mirror gently squeeze each nipple and note for discharge which may be milky, yellow, green or bloody
4.  in a lying position palpate each breast. The right hand palpates the left breast and vice versa. The first few fingers of the hand should be used, keeping the fingers flat and together. The entire breast should be palpated from collar bone to the top of the abdomen, and from armpit (including the armpit in the examination) to sternum. A repeatable pattern should be used to ensure a thorough examination
5.  the final step is the same palpating examination while in a standing position, which may be aided by keeping the arm on the side of the breast being examined raised over the patient's head. Regular examinations are generally accepted as an efficient method to maintain breast health awareness, though impact on cancer mortality is not well established.[42]

A screening mammogram for asymptomatic women, which includes the mediolateral-oblique (MLO) and craniocaudal (CC) views is recommended annually for all women 40 years of age and older, along with annual or biannual clinical breast examination. The age for beginning screening mammography is not without controversy, but is the view promoted by such organizations as the American Cancer Society, and American College of Surgeons. Screening mammography is especially important for the menopausal patient. Multiple large-scale trials researching the efficacy of screening mammography have been performed, and subset analysis performed on these trials showed the greatest effect among patients aged 50 years and older.[43] These recommendations apply to women through the extent of their lifetime, including the elderly in the geripause. Women in advanced age groups have excellent response to surgical treatment, and those aged 75 years and older at diagnosis of breast cancer have a five-year survival rate of nearly 89%.[44] After a screening mammogram is performed, if an abnormality is detected further mammograhic views should be obtained with a diagnostic mammogram. The additional views may include compression (spot view), magnification, mediolateral, and cleavage views with focus on lesions seen in the screening mammogram. Ultrasound imaging should be obtained to evaluate densities in areas of interest as needed. To properly assess the significance of mammographic findings a standardized approach has been developed (Table 19.2). Detected abnormalities must be characterized appropriately in accordance with American College of Radiology Standardized Breast Imaging Reporting and Data Systems (BI-RADS).[45–47]

Screening and diagnostic mammography are valuable tools in the fight against breast cancer, but have well-documented limitations. False-negative rates usually range from 10% to 15%. Increased breast density may also confound the sensitivity of the test. In this regard, decreased breast density may be advantageous to the menopausal patient, but this advantage may be absent in women with a history of prolonged HRT. Integral to the efficacy of the screening mammogram is appropriate storage, and availability of previous studies which are required for comparison. This creates a challenge for the medical field. Digital mammography is a new approach that may address these. This advanced form of screening allows for much more efficient computer-aided image interpretation and archiving.[48] This technique also yields increased contrast resolution over a wider range, and may enhance specificity in breast cancer imaging. The conversion to digital mammography requires a significant monetary investment and co-operation by members of the medical field. Prospective trials investigating the feasibility and effects are under way. Practicing physicians should be aware of locally available resources, and advise their patients accordingly.

Newer alternatives to screening mammography currently being utilized include whole-breast ultrasound, and MRI. The well-established use of ultrasound to evaluate the density of breast lesions may expand into a possible screening tool. Promising studies have shown that it may serve as a useful adjunct to screening mammography in radiologically dense tissue.[49] However, ultrasound is a labor-intensive procedure which is highly operator dependent, and will require further investigation before it can be recommended as a screening modality.

The use of MRI in breast imaging is proven to be beneficial in those with axillary metastases with occult primary breast cancer. The sensitivity of MRI approaches 100%, and negative MRI examination effectively excludes the imaged breast. MRI often is able to detect radiologically silent lesions and helps identify candidate patients for BCT. Another use is detection of silicon breast implant leakage. Use of MRI in other scenarios is not well established.[50] The main limitations to MRI as a screening tool are cost and high false-negative

| Table 19.2 | BI-RADS classification and likelihood of cancer | | |
|---|---|---|---|
| Category | Findings | Recommendations | Likelihood of malignancy |
| 0 | Incomplete imaging | Additional imaging required | |
| 1 | Negative; no architectural disturbance identified | No further actions recommended | <0.5% |
| 2 | Benign-appearing lesion identified; negative mammogram | No further actions recommended | <0.5% |
| 3 | Probably benign finding; lesion identified with high probability of being benign | Short-interval follow-up to establish stability of finding | 1–2% |
| 4 | Suspicious abnormality; lesion detected that is not necessarily typical of cancer. Radiologist may comment specifically on the likelihood of cancer based on the type of lesions detected (i.e. calcifications, mass, etc) | Biopsy should be considered | 2–75% |
| 5 | Highly suggestive of malignancy | Appropriate action should be taken to provide histopathological confirmation | >75% to 95% |

rate. Any hypervascular structure may enhance on MRI imaging, and specificity may range as low as 37%.[51]

## Breast cancer prevention

All menopausal women should be aware of their susceptibility to breast cancer. To better approach the screening and management of the female patient, identification of risk factors and stratification is based on present risks. Women can be classified as having average risk, elevated or high risk, and very high risk. Assessing a woman's risk may be done by several methods. The most well-known model among clinicians is the Gail model published by Mitchell Gail in 1989,[52] using data from more than 270 000 women.[52] The factors included in the model are age, age at menarche, family history of breast cancer in first-degree relatives, history of benign breast biopsies, age at first live birth, and race. The National Cancer Institue (NCI) makes available the Breast Cancer Risk Assessment tool and an online risk assessment calculator at http://www.cancer.gov/bcrisktool. Those at average risk have a relative risk of 1.5 or less. The elevated-risk patient has a relative risk of 1.5 to 5, and/or a 5-year Gail model risk greater

than 1.7%. Those at a very high risk have a relative risk of greater than 5 comprise four groups of women:

1. those with a personal history of invasive breast cancer, DCIS, or LCIS
2. those with a personal history of cellular atypia on cytology, or a breast biopsy with atypical ductal or lobular hyperplasia, and who have a first-degree relative with breast cancer
3. those with known *BRCA1* or *BRCA2* mutation
4. those with history of breast or thoracic irradiation before age 20.[53]

All women should have annual clinical breast exam and mammography beginning at age 40. Women in the menopause at elevated risk should consider enrolment into a trial involving use of selective estrogen receptor modulators (SERMs) as prophylactic treatment. This modality of treatment has shown greatest benefit in women over 50 years of age, with the least side-effects in this population.[54] Those with atypical hyperplasia show highest risk reduction, and in those with previous hysterectomy the risk–benefit ratio is most favorable. The risk of adverse effects must be weighed against possible benefits in determining management. Ductal lavage may also be recommended if the results would allow better decision making by the patient.

In the very high-risk patient, follow-up should be even more rigorous, with recommended clinical breast examination every 6 months along with yearly mammography. For this subset of patients SERM therapy or enrolment in a prophylactic trial should be strongly considered. In addition prophylactic surgery may be offered. Prophylactic mastectomy may be considered for the DCIS patients, and bilateral prophylactic mastectomy might be offered to those with LCIS and *BRCA1* or *BRCA2* mutations. In the DCIS and LCIS patient, a ductal lavage should be offered if a diagnosis of atypia may aid decision making by the patient. Prophylactic oopherectomy should also be considered for the *BRCA1* or *BRCA2* patients, as this is the prophylactic therapy most likely to improve survival.

## Work-up of suspicious lesions

In a menopausal woman with a new finding of a palpable mass, a complete physical examination should assess the mass, the rest of the breasts bilaterally, and axillary and supraclavicular lymph nodes. Ideally this is followed by bilateral diagnostic mammography and ultrasound. In some cases the decision to proceed directly to biopsy may be done with the understanding that the biopsy may affect subsequent ultrasound imaging in cases of leakage of cystic fluid or hematoma. In patients where delay of treatment may affect outcome, or who are unreliable for follow-up, immediate biopsy is reasonable.

Ultrasonography is a valuable tool in the work-up of palpable masses or radiologically suspicious lesions. In cystic lesions, sonographic appearance suspicious for malignancy contrasts to the well-defined appearance of simple cysts. The terms 'complicated 'and 'complex' are used to describe cystic masses or components that are more concerning for malignancy. A complicated cyst is one where there are some internal echoes but other features of a simple cyst, and these have a lesser degree of suspicion for malignancy. A complex cyst evidences suspicious structures such as mural nodules, thick septations, or a thick, irregular wall. Complex cysts require aspiration and probably subsequent biopsy.

Ultrasound may also help characterize a solid mass as benign or malignant. Malignant features on sonogram include spiculations, angular margins, marked hypoechogenicity, shadowing, presence of calcifications, duct extensions, microlobulations, and a branching pattern. Ultrasound increases sensitivity and specificity when combined with mammogram versus mammogram alone.[55]

Several techniques of biopsy are available. Fine needle aspiration (FNA) may be performed as an office procedure. As described before, it is performed using a 20- or 22-gauge needle with an appropriate syringe. The mass is biopsied several times, and aspirate is collected. If cystic fluid alone is aspirated, management should follow as described earlier. In solid tumors the tissue is sent for cytology. The procedure is quick, with minimal morbidity and inconvenience for the patient. A diagnosis of malignancy allows planning for definitive treatment without further biopsy. The disadvantages are that equivocal results will require a second biopsy, FNA cannot distinguish between in situ versus invasive carcinoma, and the sensitivity of results is operator dependent, with false-negative rates of up to 30%.

Large-core needle biopsy (LCNB) may also be performed as an office procedure, but differs from FNA in the amount of tissue sampled. LCNB is performed with a 14-, 16- or 18-gauge needle, or automated sampling device. LCNB provides a large enough tissue sample for histological analysis. LCNB also decreases the false-negative rate significantly as compared to FNAB. The accuracy of percutaneous biopsies can be enhanced by ultrasound guidance, provided that an experienced operator is available for sonographic guidance. Steroactic guidance has become a popular adjunct to percutaneous biopsy, where the location of the lesion is trangulated by computer analysis of mammographic images. A clinician may then perform the biopsy or employ an automated system to obtain the stereotactic-guided LCNB. In non-palpable lesions detected on survey, the stereotactic-guided LCNB has become the diagnostic method of choice for many institutions. Percutaneous biopsy is a valuable diagnostic tool for evaluation of suspected lesions, and has seen improved sensitivity with ultrasound and stereotactic techniques. However, non-diagnostic results from inaccurate or insufficient sampling may still result. When these techniques are performed, a clip is left at the site of biopsy to allow for future evaluation or excision of the area. For some patients these techniques may not be readily available, and this becomes especially pertinent for patients presenting with non-palpable masses whose chance of sampling error on percutaneous biopsy is unacceptable. Also for some cases a benign result on biopsy does not correlate with highly suspicious masses. For these cases, open surgical biopsy must be performed.

Excisional biopsy describes the complete removal of the defined lesion. It is an outpatient procedure that most commonly is performed under local anesthesia and sedation. As in cystic masses the diagnosis and management should follow a step-wise procedure (Figure 19.3). For benign disease this is definitive management. In the case of malignancy, this may serve as a therapeutic lumpectomy, and often excisional biopsy may be designed as a two-stage procedure, with the initial excision followed by a planned second procedure for removal of additional tissue as needed. Adequate imaging helps ensure appropriate margins in palpable masses, and is essential in non-palpable masses for targeted incision. The technique employed in non-palpable masses involves the placement of a localizing needle prior to the procedure, under radiological guidance. The barbed tip of the needle is placed within the area of interest, and the straight end remains protruding from the patient's breast. Excision is then performed carefully, to ensure adequate margins of tissue around the barbed tip. The biopsied sample should be marked in the operating suite to allow for oriented assessment of the borders by pathology. Also radio-opaque markers may be left in the biopsy bed if further therapy or second stage is anticipated.

Incisional biopsy describes the sampling of only a portion of the targeted lesion, and is reserved for very large lesions which are deemed too large to remove for diagnostic studies alone. Incisional biopsies are rarely used today with the advent of FNA and LCNB and better techniques to characterize tumors on cytology or core specimens.

## Breast cancer staging

Once the diagnosis of breast cancer has been determined, the patient will decide together with her physicians and surgeon on a therapeutic plan. Staging of the breast cancer is essential to formulating the appropriate treatment strategy. In 2003 the American Joint Committee on Cancer (AJCC) released the revised staging system for breast cancer. The criteria include the tumor size, lymph node status and presence of metastases. The purpose of grading the breast cancer allows clinicians and the patient to understand the severity and expected outcomes of disease. Generally, disease severity may also be staged by extent with local, regional, and distant disease being increasingly more ominous (Table 19.3).[55]

## Breast cancer treatment

The surgical treatment of breast cancer aims to provide local control of disease with excision of all malignant tissue. Historically, the radical mastectomy with removal of the breast tissue and pectoralis muscles was the treatment of choice to achieve control; after studies demonstrated no survival benefit, this procedure was completely

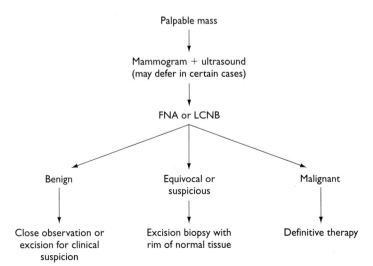

**Figure 19.3** Diagnosis and management of palpable solid breast masses. FNA, fine needle aspiration; LCNB, large-core needle biopsy.

| Table 19.3 Breast cancer staging and survival | |
|---|---|
| **Breast cancer stage** | **5-year survival (all races) (%)** |
| Localized | 98 |
| Regional | 80 |
| Distant | 26 |
| All stages | 88 |

replaced by the less disfiguring modified radical mastectomy. After the National Surgical Adjuvant Breast and Bowel Project (NSABP) B-04 was completed in the 1980s, breast-conserving surgery was found to be equivalent to mastectomy for survival, and there have been increasing trends toward breast conservation.[57,58]

Mastectomy is performed in two general ways: simple mastectomy, or modified radical mastectomy. The simple mastectomy or total mastectomy is removal of the breast including the nipple–areola complex, by an elliptical incision. The breast and underlying fascia are dissected off from the pectoralis muscle fibers. The modified radical mastectomy also includes the removal of ipsilateral axillary, and some lateral pectoral lymph nodes. The pectoralis major is always preserved. This procedure is often available in conjunction with an immediate plastic surgical reconstruction. Options available to postmenopausal women are only limited by medical comorbidities or patient preference.

BCT is the option the majority of women, including postmenopausal women, who are faced with breast cancer, would choose when eligible. BCT consists of removal of the primary tumor with a rim of normal tissue, followed by radiotherapy to provide local-regional control of disease. The three criteria to determine eligibility are:

1. capability to deliver breast irradiation
2. likelihood of achieving a cosmetically acceptable result
3. capability of removing a margin negative resection or lumpectomy.

The criteria of a cosmetically acceptable result will vary depending on the location of the tumor, but treating physicians should always defer to the patient to decide what is cosmetically 'acceptable'. Contraindications to BCT are included in Table 19.4. The standard radiation treatment involves external beam radiation daily for 5 weeks to the whole breast, followed by 1 to 2 weeks of supplemental radiation to the tumor bed. Recently, alternatives to this regimen have been investigated involving brachytherapy or implanted sources of radiation, which may be less inconvenient to the patient, providing a less rigorous schedule of outpatient or in-hospital irradiation.[59] Further testing will be evaluated to determine applicability and utility of these techniques.

Axillary dissection for lymph nodes of the ipsilateral breast is conventionally performed for breast cancer, primarily as a staging procedure. Examination of these nodes will detect metastases in 98% of patients with breast cancer. It is the most powerful prognostic tool in predicting cancer relapse. In addition, multiple studies have shown that axillary recurrence of disease nears zero when five to ten nodes are removed in the dissection.[60] Morbidity of the procedure is not insignificant, however, and risk of lymphedema of the upper extremity occurs in about 25% of patients.[61] Other complications include sensory nerve injury and, less commonly, motor nerve injury.[62]

Recently, a more selective approach to lymph node dissection has been validated and has become an acceptable standard for those without clinically evident axillary disease.[63,64] The technique identifies the first lymph node to receive drainage from the malignant tumor or the 'sentinel' node. Lymphatic mapping is performed with visible dye or radioactive markers, or a combination of both. This technique is believed to accurately identify 90% of sentinel nodes and predict the status of remaining nodes. Contraindications to sentinel node biopsy include suspected palpable adenopathy, tumor >5 cm or locally advanced, use of preoperative chemotherapy, multicentric disease, and a pregnant or lactating patient.[3] Once the sentinel node has been identified, and metastases have been confirmed, current convention is followed with a complete dissection of the remaining nodes, though several studies are investigating the alternative of observation only and therapeutic dissection for regional relapse. Results of these studies will help determine the most prudent management of axillary metastases.

### Adjuvant therapy

Adjuvant therapy aims to eradicate occult micrometastases not removed by surgical resection. Many women with nodal metastases and carcinomas larger than 1 cm in size will benefit from

**Table 19.4**   Eligibility for breast-conserving therapy

| Criteria of eligibility for BCT | Contraindications to eligibility for BCT |
| --- | --- |
| Ability to receive radiation therapy | Multicentric disease in separate quadrants of the breast predicts an excessive radiation load (multiple lesions in a single quadrant may be considered) |
| | Prior therapeutic irradiation overlapping the breast. Prohibitive increase in future breast cancer risk due to radiation exposure |
| | Pregnancy. Selected third trimester pregnancies may undergo surgical therapy and delayed radiation therapy post-partum |
| | History of collagen vascular disease (e.g. scleroderma and lupus).[a] May experience excessive radiation toxicity especially if steroid dependent |
| | Large pendulous breasts where consistent targeted irradiation dosage cannot be ensured[a] |
| Capability of obtaining negative margins or cosmetically acceptable results | Diffuse malignant-appearing microcalcifications. Predicts extensive DCIS and low likelihood of negative margins |
| | Persistent positive margins after reasonable number of surgical attempts |
| | Primary tumor size greater than 5 cm.[a] Ratio of tumor to breast size may prevent cosmetically acceptable results |

[a]Relative contraindications.

systemic chemotherapy. However, the majority of randomized trials have indicated that the benefits of systemic cytotoxic chemotherapy may be less apparent in postmenopausal women.[65] The current regimens should be reviewed by the patient in conjunction with an oncologist to provide the most appropriate therapy.

In addition to the presence of metastasis, tumors themselves may be assessed for expression of receptors which, when activated, may promote tumor growth, and when blocked may provide treatment against tumor growth. Tumors are routinely assessed for expression of estrogen receptors (ER), progesterone receptors (PR), and human epidermal growth factor receptor 2 (Her2/neu). A significant percentage of women will benefit from systemic endocrine therapy targeting these proteins. Hormone receptor expression will vary in breast cancers. In addition subtypes of estrogen receptors have been described ERα and ERβ that have different responses, anti-estrogenic therapies, and different tissue distribution.[66,67] The vascular protective effects may be predominantly mediated through ERβ, while the effects classically attributed to estrogen receptors in breast cancer and uterine stimulation may be predominantly effected by ERα. Further research is being directed into developing selective therapy that differentially targets the subtypes ERα and ERβ for optimal therapeutic profiles.

Patients with these tumors expressing estrogen or progesterone receptors, or both, have been shown to benefit significantly from tamoxifen therapy.[68] Tamoxifen belongs to a family of drugs called selective estrogen receptor modulators (SERMs), which act as estrogen antagonists in the breast, while acting as agonists in bone and liver. The best known are tamoxifen, raloxifene and toremifene The SERMs' effects are preventative against breast cancer, while protecting bone, and possibly lowering cholesterol. In women with receptor-positive tumors, they have been shown to reduce recurrence by 47% and annual odds of death by 26%. All postmenopausal women with estrogen or progesterone receptor-positive tumors should be given anti-estrogen treatment unless contraindicated. Tamoxifen's side-effects include increased incidence of endometrial cancer, stroke, and pulmonary embolism. Currently, newer drugs with decreased side-effect profiles are being investigated in postmenopausal women. The ATAC (Arimidex, Tamoxifen, Alone or in Combination) trial compared the utility of anastrazole (Arimidex™) an aromatase inhibitor, in conjunction with tamoxifen or instead of tamoxifen as adjuvant therapy to breast cancer.[69] Data have shown promising results, and we are seeing the replacement of tamoxifen with aromatase inhibitors as the treatment of choice in these women.

Immunotherapy is also being investigated as a mode of adjuvant therapy. Cancers overexpressing Her2/neu receptors have, historically, been associated with poor prognosis. Trastuzumab, an antibody targeting these protein receptors, has recently been shown by two studies to have significant benefit for women with cancers expressing Her2/neu receptors. The studies showed the use of trastuzumab in conjunction with other chemotherapy improved disease-free survival in this subpopulation of women. The most concerning adverse effect shown to the treatment was cardiac toxicity.[66,70–72]

For locally advanced disease, the use of preoperative neoadjuvant chemotherapy has become an established management. Multiple trials have shown its ability to downstage a percentage of tumors and to increase eligibility for BCT without compromising local control. It should be noted that if preoperative chemotherapy is considered, then marking of the tumor bed may be required to ensure localization of a responsive tumor at surgery.

In inflammatory breast cancer, neoadjuvant chemotherapy as initial treatment followed by surgery and radiation has seen improved survival rates in a once universally fatal disease. The response of tumors to preoperative chemotherapy may also serve as a predictor to response after removal of tumor.

## Prognosis in breast cancer

Proper treatment of breast cancer patients requires that the patient appropriately understands the prognosis of her disease and the likely effect of the various treatment modalities. Prognostic factors have been identified by the AJCC as predictive of death. Most non-invasive cancer patients can expect cure, while invasive carcinomas and subsequent metastases have a poorer outcome. Distant metastases predict cure of disease as highly unlikely, and treatment is palliative. Lymph node metastasis is the most important prognostic factor for invasive carcinoma without distant metastases. No nodes predicts a 70% to 80% 10-year survival rate, while one to three positive nodes predicts a 35% to 40% survival rate and with more

than ten positive nodes it falls to a 10% to 15% rate. Tumor size is the second most important prognostic factor, with tumors less than 1 cm having a much better outcome. Locally advanced disease negatively affects outcome, with tumors invading the skin and skeletal muscle having poor prognosis. Inflammatory carcinomas are especially concerning. Women presenting with clinical edema and skin changes have a very poor prognosis in the range of a 3% to 10% three-year survival rate.

In recurrent breast cancer the outcome is dependent on the extent of recurrent disease. In local regional recurrence or axillary node recurrence, the five-year survival rates can range as high as 76% to 92%.[73] However, recurrent metastatic disease has an almost uniformly poor outcome though subsets of patients may still benefit from systemic chemotherapy or endocrine therapy, especially in hormone receptor-positive cancers.

## SUMMARY

The health of the female breast in the menopause requires regular and appropriate care and management. A combined effort of patient and physician can help to ensure consistent evaluation and timely intervention in cases of breast disease. The management and treatment of breast cancer has been a dynamic field of interest with much activity and advances over the past two decades. Current treatments have shown excellent results for all ages from women early in the menopause to late into the geripause. The advent of BCT, sentinel node biopsy, and improved adjuvant chemotherapy and hormonal regimens have greatly advanced the treatment of breast cancer, improved disease-free survival, and prospective quality of life.

## REFERENCES

1. Moore KL, Dalley AF. Thorax. In: Moore KL, Dalley AF, eds, Clinically Oriented Anatomy, 4th edn. Philadelphia: Lippincott Williams & Wilkins, 1999: 59–173.
2. Iglehart JD, Kaelin CM. Diseases of the breast. In: Townsend CM, Beauchamp RD, Evers BM, Mattox KL, eds. Sabiston Textbook of Surgery, 17th edn. Philadelphia: Elsevier Saunders, 2004: 867–927.
3. Morrow M. Breast. In: Greenfield LJ, Mulholland MW, Oldham KT, Zelenock GB, Lillemoe KD, eds. Surgery: Scientific Principles and Practice, 3rd edn. Philadelphia: Lippincott Williams & Wilkins, 2001: 1334–72.

4. Russo J, Russo IH. Development of the human breast. Maturitas 2004; 49: 2–15.
5. Russo J, Rivera R, Russo IH. Influence of age and parity on the development of the human breast. Breast Cancer Res Treat 1992; 23: 211–18.
6. Eskin BA. The breast in the menopause. In: Eskin BA, ed. The Menopause: Comprehensive Management, 4th edn. New York: Parthenon Publishing, 2000: 185–99.
7. Morrow M. The evaluation of common breast problems. Am Fam Physician 2000; 61: 2371–8, 2385.
8. Marchant DJ. Benign breast disease. Obstet Gynecol Clin North Am 2002; 29: 1–20.
9. Marchant DJ. Benign breast disease. Obstet Gynecol Clin North Am 2002; 29: 1–20.
10. Kessler JH. The effect of supraphysiologic levels of iodine on patients with cyclic mastalgia. Breast J 2004; 10: 328–36.
11. Seltzer MH, Perloff LJ, Kelley RI, Fitts WT, Jr. The significance of age in patients with nipple discharge. Surg Gynecol Obstet 1970; 131: 519–22.
12. Cabioglu N, Hunt KK, Singletary SE et al. Surgical decision making and factors determining a diagnosis of breast carcinoma in women presenting with nipple discharge. J Am Coll Surg 2003; 196: 354–64.
13. Dooley WC, Ljung BM, Veronesi U et al. Ductal lavage for detection of cellular atypia in women at high risk for breast cancer. J Natl Cancer Inst 2001; 93: 1624–32.
14. Dooley WC, Spiegel A, Cox C, Henderson R, Richardson L, Zabora J. Ductoscopy: defining its role in the management of breast cancer. Breast J 2004; 10: 271–2.
15. Dooley WC, Francescatti D, Clark L, Webber G. Office-based breast ductoscopy for diagnosis. Am J Surg 2004; 188: 415–18.
16. Francis A, England D, Rowlands D, Bradley S. Breast papilloma: mammogram, ultrasound and MRI appearances. Breast 2002; 11: 394–7.
17. Falkenberry SS. Nipple discharge. Obstet Gynecol Clin North Am 2002; 29: 21–9.
18. Marchant DJ. Benign breast disease. Obstet Gynecol Clin North Am 2002; 29: 1–20.
19. Daskal I. Pathology of common premalignant and malignant lesions. In: Eskin BA, Asbell SO, Jardines L, eds. Breast Disease for Primary Care Physicians, 1st edn. New York: Parthenon Publishing Group, 1999: 83–102.
20. Mehta TS. Current uses of ultrasound in the evaluation of the breast. Radiol Clin North Am 2003; 41: 841–56.
21. Park SY, Oh KK, Kim EK, Son EJ, Chung WH. Sonographic findings of breast hamartoma: emphasis on compressibility. Yonsei Med J 2003; 44: 847–54.
22. Marchant DJ. Benign breast disease. Obstet Gynecol Clin North Am 2002; 29: 1–20.
23. Marchant DJ. Inflammation of the breast. Obstet Gynecol Clin North Am 2002; 29: 89–102.
24. Marchant DJ. Inflammation of the breast. Obstet Gynecol Clin North Am 2002; 29: 89–102.
25. Jemal A, Murray T, Ward E et al. Cancer statistics, 2005. CA Cancer J Clin 2005; 55: 10–30.
26. Rosen PP. The pathological classification of human mammary carcinoma: past, present and future. Ann Clin Lab Sci 1979; 9: 144–56.
27. Frykberg ER. Lobular carcinoma in situ of the breast. Breast J 1999; 5: 296–303.
28. Li CI, Anderson BO, Porter P, Holt SK, Daling JR, Moe RE. Changing incidence rate of invasive lobular breast carcinoma among older women. Cancer 2000; 88: 2561–9.
29. Yap J, Chuba PJ, Thomas R et al. Sarcoma as a second malignancy after treatment for breast cancer. Int J Radiat Oncol Biol Phys 2002; 52: 1231–7.
30. Falkenberry SS, Legare RD. Risk factors for breast cancer. Obstet Gynecol Clin North Am 2002; 29: 159–72.
31. Falkenberry SS, Legare RD. Risk factors for breast cancer. Obstet Gynecol Clin North Am 2002; 29: 159–72.
32. Breast cancer and breastfeeding: collaborative reanalysis of individual data from 47 epidemiological studies in 30 countries, including 50 302 women with breast cancer and 96 973 women without the disease. Lancet 2002; 360: 187–95.
33. Dorgan JF, Baer DJ, Albert PS et al. Serum hormones and the alcohol-breast cancer association in postmenopausal women. J Natl Cancer Inst 2001; 93: 710–15.
34. Couch FJ, Cerhan JR, Vierkant RA et al. Cigarette smoking increases risk for breast cancer in high-risk breast cancer families. Cancer Epidemiol Biomarkers Prev 2001; 10: 327–32.
35. Lee IM, Cook NR, Rexrode KM, Buring JE. Lifetime physical activity and risk of breast cancer. Br J Cancer 2001; 85: 962–5.
36. Armes JE, Venter DJ. The pathology of inherited breast cancer. Pathology 2002; 34: 309–14.
37. Chlebowski RT, Hendrix SL, Langer RD et al. Influence of estrogen plus progestin on breast cancer and mammography in healthy postmenopausal women: the Women's Health Initiative Randomized Trial. JAMA 2003; 289: 3243–53.
38. Anderson GL, Limacher M, Assaf AR et al. Effects of conjugated equine estrogen in postmenopausal women with hysterectomy: the Women's Health Initiative Randomized Controlled Trial. JAMA 2004; 291: 1701–12.
39. Breast cancer and hormone replacement therapy: collaborative reanalysis of data from 51 epidemiological studies of 52 705 women with breast cancer and 108 411 women without breast cancer. Collaborative Group on Hormonal Factors in Breast Cancer. Lancet 1997; 350: 1047–59.
40. La VC. Menopause, hormone therapy and breast cancer risk. Eur J Cancer Prev 2003; 12: 437–8.
41. La VC. Estrogen and combined estrogen-progestogen therapy in the menopause and breast cancer. Breast 2004; 13: 515–18.
42. Hackshaw AK, Paul EA. Breast self-examination and death from breast cancer: a meta-analysis. Br J Cancer 2003; 88: 1047–53.
43. Newman LA, Sabel M. Advances in breast cancer detection and management. Med Clin North Am 2003; 87: 997–1028.
44. Ries LAG, Eisner MP, Kosary CL et al. SEER Cancer statistics review, 1975–2002. Bethesda MD: National Cancer Institute Bethesda, 2005. http://seer.cancer.gov/csr/1975_2002/ (accessed 4 April 2006).
45. Liberman L, Abramson AF, Squires FB, Glassman JR, Morris EA, Dershaw DD. The breast imaging reporting and data system: positive predictive value of mammographic features and final assessment categories. Am J Roentgenol 1998; 171: 35–40.
46. Liberman L, Menell JH. Breast imaging reporting and data system (BI-RADS). Radiol Clin North Am 2002; 40: 409–30.

47. Obenauer S, Hermann KP, Grabbe E. Applications and literature review of the BI-RADS classification. Eur Radiol 2005; 15: 1027–36.

48. Pisano ED, Yaffe MJ. Digital mammography. Radiology 2005; 234: 353–62.

49. Kolb TM, Lichy J, Newhouse JH. Occult cancer in women with dense breasts: detection with screening US – diagnostic yield and tumor characteristics. Radiology 1998; 207: 191–19.

50. Morris EA. Review of breast MRI: indications and limitations. Semin Roentgenol 2001; 36: 226–37.

51. Klimberg VS, Harms SE, Henry-Tillman RS. Not all MRI techniques are created equal. Ann Surg Oncol 2000; 7: 404–5.

52. Gail MH, Brinton LA, Byar DP et al. Projecting individualized probabilities of developing breast cancer for white females who are being examined annually. J Natl Cancer Inst 1989; 81: 1879–86.

53. Hollingsworth AB, Singletary SE, Morrow M et al. Current comprehensive assessment and management of women at increased risk for breast cancer. Am J Surg 2004; 187: 349–62.

54. King MC, Wieand S, Hale K et al. Tamoxifen and breast cancer incidence among women with inherited mutations in BRCA1 and BRCA2: National Surgical Adjuvant Breast and Bowel Project (NSABP-P1) Breast Cancer Prevention Trial. JAMA 2001; 286: 2251–6.

55. Stavros AT, Thickman D, Rapp CL, Dennis MA, Parker SH, Sisney GA. Solid breast nodules: use of sonography to distinguish between benign and malignant lesions. Radiology 1995; 196: 123–34.

56. Jemal A, Murray T, Ward E et al. Cancer statistics, 2005. CA Cancer J Clin 2005; 55: 10–30.

57. Fisher B, Montague E, Redmond C et al. Findings from NSABP Protocol No. B-04-comparison of radical mastectomy with alternative treatments for primary breast cancer. I. Radiation compliance and its relation to treatment outcome. Cancer 1980; 46: 1–13.

58. Fisher B, Wolmark N, Redmond C, Deutsch M, Fisher ER. Findings from NSABP Protocol No. B-04: comparison of radical mastectomy with alternative treatments. II. The clinical and biologic significance of medial-central breast cancers. Cancer 1981; 48: 1863–72.

59. Hogle WP, Quinn AE, Heron DE. Advances in brachytherapy: new approaches to target breast cancer. Clin J Oncol Nurs 2003; 7: 324–8.

60. Fisher B, Wolmark N, Bauer M, Redmond C, Gebhardt M. The accuracy of clinical nodal staging and of limited axillary dissection as a determinant of histologic nodal status in carcinoma of the breast. Surg Gynecol Obstet 1981; 152: 765–72.

61. Erickson VS, Pearson ML, Ganz PA, Adams J, Kahn KL. Arm edema in breast cancer patients. J Natl Cancer Inst 2001; 93: 96–111.

62. Roses DF, Brooks AD, Harris MN, Shapiro RL, Mitnick J. Complications of level I and II axillary dissection in the treatment of carcinoma of the breast. Ann Surg 1999; 230: 194–201.

63. Newman LA. Lymphatic mapping and sentinel lymph node biopsy in breast cancer patients: a comprehensive review of variations in performance and technique. J Am Coll Surg 2004; 199: 804–16.

64. Schwartz GF. Clinical practice guidelines for the use of axillary sentinel lymph node biopsy in carcinoma of the breast: current update. Breast J 2004; 10: 85–8.

65. Crivellari D, Bonetti M, Castiglione-Gertsch M et al. Burdens and benefits of adjuvant cyclophosphamide, methotrexate, and fluorouracil and tamoxifen for elderly patients with breast cancer: the International Breast Cancer Study Group Trial VII. J Clin Oncol 2000; 18: 1412–22.

66. Katzenellenbogen BS, Katzenellenbogen JA. Estrogen receptor transcription and transactivation: Estrogen receptor alpha and estrogen receptor beta: regulation by selective estrogen receptor modulators and importance in breast cancer. Breast Cancer Res 2000; 2: 335–44.

67. Kraichely DM, Sun J, Katzenellenbogen JA, Katzenellenbogen BS. Conformational changes and coactivator recruitment by novel ligands for estrogen receptor-alpha and estrogen receptor-beta: correlations with biological character and distinct differences among SRC coactivator family members. Endocrinology 2000; 141: 3534–45.

68. Early Breast Cancer Trialists' Collaborative Group. Tamoxifen for early breast cancer: an overview of the randomised trials. Lancet 1998; 351: 1451–67.

69. Howell A, Cuzick J, Baum M et al. Results of the ATAC (Arimidex, Tamoxifen, Alone or in Combination) trial after completion of 5 years' adjuvant treatment for breast cancer. Lancet 2005; 365: 60–2.

70. Kraichely DM, Sun J, Katzenellenbogen JA, Katzenellenbogen BS. Conformational changes and coactivator recruitment by novel ligands for estrogen receptor-alpha and estrogen receptor-beta: correlations with biological character and distinct differences among SRC coactivator family members. Endocrinology 2000; 141: 3534–45.

71. Emens LA, Davidson NE. Trastuzumab in breast cancer. Oncology (Huntingt) 2004; 18: 1117–28.

72. Finn RS, Slamon DJ. Monoclonal antibody therapy for breast cancer: herceptin. Cancer Chemother Biol Response Modif 2003; 21: 223–33.

73. Huston TL, Simmons RM. Locally recurrent breast cancer after conservation therapy. Am J Surg 2005 February; 189(2): 229–35.

# Treatment of the menopausal woman

# Chapter 20

# Pharmacology of hormonal therapeutic agents

Bhagu R Bhavnani

## INTRODUCTION

In this chapter, the basic pharmacology of estrogens and progestins used for hormone replacement therapy (HRT, or estrogen/progestin therapy; EPT) and estrogen replacement therapy (ERT, or estrogen therapy; ET) in postmenopausal women are discussed. The structures of some of the estrogens and progestins are shown in Figures 20.1 and 20.2. The emphasis is on estrogens and on factors such as rate of absorption, enterohepatic circulation, route of administration and serum transport via serum-binding proteins, and how these factors influence the bioavailability of these steroids. The recent advances in the genomic and non-genomic mechanisms of action involved in estrogen and progestin effects are described. Differences between various preparations, and the impact these may have clinically, are presented. The antioxidant properties of various estrogens are discussed in the context of cardiovascular disease and Alzheimer's disease in postmenopausal women. The most frequently and widely prescribed estrogen preparation for postmenopausal estrogen replacement is conjugated equine estrogen (CEE). This preparation contains a number of components that are also used individually, and therefore the pharmacology of this preparation is dealt with in detail.

## GENERAL ASPECTS

Natural menopause is a normal physiological process that occurs in healthy Caucasian women at a median age between 50 and 55 years.[1] Current smokers reach menopause an average of 1.5 to 2 years earlier.[1] Menopause is associated with a cessation of ovarian function and menstrual bleeding. This normal physiological change generally takes place over a period of time (years) and is roughly divided into three phases: the perimenopause is the phase during which, in most women, ovarian function gradually declines, and may result in irregular and anovulatory menstrual cycles.[2] By definition, menopause is the absence of menstrual flow for 12 months, and is characterized by low serum 17β-estradiol and high follicle-stimulating hormone (FSH) levels. During this phase, all of the ovarian follicles have been either depleted or are unresponsive to gonadotropin stimulation; the postmenopausal years are the continuation, for the rest of the woman's life, of changes that have occurred at menopause. Although during the postmenopausal years the ovary does not secrete estrogens, its stromal cells continue to produce small amounts of androstenedione. The importance of this ovarian androgen secretion is discussed in subsequent sections.

Some authors refer to the three phases collectively as 'the climacteric', while others refer to the transitional period between perimenopause and the actual menopause as 'the climacteric'. In contrast to natural menopause, which occurs gradually over a period of time, removal of ovaries in a young woman results in a very rapid and perhaps unexpected entry into menopause.

During the past century, the world population and, more importantly, the elderly population been increasing at a rapid rate.[3] Thus, in 1900, the world population was around 2 billion people; by the year 2020, the United Nations has projected it to be 8 billion.[3] The proportion of elderly (above 65 years), will have increased from 5% in 1950 to 9% by the year 2020, and this represents an elderly

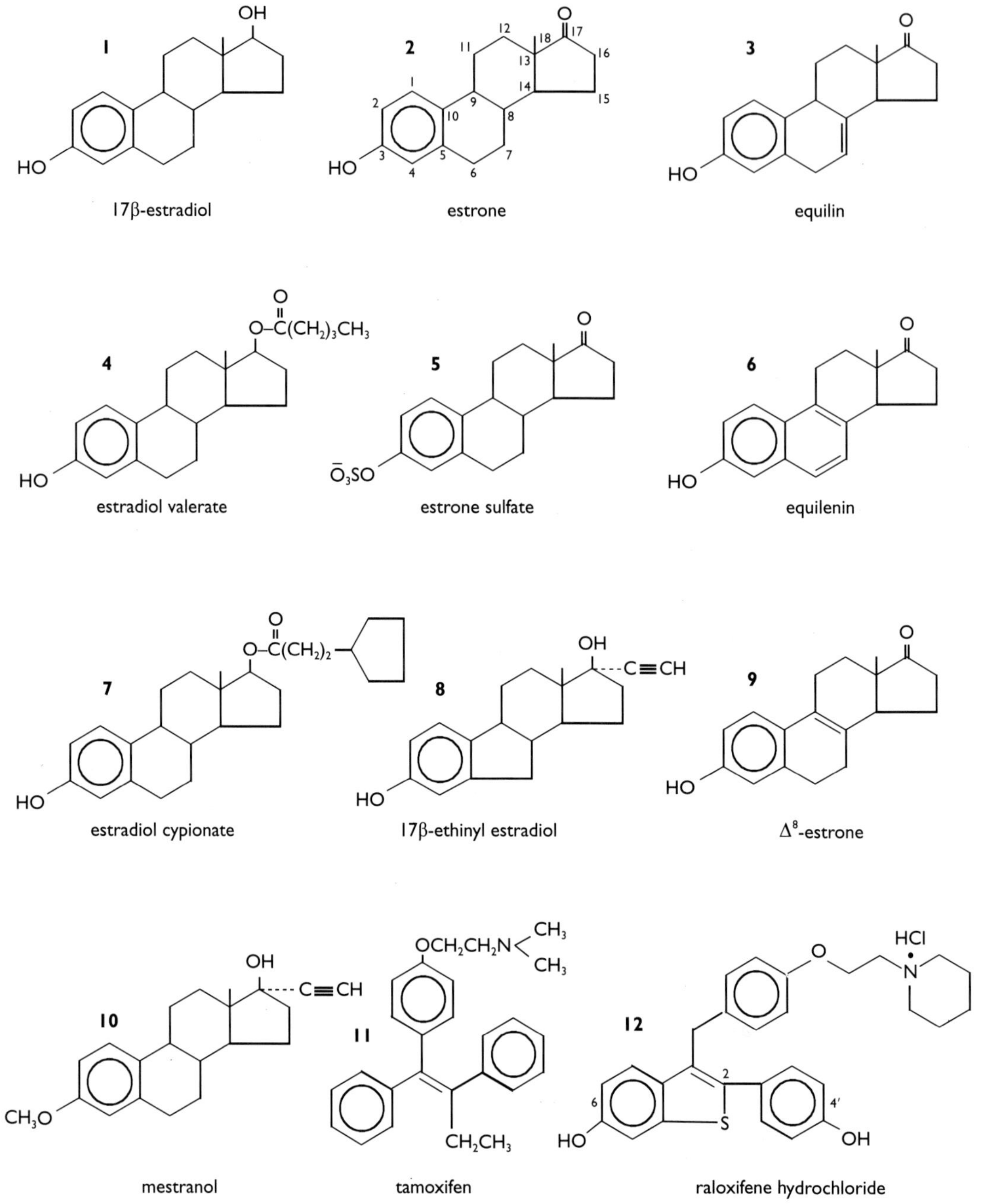

**Figure 20.1** Structure of natural and synthetic estrogens and related compounds.

population of 796 million people. Moreover, nearly 124 million are expected to be over 80 years old. The majority of this elderly population will be postmenopausal women.[3] It is estimated that the average life expectancy of women in the next decade or so is going to be 81 plus years in the US, Canada and Europe. Thus, most women can expect to live more than one-third of their lives after menopause. The demographics, health, socioeconomic and ethical implications of the soaring elderly population have been previously reviewed.[3]

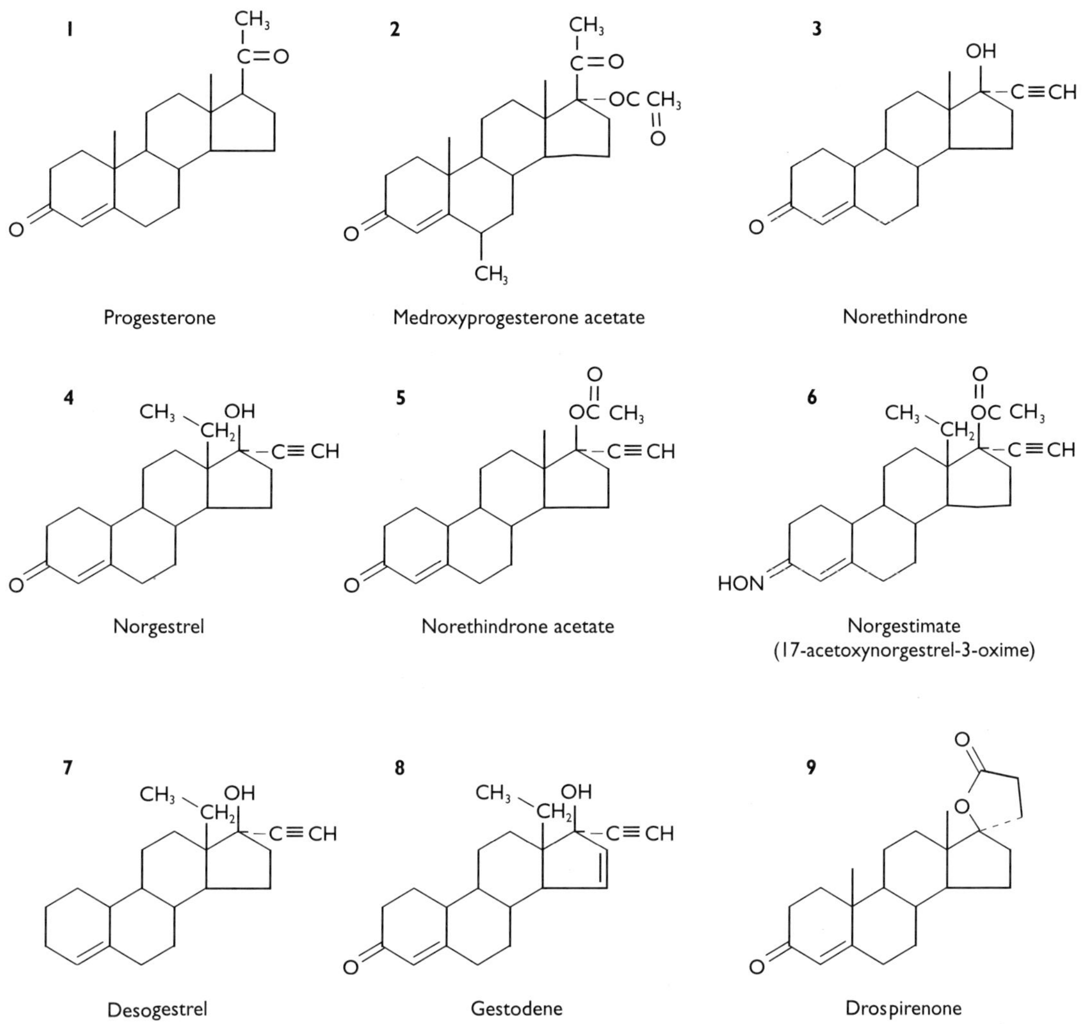

**Figure 20.2**   Structure of various progestins available for hormone replacement therapy.

Since normal aging is associated with increasing health problems such as osteoporosis, cardiovascular disease, neurodegenerative diseases and cancer, it is essential that we strive to develop preventive strategies that will assist postmenopausal women to maintain a healthy and productive quality of life.

## ESTROGEN AND PROGESTERONE PRODUCTION DURING MENOPAUSE

During the premenopausal reproductive years, the human ovaries utilize the classical pathway of steroidogenesis to biosynthesize both estrogens and progesterone from simple precursors such as acetate (Figure 20.3). In this pathway, cholesterol is the obligatory intermediate, and several enzymes and cofactors are involved.[4] In contrast to this classical pathway of steroidogenesis, an alternate pathway, where cholesterol is not an obligatory precursor, has been described for the biosynthesis of unique ring B unsaturated estrogens.[4] These estrogens are some of the known components present in the most frequently prescribed drug (CEE) for ERT. In premenopausal women, estrogen is produced by two pathways, and the precursors needed arise from the ovary and the adrenal (Figure 20.4). The predominant estrogen secreted during premenopause (reproductive life), is 17β-estradiol which is secreted by the ovary, and is formed predominantly from ovarian

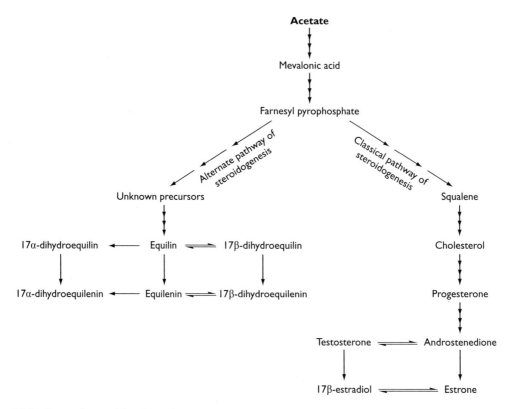

**Figure 20.3** Biosynthesis of the classical estrogens estrone and estradiol, and the ring B unsaturated estrogens equilin and equilenin.

androstenedione/testosterone.[5] The serum levels range from 40 pg/ml in the early proliferative (follicular) phase, to 250 pg/ml at mid-cycle and 100 pg/ml during the mid-secretory (mid-luteal) phase.[5] The total amount of 17β-estradiol secreted varies from 20–40 μg/day during the early proliferative and late secretory phases of the menstrual cycle to 600–1000 μg/day just prior to ovulation.[6] During premenopause, along with 17β-estradiol, a small amount of estrone is produced by the peripheral or extraglandular (extra-ovarian) aromatization of adrenal androstenedione. This extraglandular formation of estrone does not vary during the menstrual cycle, and approximately 45 μg/day of estrone is produced from this source.[6] In contrast, in postmenopausal women, the predominant estrogen is estrone, produced almost exclusively by extraglandular aromatization (Figure 20.4). The androgen precursor needed for this aromatization is circulating androstenedione, which is secreted mainly (95%) by the adrenal cortex, and to a much lesser extent (5%), by the ovarian stroma. The primary site of peripheral

aromatization is the adipose tissue, although tissues such as skin, muscle, bone, brain, and hair follicles may also be involved.[7] Obesity is associated with higher levels of circulating estrogens which arise from peripheral aromatization of androstenedione by the adipose tissue.[8]

During the perimenopausal phase, and with cessation of menstruation, the 17β-estradiol secretion declines to low levels (Table 20.1) during the first year, and these low levels (20–40 pg/ml) are maintained over the postmenopausal years.[9] During menopause, there is a decline in the ovarian secretion of androgens, particularly that of androstenedione,[9,10] yet during the transition from perimenopause to postmenopause, the levels of androgens do not decline significantly, As a result of the declining levels of estrogen during menopause, the negative feedback effect on the hypothalamic-pituitary axis is lost, and the levels of gonadotropins (Table 20.1), particularly those of FSH, increase several-fold.[9]

Although the levels of testosterone in postmenopausal women do not significantly decline,

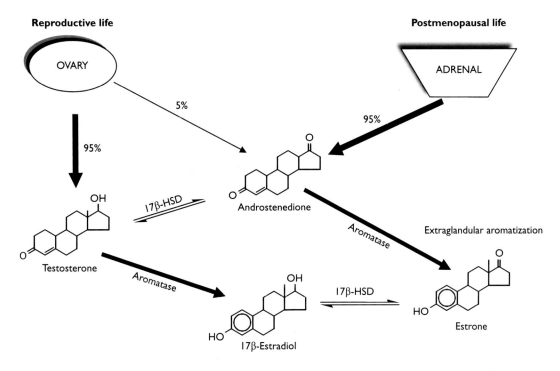

**Figure 20.4** Formation of estrogens in women during the reproductive and postmenopausal years. 17β-HSD, 17β-hydroxydehydrogenase.

peripheral aromatization of testosterone to 17β-estradiol or estrone is minimal.[9] In contrast to premenopausal women, the principal source of 17β-estradiol in postmenopausal women is from the peripheral conversion of estrone by 17β-hydrosteroid dehydrogenase (type I; 17β-HSD).[11]

It has been estimated that the conversion of androstenedione to estrone in peripheral tissues is about 2–3% and, based on the androstenedione production rate of 1500 μg/day in healthy menopausal women, approximately 30–45 μg of estrone/day is produced by this mechanism. This amount of estrone represents essentially the total amount found in these women. There is no evidence of direct secretion of estrogens by either the ovary or the adrenal gland.[6,8] In obese postmenopausal women, the amount of androstenedione secreted by the adrenal gland is the same,

**Table 20.1** Concentrations of 17β-estradiol and FSH in perimenopausal and postmenopausal women

| Months from last menses | Mean ± SEM | |
|---|---|---|
| | 17β-estradiol (pg/ml) | FSH (mIU/ml) |
| <3 | 108 ± 19 | 27 ± 4 |
| 9–12 | 26 ± 4[a] | 84 ± 16[a] |
| 12–24 | 19 ± 4[a] | 97 ± 18[a] |
| >24 | 14 ± 1[a] | 69 ± 9[a] |

SEM, standard error of the mean.

[a]$P < 0.05$, compared to value at < 3 months.

Data from Longcope et al. Maturitas 1986; 8: 189–96,[9] with permission from the publisher.

but the percentage conversion to estrone is over 11%. This then accounts for the higher level (120–130 µg/day) of estrone found in these wome.[12] Since the amount of progesterone found in postmenopausal women is extremely low, the extraglandular estrogen is considered to be unopposed estrogen, and a correlation between this estrogen and increased risk for endometrial cancer has been proposed.[12]

## IN VIVO TRANSPORT OF ESTROGENS AND PROGESTINS

The binding of steroid hormones to serum proteins such as sex hormone-binding globulin (SHBG) and corticosteroid-binding globulin (CBG) plays an important role in the transport and distribution of hormones. In the human circulation, estrogens and progestins are primarily bound non-specifically and with low affinity to albumin, and specifically with high affinity to SHBG or CBG.[13,14] Only a small fraction of these hormones circulate in the unbound or free form.[13,14] It is generally accepted that only the free steroid hormone can readily enter the target cell to exert its biological effect, or be further metabolized and excreted. Some have argued that the protein-bound form of some steroids can also enter the cell, but the physiological significance of this remains to be established.[15]

The levels of SHBG and CBG regulate the free hormone concentration, and the protein-bound hormones constitute a readily available pool of hormones. Since steroid hormones bind to serum albumin with low affinity and are easily dissociable to the free hormones, the albumin-bound hormone is considered to be also available for biological action.

In premenopausal women, approximately 60% of the 17β-estradiol in circulation is loosely (i.e. with low affinity) bound to albumin, and 38% bound to SHBG with relatively high affinity.[16] The relative affinity constants for various estrogens and androgens: estrone, equilin, 17β-dihydroequilin, 17β-estradiol, testosterone, and 5α-dihydrotestosterone are: 0.07, 0.15, 0.22, 0.29, 2.70, and $4.53 \times 10^9 M^{-1}$, respectively.[17] Although the 17β-reduced estrogens have a relatively higher affinity for SHBG than the corresponding 17-ketones, these relative binding affinities are

much lower than those observed with androgens.[17,18] In contrast to the unconjugated estrogens, the sulfate esters of estrogens do not bind to SHBG but instead bind to serum albumin with relatively high affinity ($0.9–1.1 \times 10^5$ M$^{-1}$).[17,19] Between 60% and 90% of estrogen sulfates are bound to albumin, and this is the main circulating form of estrogen sulfates in postmenopausal women. These estrogen sulfates serve as reservoirs from which the unconjugated estrogens are being continuously formed.

Oral administration of estrogen increases SHBG levels, resulting in a greater percentage of estrogen bound to SHBG, and therefore a lesser amount of the free hormone is available for biological action. Levels of SHBG are also increased during pregnancy, hyperthyroidism, and cirrhosis. In contrast, obesity, androgen excess, and hypothyroidism lower the level of SHBG, and can result in an increase in the free fraction of estrogens.[8] The extent and degree of binding of estrogen to serum proteins not only determines the amount of estrogen available for biological action, but also plays an important role in the metabolic clearance rate (MCR) of estrogens, and this aspect will be discussed in subsequent sections.

Like estrogens, progestins (Figure 20.2), also circulate primarily in a bound form. Approximately 20% of progesterone is bound to CBG, and the rest to albumin.[14] Similarly, over 90% of medroxyprogesterone is bound to albumin.[20] Progesterone and medroxyprogesterone do not appear to bind to SHBG to any significant extent, however binding of progesterone to other proteins, particularly in some species, has been noted.[13] In contrast to progesterone and medroxyprogesterone acetate, 19-norprogestins bind in substantial amounts to SHBG. Thus, the amount of norethindrone, levonorgestrel, desogestrel (3-ketodesogestrel) and gestodene bound to SHBG is 35%, 47%, 32% and 75% respectively.[21,22] Approximately 0.6% to 3.7% of these progestins is present in the free form and the remainder is bound to albumin.[21,22] Norgestimate is a 3-oximo 17-acetoxy derivative of norgestrel (levonorgestrel), and since it is metabolized to levonorgestrel,[23,24] essentially all of its biological effects are most probably a result of its first metabolism to norgestrel and/or norgestrel acetate. Its distribution in serum has not been well documented, and will essentially be similar to that of levonorgestrel.[21]

# THE GENOMIC MECHANISM OF STEROID HORMONE ACTION

The basic genomic mechanism of steroid hormone action has been known for more than three decades, and excellent detailed reviews are available.[25-30] In the following section, the genomic mechanism of action of steroid hormones with emphasis on estrogens is briefly outlined.

As discussed above, in the human, estrogens circulate in the blood bound mostly to serum proteins; the free (unbound) hormone enters the target tissues and interacts with estrogen receptors (ERs) as shown in Figure 20.5. The ER belongs to a superfamily of ligand-dependent transcription factors that regulate estrogen-responsive genes,[25] and it is by this process that the main biological effects of estrogens are exerted. Until 1995, only one specific estrogen receptor, ERα, located in the target cell nuclei had been described. However, now another gene that codes for a second estrogen receptor, ERβ, has been identified.[31] These two receptors are similar (Figure 20.6), and even though the ERβ is considerably smaller, it binds to 17β-estradiol with similar affinity. In the absence of estrogen, the ER resides in a transcriptionally inactive (latent) form associated with heat shock proteins (HSPs) in the cell nuclei (Figure 20.5).

The mechanism of estrogen hormone action involves a series of molecular steps that are schematically depicted in Figure 20.5. Briefly, the unbound (free) estrogen is lipophilic, and readily enters target tissue cells by passive diffusion through the cell membrane where it binds to its specific receptor in the nuclear compartment. This estrogen–receptor complex undergoes a series of concerted steps that includes phosphorylation, homodimerization, and allosteric conformational changes. This 'activated' estrogen–receptor complex then binds to a specific region of DNA called the estrogen response element (ERE; or hormone response element, HRE; or steroid response elements, SREs), located near the promoter of the target gene (Figure 20.5). The receptor complex then stimulates or induces transcription by yet-to-be defined mechanisms. The process involves interaction with accessory transcription factors that are needed for RNA polymerase II to bind to the promoter, and thereby initiating transcription. The pre-mRNA formed is processed, and the mRNA is exported to the cytoplasm where it is translated in the ribosomes to form a new protein. It is via the newly synthesized protein(s) that the biological effects of estrogens are expressed via autocrine, paracrine, and endocrine mechanisms (Figure 20.5).

Although the above mechanism of estrogen action is based on a substantial body of evidence and has gained general acceptance, it does not, however, explain how different target cells distinguish between different estrogens, i.e. how different estrogens interacting with the same ER display different activities in different cells.[30] The original concept proposed that the first (main) determinant of selectivity and efficacy was the binding affinity of the specific estrogen for the estrogen receptor, second, all estrogens function in the same manner in any cell that has an ER, and third, no other cellular factors were required. In this model, the biological activity of an estrogen was believed to be directly proportional to its binding affinity.[32] Similarly, the above general mechanism does not explain tissue-selective effects of estrogens and antiestrogens, for example tamoxifen's differential effect on the uterus, bone, and breast. In all three tissues, tamoxifen's action is mediated by the same estrogen receptor(s), yet the effects are profoundly different.

Three distinct mechanisms for steroid hormone selectivity for nuclear receptors at the tissue, the cell, and the gene have been proposed, and are: ligand-based selectivity; receptor-based selectivity; and effector-based selectivity.[26] To understand these mechanisms better, knowledge of the receptor structure and its interaction with DNA and the general transcription apparatus is essential, and they are briefly described here.

The ER protein and other members of this family have a modular structure, and are made up of six distinct domains that are termed A/B, C, D, E and F domains.[25,29] In Figure 20.6, these domains along with the amino- and carboxy-termini of the protein are depicted. These domains have the following functions:[29] regions A/B and E contain hormone-independent transactivation function AF-1 (or TAF-1) and the hormone-dependent transactivation function AF-2 (or TAF-2);[33] region C contains two type II zinc fingers that are involved in DNA binding (DBD) and dimerization of the receptor; region D or the 'hinge' region contains a nuclear localization signal sequence (NLS) for receptors. The DNA-binding domain (DBD)

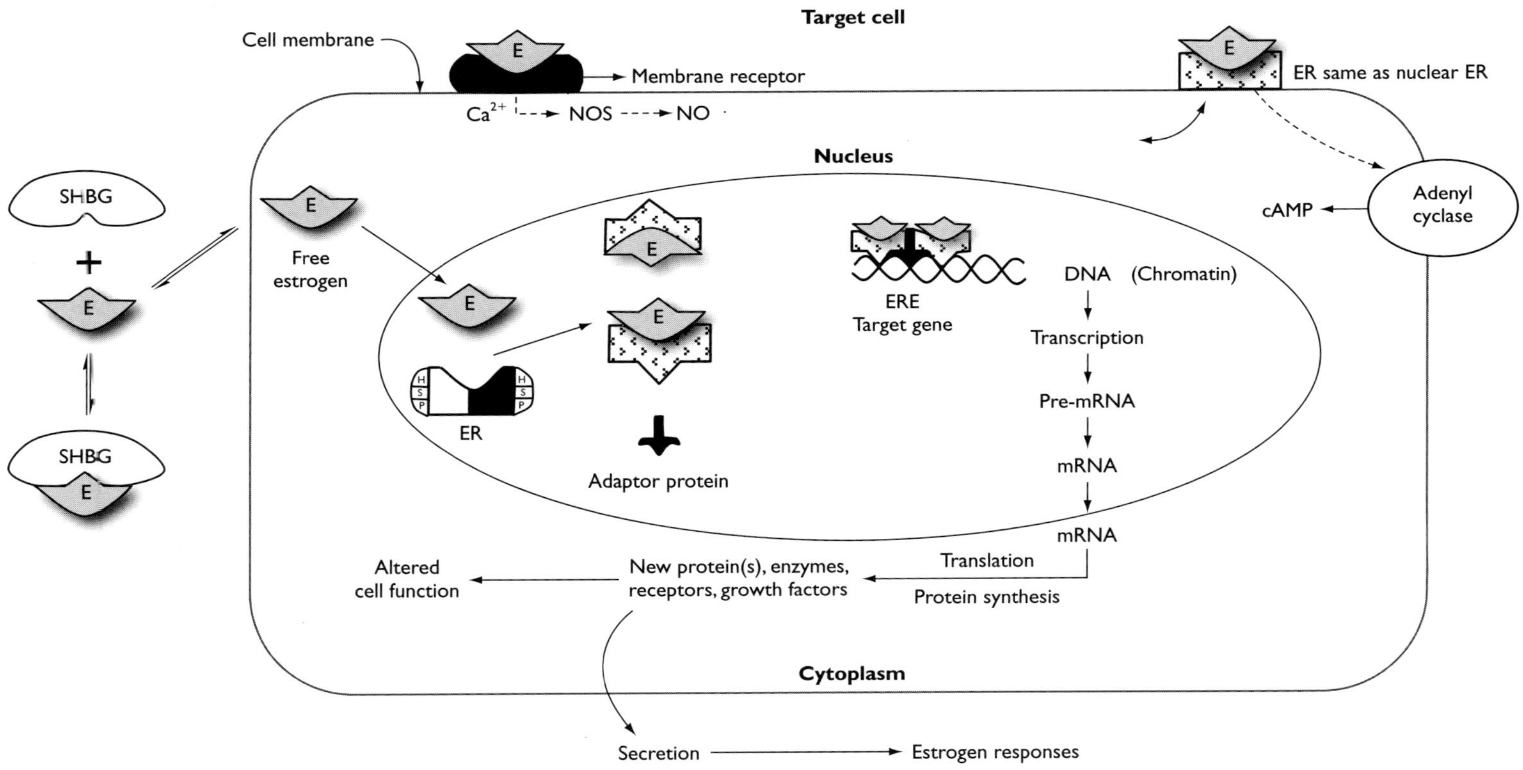

**Figure 20.5** A simplified model of estrogen action. In this model estrogen (E) in the unbound form enters the target cell by diffusion. In the absence of estrogen (ligand), the estrogen receptor (ER) resides in the nucleus associated with heat-shock proteins (HSP). Upon interaction with estrogen, a series of molecular events are initiated (removal of HSP, phosphorylation, dimerization recruitment of adapters) that permit the estrogen–receptor complex to bind to specific DNA response elements (ERE) and allows transcription to proceed. The new mRNA synthesized after processing is exported to the cytoplasm where it is translated into a new protein(s) (enzymes, growth factors) that result in altered cell function. The effects of these newly synthesized proteins are expressed by autocrine, paracrine or endocrine mechanisms. SHBG, sex hormone-binding globulin; NO, nitric oxide; NOS, nitric oxide synthase.

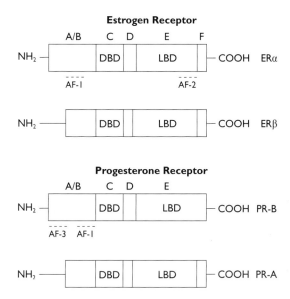

**Estrogen Receptor**

A/B   C   D   E   F

NH₂ — [ DBD | LBD ] — COOH   ERα

AF-1          AF-2

NH₂ — [ DBD | LBD ] — COOH   ERβ

**Progesterone Receptor**

A/B   C   D   E

NH₂ — [ DBD | LBD ] — COOH   PR-B

AF-3  AF-1

NH₂ — [ DBD | LBD ] — COOH   PR-A

**Figure 20.6** Functional domains of estrogen and progestin receptors. The six domains: A, B, C, D, E and F are defined in the text. AF, activation function; DBD, DNA-binding domain; LBD, ligand-binding domain; ER, estrogen receptor; PR, progesterone receptor.

also contains specific binding sequences termed steroid response elements (SREs); region E is the ligand (hormone)-binding domain (LBD) and AF-2, and is important for the hormone specificity of the receptor; region F present in ER has minimal function,[29] and is absent in the progesterone receptor (PR). The ER functions as a ligand-dependent transcription activator through the concerted action of the activation functions AF-1 and AF-2 in a tissue- and promoter-specific manner.[34,35] It has further been shown that in most cell environments both AF-1 and AF-2 participate and stimulate ER transactivation of gene expression,[36] however, in some contexts, individual activation functions can act independently. Estrogens such as 17β-estradiol act as ER agonists in cells where either, or both AFs are required. Compounds such as tamoxifen and its active metabolite trans-4-hydroxy tamoxifen function as partial agonists (bone, uterus) in cells where AF-1 alone is required. In tissues where only the hormone-dependent AF-2 is required, these triphenylethylene derivatives act as antagonists, and inhibit the activity of the AF-2.[30,36] In contrast, pure estrogen antagonists such as ICI-164 384 and ICI-182 780 inhibit the activity of AF-1 and AF-2, and this com-

pletely blocks the ER's transcriptional activity.[36] This mechanism provides a rational explanation of how some estrogenic compounds can have both agonist and antagonist activity, but more importantly, how compounds such as tamoxifen, raloxifene and other selective receptor modulators (SERMs), can manifest specific activities in different target tissues.

It has also been proposed,[28,29] and recently confirmed experimentally,[37] that different estrogens that interact with ERs produce a unique conformational form (shape) of the receptor. This specific conformation of the receptor is able to recruit a distinct protein(s) termed the co-activator (adapter) protein, that then allows contact with the target gene control region and promotes transcription.[26,29,36–39] In Figure 20.7, two different estrogens (estrogen A and estrogen B), after interaction with ER and dimerization, result in a specific estrogen–receptor configuration that can only be recognized by a specific adapter protein present in that target cell. Since several adapter proteins have been identified,[29,39] it is now possible to envision that, in the presence of two ERs and different estrogens, the estrogen–receptor complexes generated will have conformations that can be recognized differentially in various target cells, depending on the presence or absence of a specific adapter protein. Thus, depending on which estrogen (agonist, partial agonist or antagonist) binds to the ER (ERα, ERβ, or both), the receptor complex can associate with a specific co-activator which positively interacts with the gene transcription apparatus to activate target gene transcription. Since estrogens such as 17β-estradiol appear to be active in all estrogen target tissues, it is likely that the receptor conformation induced is recognized by co-activators in all target cells. Alternatively, if the conformation of ER generated can only recruit a co-repressor protein, this will have a negative impact on gene transcription,[36] and the estrogen analog acts as an anti-estrogen.

In the above model, the relative binding affinity of an estrogen for ERs is not the sole determinant of biological activity or potency, yet binding of the estrogen or anti-estrogen with ER is a prerequisite. It therefore appears that all three mechanisms proposed are involved in the overall mechanism of steroid hormone action.[26] The ligand-based selectivity also takes into consideration the pharmacokinetics of each estrogen; thus, the same receptor in different target tissues or cells is exposed to a different group of hormones, and hence mediates

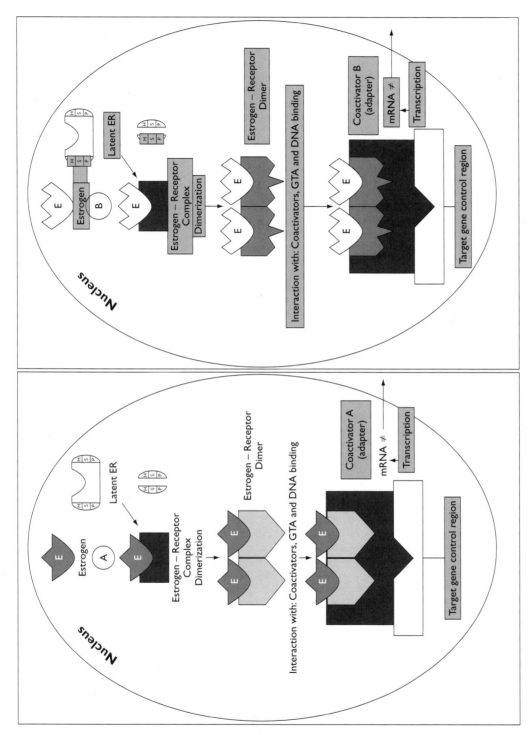

**Figure 20.7** Schematic visualization of how different estrogens can express different activities in different target tissues. Each estrogen induces a distinct conformational form (shape) in the estrogen receptor (ER). In this overly simplified figure, two different estrogens A and B and the conformations these induce in the ER are shown (white/black). Each form of ER is then able to recruit a specific adapter protein or co-activator (or co-repressor) (A and B), and the complex is then able to interact with the transcription apparatus, which ultimately results in the stimulation of transcription. Each adapter protein recognizes only specific estrogen/receptor configurations.[26–29] GTA, general transcription apparatus; HSP, heat shock protein.

responses in a tissue-selective manner.[26] Similarly, the receptor-based selectivity is plausible, as different target tissues, or cells exposed to same hormones, may react in a specific manner because they have a different composition of receptors, for example the proportion or amount of ERα and ERβ, or the A and B subtypes of PR. Although these two mechanisms are important, the evidence discussed above strongly suggests that to explain the tissue-selective actions of agonists, partial agonists, and antagonists, the effector site-based selectivity is perhaps the most important. The cell-specific factors (co-activators, co-repressors) play a key role in the overall pharmacology of steroid hormones such as estrogens and progestins.[26]

Progesterone's effects are also mediated by its nuclear receptor, and two receptor isoforms PR-A and PR-B (Figure 20.6), which are encoded by a single gene, have been identified.[40] Recent evidence indicates that these two forms are functionally different, and the ratio of PR-A and PR-B may modulate the cellular activity. PR-B appears to be a more potent activator of target genes, while PR-A acts as a dominant repressor of PR-B.[40] Since different progestins can interact with the two receptors differentially, all progestins, just like the various estrogens, may not have the same effects in different progesterone target tissues.

Although substantial evidence in support of effector site-based selectivity is based on in vitro transient transfection assays, the transfected gene construct may not fully mimic the normal physiological conditions in vivo. However, the existence of nuclear receptor coregulator complexes has been demonstrated in vivo.[41] For example, steroid receptor co-activator-1 (SRC-1) is a histone acetyltransferase,[42] which can play along with other proteins, a functional role in vivo, strongly supporting the concept discussed above.

CEE preparation is the single most prescribed drug for ERT for the treatment of vasomotor symptoms, vaginal dryness, and prevention of osteoporosis. The clinical aspects of these are dealt with in other sections of this book. The drug CEE is a complex 'natural' extract of pregnant mares' urine, and contains at least 10 different estrogens in their sulfate ester forms.[4,43] All 10 of these estrogens in their unconjugated form have been shown to bind with estrogen receptors in human endometrial and rat uterine preparations.[44] The relative binding affinities have the following order of activity: 17β-dihydroequilin ≥ 17β-estradiol > 17β-dihydroequilenin > estrone > equilin > 17α-dihydroequilin > 17α-estradiol

> Δ8-17β-estradiol > 17βα-dihydroequilenin > equilenin > Δ8-estrone.[44–46] The Δ8-17β-estradiol has not yet been shown to be present in CEE, but is an in vivo metabolite of Δ8-estrone in postmenopausal women.[46] Based on the mechanism of action of steroid hormones discussed, it would appear that each individual component of CEE can result in a specific estrogen–receptor conformation that can potentially have different or selective effects in different estrogen target tissues, i.e. act as a SERM. Therefore, the overall biological and clinical effects observed in postmenopausal women treated with CEE are the result of the sum of the individual activities of all of its estrogenic and non-estrogenic components. This is in keeping with observations that all of these estrogens are biologically active and have varying degree of uterotropic activity.[44,45]

## New developments in the genomic mechanism of estrogen action

### Knockout mice
During the past decade, both ERα and ER β knockout (ERKO and BERKO) mice have been produced.[47–49] Although the ERKO mice had normal external phenotypes and survived to adulthood, the females are infertile. The ERKO mice express ERβ, but the plasma levels of 17β-estradiol and luteinizing hormone (LH) in female ERKO mice are high compared to the wild-type animals.[50] In contrast to the ERKO mice, the BERKO females express ERα and have normal plasma levels of 17β-estradiol and LH, and are fertile but have smaller litters.[48] These observations indicate that the absence of ERβ has a much lesser impact on the reproductive system than the loss of ERα. These types of observations indicate that perhaps both ERα and ERβ are required for normal reproductive function. The availability of these knockout mice will help in understanding the role of estrogens in infertility, osteoporosis, cardiovascular disease, and Alzheimer's disease.

## DIFFERENTIAL EXPRESSION OF ESTROGEN RECEPTORS

The relative distribution and levels of ERα and ERβ in various tissues are quite different. High to moderate expression of ERα is seen in tissues such as the uterus, ovary (stroma), testis, epididymis, kidney, pituitary, brain, and adrenal. In contrast, high to moderate levels of ERβ are present in the ovarian granulose cells, prostate (epithelial cells), bladder, testis, lung, brain, and gastrointestinal tract. Not only are there differences in the levels of estrogen receptors in various tissues, but there are also inter-species differences.[51–55]

Recent data indicate that all 10 estrogens present in CEE and $\Delta^8$-17β-estradiol bind with recombinant human ERα and ERβ with high affinity.[56] Interestingly, a number of ring B unsaturated estrogens such as 17β-dihydroequilenin, equilin, equilenin, $\Delta^8$-$E_1$ have higher affinity for ERβ.[56] Cotransfection of ERα and ERβ into cells that were devoid of ERs indicated that biological (functional) activity of 17β-estradiol was not altered in the presence of the two ER subtypes, while the biological activity of ring B unsaturated estrogens such as 17β-dihydroequilin, 17β-dehydroequilenin, $\Delta^8$,17β-estradiol and equilenin was enhanced significantly.[57]

Since high levels of ERβ are present in the gastrointestinal tract of human and in some specific regions of the brain[51,54] estrogens such as equilenin, 17β-dihydroequilenin, $\Delta^8$,estrone and $\Delta^8$,17β-estradiol whose effects are primarily mediated via ERβ may help in the development of new therapeutic agents for the prevention of colon cancer and neurodegenerative disorders such as Alzheimer's disease.

## NON-GENOMIC MECHANISM OF STEROID HORMONE ACTION

Although a large number of cellular actions of estrogens and other steroid hormones can be explained by the genomic mechanism, there are a number of biological effects that occur extremely rapidly (seconds to minutes), and cannot be explained by the much slower (hours to days) genomic mechanism. These rapid effects of steroid hormones appear to be mediated via non-genomic mechanisms through cell membrane proteins (receptors).[58–60]

More than 35 years ago, Szego's group had shown the involvement of membrane receptors, cAMP and $Ca^{2+}$ as a playing a key role in the rapid and early physiological effects of estrogens and other steroids hormones.[61–63] Some of the well-known rapid effects of estrogens are: vasodilation, and alterations in glucose, water, and electrolyte metabolism.[61–63] Unfortunately this evidence was largely ignored by most investigators in this field until recently.[64] Confirmation of this hypoth-esis is now supported by demonstrations that 17β-estradiol can stimulate very rapidly the release of cAMP,[65] calcium flux,[66] and prolactin,[67] and also activates phosphalipase C in osteoblasts.[68] These and other rapid effects of 17β-estradiol can occur by direct involvement of the putative cell membrane ER.[62,69–72]

Although the membrane receptor remains to be characterized, recent data strongly indicate that at least one form of membrane receptor is very similar to nuclear ERs and can be derived from a single transcript.[73]

However, how the nuclear ER made in the cytoplasm of the cell translocates and gets inserted in the cell membrane, remains to be investigated. The physiological and clinical relevance of this mechanism, and the likelihood of 'cross-talk' between these two distinct mechanisms, remains to be established.

## NATURAL AND SYNTHETIC ESTROGENS AND PROGESTINS FOR ERT AND HRT

Estrogens and progestins used for ERT and HRT have, for simplicity, been divided into three types: natural, native/synthetic, and synthetic (Figure 20.8). The term 'natural' implies that the substance exists in nature in that form, and that it can be formulated into a drug with minimal processing and requires no chemical modification, for example CEE. Native/synthetic means that the steroid exists in nature, for example 17β-estradiol, but for it to be formulated as a drug, it has to be synthesized (several chemical steps) from a natural starting materials such as Mexican yams or soy beans. It is important to note that steroid hormones such as 17β-estradiol, estrone sulfate, or progesterone are not found in Mexican yam or the soy bean, but can be prepared from sterols and sapogenins present in these plants. For more than 55 years, most of the currently available steroid hormones have been synthesized from these plant sources.[74]

Although the steroid hormones synthesized from these plants are chemically and biologically the same as those produced by the humans or animals, there is no scientific evidence to date that indicates that the ingestion or application of topical creams containing Mexican yams, or soy beans, leads to the formation of 17β-estradiol, estrone, progesterone etc. The human body lacks the necessary enzymes to transform plant sterols and sapogenins biochemically into active steroid hormones.

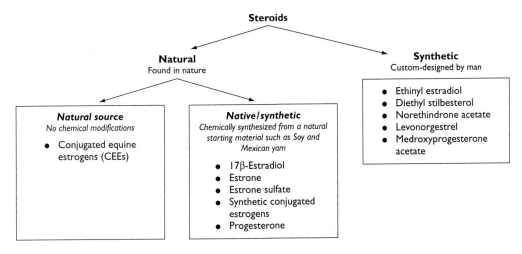

**Figure 20.8**  Examples of natural and synthetic estrogens and progestins.

The term 'synthetic' means that these steroids do not exist in nature, and are designed and chemically synthesized by man. Like the native/synthetic steroids, these can also be synthesized from the same plant sources.[74] A wide variety of these drugs are currently available, and some of the oral and parenteral forms of estrogens used for replacement therapy are given in Tables 20.2 and 20.3. The active components, and their concentrations are also indicated.

## PHARMACOKINETICS OF VARIOUS ESTROGENS: EFFECT OF ROUTE OF ADMINISTRATION

### Absorption and metabolic changes

For an estrogen to exert its biological effects, it must first be absorbed, then reach and interact with its receptors in target tissues. The rate at which these events occur depends on the route of administration. The overall metabolic fate of an estrogen (or progestin) in the human body is schematically depicted in Figure 20.9.[75]

The oral route of administration is the most frequently used method, and appears to be the route preferred by a majority of postmenopausal women. As depicted in Figure 20.9, the route and dose of administration of an estrogen can have distinct and divergent effects in postmenopausal women. Oral estrogen, by virtue of the first-pass effect, results in marked alterations in hepatic metabolism, such as increase in angiotensinogen, SHBG, CBG, high-density lipoprotein cholesterol (HDL), triglycerides, and clotting factors, and a decrease in low-density lipoprotein cholesterol (LDL), and total cholesterol levels. These changes in plasma proteins and lipids are a consequence of the initial high concentrations of estrogens in the liver after oral administration. These metabolic changes can have important clinical implications particularly for cardiovascular disease in postmenopausal women,[76,77] and these are discussed in other parts of this book.

Routes of administration whereby the liver is bypassed, such as transdermal, vaginal, and parenteral administration (Figure 20.9), do not undergo the first-pass effect, and either the changes in serum proteins and lipids are not observed, or the effects are blunted.[78–82] A comparison of the effects of oral and transdermal administration on hepatic parameters is given in Table 20.4. The improvements in lipid profiles observed with oral estrogens have recently been confirmed in a prospective prevention trial.[83] Another factor that may have an important role in cardiovascular disease is plasminogen activator inhibitor type I (PAI-1), which is an important inhibitor of fibrinolysis.[82] Changes in PAI-1 levels are the result of the first-pass effect seen with oral estrogens (Table 20.4). The increase in triglycerides seen with oral estrogens is not observed with transdermal estrogens.[78–80] Although triglycerides are considered to be a separate risk factor for cardiovascular disease, the modest increases seen with oral estrogens in normal healthy postmenopausal women do not appear to have a negative impact.[76,77,83]

**Table 20.2**  Examples of various estrogen preparations (concentration of active estrogens)

| Brand name | Active components (concentration) | Available dose(s) |
|---|---|---|
| Estrace® | Micronized 17β-estradiol (100%) | 1 mg, 2 mg |
| Ogen®) | Piperazine estrone sulfate (100%) | 0.625 mg, 1.25 mg, 2.5 mg, 5 mg |
| Premarin® | Mixture of at least 10 conjugated equine estrogens (CEE): sulfate esters of estrone (50%), equilin (22%), 17α-dihydroequilin (14%), 17α-estradiol (4.5%), Δ8-estrone (3.5%), equilenin (2%), 17β-dihydroequilin (1.7%), 17α-dihydroequilenin (1.2%), 17β-estradiol (1%), 17β-dihydroequilenin (0.5%) | 0.3 mg, 0.625 mg, 0.9 mg, 1.25 mg, 2.5 mg |
| Estratab® | Estrone sulfate (75–85%), equilin sulfate (6–15%) | 0.625 mg |
| Estinyl® | Ethinyl estradiol (100%) | 0.02 mg, 0.05 mg, 0.5 mg |
| Estraderm® | Transdermal 17β-estradiol (100%) | 0.025 mg, 0.05 mg, 0.1 mg |
| Climara® | Transdermal (matrix patch) 17β-estradiol (100%) | 0.025, 0.0375, 0.05, 0.1 mg |
| Vivelle-Dot® | Transdermal 17β-estradiol (100%) | 0.025, 0.0375, 0.05, 0.075, 0.1 mg/day |
| Premarin® vaginal cream | Mixture of 10 estrogens – CEE (see Premarin®) | 0.625 mg/g cream |
| Estring® | Vaginal ring containing 17β-estradiol (100%) | 2 mg/90 days, (7.5 μg/day release) |
| Femring® | Vaginal ring containing 17β-estradiol acetate (100%) | 2.5 mg/2 g |
| Del Estrogen® | 17β-Estradiol valerate (100%) | 10 mg/ml (sesame oil for IM administration) |
| Estrasorb® | Topical emulsion containing 17β-estradiol hemihydrate (100%) | 2.5 mg/2 g (0.05 mg 17β-estradiol/day) |
| Estrogel® | Gel containing 17β-estradiol | 0.75 mg/1.25 g gel |

IM, intramuscular.

Apart from differences between oral and non-oral estrogen, there are important differences between various oral estrogens. In general, oral estrogen sulfates, for example equilin sulfate (a major ring B unsaturated component of CEE), after oral administration, is directly absorbed to some extent from the gastrointestinal tract without prior hydrolysis.[84] However, a substantial portion of the ingested estrogen sulfate is absorbed after the removal of the sulfate ester by hydrolysis.[84] The unconjugated estrogen after absorption is rapidly resulfated as the result of the first-pass effect (Figure 20.9). The estrogen sulfates such as estrone sulfate and equilin sulfate are the main (>90%) circulating forms of estrogens in postmenopausal women on ERT.[84–86] Similarly, inges-

tion of 10 mg CEE, containing approximately 4.5 mg estrone sulfate and 2.5 mg of equilin sulfate, results in maximum levels of equilin (560 pg/ml) and estrone (1400 pg/ml) after 3 and 5 h, respectively. Plasma levels decline gradually, and only small amounts of both estrogens are detectable after 24 h.[87] Similar rates of appearance and disappearance of estrogens are also observed when smaller doses of CEE are administered. In contrast, intravenous administration of 10 mg CEE result in maximum concentrations of equilin (4000 pg/ml) and estrone (11200 pg/ml) within 10 min.[87] Oral administration of estrone sulfate also results in rapid appearance of unconjugated 17β-estradiol and estrone in the blood.[88,89] Micronization of aqueous insoluble steroids

**Table 20.3**  Examples of various estrogen plus progestins (concentration of active estrogens)

| Brand name | Active components (concentration) | Available dose(s) |
|---|---|---|
| **Continuous combined HRT** | | |
| Prempro® | CEE/medroxy progesterone acetate (MPA) | 0.3 mg/1.5 mg, 0.45 mg/1.5 mg, 0.625 mg/2.5 mg |
| Femhrt® | Ethinyl/estradiol/norethindrone acetate | 5 μg/1 mg |
| ClimaraPro® | Transdermal 17β-estradiol/levonorgestrel | 4.4 mg/1.39 mg |
| Prefest® (progestin every 3 days for 3 days) | 17β-estradiol/norgestimate | 1 mg/0.09 mg |
| Combipack® | Transdermal 17β-estradiol/norethindrone acetate | 0.62 mg/2.7 mg, 0.51 mg/4.8 mg |
| **Cyclic HRT** | | |
| Premphase® (Premia®) | CEE plus cyclic MPA (2 weeks) | 0.625 mg/5.0 mg, 0.625 mg/2.5 mg |

increases the surface area and results in increased absorption and thus oral administration of micronized 17β-estradiol (Estrace®) has also been shown to be efficacious, provided sufficiently high doses are administered.[90] Although oral micronized 17β-estradiol is absorbed, a substantial amount of it is metabolized in the gastroin-

**Table 20.4**  Effect of oral and transdermal estrogens on hepatic parameters

| Hepatic parameter | Oral estrogens | Transdermal estradiol |
|---|---|---|
| SHBG | ↑ | → |
| CBG | ↑ | → |
| Renin substrate angiotensinogen | ↑ | → |
| IGF-I | ↓ | ↓ |
| Total cholesterol | ↓ | ↓ |
| HDL cholesterol | ↑ | → |
| | | ↓ |
| LDL cholesterol | ↓ | ↓ |
| Triglycerides | ↑ | → |
| | | ↓ |
| PAI–I | ↓ | → |

SHBG, sex hormone-binding globulin; CBG, corticosteroid-binding globulin; IGF, insulin-like growth factor; HDL, high-density lipoprotein; LDL, low-density lipoprotein; PAI, plasminogen activator inhibitor; ↑, increase; ↓, decrease; →, no change.

testinal tract prior to it reaching the liver, where it is further metabolized and inactivated (Figure 20.9). The main metabolites that enter the circulation are estrone and estrone sulfate. These observations indicate that not only are estrogen sulfates highly water soluble and easily absorbable, but also the sulfation protects the estrogen from rapid metabolism in the gastrointestinal tract.

The synthetic estrogens such as ethinylestradiol are infrequently used in North America for ERT, and are also readily absorbed from the gastrointestinal tract. Peak serum levels are observed between 1 h and 4 h.[91] This estrogen, because of its structure (17-ethinyl group), is not readily deactivated in the liver, and therefore it has a profound and prolonged effect on hepatic protein synthesis (Table 20.5).

Although all oral estrogens undergo the first-pass effect, the amounts that are bioavailable are quite variable, and this is reflected in their potencies. Comparison of the relative potencies of four oral estrogens: piperazine estrone sulfate, micronized estradiol, CEE, and ethinylestradiol, in terms of suppression of serum FSH and increase in hepatic protein synthesis (Table 20.5), indicates that on weight basis, ethinylestradiol is far more potent than the other three oral estrogens. The CEE are up to three times more potent in inducing hepatic proteins than micronized estradiol and estrone sulfate.[92] As discussed under 'In vivo transport of estrogens', the significantly higher levels of SHBG will result in a lower level of the physiologically active free form of estrogen available for biological action.

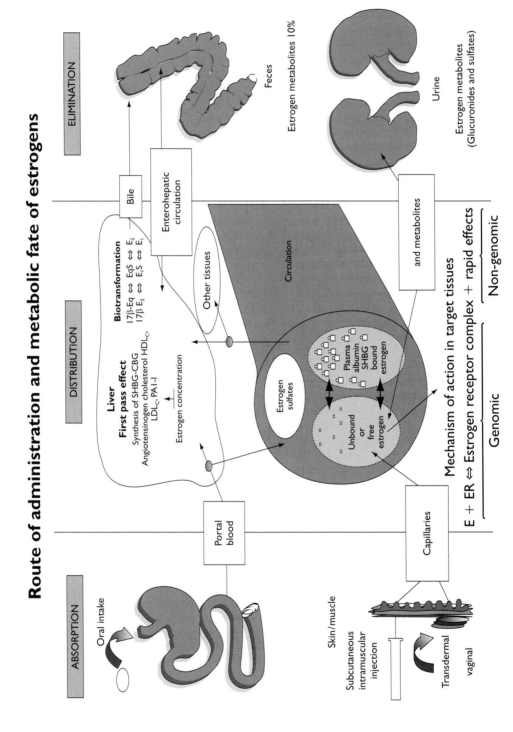

**Figure 20.9**   Effect of route of administration on the metabolic fate of estrogens. SHBG, sex hormone-binding globulin; CBG, corticosteroid-binding globulin; HDLC, high-density lipoprotein cholesterol; LDLC, low-density lipoprotein cholesterol; PAI, plasminogen activator inhibitor; $17\beta$-Eq, $17\beta$-dihydroequilin; EqS, equilin sulfate; Eq,equilin; $17\beta$-$E_1$, $17\beta$-estradiol; $E_1$, estrone; $E_1S$, estrone sulfate; E, estrogen; ER, estrogen receptor.

**Table 20.5**   Differences in the relative potency of oral estrogens according to some serum parameters of estrogenicity

| Estrogen preparation | SHBG-BC | CBG-BC | Angiotensinogen | FSH |
|---|---|---|---|---|
| Ogen® (piperazine estrone sulfate) | 1.0 | 1.0 | 1.0 | 1.1 |
| Estrace® (micronized estradiol) | 1.0 | 2.0 | 0.7 | 1.3 |
| Premarin® (conjugated equine estrogens) | 3.2 | 2.5 | 3.5 | 1.4 |
| Estinyl® (ethinyl estradiol) | 614 | 1000 | 232 | 80–200 |

SHBG-BC, sex hormone-binding globulin binding capacity; CBG-BC, corticosteroid-binding globulin binding capacity; FSH, follicle-stimulating hormone. Modified from Mashchak et al. Am J Obstet Gynecol 1982: 144; 511–18[92] with permission from Elsevier.

A large prospective study of postmenopausal women showed a significant association between a lower percentage of endogenous 17β-estradiol, and a higher risk for breast cancer.[93] Thus, estrogen formulations for ERT or HRT that increase the levels of SHBG to a greater extent may be preferable. Even though, as discussed above, ethinylestradiol compared to other oral estrogens stimulated the synthesis of SHBG by over 600 times (Table 20.5), this estrogen may not be an ideal one for ERT (at least in concentrations used in oral contraceptives); it does not bind to SHBG, and therefore most of it is essentially in a bioavailable form, which is reflected in its much higher stimulatory hepatic activity.

The notion that dosages of various estrogens which result in comparable serum levels of unconjugated 17β-estradiol, or the assumption that all of the estrogenic effects of natural estrogens are solely dependent on levels of 17β-estradiol, is not supported by firm scientific data. On the contrary: a recent prospective study of menopausal women compared the effects of CEE, micronized estradiol and transdermal 17β-estradiol on serum SHBG, and correlated this with serum levels of 17β-estradiol, estrone and free 17β-estradiol.[94] The data indicated that the levels of unconjugated 17β-estradiol were the lowest after CEE therapy (4 months), yet the levels of SHBG were the highest. In contrast, levels of 17β-estradiol following administration of micronized estradiol and transdermal estradiol were significantly higher, yet compared to CEE, the effect on SHBG was only 50% and 14% respectively. The increase in SHBG levels following CEE were associated with a corresponding decrease in the free form of 17β-estradiol. Therefore, the estrogenic effects of various ERT modalities are dependent on factors besides serum levels of unconjugated estradiol.[94] Moreover, the same drug in different formulation can also give rise to differences in the rate of absorption and biological effects. For example vaginal CEE cream is rapidly absorbed, but the serum levels of estrogens attained are approximately one-quarter of those obtained with similar oral doses.[95,96] However, even though the serum levels of estrogens following 0.3 mg vaginal CEE are low, this dose is sufficient to provide physiological replacement to the vaginal epithelium, but no effects on hepatic proteins are observed.[96] In contrast, after 25 mg vaginal CEE, systemic effects comparable to 0.625 mg oral CEE are observed.[96,97] Similarly, comparison of the rate and extent of absorption following administration of 0.625 mg CEE or 0.625 mg of a mixture of estrone sulfate and equilin sulfate (Estratab) indicate significant differences in the relative bioavailability of estrogens.[98,99] Since osteoporosis and coronary heart disease are silent diseases, it seems prudent to require at least some clinical evidence of efficacy for each different estrogen formulation. Recent data indicate the low dose of estrogen, i.e. lower than doses used previously for prevention of osteoporosis, also reduced bone turnover or remodeling to a similar extent as seen with standard dose of 1 mg/day 17β-estradiol or 0.625 mg of CEE.[100–102]

These low doses of estrogen increase the circulatory levels of biologically active estrogens that appear to be sufficient to protect the bone. Whether these low-dose forms of estrogen can prevent fractures has however, not been demonstrated.

## Metabolic clearance rate of conjugated and unconjugated estrogens

The metabolic clearance rate (MCR) of a steroid is defined as the volume of plasma (blood) from which the steroid is totally and irreversibly cleared in unit time (liters per day or liters per day per m²), and provides information regarding the overall in vivo metabolic fate of the steroid.[103] The

MCR of some sulfate-conjugated and -unconjugated estrogens have been reported (Table 20.6). The elimination from plasma of equilin sulfate, 17β-dihydroequilin sulfate, and estrone sulfate is described as a function of two exponentials, and examples of these are shown in Figure 20.10.[104,105] The initial fast component for the three estrogens has a half-life ($t\frac{1}{2}$) of 3 to 5 minutes, while the $t\frac{1}{2}$ of the slower component of equilin sulfate, 17β-dihydroequilin sulfate and estrone sulfate is 190 ± 23, 147 ± 15, and 300–500 min respectively.[85,86,104,105] The initial volumes of distribution ($V_1$) for equilin sulfate, 17β-dihydroequilin sulfate, and estrone sulfate are 12.4 ± 1.6, 6.0 ± 0.5 and 7.2 ± 0.6 respectively. The $V_1$ of estrogen sulfates depends on their relative binding affinities to plasma proteins. However, since the apparent $V_1$ is higher than plasma volume, these sulfates bind to plasma proteins such as albumin with relatively low affinity, as has been discussed.[17] The MCR of estrone sulfate (80–105 l/(day × m²)), equilin sulfate (170–176 l/(day × m²)), and 17β-dihydroequilin sulfate (376–460 l/(day × m²)) (Table 20.6), indicates that ring B unsaturated estrogens are cleared from the circulation at a faster rate than the ring B saturated estrogen estrone sulfate.[85,86,104–108] The MCRs of these sulfates compared to their unconjugated forms is low (Table 20.6), and this is due to their relatively higher binding affinity for serum albumin compared to unconjugated forms.[16–19] The ionic nature of the steroid sulfates may also play a role in the overall clearance of the estrogen sulfates. The low MCR can also result only if a small fraction of these estrogen sulfates is being metabolized. This appears to be the case as only 11%, 16% and 35% estrone sulfate, equilin sulfate and 17β-dihydroequilin sulfate are metabolized respectively.[85,86,99,104–107] The 2- to 5-fold higher MCR of 17β-dihydroequilin sulfate compared to equilin sulfate and estrone sulfate is in keeping with its higher rate of metabolism.[105]

The MCRs of unconjugated equilin (2641 l/(day × m²)), 17β-dihydroequilin (1252 l/(day × m²)), estrone (1050 l/(day × m²)), and 17β-estradiol (580 l/(day × m²)), are several-fold higher than their corresponding sulfate forms (Table 20.6). The patterns of disappearance of equilin (Figure 20.10) and estrone are consistent with a one-component model,[104,108] whereas, those of 17β-dihydroequilin and Δ⁸-estrone exhibit two components.[46,105] The 17β-reduced estrogens such as 17β-estradiol and 17β-dihydroequilin have a much higher affinity for SHBG, and therefore are cleared more slowly

| Table 20.6 | Metabolic clearance rate (MCR) of estrogens | |
|---|---|---|
| Estrogen | MCR (L/day/m² ± SEM) | Reference(s) |
| Estrone sulfate | 80 ± 10ᵃ; 105 ± 20 | 85, 86 |
| Equilin sulfate | 176 ± 44ᵃ; 170 ± 18 | 104, 106 |
| 17β-Dihydroequilin sulfate | 376 ± 53ᵃ; 460 ± 60 | 105, 107 |
| Estrone | 1050 ± 70 | 108 |
| 17β-Estradiol | 580 ± 30 | 108 |
| Equilin | 2641ᵃ | 104 |
| 17β-Dihydroequilin | 1252 ± 103ᵃ | 105 |
| Δ⁸-Estrone | 1711 ± 252ᵃ | 46 |

SEM, standard error of the mean.
ᵃMCR measured by the single injection technique.

(two times) than their corresponding 17-keto forms estrone and equilin.

The pharmacokinetics of estrogen sulfate compared to their unconjugated (non-sulfated) forms further indicate that the sulfate-conjugated forms of estrogens are cleared from the circulation at a much slower rate (Table 20.6). These data support the general hypothesis that sulfate-conjugated steroids act as reservoirs from which the unconjugated steroids are being formed as needed. Not only are there pharmacokinetic differences between various estrogens, but, more importantly, major differences were also observed between natural form of CEE (Premarin® Wyeth, Canada) and CES (ICN, Canada), a synthetic mixture of some of the components of CEE. These two formulations were shown not to be bioequivalent or therapeutically equivalent.[109] Since these types of pharmacokinetic differences between various estrogen preparations may translate into long-term clinical differences, detailed pharmacokinetic comparison studies are necessary to establish bioequivalence.

## Interconversions between estrogens under steady-state conditions

In postmenopausal women, estrone, Δ⁸-estrone and equilin are metabolized to circulating 17β-estradiol, Δ⁸-17β-estradiol, and 17β-dihydroequilin respectively.[46,85,86,104,105] The precise conversion ratios for the formation of some of these metabolites have been determined under steady-state conditions (Figure 20.11). The transfer constants (ρ or rho values) for the conversion of equilin

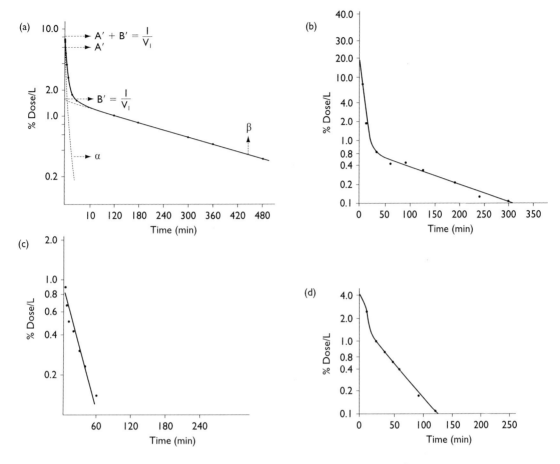

**Figure 20.10** Disappearance of radioactivity from plasma as [³H]equilin sulfate (a), [³H]17β-dihydroequilin sulfate (b), [³H]equilin (c), and [³H]17β-dihydroequilin (d) plotted as a percentage of the administered dose versus time of blood sampling.[77,78]

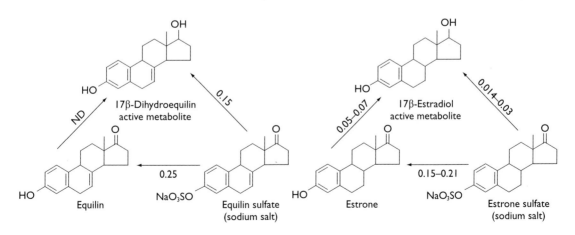

**Figure 20.11** Extent of in vivo activation of two main components of conjugated equine estrogens by 17β-hydroxysteroid dehydrogenase. The values shown are transfer (ρ values). ND, not determined.

sulfate to equilin and 17β-dihydroequilin are 0.25 and 0.15 respectively.[106] The corresponding ρ values for the conversion of estrone sulfate to estrone and 17β-estradiol are 0.15–0.21 and 0.014–0.03 respectively (Figure 20.11).[85,86] Recent data also indicate that, like equilin sulfate and estrone sulfate, the main circulating forms of $\Delta^8$-estrone are $\Delta^8$-estrone sulfate and $\Delta^8$,17β-estradiol sulfate.[46] Moreover, the amounts of these $\Delta^8$-metabolites are almost equal.[46] This pattern of metabolism, i.e. formation of equal amounts of 17-oxidized and 17β-reduced metabolites, is not observed with other estrogens. The oxidative pathway is generally preferred compared to the reductive pathway.[110] The 17β-reduced estrogens are considered to be the active metabolites, and the activation by 17β-reduction is several-fold higher for the ring B unsaturated estrogens compared to the ring B saturated estrogens. These types of metabolic differences between various types of estrogens may impact on the overall biological and clinical activity of different estrogens. The increased estrogenicity (Table 20.5), associated with CEE may in part be due to the higher level of 17β-activation.

## Estrogen metabolism

Apart from the metabolic interconversions, estrogens ultimately undergo irreversible metabolism primarily in tissues such as the liver, kidney, and to some extent in target tissues such as the endometrium and brain.[45,90] The major irreversible metabolic transformations of estrogens occur in the A and D ring, yielding mainly the 2, 4 and 16α-hydroxylated metabolites (Figure 20.12). The 16α-hydroxylated metabolites will be discussed separately under urinary excretion of estrogens.

## Catechol estrogens

Both 2- and 4-hydroxyestrogen metabolites (catechol estrogens) are formed in the human, and it has been suggested that the oncogenic potential of endogenous estrogens estrone and 17β-estradiol and synthetic estrogens depends on the extent of their metabolism to catechol estrogens.[111,112] Thus, in the Syrian hamster kidney model, 17β-estradiol, estrone, and equilin induce kidney tumors in the majority of animals, however, 2-hydroxyestrone and 2-hydroxy, 17β estradiol are inactive, while the corresponding 4-hydroxylated metabolites, 4-hydroxyestrone and 4-hydroxy, 17β-estradiol induce tumors in 100% of animals.[113,114] In contrast,

4-hydroxyequilenin is devoid of any carcinogenic activity in the hamster kidney.[114,115] Conflicting data have been reported by the same group of investigators,[113,114] and the relevance of these observations in postmenopausal women taking exogenous estrogens has not been established.

In the human endometrium, equilin forms mostly 2-hydroxyequilin, and small amounts of 4-hydroxy equilin.[114] In contrast, 2-hydroxy, 17β-estradiol and 4,hydroxy-17β-estradiol are formed in equal amounts by the proliferative human endometrium.[115,116] Thus, the extent of 2- and 4-hydroxylation depends on the structure of the estrogen. The role of catechol estrogen formed in vivo by the endometrium in postmenopausal women is not known. Whether the catechol derivatives of ring B unsaturated estrogens serve as substrates for redox cycling, and generate free radicals that may subsequently cause cell damage in a manner proposed for the classical estrogens, remains to be established. Alternatively, catechol equilin derivatives and those of other estrogens can play a protective role in the endometrium and other estrogen target tissues as free radical scavengers and antioxidants.[45] Moreover, the formation of these types of catechol estrogen metabolites can also decrease the amount of active estrogens available for metabolism to the more potent 17β-reduced products (Figure 20.12). CEE has been in use by millions of postmenopausal women for over 65 years, and to date there is no rigorous scientific evidence that indicates either CEE or its novel components are carcinogenic to the human. Its safety and efficacy are well established.

## Urinary excretion of ring B unsaturated estrogens

In postmenopausal women, ring B unsaturated estrogens equilin sulfate, equilin, 17β-dihydroequilin sulfate, and 17β-dihydroequilin are extensively metabolized. Approximately 50% of the administered dose is excreted in the urine,[43,45,115,117] and of this, approximately 60–75% is in the form of glucuronides and 15–20% as sulfate metabolites. Only 1–2% is excreted as unconjugated metabolites. These data indicate that although estrogens circulate mainly in the form of estrogen sulfates in postmenopausal women, before excretion, these estrogens are further metabolized to the corresponding glucuronides. In the urine of women small amounts of equilin, equilenin, 17β-dihydroequilin, and 17β-dihydroequilenin are excreted in the urine following administration of equilin or equilin sulfate.[43,45,115,117]

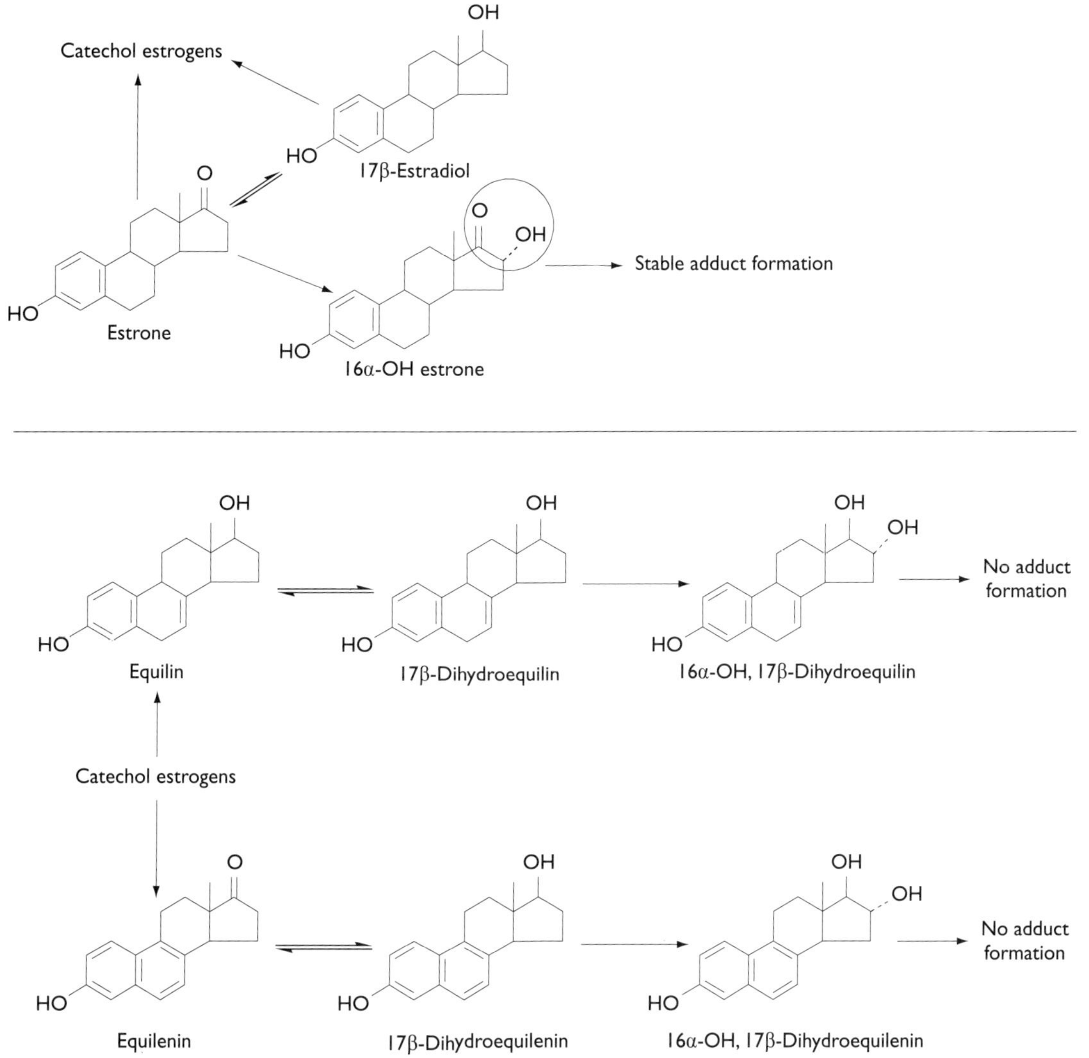

**Figure 20.12** In vivo and in vitro metabolism of estrone and equilin via catechol estrogen and 16α-hydroxylation. The potential for adduct formation with macromolecules is indicated. The α-ketol structure is circled. (Reproduced from Bhavnani. Proc Soc Exp Biol Med 1998; 217: 6–16,[45] with permission from Blackwell Publishing.)

In postmenopausal women and men, the bulk of equilin metabolites formed and excreted in the urine following administration of equilin, or equilin sulfate, or 17β-dihydroequilin sulfate are two extremely polar metabolites.[4,43,45,117] These metabolites were recently[45,118] identified as being 16α-hydroxy,17β-dihydroequilin and 16α-hydroxy, 17β-dihydroequilenin (Figure 20.12).[45,118] The corresponding 17-keto metabolites 16α-hydroxyequilin and 16α-hydroxyequilenin were not present in the urine. Recently, the two 17β-reduced and 16α-hydroxylated metabolites of equilin and equilenin were identified in pregnancy urine from women

carrying a Smith-Lemli-Opitz Syndrome (SLOS) fetus.[119] This syndrome is a birth disorder caused by a defect in 7-dehydrocholesterol conversion to ($\Delta^7$-cholesterol) to cholesterol.[119] These observations support the hypothesis that under certain pathological conditions, ring B unsaturated estrogen can be formed from $\Delta^7$-steroids and $\Delta^7$-androgens.[4,115]

Earlier studies with classical estrogens, indicate the potential involvement of 16α-hydroxylated estrogens in the oncogenic process.[120,121] The hypothesis is based on the demonstration that 16α-hydroxyestrone, a major urinary metabolite of

17β-estradiol and estrone can form stable covalent adducts with macromolecules (proteins, DNA). They propose that the covalent adduct formation (Figure 20.12), between 16α-hydroxyestrone, a major urinary metabolite of estrone can lead to the formation of stable covalent adducts with macromolecules (proteins, DNA) involved in diseases such as breast cancer.[122,123] They further propose that the covalent adduct formation (Figure 20.12), between 16α-hydroxyestrone and macromolecules occurs because of the presence of the D ring α-ketol (i.e. 16α-hydroxy-17-ketone structure, Figure 20.12, circled).[123] These investigators have further suggested that metabolism favoring 16α-hydroxylation leads to an increase cancer risk in postmenopausal women.[124] Based on the observation that 16α-hydroxyestrone is a potent estrogen, while 2-hydroxyestrone is relatively inactive, they further propose that the ratio of urinary 2-hydroxyestrone to 16α-hydroxyestrone is a predictor of cancer risk, and that this ratio is inversely correlated with risk for breast and cervical cancer.[124] A recent pilot study did not find a significant correlation between the ratio of urinary 2-hydroxyestrone and 16α-hydroxyestrone in postmenopausal women with and without breast cancer.[125] Careful analysis of these data indicate that the association observed previously, is most likely an 'artifact' of subgroup analysis, a result of the disease process itself, or of the treatment the women with breast cancer received.[125] The results of this study have been further substantiated, and inclusion of data from 66 patients with breast cancer and 76 control subjects has indicated that the ratios of 2-hydroxyestrone and 16α-hydroxyestrone were nearly identical in the two groups. These observations do not support the hypothesis that the ratio of the two hydroxylated estrogen metabolites (2-hydroxyestrone/16α-hydroxyestrone) is an important risk factor for breast cancer, or that it can predict women who are of risk for cancer.[126]

Interestingly, the two 16α-hydroxylated metabolites of ring B unsaturated estrogens isolated from the human urine lack the α-ketol structure (Figure 20.12), it is therefore, highly unlikely that these 16α-hydroxylated metabolites of equilin can form the potentially carcinogenic stable adducts, by the proposed mechanism.[115,120–124] The absence of 17-keto,16α-hydroxylated derivatives of equilin in human urine following administration of equilin, equilin sulfate, 17β-dihydroequilin, and 17β-dihydroequilin sulfate, support the previous conclusions that 17β-reduction occurs at a much higher extent with ring B unsaturated estrogens than with the classical estrogen estrone (Figure 20.11). Based on these observations, it appears that 17β-reduction of ring B unsaturated estrogens occurs not only at a higher rate, but also prior to 16α-hydroxylation as depicted in Figure 20.12. Whether these differences in metabolism between various estrogens determine if an estrogen play a role in carcinogenicity in the human remains to be investigated.

The fact that some of those estrogens (CEE) have been in use for more than six decades, and the increased risk for breast cancer in women taking these estrogens is barely detectable, contradicts the hypothesis that exogenous estrogens or their catechol or 16α-hydroxylated metabolites play a significant role in the etiology of breast cancer. Recent data from the Women's Health Initiative (WHI) randomized control trial dealing with the use of CEE alone in hysterectomized postmenopausal women demonstrated no increase in the risk for breast cancer, and this has recently been discussed in detail.[127]

## PHARMACOKINETICS OF PROGESTINS

The doses of estrogen used for ERT to prevent bone loss can result in endometrial hyperplasia in 15–30% of non-hysterectomized postmenopausal women.[83] Various progestins are available to prevent endometrial hyperplasia and thus reduce or eliminate the risk for endometrial adenocarcinoma.[128,129] Uterine protection requires that progestin be given in sufficient amounts for 10 to 14 days per month (sequential estrogen–progestin) or with each dose of estrogen (continuous combined). The former regimen causes monthly bleeding, and the latter may result in spotting or bleeding for the first few months of therapy. All progestins attenuate some of the estrogens' favorable effects on lipoproteins.[83] Progesterone and hydroxyprogesterone derivatives appear to have a less negative impact than the more androgenic 19-nortestosterone derivatives (Figure 20.2).

There are little published pharmacokinetic data of various progestins in postmenopausal women. Most of the pharmacokinetic data regarding progestins are derived from studies of oral contraceptives (OCs) in young women. Moreover, these data are also based on studies where the pharmacokinetics of the progestin were determined in the presence of a relatively high dose of an extremely potent oral estrogen ethinyl estradiol. This estrogen has profound effects on hepatic protein synthesis that can have a major impact on the amount of bioavailable progestin, as has been discussed above. The 'ideal' progestin, i.e. a progestin that can selectively antagonize the effect of estrogen only at the endometrium is not yet available; however, a number of progestins have been shown to be effective in protecting the endometrium.[128–130] Medroxyprogesterone acetate (MPA) is the most frequently used progestin in North America, while others such as norethindrone acetate, norethisterone, norgestrel etc are used more frequently in Europe.

Medroxyprogesterone acetate is readily absorbed after oral administration, and peak levels (3–5 ng/ml) are observed between 1 h and 4 h. Its MCR is approximately 21 l/day/kg, and it has a $t^{1/2}$ of 24 h.[20,131,132] Over 90% of MPA circulates bound to serum albumin, and is metabolized to 3, 6, and 20-hydroxy-5α- and 5β-reduced compounds. These metabolites are excreted in urine in the form of glucuronides.[131] The usual effective dose when given over the last 10–14 days of each monthly cycle is 10 mg, however, 2.5 mg given daily in combination with estrogen is as effective in protecting the endometrium in most postmenopausal women.[83,128,130]

Oral crystalline progesterone is poorly absorbed, and is rapidly inactivated in the gastrointestinal tract and during the first pass through the liver. However, sufficient amounts of micronized progesterone (200 mg) are absorbed and escape the first-pass hepatic metabolism, such that levels of approximately 4–12 ng/ml are observed within 4 h. This dose of micronized progesterone is sufficient to protect the endometrium, and does not appear to reduce the benefits of estrogens on lipids.[83] Progesterone circulates primarily bound to albumin, and approximately 20% is bound to CBG. Progesterone is rapidly metabolized to its 3, 5 and 20-reduced (α and β) metabolites, which are excreted mainly as glucuronides.

The detailed pharmacokinetics of synthetic progestins such as norethindrone, leveonorgesterol, norgestimate, desogesterel, and gestodene have been determined in young premenopausal women, and usually in combination with ethinyl estradiol. The comparative data indicate that the plasma $t^{1/2}$ of these progestins is between 8 and 12 h. Maximum plasma levels were attained within 1–2 h. Gestodene was cleared at a slower rate (48 ml/h/kg) compared to levonorgesterel (105 ml/r/kg), 3-ketodesogestrel (174 ml/h/kg), and norethindrone (355 ml/h/kg).[133–136] Recently, a new progestin, drospirenone (Figure 20.2), a spironolactone analog, has been described to have a unique pharmacological profile that is similar to that of progesterone. It has antimineralocorticoid, progestogenic activity, and no apparent androgenic activity. This progestin is at present being used as a component of an OC. Data from studies in reproductive-age women indicate that in combination with estrogen, this OC, unlike the earlier OCs, reduced body weight and blood pressure secondary to water retention (bloating) induced by estrogen. These beneficial effects are probably due to its antimineralocorticoid activity.[137] This new OC was shown to be useful in ameliorating the clinical and hormonal features of polycystic ovary syndrome.[138] The pharmacological profile of drospirenone may warrant testing the suitability of this progestin as a component of HRT in postmenopausal women.

Studies are also needed to determine the pharmacokinetics, the efficacy, and the minimum doses of these newer progestins that are required to protect against endometrial hyperplasia in postmenopausal women on ERT. Long-term comparative trials of these progestins versus progesterone and medroxyprogesterone acetate are also needed to determine whether there are any advantages in using these $C_{19}$-nortestosterone derivatives.

## ANTIOXIDANT PROPERTIES OF ESTROGENS

LDL cholesterol is a risk factor for atherogenesis.[139] Several observational studies indicate that ERT andHRT in postmenopausal women are cardioprotective.[83,140–143] However, the results from observational studies have been questioned by the recent publication of two randomized clinical trials: The WHI, a primary prevention trial,[144] and the Heart and Estrogen Replacement Study (HERS), a secondary prevention trial.[145] These studies were carried out in predominantly overweight and older (63 to 71 years) women who had been in an estrogen-deficient state for more than 10 years prior to initiation of the study. Both of these studies have serious flaws such that the results are generally not directly applicable to most healthy and younger (<60 years) postmenopausal women. Since these studies have been recently discussed in detail,[127] review of these is beyond the scope of this chapter. The mechanism(s) by means of which these estrogens exert their beneficial effects is not known. An earlier hypothesis proposed that changes in total cholesterol, LDL and HDL cholesterol are key factors. Recent observations suggest that these types of lipid changes account for only 25–35% of the cardioprotective benefits associated with ERT.[140] Recent studies suggest that excess free radicals may initiate atherosclerosis by damaging blood vessel walls, and that oxidized LDL that can be formed in vivo, is more atherogenic than native LDL.[146] Inhibition of this free radical-initiated LDL oxidation can be one of the mechanisms by means of which antioxidants such as vitamin E and phenolic compounds such as estrogens exert their beneficial effects. Indeed, in vivo and in vitro studies have demonstrated that estrogens can inhibit oxidation of LDL.[147–152] In vitro studies have demonstrated that all estrogens are potent antioxidants (Figure 20.13) with $\Delta^8$-estrone, 17β-dihydroequilenin, and 17α-dihydroequilenin being the most potent.[150] From the dose–response data, the quantity of each compound required to double the length of the lag phase of LDL oxidation indicated that the minimum dose of $\Delta^8$-estrone, 17β-dihydroequilenin, and 17α-dihydroequilenin was 0.47 nmoles; for $\Delta^8$,17β-estradiol, and equilenin, it was 0.7 nmoles; for 17β-dihydroequilin, and 17α-dihydroequilin it was 0.9 nmoles; and for equilin, estrone, 17β-estradiol, and 17α-estradiol, 1.3 nmoles. In comparison to estrogens, antioxidants such as two red wine components trans-resveratrol (4,3',5'-trihydroxy stilbene) and quercetin (3,3',4',5,7-pentahydroxyflavone), vitamin E, and a serum

cholesterol-lowering drug Probucol are, with the exception of quercetin, much weaker antioxidants (Figure 20.13).

All of the estrogens tested appear to act directly, as no metabolism of any of these estrogens to more potent antioxidant occurs under the conditions used. These results further indicate that all of the estrogenic components of CEE are potent antioxidants.[150] Interestingly, the most potent estrogenic antioxidants are relatively weak uterotropic agents.[45] These types of weak estrogens can serve as models for development of SERMs that may be useful in reducing the risk of cardiovascular disease not only in postmenopausal women but also in men. Since the cardioprotective effects are to some extent due to the ability of these estrogens to protect LDL against oxidative modification(s), the mechanisms involved are most likely non-genomic.

The ability of these estrogens to protect in vivo the oxidation of LDL in postmenopausal women has also been demonstrated both when given individually ($\Delta^8$-estrone sulfate) and after long-term (>1 year) treatment of postmenopausal women with CEE.[150–152] Addition of medroxyprogesterone acetate in the long-term study did not reduce the antioxidant effect of estrogens,[150] however, in a short-term (30 days) study, the addition of progestin given either continuously or in a cyclic manner, caused the effect of CEE on LDL oxidation to be blunted or absent.[152]

The precise mechanism(s) by which estrogens inhibit LDL oxidation remains to be established; however, a number of potential mechanisms can be proposed: estrogens may get incorporated into the LDL particle in a manner similar to that described for the incorporation of vitamin E into LDL. This incorporation of estrogen may change the conformation of LDL such that it is protected from oxidation. Alternatively, estrogens can function as free radical scavengers and thereby inhibit the lipid peroxidation process. Estrogens may also act by directly sequestering endogenous metal ions such as copper and iron, or by donating a proton to reduce the peroxyl free radical.[153] Estrogens may also function synergistically with endogeneous antioxidants associated with LDL. Along with the above possibilities, a number of other possible mechanisms involving effects of estrogens on arachidonic acid-induced DNA damage, have been proposed and recently reviewed.[154,155]

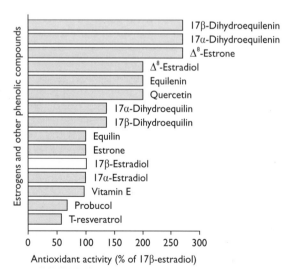

**Figure 20.13** Antioxidant activity of various estrogens and other phenolic compounds.

## THE ROLE OF HDL CHOLESTEROL IN ATHEROSCLEROSIS

In contrast to the impact of high plasma LDL levels, epidemiological data indicate a strong inverse correlation between plasma HDL concentrations and the incidence of coronary and cerebral atherosclerosis.[156,157] Traditionally, this relationship has been proposed to be due in part to the involvement of HDL in reverse cholesterol transport, however, recent studies have shown that HDL can prevent the oxidation of LDL.[158] This prevention of LDL oxidation by HDL contributes to a decrease in the formation of lipid peroxides, foam cell formation and cytotoxicity otherwise caused by oxidized LDL.[159–161] Although HDL-associated enzymes such as paroxonase, may play a critical role in the protective effect,[162,163] HDL itself can get oxidized, and the ability of oxidized HDL in reverse cholesterol transport is impaired.[164] Furthermore, oxidized HDL is neurotoxic, and has been postulated to play a role in the genesis of coronary artery spasm that contributes to the process of coronary heart disease.[165] Interestingly, it was recently demonstrated that not only can HDL delay or inhibit LDL oxidation, but that all 11 equine estrogens present in CEE protected HDL from oxidation in a concentration-dependent manner.[166] Equilenin, 17β-dihydroequilenin, 17α-dihydroequilenin, $\Delta^8$-17β-estrone, and $\Delta^8$,17β-estradiol were 2.5 to 4 times more potent inhibitors of HDL oxidation than 17β-estradiol. More importantly, the prevention of LDL oxidation by HDL is further enhanced in the presence of equine estrogens.[166] Thus, estrogen therapy in postmenopausal women not only results in a favourable lipid profile (Table 20.4), but some of the beneficial effects of estrogen may impact more directly the prevention of the oxidation of LDL cholesterol and HDL cholesterol. A number of potential molecular mechanisms have been suggested and have been reviewed.[166]

## NEUROPROTECTIVE EFFECTS OF ESTROGENS

Alzheimer's disease, other neurodegenerative diseases, and dementia are projected to quadruple over the next 50 years, and with higher incidence in women. Risk factors include head injury, cardiovascular disease, obesity (overweight), diabetes, hypertension, angina, stroke, history of myocardial infarction, and estrogen deficiency.

These have been recently discussed in detail and will not be reviewed here.[127]

A number of observational studies indicate that ERT in postmenopausal women significantly reduces the risk or delays the onset of Alzheimer's disease.[167–169] Recent meta-analyses indicated a 29–56% reduction in risk of Alzheimer's disease in women taking estrogens or estrogen plus progestin.[170–172] However, estrogen replacement in women who have Alzheimer's disease had no beneficial effect.[173,174] Similarly, the Women's Health Initiative Memory Study (WHIMS) found in predominantly overweight women with an average age of 71 years, HRT increased the incidence of dementia.[174,175] This randomized control trial study, like the main WHI trial was also prematurely stopped, and suffers from the same flaws, which have been reviewed previously.[127] The results from WHIMS provide no information regarding the ability of ERT or HRT to prevent or delay the onset of Alzheimer's disease in women between the age of 50 and 65 years. Therefore extrapolation of WHIMS data to younger menopausal women is unwarranted.

A large body of experimental studies indicate that pharmacological and physiological doses of estrogens have numerous effects that include vascular and neuronal changes, enhancement of nitric oxide production, endothelial protection, vasodilatation, increased blood flow, angiogenesis, antioxidant protection, and improvement in lipid profile, neurotransmitter function, axonal regeneration etc (see reference 127 for review). Studies in a number of neuronal cells also indicate that equine estrogens can differentially protect neurons against oxidative stress, and excitotoxicity, with $\Delta^8$-estrogens being significantly better neuroprotectors than 17β-estradiol.[176–178] Although a number of mechanisms have been proposed to explain the mechanisms involved in neuroprotective effects of estrogens, one important mechanism appears to be the ability of estrogens to inhibit the process of apoptosis induced by neurotoxins such as oxidized LDL, high concentrations of glutamate, and β amyloid.[179–182] The molecular mechanisms involved remain to be elucidated.[179,180–182]

## SUMMARY AND FUTURE DIRECTIONS

Most menopausal women can expect to live more than one-third of their lives in the postmenopausal years. This period of life is associated with an estrogen- and progesterone-deficient state, and as a result, women often experience a series of menopausal symptoms. The most frequent early symptoms are hot flushes, dyspareunia, atrophic vaginitis, insomnia, and mood disturbances. Some of the long-term and potentially fatal consequences of estrogen loss are osteoporosis, cardiovascular disease, and Alzheimer's disease. Estrogen replacement or estrogen/progestin replacement can ameliorate and/or decrease the risk of these debilitating disorders.

Both the structure of the estrogen and the route of administration play an important role in the absorption, metabolism, and the type of pharmacological effects observed. Currently, several types of estrogen preparations such as oral, transdermal patches, percutaneous gels, subcutaneous implants, vaginal rings, impregnated pessaries etc are available. At equivalent doses, these estrogens are effective in controlling vasomotor symptoms and some such as the oral (CEE) and transdermal (Estraderm) forms prevent osteoporosis.

Regarding cardiovascular disease, different types of estrogens, administered by different routes, for example oral versus transdermal, can have profoundly different effects on lipid metabolism and other risk factors. Most of the long-term studies showing a reduced risk for cardiovascular disease were in postmenopausal women who had used oral estrogens and in particular CEE. In view of the conflicting results from recent studies carried out in generally older postmenopausal women (63–71 years),[144,145,175] there is an urgent need to carry out similar randomized control trials in healthy and younger postmenopausal women.

## Acknowledgements

The work in the author's laboratory was supported by the Medical Research Council of Canada Grant MT-11929, and by a basic research grant from Wyeth, Philadelphia, USA. I would like to express my sincere thanks to Mrs. Francine Bhavnani for the preparation of the figures and manuscript.

## REFERENCES

1. Shier MR, Strickler R. The ovaries and related reproductive endocrinology. In: Ezrin C, Godden JO, Volpe R, eds. Systemic Endocrinology. New York: Harper and Row, 1979: 258–331.
2. McKinlay SM. The normal menopause transition: an overview. Maturitas 1996; 23: 137–45.
3. Diczfalusy E, Benagiano G. Women and the third and fourth age. Int J Gynecol Obstet 1997; 58: 177–88.
4. Bhavnani BR, The saga of the ring B unsaturated equine estrogens. Endocr Rev 1988; 9: 396–416.
5. Kletzky OA, Nakamura RM, Thorneycroft IH, Mishell DR Jr. Log normal distribution of gonadotropins and ovarian steroid values in the normal menstrual cycle. Am J Obstet Gynecol 1975; 121: 688–94.
6. Siiteri PK, MacDonald PC. Role of extraglandular estrogen in human endocrinology. In: Greep RO, Astwood EB, eds. Handbook of Physiology. Washington DC: American Physiological Society, 1963: Section 7: Endocrinology, 615–29.
7. Casey ML, MacDonald PC. Origin of estrogen and regulation of its formation in postmenopausal women. In: Bushsbaum HJ, eds. The Menopause, New York: Springer-Verlag 1983: 1–8.
8. Siiteri PK. Adipose tissue as a source of hormones. Am J Clin Nutr 1987; 45: 277–82.
9. Longcope C, Franz C, Morello C, Baker R, Johnston CC Jr. Steroid and gonadotropin levels in women during the peri-menopausal years. Maturitas 1986; 8: 189–96.
10. Longcope C. Adrenal and gonadal androgen secretion in normal females. J Clin Endocrinol Metab 1986; 15: 213–28.
11. Judd HL, Shamonki IM, Frumar AM, Lagasse LD. Origin of serum estradiol in postmenopausal women. Obstet Gynecol 1982; 59: 680–6.
12. Siiteri PK. Non glandular production of estrogen. In: Givens JR, ed. Gynecologic Endocrinology. Chicago: Year Book Medical Publishers, Inc, 1977: 171–82.
13. Siiteri PK, Murai JT, Hammond GL, Nisker JA, Raymoure WJ, Kuhn RW. The serum transport of steroid hormones. Recent Prog Horm Res 1982; 38: 457–510.
14. Westphal U. Steroid-protein interactions II. New York: Springer-Verlag, 1986: 259.
15. Partridge WM. Transport of protein-bound hormones into tissues in vivo. Endocr Rev 1981; 2: 103–23.
16. Wu CH, Motohashi T, Abdel-Rahman HA, Flickinger GL, Mikhail G. Free and protein bound plasma 17β-estradiol during the menstrual cycle. J Clin Endocrinol Metab 1976; 43: 436–45.
17. Pan CC, Woolever CA, Bhavnani BR. Tansport of equine estrogens: binding of conjugated and unconjugated equine estrogens with human serum proteins. J Clin Endocrinol Metab 1985; 61: 499–507.
18. Dunn JF, Nisula BC, Rodbard D. Transport of steroid hormones: binding of 21 endogenous steroids to both testosterone-binding globulin and corticosteroid-binding globulin in human plasma. J Clin Endocrinol Metab 1981; 53: 58–68.
19. Rosenthal HE, Pietrzak E, Slaunwhite WR Jr, Sandberg AA. Binding of estrone sulfate in human plasma. J Clin Endocrinol Metab 1972; 34: 805–13.
20. Mathrubutham M, Fotherby K. Medroxyprogesterone acetate in human serum. J Steroid Biochem 1981; 14: 783–6.
21. Hammond GL, Lahteenmaki PL, Lahteenmaki P, Luukkainen T. Distribution and percentages of non-protein bound contraceptive steroids in human serum. J Steroid Biochem 1982; 17: 375–80.
22. Kuhnz W, Pfeffer M, al-Yacoub G. Protein binding of the contraceptive steroids gestodene, 3-keto-desogestrel and ethinylestradiol in human serum. J Steroid Biochem 1990; 35: 313–18.

23. Alton KB, Hetyei NS, Shaw C, Patrick JE. Biotransformation of norgestimate in women. Contraception 1984; 29: 19–29.

24. McGuire JL, Phillips A, Hahn DW, Tolman EL, Flor S, Kafrissen ME. Pharmacologic and pharmacokinetic characteristics of norgestimate and its metabolites. Am J Obstet Gynecol 1990; 163: 2127–31.

25. Evans RM. The steroid and thyroid hormone receptor superfamily: transcriptional regulators of development and physiology. Science 1988; 240: 889–95.

26. Katzenellenbogen JA, O'Malley BW, Katzenellenbogen BS. Tripartite steroid hormone receptor pharmacology: interaction with multiple effector sites as a basis of the cell- and promoter-specific action of these hormones. Mol Endocrinol 1996; 10: 119–31.

27. Beato M, Sanchez-Pacheco A. Interaction of steroid hormone receptors with the transcription initiation complex. Endocr Rev 1996; 17: 587–609.

28. Vegeto E, Wagner BL, Imhof MO, McDonnell DP. The molecular pharmacology of ovarian steroid receptors. Vitam Horm 1996; 52: 99–128.

29. Shibata H, Spencer TE, Onate SA et al. Role of co-activators and co-repressors in the mechanism of steroid/thyroid receptor action. Recent Prog Horm Res 1997; 52: 141–64.

30. McDonnell DP. The molecular determinants of estrogen receptor pharmacology. Maturitas 2004; 48 (Suppl 1): S7–12.

31. Kuiper GG, Enmark E, Pelto-Huikko M, Nilsson S, Gustafsson JA. Cloning of a novel estrogen receptor expressed in rat prostate and ovary. Proc Natl Acad Sci U S A 1996; 93: 5925–30.

32. Clark JH, Peck EJ Jr. Female sex steroids: receptors and function. Berlin: Springer-Verlag, 1979: 14.

33. Tora L, White J, Brou C et al. The human estrogen receptor has two independent nonacidic transcriptional activation functions. Cell 1989; 59: 477–87.

34. Berry M, Metzger D, Chambon P. Role of the two activating domains of the estrogen receptor in the cell-type and promoter-contex dependent agonistic activity of the anti-oestrogen 4-hydroxytamoxifen. EMBO J 1990; 9: 2811–18.

35. Fan JD, Wagner BL, McDonnell DP. Identification of the sequences within the human complement 3 promoter required for estrogen responsiveness provides insight into the mechanism of tamoxifen mixed agonist activity. Mol Endocrinol 1996; 10: 1605–16.

36. Smith CL, Nawaz Z, O'Malley BW. Coactivator and corepressor regulation of the agonist/antagonist activity of the mixed antiestrogen, 4-hydroxytamoxifen. Mol Endocrinol 1997; 11: 657–66.

37. Paige LA, Christensen DJ, Gron H et al. Estrogen receptor (ER) modulators each induce distinct conformational changes in ER alpha and ER beta. Proc Natl Acad Sci U S A 1999; 90: 3999–4004.

38. McInemey EM, Tsai MJ, O'Malley BW, Katzenellenbogen BS. Analysis of estrogen receptor transcriptional enhancement by a nuclear hormone receptor coactivator. Proc Natl Acad Sci U S A 1996; 93: 10069–73.

39. Onate SA, Boonyaratanakornkit V, Spencer TE et al. The steroid receptor coactivator-1 contains multiple receptor interacting and activation domains that cooperatively enhance the activation function 1 (AF1) and AF2 domains of steroid receptors. J Biol Chem 1998; 273: 12101–8.

40. Graham JD, Clarke CL. Physiological action of progesterone in target tissues. Endocr Rev 1997; 18: 502–19.

41. McKenna NJ, Nawaz Z, Tsai SY, Tsai MJ, O'Malley BW. Distinct steady-state nuclear receptor coregulator complexes exist in vivo. Proc Natl Acad Sci U S A 1998; 95: 11697–702.

42. Spencer TE, Jenster G, Burcin MM et al. Steroid receptor coactivator-1 is a histone acetyl transferase. Nature 1997; 389: 194–8.

43. Bhavnani BR, Woolever CA. The metabolism of equilin in normal men. J Steroid Biochem 1982; 17: 217–23.

44. Bhavnani BR, Woolever CA. Interaction of ring B unsaturated estrogens with estrogen receptors of human endometrium and rat uterus. Steroids 1991; 56: 201–10.

45. Bhavnani BR. Pharmacokinetics and pharmacodynamics of conjugated equine estrogens: chemistry and metabolism. Proc Soc Exp Biol Med 1998; 217: 6–16.

46. Bhavnani BR, Cecutti A, Gerulath A. Pharmacokinetics and pharmacodynamics of a novel estrogen $\Delta^8$-estrone in postmenopausal women and men. J Steroid Biochem Mol Biol 1998; 67: 119–31.

47. Lubahn DB, Moyer JS, Golding TS, Couse JF, Korach KS, Smithies O. Alteration of reproductive function but not prenatal sexual development after insertional disruption of the mouse estrogen receptor gene. Proc Natl Acad Sci U S A 1993; 90: 11162–6.

48. Krege JH, Hodgin JB, Couse JF, Warner M, Mahlor JF, Smithies O. Generation and reproductive phenotypes of mice lacking estrogen receptor beta. Proc Natl Acad Sci U S A, 1998; 95: 15677–82.

49. Couse JF, Korach KS. Estrogen receptor null mice: what have we learned and where will they lead us? Endocr Rev 1999; 20: 358–417.

50. Schomberg DW, Couse JF, Mukherjee A et al. Targeted disruption of the estrogen receptor-α gene in female mice: characterization of ovarian responses and phenotype in the adult. Endocrinology 1999; 140: 2733–44.

51. Shughrue PJ, Komm B, Merchenthaler I. The distribution of estrogen receptor-β mRNA in the rat hypothalamus. Steroids 1996; 61: 678–81.

52. Kuiper GG, Carlsson B, Grandien K et al. Comparison of the ligand binding specificity and transcript tissue distribution of estrogen receptor α and β. Endocrinology 1997; 138: 863–70.

53. Enmark E, Pelto-Huikko M, Grandien K et al. Human estrogen receptor beta-gene structure, chromosomal localization, and expression pattern. J Clin Endocrinol Metab 1997; 82: 4258–65.

54. Shughrue PJ, Lane MV, Scrimo PJ, Merchenthaler I. Comparative distribution of estrogen receptor-α (ER-α) and β (ER-β) mRNA in the rat pituitary, gonad, and reproductive tract. Steroids 1998; 63: 498–504.

55. Nilsson S, Gustafsson JA. Biological role of estrogen and estrogen receptors. Crit Rev Biochem Mol Biol 2002; 37: 1–28.

56. Bhavnani BR, Lu XF. Differential interaction of equine estrogens with recombinant human estrogen receptors alpha (ERα) and beta (ERβ). J Soc Gynecol Invest 2003; 10: 298: 626A.

57. Tam SP, Bhavnani BR. Different effects of various equine estrogens mediated via estrogen receptors and β in HepG2 cells. The Endocrine Society's 85th Annual Meeting, Philadelphia, 2003: 104A.

58. Wehling M. Specific, nongenomic actions of steroid hormones. Annu Rev Physiol 1997; 59: 365–93.

59. Revelli A, Massobrio M, Tesarik J. Nongenomic actions of steroid hormones in reproductive tissues. Endocr Rev 1998; 19: 3–17.

60. Norman AW, Wehling M. Baldi E, Forti G. Proceedings of the Third International Meeting on Rapid Responses to Steroid Hormones. Steroids 2004; 515–97.

61. Szego CM. The lysosome as a mediator of hormone action. Recent Prog Horm Res 1974; 30: 171–233.

62. Pietras RJ, Szego CM. Specific binding sites for oestrogen at the outer surfaces of isolated endometrial cells. Nature 1977; 265: 69–72.

63. Pietras RJ, Szego CM. Partial purification and characterization of oestrogen receptors in subfractions of hepatocyte plasma membranes. Biochem J 1980; 191: 743–60.

64. Bhavnani BR. Pharmacology of estrogens – basic aspects. Menopause Review 2000; V: 1–14.

65. Aronica SM, Kraus WL, Katznellenbogen BS. Estrogen action via the cAMP signaling pathway: stimulation of adenylate cyclase and cAMP-regulated gene transcription. Proc Natl Acad Sci U S A 1994; 91: 8517–21.

66. Tesarik J, Mendoza C. Nongenomic effects of 17β-estradiol on maturing human oocytes: relationship to oocyte developmental potential. J Clin Endocrinol Metab 1995; 80: 1438–43.

67. Pappas TC, Gametchu B, Yannariello-Brown J, Collins TJ, Watson CS. Membrane estrogen receptors in GH3/B6 cells are associated with rapid estrogen-induced release of prolactin. Endocrine 1994; 2: 813–22.

68. Lieberherr M, Grosse B, Kachkache M, Balsan S. Cell signaling and estrogens in female rat osteoblasts: a possible involvement of unconventional nonnuclear receptors. J Bone Miner Res 1993; 8: 1365–76.

69. Pappas TC, Gametchu B, Watson CS. Membrane estrogen receptors identified by multiple antibody labeling and impeded-ligand binding. FASEB J 1995; 9: 404–10.

70. Morey AK, Pedram A, Razandi M, Prins BA, Hu RM, Biesiada E, Levin ER. Estrogen and progesterone inhibit human vascular smooth muscle proliferation. Endocrinology 1997; 138: 3330–9.

71. Morey AK, Razandi M, Pedram A, Hu RM, Prins BA, Levin ER. Oestrogen and progesterone inhibit the stimulated production of endothelin-1: differential positive and negative regulatory mechanisms. Biochem J 1998; 330: 1097–105.

72. Watters JJ, Campbell JS, Cunningham MJ, Krebs EG, Dorsa DM. Rapid membrane effects of steroids in neuroblastoma cells: effects of estrogen on mitogen activated protein kinase signalling cascade and c-fos immediate early gene transcription. Endocrinology 1997; 138: 4030–3.

73. Ranzandi M, Pedram A, Greene GL, Levin ER. Cell membrane and nuclear estrogen receptors (ERs) originate from a single transcript: studies of ERα and ERβ expressed in Chinese hamster ovary cells. Mol Endocrinol 1999; 13: 307–19.

74. Bradlow LH. A history of steroid chemistry. Part II. Steroids 1992; 57: 577–664.

75. Kalant H, Roschlau WHE. Principles of Medical Pharmacology. Toronto: BC Decker Inc, 1989.

76. Gerhard M, Ganz P. How do we explain the clinical benefits of estrogen? Circulation 1995; 92: 5–8.

77. Sullivan JM. Hormone replacement therapy in cardiovascular disease: The human model. Br J Obstet Gynaecol 1996; 103 (Suppl 13): 50–67.

78. Chetkowski RJ, Meldrum DR, Steingold KA et al. Biologic effects of transdermal estradiol. N Engl J Med 1986; 314: 1615–20.

79. De Lignieres B, Basdevant A, Thomas G et al. Biological effects of estradiol-17β in postmenopausal women: oral versus percutaneous administration. J Clin Endocrinol Metab 1986; 62: 536–41.

80. Crook D, Cust MP, Gangar KF et al. Comparison of transdermal and oral estrogen-progestin replacement therapy: effects on serum lipids and lipoproteins. Am J Obstet Gynecol 1992; 166: 950–5.

81. Friend KE, Hartman ML, Pezzoli SS, Clasey JL, Thorner MO. Both oral and transdermal estrogen increase growth hormone release in postmenopausal women – a clinical research center study. J Clin Endocrinol Metab 1996; 81: 2250–6.

82. Koh KK, Cardillo C, Bui MN et al. Vascular effects of estrogen and cholesterol-lowering therapies in hypercholesterolemic postmenopausal women. Circulation 1999; 99: 354–60.

83. The writing group for the PEPI Trial. Effects of estrogen or estrogen/progestin regimens on heart disease risk factors in postmenopausal women. JAMA 1995; 273: 199–208.

84. Bhavnani BR, Woolever CA, Wallace D, Pan CC. Metabolism of [³H]equilin-[³⁵S]sulfate and [³H]equilin sulfate after oral and intravenous administration in normal postmenopausal women and men. J Clin Endocrinol Metab 1989; 68: 757–65.

85. Ruder HJ, Loriaux L, Lipsett MB. Estrone sulfate: production rate and metabolism in man. J Clin Invest 1972; 51: 1020–33.

86. Longcope C. The metabolism of estrone sulfate in normal males. J Clin Endocrinol Metab 1972; 34: 113–22.

87. Bhavnani BR, Sarda IR, Woolever CA. Radioimmunoassay of plasma equilin and estrone in postmenopausal women after the administration of premarin. J Clin Endocrinol Metab 1981; 52: 741–7.

88. Englund DE, Johansson ED. Plasma levels of oestrone, oestradiol and gonadotrophins in postmenopausal women after oral and vaginal administration of conjugated equine oestrogens (Premarin). Br J Obstet Gynaecol 1978; 85: 957–64.

89. Anderson AB, Sklovsky E, Sayers L, Steele PA, Turnbull AC. Comparison of serum oestrogen concentrations in post-menopausal women taking oestrone sulphate and oestradiol. BMJ 1978; 1: 140–2.

90. Quirk JG, Wendel GD. Biologic effects of natural and synthetic estrogens. In: Buchsbaum HJ, ed. The Menopause. New York: Springer-Verlag, 1983: 55–75.

91. Bhavnani BR. Analytical methodology for estimation of ethinyl estradiol following ingestion of oral contraceptives. Adv Contracept 1991; 7 (Suppl 3): 116–39.

92. Mashchak CA, Lobo RA, Dozono-Takano R et al. Comparison of pharmacodynamic properties of various estrogen formulations. Am J Obstet Gynecol 1982; 144: 511–18.

93. Toniolo PG, Levitz M, Zeleniuch-Jacquotte A et al. A prospective study of endogenous estrogens and breast cancer in postmenopausal women. J Natl Cancer Inst 1995; 87: 190–7.

94. Nachtigall LE, Raju U, Banerjee S, Wan L, Levitz M. Serum estradiol-binding profiles in postmenopausal women undergoing three common estrogen replacement therapies: associations with sex hormone-binding

globulin, estradiol, and estrone levels. Menopause 2000; 7: 243–50.

95. Deutsch S, Ossowski R, Benjamin I. Comparison between degree of systemic absorption of vaginally and orally administered estrogens at different dose levels in postmenopausal women. Am J Obstet Gynecol 1981; 139: 967–8.

96. Mandel FP, Geola FL, Meldrum DR et al. Biological effects of various doses of vaginally administered conjugated equine estrogens in postmenopausal women. J Clin Endocrinol Metab 1983; 57: 133–9.

97. Lobo RA. Absorption and metabolic effects of different types of estrogens and progestogens. Obstet Gynecol Clin North Am 1987; 14: 143–67.

98. Troy SM, Hicks DR, Parker VD, Jusko WJ, Rofsky HE, Porter RJ. Differences in pharmacokinetics and comparative bioavailability between Premarin® and Estratab® in healthy postmenopausal women. Curr Ther Res 1994; 55: 359–72.

99. Bhavnani BR, Cecutti A. Estratab, Estratest, and Premarin are not bioequivalent. Am J Obstet Gynecol 1993; 169: 234–5.

100. Prestwood KM, Kenny AM, Unson C, Kulldorff M. The effect of low dose micronized 17β-estradiol on bone turnover, sex hormone levels, and side effects in older women: a randomized, double blind, placebo-controlled study. J Clin Endocrinol Metab 2000; 85: 4462–9.

101. Lindsay R, Gallagher JC, Kleerekoper M, Pickar JH. Effect of lower doses of conjugated equine estrogens with and without medroxyprogesterone acetate on bone in early postmenopausal women. JAMA 2002; 287: 2668–76.

102. Lindsay R. Hormones and bone health in postmenopausal women. Endocrine 2004; 24: 223–30.

103. Tait JF, Burstein S. In vivo studies of steroid dynamics in man. In Pincus G, Thimann KV, Astwood EB, eds. The Hormones. New York: Academic Press, 1964: 441–557.

104. Bhavnani BR, Woolever CA, Benoit H, Wong T. Pharmacokinetics of equilin and equilin sulfate in normal postmenopausal women and men. J Clin Endocrinol Metab 1983; 56: 1048–56.

105. Bhavnani BR, Cecutti A. Pharmacokinetics of 17β-dihydroequilin sulfate and 17β-dihydroequilin in normal postmenopausal women. J Clin Endocrinol Metab 1994; 78: 197–204.

106. Bhavnani BR, Cecutti A. Metabolic clearance rate of equilin sulfate and its conversion to plasma equilin, conjugated and unconjugated equilenin, 17β-dihydroequilin, and 17β-dihydroequilenin in normal postmenopausal women and men under steady state conditions. J Clin Endocrinol Metab 1993; 77: 1269–74.

107. Bhavnani BR, Cecutti A, Gerulath AH. 17β-dihydroequilin sulfate dynamics in postmenopausal women and man under steady state conditions. J Soc Gynecol Invest 1997; 4 (Suppl 1): 177.

108. Longcope C. Metabolic clearance and blood production rates of estrogens in postmenopausal women. Am J Obstet Gynecol 1971; 111: 778–81.

109. Bhavnani BR, Nisker JA, Martin J, Aletebi F, Watson L, Milne JK. Comparison of pharmacokinetics of a conjugated equine estrogen preparation (premarin) and a synthetic mixture of estrogens (CES) in postmenopausal women. J Soc Gynecol Investig 2000; 7: 175–83.

110. Baird DT, Horton R, Longcope C, Tait JF. Steroid dynamics under steady-state conditions. Recent Prog Horm Res 1969; 25: 611–64.

111. Purdy RH, Goldzieher JW, Le Quesne PW, Abdel-Baky S. Active metabolites and carcinogenesis. In: Kono S, Merriam GR, Brandon DD, eds. Catechol Estrogens. New York: Raven Press, 1983; 123–40.

112. Zhu BT, Roy D, Liehr JG. The carcinogenic activity of ethinyl estrogens is determined by both their hormonal characteristics and their conversion to catechol metabolites. Endocrinology 1993; 132: 577–83.

113. Li JJ, Li SA. Estrogen carcinogenesis in hamster tissues: a critical review. Endocr Rev 1990; 11: 524–31.

114. Li JJ, Li SA, Oberley TD, Parsons JA. Carcinogenic activities of various steroidal and nonsteroidal estrogens in the hamster kidney: relation to hormonal activity and cell proliferation. Cancer Res 1995; 55: 4347–51.

115. Bhavnani BR. Pharmacology of conjugated equine estrogens. Menopause Review 2000; V: 1–24.

116. Reddy VV, Hanjani P, Rajan R. Synthesis of catechol estrogens by human uterus and leiomyoma. Steroids 1981; 37: 195–203.

117. Bhavnani BR, Cecutti A, Wallace D. Metabolism of [³H]17β-dihydroequilin and [³H]17β-dihydroequilin sulfate in normal postmenopausal women. Steroids 1994; 59: 389–94.

118. Bhavnani BR, Cecutti A. Identification of a novel 16α-hydroxylated ring B unsaturated estrogens following administration of equilin to postmenopausal women and men. J Soc Gynecol Investig 1996; 3 (Suppl 2): 365.

119. Shackleton CH, Roitman E, Kratz LE, Kelley RI. Equine type estrogens produced by a pregnant woman carrying a Smith-Lemli-Opitz syndrome fetus. J Clin Endocrinol Metab 1999; 84: 1157–9.

120. Schneider J, Kinne D, Fracchia A et al. Abnormal oxidative metabolism of estradiol in women with breast cancer. Proc Natl Acad Sci U S A 1982; 79: 3047–51.

121. Bradlow HL, Hershcopf RJ, Martucci CP, Fishman J. Estradiol 16α-hydroxylation in the mouse correlates with mammary tumor incidence and presence of murine mammary tumor virus: a possible model for the hormonal etiology of breast cancer in humans. Proc Natl Acad Sci U S A 1985; 82: 6295–9.

122. Yu SC, Fishman J. Interaction of histones with estrogens. Covalent adduct formation with 16α-hydroxyestrone. Biochemistry 1985; 24: 8017–21.

123. Swaneck GE, Fishman J. Covalent binding of the endogenous estrogen 16α-hydroxyestrone to estradiol receptor in human breast cancer cells: characterization and intranuclear localization. Proc Natl Acad Sci U S A 1988; 85: 7831–5.

124. Kabat GC, Chang CJ, Sparano JA et al. Urinary estrogen metabolites and breast cancer: a case-control study. Cancer Epidemiol Biomarkers Prev 1997; 6: 505–9.

125. Ursin G, London S, Stanczyk FZ et al. A pilot study of urinary estrogen metabolites (16alpha-OHE1 and 2-OHE1) in postmenopausal women with and without breast cancer. Environ Health Perspect 1997; 105 (Suppl 3): 601–5.

126. Ursin G, London S, Stanczyk FZ et al. Urinary 2-hydroxyestrone/16α-hydroxyestrone ratio and risk of breast cancer in postmenopausal women. J Natl Cancer Inst 1999; 91: 1067–72.

127. Bhavnani BR, Strickler RC. Menpausal hormone therapy. J Obstet Gynaecol Can 2005; 27: 137–62.

128. Stevenson JC. Do we need different galenic forms of estrogens and progestogens? Menopause 1996; 243: 25–8.

129. Pike MC, Peters RK, Cozen W et al. Estrogen-progestin replacement therapy and endometrial cancer. J Natl Cancer Inst 1997; 89: 1110–16.

130. Barrett-Connor E. Hormone replacement therapy. BMJ 1998; 317: 457–61.

131. Gupta C, Musto NA, Bullock LP. In vivo metabolism of progestins. In: Garattini S, Berendes HW, eds. Pharmacology of Steroid Contraceptive Drugs. New York: Raven Press, 1977: 131–6.

132. Hiroi M, Stanczyk FZ, Goebelsmann U, Brenner PF, Lumkin ME, Mishell DR Jr. Radioimmunoassay of serum medroxyprogesterone acetate (Provera) in women following oral and intravaginal administration. Steroids 1975; 26: 373–86.

133. Back DJ, Breckenridge AM, Crawford FE et al. Kinetics of norethindrone in women. II. Single-dose kinetics. Clin Pharmacol Ther 1978; 24: 448–53.

134. Back DJ, Bates M, Breckenridge AM et al. The pharmacokinetics of levonorgestrel and ethynylestradiol in women – studies with Ovran and Ovranette. Contraception 1981; 23: 229–39.

135. Back DJ, Grimmer SF, Shenoy N, Orme ML. Plasma concentrations of 3-keto-desogestrel after oral administration of desogestrel and intravenous administration of 3-keto-desogestrel. Contraception 1987; 35: 619–26.

136. Tauber U, Tack JW, Matthes H. Single dose pharmacokinetics of gestodene in women after intravenous and oral administration. Contraception 1989; 40: 461–79.

137. Oelkers W, Foidart JM, Dombrovicz N, Welter A, Heithecker R. Effects of a new oral contraceptive containing an antimineralocorticoid progestogen, drospirenone, on the renin-aldosterone system, body weight, blood pressure, glucose tolerance, and lipid metabolism. J Clin Endocrinol Metab 1995; 80: 1816–21.

138. Guido M, Romualdi D, Giuliani M et al. Drospirenone for the treatment of hirsute women with polycystic ovary syndrome: a clinical, endocrinological, metabolic pilot study. J Clin Endocrinol Metab 2004; 89: 2817–23.

139. Goldstein JL, Brown MS. The low-density lipoprotein pathway and its relation to atherosclerosis. Annu Rev Biochem 1977; 46: 897–930.

140. Bush TL, Barrett-Connor E, Cowan LD et al. Cardiovascular mortality and noncontraceptive use of estrogen in women: results from the Lipid Research Clinics Program Follow-up Study. Circulation 1987; 75: 1102–9.

141. Stampfer MJ, Colditz GA, Willett WC et al. Postmenopausal estrogen therapy and cardiovascular disease. Ten-year follow-up from the nurses' health study. N Engl J Med 1991; 325: 756–62.

142. Sullivan JM, Fowlkes LP. The clinical aspects of estrogen and the cardiovascular system. Obstet Gynecol 1996; 87 (Suppl 2): 36S–43S.

143. Grodstein F, Stampfer MJ, Manson JE et al. Postmenopausal estrogen and progestin use and the risk of cardiovascular disease. N Engl J Med 1996; 335: 453–61.

144. Rossouw JE, Anderson GL, Prentice RL et al. Writing Group for the Women's Health Initiative Investigators. Risks and benefits of estrogen plus progestin in healthy postmenopausal women: principal results from the Women's Health Initiative randomized controlled trial. JAMA 2002; 288: 321–33.

145. Hulley S, Grady D, Bush T et al. Randomized trial of estrogen plus progestin for secondary prevention of coronary heart disease in postmenopausal women. Heart and Estrogen/progestin Replacement Study (HERS) Research Group. JAMA 1998; 280: 605–13.

146. Steinberg D, Parthasarathy S, Carew TE, Khoo JC, Witztum JL. Beyond cholesterol. Modifications of low-density lipoprotein that increase its atherogenicity. N Engl J Med 1989; 320: 915–24.

147. Subbiah MT, Kessel B, Agrawal M, Rajan R, Abplanalp W, Rymaszewski Z. Antioxidant potential of specific estrogens on lipid peroxidation. J Clin Endocrinol Metab 1993; 77: 1095–7.

148. Sack MN, Rader DJ, Cannon RO 3rd. Oestrogen and inhibition of oxidation of low-density lipoproteins in postmenopausal women. Lancet 1994; 343: 269–70.

149. Wilcox JG, Hwang J, Hodis HN, Sevanian A, Stanczyk FZ, Lobo RA. Cardioprotective effects of individual conjugated equine estrogens through their possible modulation of insulin resistance and oxidation of low-density lipoprotein. Fertil Steril 1997; 67: 57–62.

150. Bhavnani BR, Cecutti A, Gerulath A, Woolever AC, Berco M. Comparison of the antioxidant effects of equine estrogens, red wine components, vitamin E, and probucol on low-density lipoprotein oxidation in postmenopausal women. Menopause 2001; 8: 408–19.

151. Bhavnani BR, Cecutti A, Dey MS. Biologic effects of delta8-estrone sulfate in postmenopausal women. J Soc Gynecol Investig 1998; 5: 156–60.

152. Wilcox JG, Hwang J, Gentzschein EK et al. Effect of combined estrogen and progestin therapy in postmenopausal women on endothelium levels and oxidation of LDL. J Soc Gynecol Invest 1996 (Suppl 2): 69A.

153. Lacort M, Leal AM, Liza M, Martin C, Martinez R, Ruiz-Larrea MB. Protective effect of estrogens and catecholestrogens against peroxidative membrane damage in vitro. Lipids 1995; 30: 141–6.

154. Tang MX, Jacobs D, Stern Y et al. Effect of oestrogen during menopause on risk and age at onset of Alzheimer's disease. Lancet 1996; 348: 429–32.

155. Subbiah MTR. Mechanisms of cardioprotection by estrogens. Proc Soc Exp Biol Med 1998; 217: 23–9.

156. Stampfer MJ, Sacks FM, Salvini S, Willett WC, Hennekens CH. A prospective study of cholesterol, apolipoproteins, and the risk of myocardial infarction. N Engl J Med 1991; 325: 373–81.

157. Durrington PN. High-density lipoprotein cholesterol: methods and clinical significance. Crit Rev Clin Lab Sci 1982; 18: 31–78.

158. Bonnefront-Rousselot D, Therond P, Beaudeux JL, Peynet J, Legrand A, Delattre J. High density lipoprotein (HDL) and the oxidative hypothesis of atherosclerosis. Clin Chem Lab Med 1999; 37: 939–48.

159. Chung BH, Segrest JP, Smith K, Griffin FM, Brouillette CG. Lipolytic surface remnants of triglyceride-rich lipoproteins are cytotoxic to macrophages but not in the presence of high density lipoprotein. A possible mechanism of atherogenesis? J Clin Invest 1989; 83: 1363–74.

160. Ohta T, Takata S, Morino Y, Matsuda I. Protective effect of lipoproteins containing apoprotein A-I on Cu2+-catalyzed oxidation of human low density lipoprotein. FEBS Lett 1989; 257: 435–8.

161. Parthasarthy S, Barnett J, Fong LG. High-density lipoprotein inhibits the oxidative modification of low-density lipoprotein. Biochim Biophys Acta 1990; 1044: 275–83.

162. Sangvanich P, Mackness B, Gaskell SJ, Durrington P, Mackness M. The effect of high-density lipoproteins on the formation of lipid/protein conjugates during in vitro oxidation of low density lipoprotein. Biochem Biophys Res Comm 2003; 300: 501–6.

163. Mackness MI, Arrol S, Abbott C, Durrington PN. Protection of low-density lipoprotein against oxidative modifications by high-density lipoprotein associated paraoxonase. Atherosclerosis 1993; 104: 129–35.

164. Nagano Y, Arai H, Kita T. High density lipoprotein loses its effect to stimulate efflux of cholesterol from foam cells after oxidative modification. Proc Natl Acad Sci U S A 1991; 88: 6457–61.

165. Ohmura H, Watanabe Y, Hatsumi C et al. Possible role of high susceptibility of high-density lipoprotein to lipid peroxidative modifications and oxidized high-density lipoprotein in genesis of coronary artery spasm. Atherosclerosis 1999; 142: 179–84.

166. Perrella J, Berco M, Cecutti A, Gerulath A, Bhavnani BR. Potential role of the interaction between equine estrogens, low-density lipoprotein (LDL) and high-density lipoprotein (HDL) in the prevention of coronary heart and neurodegenerative diseases in postmenopausal women. Lipids Health Dis 2003; 2: 1–10.

167. Paganini-Hill A, Henderson VW. Estrogen deficiency and risk of Alzheimer's disease in women. Am J Epidemiol 1994; 140: 256–61.
    Henderson VW, Paganini-Hill A, Emanuel CK, Dunn ME, Buckwalter JG. Estrogen replacement therapy in older women. Comparisons between Alzheimer's disease cases and nondemented control subjects. Arch Neurol 1994; 51: 896–900.

168. Tang MX, Jacobs D, Stern Y et al. Effect of oestrogen during menopause on risk and age at onset of Alzheimer's disease. Lancet 1996; 348: 429–32.

169. Hogervorst E, Williams J, Budge M, Riedel W, Jolles J. The nature of the effect of female gonadal hormone replacement therapy on cognitive function in postmenopausal women: a meta-analysis. Neuroscience 2000; 101: 485–512.

170. Nelson HD, Humphrey LL, Nygren P, Teutsch SM, Allan JD. Postmenopausal hormone replacement therapy: scientific review. JAMA 2002; 288: 872–81.

171. LeBlanc ES, Janowsky J, Chan BK, Nelson HD. Hormone replacement therapy and cognition: systematic review and meta-analysis. JAMA 2001; 285: 1489–99.

172. Henderson VW, Paganini-Hill A, Miller BL et al. Estrogen for Alzheimer's disease in women: randomized, double-blind, placebo-controlled trial. Neurology 2000; 54: 295–301.

173. Mulnard RA, Cotman CW, Kawas C et al. Estrogen replacement therapy for treatment of mild to moderate Alzheimer disease: a randomized controlled trial. Alzheimer's Disease Cooperative Study. JAMA 2000; 283: 1007–15.

174. Shumaker SA, Legault C, Rapp SR et al. WHIMS Investigators. Estrogen plus progestin and the incidence of dementia and mild cognitive impairment in postmenopausal women: the Women's Health Initiative Memory Study: a randomized controlled trial. JAMA 2003; 289: 2651–62.

175. Espeland MA, Rapp SR, Shumaker SA et al. Conjugated equine estrogens and global cognitive function in postmenopausal women. JAMA 2004; 291: 2959–68.

176. Berco M, Bhavnani BR. Differential neuroprotective effects of equine estrogens against oxidized low density lipoprotein-induced neuronal cell death. J Soc Gynecol Investig 2001; 8: 245–54.

177. Bhavnani BR, Berco M, Binkley J. Equine estrogens differentially prevent neuronal cell death induced by glutamate. J Soc Gynecol Investig 2003; 10: 302–8.

178. Behl C, Davis JB, Lesley R, Schubert D. Hydrogen peroxide mediates amyloid beta protein toxicity. Cell 1994; 77: 817–27.

179. Rhodin JA, Thomas TT, Clark L, Garces A, Bryant M. In vivo cerebrovascular actions of amyloid β-peptides and the protective effect of conjugated estrogens. J Alzheimer's Disease 2003; 5: 275–86.

180. Zhang YM, Lu XF, Bhavnani BR. Equine estrogens differentially inhibit DNA fragmentation induced by glutamate in neuronal cells by modulation of regulatory proteins involved in programmed cell death. BMC Neuroscience 2003; 4: 32.

181. Zhang YM, Bhavnani BR. Glutamate-induced apoptosis in primary cortical neurons is inhibited by equine estrogens via down-regulation of caspase-3 and prevention of mitochondrial cytochrome c release. BMC Neurosci 2005; 6: 13.

182. Zhang YM, Bhavnani BR. Glutamate-induced apoptosis in neuronal cells is mediated via caspase-dependent and independent mechanisms involving calpain and caspase-3 proteases as well as apoptosis inducing factor (AIF) and this process is inhibited by equine estrogens. BMC Neurosci 2006; 7: 49.

# Chapter 21

# Medications for the menopausal woman: general and replacement

Bernard A Eskin

## INTRODUCTION

A major objective for this chapter is to present the medications given to menopausal women and how the types, uses, and doses may differ from those given to younger patients. Detailed general and basic concepts of the pharmacology of menopause and aging are clearly detailed in Chapter 20. Apparently, aging is not gender-driven; however, this chapter pertains specifically to aging women who are menopausal. In males, there is no evident acute reproductive loss in the early 50s age group. However, in women cessation of reproduction and severe reductions of an essential steroid, estrogen, have major general and specific effects on her growth, development, quality of health, and metabolism. In the perimenopause, postmenopause, geripause, women have minimal estrogen, and sex differences are evident.

Hence, this chapter concerns varied therapies, given to women during the menopause, as they relate to both her aging and sex hormonal losses. Pertinent medications and replacement hormones and modifications that may be useful will be discussed.

## GENERAL THERAPEUTICS

Until recently, medical treatments for menopausal women have not differed from those given to younger patients. Therapeutic requirements for cardiac, pulmonary, gastrointestinal, and neurological diseases are being carefully re-assessed by many gynecologists, internists, cardiologists and gerontologists.[1] Most physicians have preferred to undertreat women in their menopause, and particularly those over 65 years of age.[2,3] There was the belief that in similar disease states, older patients require a lower dose than younger patients. This concept, which has been acceptable for a majority of therapies, was certainly not universal. Undertreatment, which has been casually used, may have resulted in serious chronicity and complications.[4] Outdated life charts are still employed, which result in improper expectations for the aging patient, and, often, cause the physician to use low and inadequate dose levels.[5]

Evaluating specific changes in therapy in much of general medicine in the aging patient is beyond the scope of this textbook. Several of the contributors have described treatments in their chapters to which they adhere, and special methods they use for medical conditions. Most difficult is to decide the dose values for same-age elderly patients in today's upscale environment.

### Inappropriate medical use[6]

There has been growing evidence that some medications are not effective for the postmenopausal patient and may be an actual health hazard. Inappropriate medication use is a major patient safety concern, especially in the elderly population.[7-10] Many researchers have documented widespread unacceptable medication use by postmenopausal persons in hospitals,[11] nursing homes,[12-14] board and care facilities,[15] physician office practices,[16,17] hospital outpatient departments,[18] and homebound elderly,[19] with the estimated prevalence of potentially improper use ranging from 12% to 40%. Two studies have examined inappropriate medication use in the community-dwelling elderly, using population-based nationally representative surveys. Using the National Medical Expenditure Survey

(NMES),Wilcox et al estimated that 23.5% of the community-dwelling elderly in the US (6.64 million people) used at least 1 of 20 inappropriate medications in 1987.[20] Since then, using the Medicare Current Beneficiary Survey (MCBS), the General Accounting Office estimated that 17.5% (5.2 million) of the community-dwelling elderly used at least 1 of the same 20 inappropriate medications in 1992.[21] Reassessed in 2005, unacceptable treatments for the elderly still exist.[6,22] New medications cause much of the difficulty, since a long observation period is needed to quantitate the drug doses required.[22]

Studies of inappropriate medication use in elderly patients, including the two nationally representative studies, use explicit criteria developed in 1991 by Beers et al for nursing home patients.[23] Although generally accepted by the medical community and expert opinion,[8] the Beers criteria continue to be questioned. The explicit criteria expressed cannot completely capture all factors that define appropriate prescription decision making.[24] Some drugs on the Beers criteria may be justified in a given circumstance because the benefits outweigh the risk for a specific patient. Beers et al have agreed that there are limitations to both the sensitivity and specificity of the criteria presented;[25] however, these criteria may be considered a screening test for assessing inappropriate use.

The available national estimates from the Medical Expenditure Panel Surgery (MEPS) of 1996 and 2003 of potentially inappropriate medication use among the community-dwelling elderly population have been reported.[6,22] These estimates use updated criteria specifically designed to be applied to community-dwelling individuals.[19] Because of ongoing controversy surrounding the Beers criteria,[18] a panel was convened with expertise in geriatrics, pharmacoepidemiology, and pharmacy, to identify a subset of these drugs that should be avoided. The panel was instructed to identify any clinical indications for use of the listed drugs as of 1996 and after. In comparing previously published findings with their own data, they examined trends over a 10-year period. Only those factors that could be associated with inappropriate medication use among elderly patients were considered. Most of the products that were selected by these expert panels are relevant to general gerontological and medical practices, as noted in Table 21.1.[6] Although some hormonal therapies are included in this report, details of hormone replacement therapies that are more appropriate for postmenopausal and geripausal women will be presented in this chapter.[26]

The utilization of prescriptions, medication, and therapies is influenced by diagnoses. However, the quantity of therapy given is a decision by the physician on the basis of intensity of

**Table 21.1**   National US estimates of potentially inappropriate medication use by expert panel by generic name

| Always avoid | Rarely appropriate | Some indications |
|---|---|---|
| Barbiturates[a] | Chlordiazepoxide | Amitriptyline |
| Flurazepam | Diazepam | Doxepin |
| Meprobamate | Propoxyphene | Indometacin |
| Chlorpropamide | Carisoprodol | Dipyridamole |
| Meperidine | Chlorzoxazone | Ticlopidine |
| Pentazocine | Cyclobenzaprine | Methyldopa |
| Trimethobenzamide | Metaxalone | Reserpine |
| Belladonna alkaloids | Methocarbamol | Disopyramide |
| Dicycloverine | | Oxybutynin |
| Hyoscyamine | | Chlorpheniramine |
| Propantheline | | Cyproheptadine |
| | | Diphenhydramine |
| | | Hydroxyzine |
| | | Promethazine |

[a]Includes butabartibal, secobarbital, and pentobarbital.
Abridged from Drugs (1997) Beers Criteria and Classification by Expert Panel.

the illness and other more personal aspects such as weight, health level, and responses to medication. While women in early menopause usually respond closely to premenopausal adults, post-menopausal women vary as the patient ages, and require observation. Response then becomes a mixture of the hormone aging of the woman, and gerontological rules of dosage combined. Much improvement in this aspect of care is needed, and is being considered in government-directed programs, especially through the Agency for Healthcare Research and Quality (AHRQ). Good information is available online from this program and similar bureaus around the world.[22]

## Replacement therapies

Replacement therapies are given as substitutes for biological or hormonal secretions that are reduced or lost during the aging process. A deficiency or inadequacy may result from this loss and eventually result in an abnormality or disease process.

Many replacement therapies are available for use. The most evident are those needed for hormone deficiencies (i.e. insulin, thyroid hormone). These dysfunctions occur either through aging, reduction of secretion, or atrophy of endocrine glands. If tissue and cellular growth does continue, there is often a quantitative reduction in the effectiveness of the secretions as shown by decreased metabolic function at target tissues. This is caused often by reduced receptor availability or response at the target organs. Additionally, some endocrine gland stimulators produce an inadequate effectiveness because of transport reduction into the cells. These can be remedied only by direct stimulation or by exogenous replacement.

Supplements, such as vitamins, elements and macronutrients have been used to replace or maintain tissue staying within recommended dietary allowances established by medical and governmental agencies. Specific US recommendations made for vitamin and mineral replacement are presented in Table 21.2. A popular source of desired food intake is described in the new food pyramid (Chapter 23) showing the daily dietary requirements suggested by the United States Department of Agriculture (USDA).

## ENDOCRINE REPLACEMENT THERAPY

Most theories of aging describe intracellular changes that are appropriate throughout the body. Actually, most scientific matter on aging characterizes only those tissues we associate with clinical senescence; i.e. skin, neurological and vascular tissues, muscle, and bone. In these specific areas, anatomical and physiological modifications have been presented and hypothetical models established.

However, the endocrine system is unique in that, besides apparent losses of tissue growth and metabolism, secretory activity may in some cases be inhibited, modified, or even completely reversed during the aging process. Essential hormones generally required for normal physiological functioning of other parts of the body may be lost.[2] Particularly applicable is a reduction in muscle strength, which leads eventually to frailty.[3,4]

A series of histological modifications, which are not unique, occurs in the endocrine glands due to aging.[2] Connective tissue increases in the gland capsule, and connective tissue elements replace secretory cells. In the endocrine cell, mitotic rate decreases, and fragmentation of mitochondria and nuclear damage often appear. Thus, alterations in the endocrine tissues with aging relate to both secretory and target organ functions.[5] The changes are:

1.  primary loss of functional tissue by hypoplastic or atrophic changes in secreting cells
2.  decrease in secretory rate as a result of these cellular changes
3.  decrease of metabolic clearance of hormones produced
4.  decrease in end-organ response to the hormones.

Most of the changes are gradual, except for those related to ovarian demise. Clinically, the most evident and important modifications are hormonal, but age-related factors are present and often difficult to factor out. Those hormones considered most evident and present are: gonadal hormones; thyroid hormones; pancreatic hormones in diabetes mellitus; adrenal hormones; and the neurological and secretory hormonal controls in the brain. Our discussion entails those that are considered most affected by the postmenopause and geripause. Most evident are the gonadal and thyroid hormones; however, some information has

**Table 21.2**   Dietary reference intakes for older adults (compiled by the National Policy and Resource Center on Nutrition and Aging, Florida International University; revised 18 December 2001. Values excerpted with permission from Institute of Medicine. *Dietary Reference Intakes: Applications in Dietary Assessment, 2000*[25])

| Vitamins and elements | | | | | | | | | | |
|---|---|---|---|---|---|---|---|---|---|---|
| | Vitamin A (µg)[b,c] | Vitamin C (mg) | Vitamin D (µg)[d,e] | Vitamin E (mg)[f,g,h] | Vitamin K (µg) | Thiamin (mg) | Riboflavin (mg) | Niacin (mg)[h,i] | Vitamin B₆ (mg) | Folate (µg)[h,i] |
| *RDA or AI\** | | | | | | | | | | |
| *Age 51–70* | | | | | | | | | | |
| Male | 900 | 90 | 10* | 15 | 120* | 1.2 | 1.3 | 16 | 1.7 | 400 |
| Female | 700 | 75 | 10* | 15 | 90* | 1.1 | 1.1 | 14 | 1.5 | 400 |
| *Age 70+* | | | | | | | | | | |
| Male | 900 | 90 | 15* | 15 | 120* | 1.2 | 1.3 | 16 | 1.7 | 400 |
| Female | 700 | 75 | 15* | 15 | 90* | 1.1 | 1.1 | 14 | 1.5 | 400 |
| *Tolerable upper intake levels (UL)[a]* | | | | | | | | | | |
| *Age 51–70* | | | | | | | | | | |
| Male | 3000 | 2000 | 50 | 1000 | ND | ND | ND | 35 | 100 | 1000 |
| Female | 3000 | 2000 | 50 | 1000 | ND | ND | ND | 35 | 100 | 1000 |
| *Age 70+* | | | | | | | | | | |
| Male | 3000 | 2000 | 50 | 1000 | ND | ND | ND | 35 | 100 | 1000 |
| Female | 3000 | 2000 | 50 | 1000 | ND | ND | ND | 35 | 100 | 1000 |

| | Vitamin B₁₂ (µg)[k] | Pantothenic acid (mg) | Biotin (µg) | Choline (mg)[l] | Boron (mg) | Calcium (mg) | Chromium (µg) | Copper (µg) | Fluoride (mg) | Iodine (µg) |
|---|---|---|---|---|---|---|---|---|---|---|
| *RDA or AI\** | | | | | | | | | | |
| *Age 51–70* | | | | | | | | | | |
| Male | 2.4 | 5* | 30* | 550* | ND | 1200* | 30* | 900 | 4* | 150 |
| Female | 2.4 | 5* | 30* | 425* | ND | 1200* | 30* | 900 | 3* | 150 |
| *Age 70+* | | | | | | | | | | |
| Male | 2.4 | 5* | 30* | 550* | ND | 1200* | 30* | 900 | 4* | 150 |
| Female | 2.4 | 5* | 30* | 425* | ND | 1200* | 30* | 900 | 3* | 150 |
| *Tolerable upper intake levels\** | | | | | | | | | | |
| *Age 51–70* | | | | | | | | | | |
| Male | ND | ND | ND | 3500 | 20 | 2500 | ND | 10000 | 10 | 1100 |
| Female | ND | ND | ND | 3500 | 20 | 2500 | ND | 10000 | 10 | 1100 |
| *Age 70+* | | | | | | | | | | |
| Male | ND | ND | ND | 3500 | 20 | 2500 | ND | 10000 | 10 | 1100 |
| FemaleND | ND | ND | ND | 3500 | 20 | 2500 | ND | 10000 | 10 | 1100 |

| Elements and macronutrients | | | | | | | | | |
|---|---|---|---|---|---|---|---|---|---|
| | Iron (mg) | Magnesium (mg)[m] | Manganese (mg) | Molybdenum (mg) | Nickel (mg) | Phosphorus (mg) | Selenium (µg) | Vanadium (mg)[n] | Zinc (mg)[n] |
| *RDA or AI\** | | | | | | | | | |
| *Age 51–70* | | | | | | | | | |
| Male | 8 | 420 | 2.3* | 45 | ND | 700 | 55 | ND | 11 |
| Female | 8 | 320 | 1.8* | 45 | ND | 700 | 55 | ND | 8 |
| *Age 70+* | | | | | | | | | |
| Male | 8 | 420 | 2.3* | 45 | ND | 700 | 55 | ND | 11 |
| Female | 8 | 320 | 1.8* | 45 | ND | 700 | 55 | ND | 8 |
| *Tolerable upper intake levels (UL)* | | | | | | | | | |
| *Age 51–70* | | | | | | | | | |
| Male | 45 | 350 | 11 | 2000 | 1 | 4000 | 400 | 1.8 | 40 |
| Female | 45 | 350 | 11 | 2000 | 1 | 4000 | 400 | 1.8 | 40 |
| *Age 70+* | | | | | | | | | |
| Male | 45 | 350 | 11 | 2000 | 1 | 3000 | 400 | 1.8 | 40 |
| Female | 45 | 350 | 11 | 2000 | 1 | 3000 | 400 | 1.8 | 40 |

|  | Energy (Kcal) | Protein (g) | Carbo-hydrates[2] | Total fat[2] | Saturated fat[2] | Cholesterol (mg) | Sodium (mg) | Fiber (g)[3] |
|---|---|---|---|---|---|---|---|---|
| 1989 RDAs for age 51+ | | | | | | | | |
| Male | 2300 | 63 | > 55% | < 30% | < 10% | < 300 | < 2400 | 20–35 |
| Female | 1900 | 50 | > 55% | < 30% | < 10% | < 300 per day | < 2400 per day | 20–35 |

[1]The 1989 RDAs are used as no new Dietary Reference Intakes have been established for energy and protein, and other macronutrients.
[2]The Food and Nutrition Board's Committee on Diet and Health recommendations base intake on the per cent of total calories in the diet (NCR, 1989).
[3]The National Cancer Institute and American Dietetic Association recommend 20–35 g dietary fiber daily (ADA, 1997).
ND, values not determined. This table (taken from the DRI reports, see www.nap.edu) presents the recommended dietary allowances (RDAs) in bold type and adequate intakes (AIs) in ordinary type followed by an asterisk (*). RDAs and AIs may both be used as goals for individual intake. RDAs are set to meet the needs of almost all (97–98%) individuals in a group. The AI for life stage and gender groups (other than healthy, breast-fed infants) is believed to cover needs of all individuals in the group, but lack of data or uncertainty in the data prevent being able to specify with confidence the percentage of individuals covered by this intake.
[a]UL = The maximum level of daily nutrient intake that is likely to pose no risk of adverse effects. Unless otherwise especified, the UL represents total intake from food, water, and supplements. Owing to lack of suitable data, ULs could not be established for vitamin K, thiamin, riboflavin, vitamin B$_{12}$, pantothenic acid, biotin, or carotenoids. In the absence of ULs, extra caution may be warranted in consuming levels above recommended intakes.
[b]As retinal activity equivalents (RAEs). 1 RAE = 1 μg retinal, 12 μg β-carotene, or 24 μg β-cryptoxanthin. To calculate RAEs from the REs of provitamin A carotenoids in foods, divide the REs by 2. For performed vitamin A in foods or supplements and for provitamin A carotenoids in supplements, 1 RE = 1 RAE.
[c]ULs – As preformed vitamin A only.
[d]Cholecalciferol. 1 μg cholecalciferol = 40 IU vitamin D.
[e]In the absence of adequate exposure to sunlight.
[f]As alpha-tocopherol. Alpha-tocopherol includes RRR-alpa-tocopherol, the only form of alpha-tocopherol that occurs naturally in foods, and the 2R-steroisomeric forms of alpha-tocopherol (RRR-, RSR-, RRS- and RSS-alpha-tocopherol) that occur in fortified foods and supplements. It does not include the 2S-stereoisomeric forms fo alpha-tocopherol (SRR-, SSR-, SRS-, SSS-alpha-tocopherol), also found in fortified foods and supplements.
[g]ULs – as alpha-tocopherol; applies to any form of supplemental alpha-tocopherol.
[h]The ULs for vitamin E, niacin, and folate apply to synthetic forms obtained from supplements, fortified foods, or a combination of the two.
[i]As niacin equivalents (NE). 1 mg of niacin = 60 mg of tryptophan: 0–6 months = performed niacin (not NE).
[j]As dietary folate equivalents (DFE). 1 DFE = 1 μg food folate = 0.6 μg of folic acid from fortified food or as a supplement consumed with food = 0.5 μg of a supplement taken on an empty stomach.
[k]Because 10–30% of older people may malabsorb food-bound B$_{12}$, it is advisable for those older than 50 years to meet their RDA mainly by consuming foods fortified with B$_{12}$ or a supplement containing B$_{12}$.
[l]Although AIs have been set for choline, there are few data to assess whether a dietary supply of choline is needed at all stages of the life cycle, and it may be that the choline requirement can be met by endogenous synthesis at some of these stages.
[m]The ULs for magnesium represent intake from a pharmacological agent only and do not include intake from food and water.
[n]Although vanadium in food has not been shown to cause adverse effects in humans, there is no justification for adding vanadium to food and vanadium supplements should be used with caution. The UL is based on adverse effects in laboratory animals and these data could be used to set a UL for adults but not children or adolescents.
Reproduced from Eskin BA, Troen BR. The Geripause: Medical Management During the Late Menopause. London: Parthenon Publishing, 2003, pp96–98 with permission from Informa UK Ltd.

become available concerning other post-menopausal endocrinopathies, which are described briefly. Perhaps future research will uncover other useful relationships for endocrine entities in the maintenance of good health status during the longevity that has been proposed (Chapter 2).

*Diabetes*
The subject of diabetes mellitus can be only briefly mentioned here. Although it is an omnipresent endocrinopathy, particularly from the late 40s, the complexity of the topic of pancreatic hormones and carbohydrate metabolism deserves a fully dedicated book. Most women in the post-menopause, not already diagnosed with insulin-dependent diabetes mellitus (IDDM; DM1), will fall into the second category of non-insulin-dependent diabetes mellitus (NIDDM; DM2), which commonly occurs after 40 years of age.

Although estrogen may already be decreasing, this decisive division is not gender-affected.[27,28]

Approximately 22% of individuals 51–65 years of age, 40% of individuals 65–74 years of age, and 50% of individuals older than 80 years have impaired glucose tolerance or a form of diabetes mellitus in the US.[29] Nearly half of elderly diabetics are undiagnosed.[29,30] These persons are at risk of developing secondary, mainly macrovascular, complications at an accelerated rate.[31] Pancreatic, insulin receptor, and post-receptor changes associated with aging are critical components of the endocrinology of aging. Apart from decreased (relative) insulin secretion by the beta-cells, peripheral insulin resistance related to poor diet, physical inactivity, increased abdominal fat mass, and decreased lean body mass contribute to the deterioration of glucose metabolism.[31]

Therapy may be more difficult for IDDM patients and re-evaluation is usually required for these women entering the menopause. Most of the new cases will be considered as NIDDM, because the age of onset of disease was much later in life. Dietary management, exercise, oral hypoglycemic agents, and insulin are the four components of treatment of these patients, although the medical care is costly and intensive.[32] These changes in insulin sensitivity that occur in the aging population are of clinical importance, and are recognized and seriously treated as diseases.

## Adrenal hormones

Aging of the adrenal gland has been shown to occur primarily in the cortex. The secretory aspects most affected by postmenopause are related to 'sex hormones' and their precursor steroids. A deficiency of aromatizing enzyme has been suggested, but not proven, which accounts for a modest reduction in estrogen (as estrone), and similarly, the adrenal as a source for androgens is slightly decreased. This occurs even though gonadotropins increase and cross-stimulation by luteinizing hormone (LH) has been described.

Age-related changes in the circulating levels of the most representative adrenal androgen, dehydroepiandrosterone (DHEA), and it sulfate (DHEAS), show a gradual decline, presenting a change in steroidogenesis.[33–35] Adrenal secretion of DHEA diminishes progressively over the last decades of life, whereas adrenocorticotropin (ACTH) secretion, which is physiologically linked to plasma cortisol levels, remains largely unchanged.[36] The decline in DHEA(S) levels in the postmenopausal woman contrasts with those of plasma cortisol, which remains at the premenopausal levels. The decline of both DHEA and DHEAS seems to be caused by a selective decrease in the number of functional zona reticularis cells in the adrenal cortex rather than through deregulation by the hypothalamus.[34] Recent studies have shown that levels of these $\Delta^5$-steroids at age 70 and 80 years are only 20–30% of those obtained between age 20 and 30 years.[35–37] There may be anatomical changes in the adrenal medulla that may also modulate this steroidogenesis.[38] However, treatment with DHEA and DHEAS fails to show any remarkable reduction in aging when given as replacement to aging seniors.

Interestingly, stimulation of the adrenal cortex with exogenous or endogenous ACTH consistently results in decreased DHEA responses in older individuals as compared to premenopausal controls.[39,40] Corticosteroid production except for androgens remains adequate during normal physiological aging, although it is possibly upregulated for glucosteroids and downregulated for mineralocorticoids.[39]

Clinically, these changes are not evident, and usually a need for replacement has not been suggested. Conditions that have shown relative risk evidence when there are enhanced levels of cortisol with decreased levels of DHEA are Alzheimer's disease and adrenal hypoplasia. Several important clinical trials have been undertaken to evaluate these findings. Enhancement of the immune system and of the growth hormone axis with replacement of DHEA has been described in some studies.[41,42]

Basically, adrenal activity with aging has been insufficiently studied in postmenopausal and geripausal women. This complex area needs further clarification.

## Growth hormone

The growth hormone (GH)-insulin-like growth factor I (IGF-I) axis gradually declines in activity during aging.[43,44] Mean pulse amplitude, duration and fraction of GH secreted, but not pulse frequency, have been seen to decrease gradually during aging. Similarly, there is a progressive fall in circulating IGF-I levels in both sexes.[44] GH is secreted by the pituitary, but is stimulated primarily by hypothalamic hormone. Pituitary somatotropes, regardless of age, can be restored to premenopausal secretory capacity when treated with GH-releasing pulsatile peptides.

The hormone secretions that might be reduced because of an aging brain seem to be difficult at this time to implicate. The central pacemaker of aging has been considered to be the hypothalamus.[35] Although studies using the hypothalamic peptide GH show an effect on pituitary release, this is not universal and not understood. Gonadotropin-releasing hormone (GnRH) responses indicate that the thermal change that occurs in menopause may at least partially be due to hypothalamic dysfunction because of the proximity of GnRH secretion to the thermal control area.[45] Use of GnRH therapy is independent of the total function of the hypophysial-pituitary-ovarian axis, and appears to restore some gonadotropin effects, but fails with complete ovarian failure.

## Thyroid hormone and iodine metabolism

Perhaps the thyroid is most influenced by aging. The thyroid gland and its complex relationship with woman's health and especially reproductive aging has been detailed in Chapter 12. Extrathyroidal iodine effects have been related to several organs and secretions.

### Sex hormone replacement therapy

### Hormone replacement therapy and estrogen replacement therapy

By the time a woman enters the menopause she has been well initiated into the many problems that a decreasing estrogen level (Table 21.3) can cause. In the premenopause these problems have included dysfunctional uterine bleeding with cyclic uterine cramps and depression. Hot flushes or vascular instability, generally considered a hypothalamic effect, may begin in the 30s, and may be reduced or minimized by 65 years. Osteoporosis or osteopenia should be monitored by dual-energy X-ray absorptiometry (DEXA) and/or other examinations from the onset of the menopause.[46,47] Atrophic vulvovaginitis and severe dryness of the perineum may become uncomfortable, with itching and burning or sexual pain (dyspareunia) as a woman reaches late post-menopause.[48,49] Reduced cognition is the first sign of neurological change, and becomes evident during early premenopause. However, later in the perimenopause the loss becomes consistent and relentless through postmenopause and geripause.[27,50]

In most cases, general menopausal symptoms due to reduced estrogen are inseparable from those seen in aging. Many women discuss initial interest and make decisions concerning the use of estrogen replacement therapy while undergoing estrogen transitions. Initially, short-term estrogen (ERT) or combined sex hormones (HRT) in a given population may be started; however, those continuing estrogen replacement are reduced to less than

5% by the onset of geripause.[29] Either complications or side-effects reduce the numbers; while other patients are satisfied with other treatments or are able to defy the symptoms that they are having in light of possible complications. Therefore, each woman singularly tries to maintain her own level of expectation.

As previously described throughout this textbook the medical need for any therapy during menopause differs with the intensity of the symptoms. Most relevant are those concerning the skin, breast and perineal atrophy, bone loss leading to frailty in the geripause,[51] neurological deficits, and cognitive failures.[52,53] Reconsiderations of extremely low-dose estrogen during the geripause as replacement therapy have found a level of interest. Recent modifications have been made concerning the dosage and delivery of the hormones used.[30,54] More specific tissue responses have been noted with certain combinations and pharmaceuticals. Alternative medications have become available and may be suitable. This entire formulation of therapies has been markedly improved and is being constantly upgraded.

### Estrogen physiology

Estradiol, estrone, and estriol are the only three natural estrogens present in significant quantities in the human female. The action of estrogens is measured by the level of receptor responses on the alpha ($\alpha$)-estrogen receptor. Estradiol is the most potent, naturally occurring ovarian and placental estrogen in humans; estrone is an oxidation product of estradiol; and estriol (much weaker) is produced by hydroxylation of estrogen and primarily identified with pregnancy and placental release. Comparing these basic steroids, estradiol is three to four times more chemically active than estrone and estriol. The biological estrogenic potency of estradiol is about 12 times that of estrone, and 80 times that of estriol (Chapter 8).

In the postmenopause, estrogen continues to be produced in peripheral tissue by chemical transformation of androgens while meager progesterone release occurs. As presented in Table 21.3, estrogen loss is gradual during the perimenopause, and then rapidly decreases in the postmenopause. Significant changes in the gonadotropins are evident with follicle-stimulating hormone (FSH) persistently high throughout the early postmenopause, and decreasing with the onset of geripause. LH remains moderately elevated after FSH has risen, but never reaches the elevations seen during the ovulatory surge in

**Table 21.3** Average estrogen levels from transition (approximate)

| Age (years) | Average estrogen levels (pg/ml) |
|---|---|
| 36–42 | 30–600 pg/ml[a] |
| 42–52 | 0–200 pg/ml |
| 52–65 | <20 pg/ml |
| >65 | <10 pg/ml |

[a]Dependent on ovulatory activity.

Data averaged from data available from multiple laboratory sources.

reproductive women. LH also decreases after geri-pause. This drop in both gonadotropins symbol-izes and defines the change of phase to geripause. The full endocrine significance of these reductions remain unknown. They may represent a failing or aging hypophyseal-pituitary axis, as described in basic neuroendocrine research.[31]

Therefore, the use of estrogen replacement dur-ing premenopause, postmenopause/geripause requires further analysis. A need for use of estro-gen for reproduction after 50 years of age seems redundant, since the inactive ovaries usually pres-ent do not produce required functional ova. However, the presence of active estrogen recep-tors in many target organs throughout the body appears to make the total loss of estrogen seem premature.[32] Whether this loss of estrogen is pro-tective or prematurely destructive in women remains a point for conjecture.[55,56]

The loss of menses is considered by many as a measure of aging in women. Menopause itself is the termination of reproduction and the deactiva-tion of the gonads, and not related to the general aging process. Geriatric aging, which is readily recognized by 65 years, is similar in men and women with no advantage evident to men. Since estrogen is the prime sex steroid that is deficient in women, the unanswered questions remain: 'What effect does estrogen loss have on women post-menopausally and into the geripause?' and also 'What evidence is there that replacement of the estrogen delays the aging process?'

**Key benefits of HRT: known and conditional**
Numerous commercially available estrogen replacement agents have achieved US regulatory approval, based on significant scientific evidence (Table 21.4), and are indicated for alleviation of vasomotor dysfunctions (hot flushes),[48] improve-ment of genital atrophy,[26] and prevention of bone demineralization.[33,34,47,51] Prevention of bone loss has been shown to be exceptionally effective in older patients, but only when the hormone is being given.[51] Positive statistical findings have been obtained in experimental clinical trials, and hormone replacement is given to patients to pri-marily treat, or often prevent those symptoms. There are published side-effects, contraindica-tions, and complications described for these drug therapies (Tables 21.5 and 21.6). There may be additional potential risks associated with estrogen replacement, including thromboembolism,[35–37] endometrial cancer,[38] breast cancer,[32,39,40] and ovarian cancer.[41]

Particularly difficult to assess is the effect of HRT/ERT on breast cancer. Since breast cancer increases with age in all women, evaluation of the effects with hormone therapies require care-ful statistical review.[42] Recent studies have shown dose–response evidence that lower doses

---

**Table 21.4** Assumed benefits of hormone replacement therapy

*Known*

1. Improves osteopenia/osteoporosis
2. Reduces genitourinary atrophy
3. Decreases hot flushes
4. Reduces colon cancer risk
5. Improves vulvovaginal atrophy

*Evidence from clinical trials*

1. Reduces acute coronary disease risk
2. Psychiatric illnesses are controlled
3. Improvement of lipoprotein profile
4. Improves sleep disturbances
5. Reduces tooth loss
6. Reduces age-related macular degeneration
7. Lessening of Alzheimer's disease
8. Reduces cataracts
9. Improves CNS function

---

**Table 21.5** Contraindications to hormone replacement therapy

Progestogens/estrogens should not be used in individuals with any of the following conditions or circumstances:

- known or suspected pregnancy, including use for missed abortion or diagnostic test for pregnancy. Progestin or estrogen may cause fetal harm when administered to a pregnant woman
- known or suspected cancer of the breast
- known or suspected estrogen-dependent neoplasia
- undiagnosed abnormal genital bleeding
- active or past history of thrombophlebitis or thromboembolic disorders
- known sensitivity to estrogen- and/or progestin-containing products
- stroke or heart attack in the last year
- current liver problems

**Table 21.6**   Complications of hormone replacement therapy

*Induction of malignant neoplasms*

**Endometrial cancer**

The reported endometrial cancer risk among users of unopposed estrogen is about 2- to 14-fold greater than in non-users, and appears dependent on the duration of treatment and estrogen dose. Most studies show no significant increased risk associated with the use of estrogens for less than 1 year. The greatest risk appears to be associated with prolonged use, with increased risks of 15- to 24-fold for use of 5 to 10 years or more, and this risk has been shown to persist for at least 15 years after cessation of estrogen treatment.

**Breast cancer**

While the majority of studies have not shown an increased risk of breast cancer in women who have ever used estrogen replacement therapy, some have reported a moderately increased risk (relative risks of 1.3–2.0) in those taking higher doses, or those taking lower doses for prolonged period of time, especially in excess of 10 years. The effect of added progestins on the risk of breast cancer is unknown.

*Gall bladder disease*

A 2- to 4-fold increase in the risk of gall bladder disease requiring surgery in women receiving postmenopausal estrogen has been reported.

*Hypercalcemia*

Administration of estrogens may lead to severe hypercalcemia in patients with breast cancer and bone metastases.

*Pregnancy*

Use in pregnancy is not recommended.

*Venous thromboembolism*

Five epidemiological studies have found an increased risk of venous thromboembolism (VTE) in users of estrogen replacement therapy (ERT) who did not have predisposing conditions for surgery, trauma, or serious illness. The increased risk was found only in current ERT users; it did not persist in former users. The risk appeared to be higher in the first year of use, and decreased thereafter. The findings were similar for ERT alone or with added progestin, and pertain to commonly used oral and transdermal doses, with a possible dose-dependent effect on risk. The studies found the VTE risk to be about one case per 10 000 women per year among women not using ERT and without predisposing conditions. The risk in current ERT users was increased to 2–3 cases per 10 000 women per year.

*Visual disturbances*

Medication should be discontinued pending examination if there is a sudden partial or complete loss of vision, or if there is a sudden onset of proptosis, diplopia or migraine. If examination reveals papilledema or retinal vascular lesions, medication should be withdrawn.

reduced breast disease. Additionally, the use of estrogen–progestin appears to increase the risk beyond that seen with estrogen alone.[43]

Long-term government-sponsored trials particularly directed at hormone replacement are HERS (Heart and Estrogen Replacement Study),[44,57,58] ERA (Estrogen Replacement and Arteriosclerosis),[45] and the WHI (Woman's Health Initiative).[59] Those results that have been published report conflicting results concerning long-term cardioprotective effects with replacement therapy. Both ERA and HERS deal with the response to already existing heart disease and provide some consistent evidence of a prophylactic effect for coronary heart disease after the patient has been on an acceptable dosage of HRT for more than two years. Similar studies since show later cardiovascular events in women may occur still in the postmenopause if the treatment is extended.[60]

Unproven general benefits of hormone replacement that have been derived from trials include improved cognitive function,[61–64] protection against colorectal cancer,[27] cardiovascular diseases,[65] lessening of psychiatric illnesses (including Alzheimer's disease),[50] improvement of lipoprotein profile, and protection against cataracts.[66] These findings showed that the relative risks (RR) for the diseases stated was reduced in the various clinical trials. While ideal results, they have not been considered to be clinically proven.

## The Women's Health Initiative

In 1993 the National Institutes of Health (NIH) began the Woman's Health Initiative (WHI). This is described as a major program to determine the putative protective effects of hormone therapy on the common chronic diseases of aging. This program was funded by the NIH for a projected 12-year duration. Other studies, previously mentioned, the HERS was concluded.[57,58]

The grant had several milestones for termination if therapeutic risk became greater than benefit – most evidently coronary heart disease and breast cancer. The HRT used was a combination of conjugated equine estrogen and medroxyprogesterone acetate (Prempro®). These were given to healthy postmenopausal women. The results obtained began to show that with the combined HRT, in this population, the risks outweighed the benefits. The HRT program was halted in July 2002.[67,68]

In March 2004, the second arm of the WHI, which evaluated the effect of unopposed estrogen on women with hysterectomies was discontinued.[69] Again, estrogen was not protective for heart disease and, in addition, there was a persistent increased risk of stroke.[70,71] However, unopposed estrogen in the WHI did not result in an increased risk of breast cancer or heart disease.[69]

Results of the benefits derived and the risks evaluated by several writing groups for the WHI have since been published. These are briefly summarized, and references given where appropriate, in Table 21.7. Additionally, several authors and groups connected to the WHI have issued various reports on women's health problems.[72]

The WHI was a disappointment to everyone, as the risk of stroke and thromboembolic disease was increased with HRT and ERT. Countless journal articles have been written for and against the study and its results.[56,73] Several articles refer to the return of undesirable symptomatology in the patients when the hormones are discontinued.[74] The decrease in use of the replacement therapies has caused a new focus on alternative medications for the symptoms of the menopause and the onset of aging that occurs. New and more cautious uses of hormone replacements are being considered instead of the older doses when considered necessary.[74] These therapies are being prescribed for shorter periods when disturbing symptoms are present.

**Table 21.7** Summary of Women's Health Initiative of menopausal complaints and diagnoses

| | Estrogen alone[a] | Estrogen + progesterone |
|---|---|---|
| **Beneficial effects – relief of:** | | |
| vasomotor symptoms | ++ | + |
| sexual dysfunction | – | – |
| skin changes | + | – |
| genitourinary tract complaints | + | – |
| depression[52] | – | – |
| cognition impairment[52,53,75] | – | – |
| osteoporosis[5] | ++ | + |
| vulvovaginal atrophy | ++ | + |
| **Risks – presence of:** | | |
| breast cancer | –? | + |
| thromboembolic disease[70–72] | + | + |
| stroke[72,76] | + | + |
| pancreatitis and cholecystitis[77] | + | + |
| weight changes | – | – |
| insulin resistance | – | – |
| osteoarthritis | ? | ? |
| cancer – ovarian[78] | + | + |
| cancer – endometrium | | + |
| cancer – colorectum | – | – |

A statistical summary of benefits and risks is listed. The effects found in the WHI or subsequent journal publications are listed as (+) positive, (−) negative or (?) still not statistically evident. This listing is adapted from the summary provided by the American College of Gynecologists Task Force on Hormone Therapy. Obstetrics and Gynecology 2004; 4 (Suppl): 1S–129S.
[a]Hysterectomized patients.

## Pharmacological replacement options with sex hormones

There is no one standard therapeutic regimen that is ideal for hormone replacement throughout the menopausal transition. In addition, there is a variety of estrogen or estrogen and progestin compounds available that may be used as single agents or in combination. The doses vary, and they are administered by several routes (oral, transdermal, and vaginal).[56] The commonly used and commercially available estrogen agents are listed in Table 21.8. This is a current sampling of the many pharmaceutical products by prescription. Table 21.9 provides a number of the alternative medications and catalogued therapies that can be purchased by the patient. Evidently, there has been some difficulty in terminology for describing 'natural' estrogen from plant or animal sources. Most pharmacologists consider 'natural' estrogens as those that are produced endogenously. The final usefulness of an estrogen preparation is generally considered to be based on its biological effectiveness.

In singling out the postmenopausal/geripausal woman, a serious consideration is the dose of the hormone that is given.[15] Several reviews present the problems involved as the woman ages. Particularly appealing would be the reduction in incidence of thromboses, breast tenderness, and dysfunctional uterine bleeding that would occur by minimizing the dose.[15,30,79,80] As a woman goes through the postmenopause and geripause, the incidence of chronic diseases such as diabetes, cardiovascular disease, and neurological problems increases. Thus, the patient should be given the lowest effective dose that alleviates her chronic menopausal symptoms and doesn't interfere with therapy for her other medical conditions. The recent availability of many dose levels to choose from is an asset for the prescribing physician.[54]

During the last several years, a considerable amount of time and effort was spent studying single pharmaceutical products for evidence of effectiveness for specific symptoms. Generally most of the medications used have relatively similar responses but vary only according to dosage and delivery system. Clinicians should choose drugs at doses that accommodate the needs of the individual postmenopausal or geripausal woman according to the accepted standards such as height and weight (body mass index (BMI)) or dose–response expectations. The variable doses of replacement medications now available make dosing levels easier to follow. Treatment can be limited to the personal needs of the patient; therapy can be adjusted for the patient according to the endpoint that results in comfort.

The use of combination estrogen with progestogen therapies is generally required for those women who still have a functional uterus; otherwise abnormal endometrial responses might occur. Hyperplasia or adenosis of the endometrial cells is often seen with irregular bleeding or shedding. This was particularly evident when unopposed estrogen was given. Cyclic or combination medications prevent these changes, and the endometrial carcinoma rate in women on HRT is below that in untreated controls.[17]

### Androgens (testosterone)

The use of testosterone 'replacement' still seems improbable to most clinicians. However, several journal articles on sexuality have indicated that increased desire and satisfaction occur with androgen (testosterone) therapy.[62] Particular attention has been drawn to the use of testosterone therapy for use in women with hypoactive sexual desire.[81–85] The use of androgens in surgical menopausal patients has been described as successful with and without estrogen.[81,85] General information indicates that while serum testosterone levels in women may remain at the premenopausal level, other androgens decrease after the menopause.[86] The authors have found no substantial link that substantiated some of the described usefulness of these androgens in menopausal women.[86]

Side-effects for androgens are cosmetic, i.e. masculinizing changes in skin (acne), hirsutism, and virilism. Other side-effects often seen include fluid retention, breast hypoplasia, sleep apnea, polycythemia, hepatic injury, endometrial hyperplasia, and emotional instability.

Androgens as metabolic steroids may increase musculoskeletal hyperactivity and tone, a factor not fully understood in aging, that is under investigation for elderly women. Sexuality and the use of replacement hormones are discussed in Chapter 6.

### Delivery systems

The delivery systems used are of prime importance. Often, drug delivery techniques have been varied to provide an improvement in personal convenience. Oral medications can be given singly or in a combination daily regimen with elimination of monthly bleeding. New patches have an extended effective life of one or two weeks, and some contain both estrogen and progesterone simultaneously, thus eliminating awkward cyclic therapy. Vaginal rings and body creams/gels/oils containing adequate therapeutic levels have become available. Long-acting rings are placed in the vagina and provide timed sex steroid release as replacement therapy. Each of these methods may permit a desirable effect with therapeutic efficiency.

There has been evidence that women taking oral HRT/ERT may experience a greater risk of gall bladder disease than with dermal patches. This statistical reduction with patches is probably due to the reduction in concentration of estrogen

**Table 21.8**   Hormone replacement/osteoporosis therapies

| Drug name | Generic name | Dose |
|---|---|---|
| **Hormone replacement:** | | |
| **transdermal system** | | |
| Alora® | Estradiol | 0.05 mg 2×/week |
| Esclim® | | |
| Estraderm® | | |
| Vivelle® | | |
| Vivelle-DOT® | | 0.0375 mg 2×/week |
| | | 0.05 mg 2×/week |
| | | 0.075 mg 2×/week |
| | | 0.1 mg 2×/week |
| Climara® | | 0.025 mg/week |
| | | 0.05 mg/week |
| | | 0.075 mg/week |
| | | 0.1 mg/week |
| Menostar® | | 0.014 mg/week |
| Combipatch® | Estradiol + norethindrone | 0.05 mg/0.14 mg 2×/week |
| | | 0.05 mg/0.25 mg 2×/week |
| **Oral therapy/estrogen: cyclic** | | |
| Cenestin® | Synthetic conjugated estrogens | 0.625 mg qd |
| | | 1.25 mg qd |
| Estinyl® | Ethinyl estradiol | 0.02 mg qd |
| | | 0.05 mg qd |
| Estrace® | Estradiol | 1 mg qd |
| | | 2 mg qd |
| Estratab® | Esterified estrogens | 0.625 mg qd |
| Ogen® | Estropipate | 0.625 mg qd |
| Ortho-Est® | | 1.25 mg qd |
| Premarin® | Conjugated estrogens | 0.625 mg qd |
| | | 1.25 mg qd |
| | | 0.3 mg qd |
| **Progestins: cyclic/combo** | | |
| Prometrium® | Progesterone | 200 mg HS/12 day/cycle |
| | | 100 mg/qd/cycle |
| Provera® | Medroxyprogesterone | 2.5 mg qd/combo |
| | | 5 mg qd/combo |
| | | 10 mg qd/12 day/cycle |
| Agestin® | Norethindrone acetate tablets | 5 mg qd |
| **Oral combination products** | | |
| Activella® | Estradiol/norethindrone | 1 mg/0.5 mg qd |
| Estratest® | Esterified estrogens | 1.25 mg/2.5 mg qd |
| Estratest HS® | Methyltestosterone | 0.625 mg/1.25 mg qd |
| Ortho-Prefest® | Estradiol/norgestimate | 1 mg/0 mg QD ×3 alternated with |
| | | 1 mg/0.9 mg qd ×3 |

| Premphase® (cyclic) | Conjugated estrogens/ medroxyprogesterone (2 pills) | 0.625 mg qd ×28 12.5 mg qd ×final 14 0.625 mg qd ×28 1 5 mg qd ×final 14 0.3 mg qd ×28 1 1.5 mg qd ×final 14 0.45 mg qd ×28 1 1.5 mg qd ×final 14 |
| Prempro® (continuous) | Conjugated estrogens/ medroxyprogesterone (1 pill) | 0.3 mg/1.5 mg qd 0.45 mg/1.5 mg qd 0.625 mg/2.5 mg qd 0.625 mg/5 mg qd |

**Vaginal estrogens: creams**

| Estrace® 0.1 mg/g | Estradiol | 1 g 1–3×/week |
| Ogen® | Estropipate 1.5 mg/g | 1 g 1–3×/week |
| Premarin® | Conjugated estrogens 0.625 mg/g | 1 g 1–3×/week |
| Estring® | Estradiol | 1 ring every 3 months 0.0075 mg/24 h |
| Vagifem® | Estradiol 1 tablet vaginally 2×/week | 0.025 mg/tablet |

**Osteoporosis therapy/prevention**

| Actonel® | Risedronate | 5 mg qd |
| Fosamax® | Alendronate | 5 mg qd 10 mg qd 35 mg 1×/week 70 mg 1×/week |
| Boniva® | Ibandronate | 150 mg 1×/month |
| Evista® | Raloxifene | 60 mg qd |
| Miacalcin® | Calcitonin-salmon | 100 IU sc or im daily 200 IU nasally qd |
| Citracal + D® | Calcium citrate + vitamin D | 5 tablets qd |
| Oscal 500 + D® | Calcium carbonate + vitamin D | 3 tablets qd |

Combo, daily with estrogen; cycle, cyclically, last 12 days with estrogen; im, intramuscular. qd, once daily; qhs, one, hour of sleep, sc, subcutaneous.

degradation by the liver and gall bladder during initial venous bypass after absorption.

## Alternative medications in the menopause

Many complimentary and alternative therapies have been suggested medically and by health advocates for postmenopausal and geripausal women, particularly those with specific symptoms that may be related to sex hormone loss (Chapter 22). A short list of the natural estrogens that can be taken appears in Table 21.9.

Other menopausal women may elect to seek relief using alternative medications which may be herbal or plant derived. These forms may also carry contraindications or side-effects, which need to be explained to the woman. The isoflavones as well as certain phytoestrogens have been utilized with some success.[27] The botanicals (herbs) may evidence severe side-effects, and need careful patient directions and dosage adjustment. In most cases, purity of product must be carefully investigated as well.

While not considered an alternative type of medication, several drugs are appropriately recommended for use of certain menopausal symptoms. Those included as effective medications for osteoporosis treatment and prevention are listed in Table 21.8. Some have shown successful responses when used as indicated, and even when administered in intervals up to a year.[76] Osteoporosis and bone problems are discussed in Chapter 14. Exercise has been recommended for menopausal symptomatology (Chapter 24), and in some studies for amelioration of endothelial dysfunction.[87]

**Table 21.9** Alternative menopausal medications

*Creams, gels*
- Pro-Gest: progesterone cream
- Phytoestrogen cream: isoflavones in gel base

*Oral*
- Phytoestrogens (generic): isoflavones
  - genisstein
  - biochanin
  - daidazin
  - formononetin
- Promensil

*Botanicals*
- St John's wort
- Black cohosh
- Ginkgo biloba
- Ginseng
- Chasteberry (monk's pepper)
- Evening primrose
- Dong quai
- Valerian root
- Ginseng

Often patients who may not be candidates for HRT may choose selective estrogen receptor modulators (SERM) therapy. SERMs are specifically effective in treating the bone loss in menopausal women that results in osteopenia. Other uses have been suggested for these prescribed medications since they act as anti-estrogens by modulating the α-estrogen receptors. Full relief from targeted symptoms in the menopause has not yet been indicated.

Therapies for vascular instability (hot flushes) include some of those listed in Table 21.8 as well as psychopharmaceutical products. Limited use of these medications seems indicated except in unusual circumstances. Many women in the late menopause and geripause did not suffer from troublesome hot flushes. If the symptom recurs later, a medical evaluation by a neurologist is often useful. Recently, some of the SERM medications listed have recently been described as providing clinical relief from the discomfort of the flushes in preliminary trials. It is projected that SERM therapy for the menopause, with and without added estrogen, will become available during the next few years.

### The downside of any replacement

Like most therapies, there are specific contraindications, side-effects, and complications when any sex hormones are administered. Tables 21.5 and 21.6 list these briefly, as they are stated in many of the medicine inserts. These facts can be clearly explained to the patient before prescribing. Careful screening is recommended, with physician office visits at least twice a year in most circumstances. When deciding the best care, the likelihood of complications occurring in the patient, from her history, must be weighed against the value of the treatment.[88]

The possibility has been described of reducing doses of both ERT and HRT while maintaining a most effective replacement for certain of the accepted and non-labeled uses. Most desirable is the potential of lower incidences of side-effects, mainly bleeding and breast discomfort. The benefits of these lower doses in retaining bone mineral density (BMD), favoring lipid-cholesterol metabolism, preventing dysfunctional uterine bleeding and breast pain, controlling vasomotor symptoms, and reducing vulvovaginal atrophy continue to be evaluated by clinical trials.

This provides an important area for specificity of symptoms. Since the menopausal problems are not universal in women, both the dosage and product employed should be tailored to the need. Certainly both side-effects and complications can be reduced.

### The use of estrogen in postmenopausal–geripausal women

Throughout this textbook, references have been made to the increased longevity for women found in all developed countries in this 21st century. Projections for 2010 show that a life expectancy of 81 years for women and 74 years for men is likely. However, quality of life reports have shown that women have twice as many medical disorders as men, prior to their deaths requiring care. This accounts for major healthcare utilization for older women. The number of postmenopausal women will reach 1.2 billion worldwide by 2030, with 47 million new menopausal women each year.[59] The size of the geripause population grows by leaps and bounds as the years go on.

Prescription plan data reveal that the percentage of women aged 40–60 years who were most likely to start HRT stood at 20% during 2005. This level saw a decline in those older than 65 years (the geripause) to 15%, and a further fall in women older than 80 years, to 7%. Improving the hormone dosage given by reducing the medication to the minimum needed for the individual is a reasonable trial. The reason for the change in interest is fear of any potential medical problems combined with aging, which might further complicate a woman's life. Thus, the weight of evidence on benefits versus difficulties in this aging population becomes complex.[89]

## QUALITY OF LIFE

Recent studies on quality of life (QOL) during aging have been connected with several projects. The HERS study group used a 'QOL questionnaire' that uniquely assessed functional capacity, emotional health, vitality and depression. Hormone therapy seemed to have mixed results in these women (50–80 years). The effects on improving their QOL depended on the presence of existing menopausal symptoms.[66] Unfortunately, the HERS population was an unhealthy population since all its members had survived a cardiovascular incident.

Editorials have indicated that no final rules can be made at this time. Few of the controlled programs include the QOL or emotional status of women on estrogen therapy. No large prolonged study has obtained results that are statistically suitable to postulate an overall safe therapeutic regimen.

## CONCLUSIONS

Physicians and clinical scientists have provided medical care that has successfully resulted in longevity and an improving physical health. Maintaining a desirable quality of life continues to be an exceptional goal. Individualized therapies are the potential mechanisms for maintaining desirable levels of function for menopausal women, and should continue to be tenaciously investigated.

## REFERENCES

1. Gerwitz JH. Incidence and preventability of adverse drug events among older persons in the ambulatory setting. JAMA 2003; 289: 1107–16.
2. Rochon PA, Gurwitz JH. Prescribing for seniors, neither too much or too little. JAMA 1999; 252: 113–15.
3. Rochon PA, Anderson GM, Tu JM et al. Age and gender-related use of low dose drug therapy: the need for manufacture 'seniors' doses. J Am Geriatr Soc 1999; 47: 954–9.
4. Barron HV, Viskin S, Lundstrom RJ et al. Beta-blocker dosage and mortality after myocardial infarction. Arch Intern Med 1998; 158: 449–53.
5. US. Food and Drug Administration. Guideline for the Study of Drugs Likely to be Used in the Elderly. Rockville, MD: Food and Drug Administration Center for Drug Evaluation and Research, 1999.
6. Zhan C, Sangl J, Bierman AS et al. Potentially inappropriate medication use in the community-dwelling elderly. JAMA 2002; 286: 2823–9.
7. Lindley C, Tuly M, Parmasothy V, Tallis R. Inappropriate medication is a major cause of adverse drug reactions in elderly patients. Age Aging 1992; 21: 294–30.
8. Gurwitz J. Suboptimal medication use in the elderly, the tip of the iceberg. JAMA 1994; 272: 316–17.
9. Nash D. Keonig J, Chatterton M. Why the Elderly Need Individual and Pharmaceutical Care. Philadelphia PA: Office of Health Policy and Clinical Outcomes. Thomas Jefferson University, 2000.
10. Institute of Medicine. To Err is Human: Building a Safer Health System. Washington, DC: National Academy Press, 1999.
11. Gosney W, Tallis R. Prescription of contraindicated and interacting drugs in elderly patients admitted to the hospital. Lancet 1984; 1: 564–7.
12. Ray W. Federspie C, Schaffner W. A study of antipsychotic drug use in nursing homes. epidemiologic evidence suggesting misuse. Am J Public Health 1980; 70: 485–91.
13. Beers MH, Ouslander JH, Fingold SF et al. Inappropriate medication prescribing in skilled nursing facilities. Ann Intern Med 1992; 117: 684–9.
14. Williams B, Betley C. Inappropriate use of nonpsychotrophic medications in nursing homes. J Am Geriatr Soc 1995; 43: 513–19.
15. Spore D, Mor V, Larrat P, Hawes C, Hiris J. Inappropriate drug prescriptions for elderly residents of board and care facilities. Am J Public Health 1997; 87: 404–9.
16. Aparasu R, Fliginger S. Inappropriate medication prescribing for the elderly by office-based physicians. Ann Pharmacother 1997; 31: 823–9.
17. Mort JR, Aparasu RR. Prescribing potentially inappropriate psychotropic medications to the ambulatory elderly. Arch Intern Med 2000; 160: 2825–31.
18. Aparasu R, Sitzman S. Inappropriate prescribing for elderly outpatients. Am J Health Syst Pharm 1999; 56: 433–9.
19. Golden A, Preston R, Barnet S et al. Inappropriate medication prescribing in homebound older adults. J Am Geriatr Soc 1999; 47: 948–53.
20. Wilcox SW, Himmelstein D, Woolhandler S. Inappropriate drug prescribing for the community-dwelling elderly. JAMA 1994; 47: 948–53.
21. US General Accounting Office. Prescription Drugs and the Elderly. Many Still Received Potentially Harmful Drugs Despite Recent Improvement. Washington, DC: US General Accounting Office, 1995.
22. Stagnitti MN. The top five therapeutic classes of outpatient prescription drugs ranked by total expense for the Medicare population age 65 and older in the US civilian non-institutionalized population, 2003. Medical Expenditure Panel Survey. Baltimore, MD: Agency for Healthcare Research and Quality. Jan 2006; Statistical Brief #109.
23. Beers MH, Ouslander JC, Rolingher I, Reuben D, Brooks J. Explicit criteria for determining inappropriate

medication use in nursing homes. Arch Intern Med 1991; 151: 1825–32.

24. Anderson G, Beers M, Kerkuk K. Auditing prescription practice using exploit criteria and computerized drug benefit claims data. J Eval Clin Pract 1997; 3: 283–94.

25. Beers MH. Exploit criteria for determining potentially inappropriate medication use by the elderly: an update. Arch Intern Med 1997; 157: 1531–6.

26. Gambrell RD, Natrajan PK. Hormone replacement therapy. In: Eskin BA, ed. The Menopause: Comprehensive Management, 4th edn. New York and London: Parthenon Publishing, 2000: 257–73.

27. Henderson VW, Paganimi-Hill A, Emanuel CK, Dunn ME et al. Estrogen replacement therapy in older women. Arch Neurol 1994; 51: 896–900.

28. Sites CK, L'Hommedieu GD, Toth MJ, Brochu M, Cooper BC, Fairhurst PA. The effect of hormone replacement therapy on body composition, body fat distribution and insulin sensitivity in menopausal women: a randomized, double-blind, placebo-controlled trial. J Clin Endocrinol Metab 2005; 90: 2701–7.

29. Carr BR. HRT management: the American experience. Eur J Obstet Gynecol Reprod Biol 1996; 64 (Suppl): S17–S20.

30. Andrews WC. Trend to lower doses of ERT/HRT for the management of menopause [Review]. ACLG Clinical Review 2001; 6: 1–16.

31. Eskin BA, Trivedi RA, Weideman CA, Walker RF. Positive feedback disturbances and infertility in women over thirty. Am J Gynecol Health 1988; 2: 110.

32. Roth GS. Hormone receptor changes during adulthood and senescence: significance for aging research. Fed Proc 1979; 38: 910.

33. Campbell S, Whitehead M. Oestrogen therapy and the menstrual syndrome. Clin Obstet Gynaecol 1977; 4: 31–47.

34. Vellareal DT. Osteopenic effects of HRT in physically frail, elderly women. JAMA 2001; 286: 815–20.

35. Daly E, Vessey MP, Hawkins MM, Caarson JL, Gough P, March S. Risk of venous thromboembolism in users of hormone replacement therapy. Lancet 1996; 348: 977–80.

36. Grodstein F, Stampfer MJ, Goldhaber SZ et al. Prospective study of exogenous hormones and risk of pulmonary embolism in women. Lancet 1996; 348: 983–7.

37. Jack H, Derby LE, Mters MW, Vassalages C, Newton KM. Risk of hospital admission for idiopathic venous thromboembolism among users of postmenopausal oestrogens. Lancet 1996; 348: 981–3.

38. The Writing Group for the PEPI Trial. Effects of hormone replacement therapy on endometrial histology in postmenopausal women. JAMA 1996; 275: 370–5.

39. Colditz GA, Hankinson SE, Hunter DJ et al. The use of estrogens and progestins and the risk of breast cancer in postmenopausal women. N Engl J Med 1995; 332: 1589–93.

40. Cauley JA, Seeley DJ, Ensrud K et al. Estrogen replacement therapy and fractures in older women. Ann Intern Med 1995; 122: 9–16.

41. Altkorn D, Vokes T. Treatment of postmenopausal osteoporosis [Review]. JAMA 2001; 285: 1415–17.

42. Eskin BA. Endocrinology of the breast. In: Eskin BA, Asbell SO, Jardines L, eds. Breast Disease for the Primary Care Physician. New York and London: Parthenon Publishing Group, 1999.

43. Schairer C, Lubin J, Troisi R et al. Menopausal estrogen and estrogen-progestin replacement therapy and breast cancer risk. JAMA 2000; 283: 485–91.

44. Hulley S, Grady D, Bush T et al. Randomized trial of estrogen plus progestin for secondary prevention of coronary heart disease in postmenopausal women. JAMA 1985; 280: 608–13.

45. Herrington DM, Reboussin DM, Brosnilian KB et al. Effects of estrogen replacemen on the progression of coronary artery atherosclerosis. N Engl J Med 2000; 343: 522–9.

46. Siris ES, Miller PD, Barrett-Conner E et al. Identification and fracture outcomes of undiagnosed low BMD in postmenopausal women. National Osteoporosis Risk Assessment. JAMA 2001; 286: 2815–22.

47. Cauley JA, Seeley DJ, Ensrud K et al. Estrogen replacement therapy and fractures in older women. Ann Intern Med 1995; 122: 9–16.

48. American College of Obstetricians and Gynecologists. RCOG Educational Bulletin No. 247. Washington DC: American College of Obstetricians and Gynecologists, May 1998.

49. Campbell S, Whitehead M. Oestrogen therapy and the menstrual syndrome. Clin Obstet Gynaecol 1977; 4: 31–47.

50. Honjo H, Tanaka K, Kashiwagi T. Senile dementia – Alzheimer's type and estrogen. Horm Metab Res 1995; 27: 204–7.

51. Banks E, Beral V, Reeves G, Balkwill A, Barnes I (for the Million Women Study Collaborators). Fracture incidence in relation to the pattern of use of hormone therapy in postmenopausal women. JAMA 2004; 291: 2212–20.

52. Espeland MA, Rapp SR, Shumaker SA et al (for the Women's Health Initiative Memory Study Investigators). Conjugated equine estrogens and global cognitive function in postmenopausal women. JAMA 2004; 291: 2959–68.

53. Shumaker SA, Legault C, Kuller L et al. (for the Women's Health Initiative Memory Study Investigators). Conjugated equine estrogens and incidence of probable dementia and mild cognitive impairment in postmenopausal women: WHI Memory Study. JAMA 2004; 291: 2947–58.

54. Utian WH, Shoupe D, Bachmann G et al. Relief of vasomotor symptoms and vaginal atrophy with lower doses of conjugated equine estrogens and medroxyprogesterone acetate. Fertil Steril 2001; 75: 1065–79.

55. Sowers MR, Matthews KA et al. Hemostatic factors and estrogen during the menopausal transition. J Clin Endocrinol Metab 2005; 90: 5942–8.

56. Hickey M, Davis SR, Sturdee DW. Treatment of menopausal symptoms: what shall we do now? Lancet 2005; 366: 409–21.

57. Hulley S, Grady D, Bush T et al. Randomized trial of estrogen plus progestin for secondary prevention of coronary heart disease in postmenopausal women. Heart and Estrogen/progestin Replacement Study (HERS) Research Group. JAMA 1998; 280: 605–13.

58. Grady D, Herrington D, Bittner V et al, HERS Research Group. Cardiovascular disease outcomes during 6.8 years of hormone study. Heart and Estrogen/progestin Replacement Study follow-up (HERS II). JAMA 2002; 288: 41064.

59. The Women's Health Initiative Study Group. Design of the Women's Health Initiative Clinical Trial and Observational Study. Control Clin Trials 1998; 19: 61–109.

60. Mackey RH, Kuller LH, Sutton-Tyrrell K, Evans RW, Holubkov R, Matthews KA. Hormone therapy lipoprotein subclasses, and coronary calcification: the Healthy Women Study. Arch Int Med 2005; 165: 510–15.

61. Kampen DL, Sherwin BB. Estrogen use and verbal memory in healthy postmenopausal women. Obstet Gynecol 1994; 83: 979–83.

62. Sherwin BB. Estrogen and/or androgen replacement therapy and cognitive functioning in surgically menopausal women. Psychoneuroendocrinology 1988; 13: 345–57.

63. Fillit H, Weinreb H, Cholst I et al. Observations in a preliminary open trial of estradiol therapy for senile dementia-Alzheimer's type. Psychoneuroendocrinology 1986; 11: 337–45.

64. Funk JL, Mortel KF, Meyer JS. Effects of estrogen replacement therapy on cerebral perfusion and cognition among postmenopausal women. Dementia 1991; 1: 268–72.

65. Grodstein F, Manson JE, Colditz GA, Willett WC, Speizer FE, Stampfer MJ. A prospective observational study of postmenopausal hormone therapy and primary prevention of cardiovascular disease. Ann Intern Med 2000; 133: 933–41.

66. Freeman EE, Munoz B, Schain OD, West SK et al. Hormone replacement may protect against cataracts. Arch Ophthalmol 2001; 199: 1687–92.

67. US Preventive Services Task Force. Hormone therapy for the prevention of chronic conditions in postmenopausal women: recommendations from the US Preventive Services Task Force. Ann Intern Med 2005; 142: 855–60.

68. Rossouw JE, Anderson GL, Prentice RL et al. Writing Group for the Women's Health Initiative Investigators. Risks and benefits of estrogen plus progestin in healthy postmenopausal women: principal results from WHI randomized control trial. JAMA 2002; 288: 321–33.

69. Anderson GL, Limacher M, Assef AR et al. (WHI Steering Committee). Effects of conjugated equine estrogen in postmenopausal women with hysterectomy: the WHI trial. JAMA 2004; 291: 1701–12.

70. Smith NL, Heckbert SR, Lemaitre RN et al. Esterified estrogens and conjugated equine estrogens and the risk of venous thrombosis. JAMA 2004; 292: 1581–7.

71. Cushman M, Kuller LH, Prentice R et al. (for the Women's Health Initiative Investigators). Estrogen plus progestin and risk of venous thrombosis: for the Women's Health Initiative Investigators. J Am Med Assoc 2004; 292: 1573–1580.

72. Howard BW, Manson JE (Writing Group for the WHI). Low-fat dietary pattern and weight change over 7 years: The WHI Dietary Modification Trial. JAMA 2006; 295: 39–49.

73. Ostrzenski A, Ostrzenska KM. WHI clinical trial revisit: imprecise scientific methodology disqualifies the study's outcome. Am J Obstet Gynecol 2005; 193: 1599–606.

74. Ockene JK, Barad DH Cochrane BB et al. Symptom experience after discontinuing use of estrogen plus progestin. JAMA 2005; 294: 183–93.

75. Kang JH, Weuve J, Grodstein F. Postmenopausal hormone therapy and risk of cognitive decline in community-dwelling aging women. Neurology 2004; 63: 101–7.

76. Bath PM, Gray LJ. Association between hormone replacement therapy and subsequent stroke: a meta-analysis. BMJ 2005; 330: 342.

77. Cirillo DJ, Wallace RB, Rodabough RG. Effect of estrogen therapy on gallbladder disease. JAMA 2005; 293: 330–9.

78. Glud E, Kjaer SK, Thomsen BL et al. Hormone therapy and the impact of estrogen intake on the risk of ovarian cancer. Arch Int Med 2004; 164: 2253–9.

79. Speroff L, Whitcomb RW, Kempfers NJ et al. Efficacy and local tolerance of a low-dose 7-day matrix estradiol transdermal system in the treatment of menopausal vasomotor symptoms. Obstet Gynecol 1996; 88: 587–92.

80. Reid IR, Brown JP, Burckhardt P et al. Intravenous zoledronic acid in postmenopausal women with low bone mineral density. N Engl J Med 2002; 346: 653–61.

81. Shifren JL, Braunstein GD, Simon JA et al. Transdermal testosterone treatment in women with impaired sexual function after oophorectomy. N Engl J Med 2000; 343: 682–8.

82. Lobo RA, Rosen RC, Yang HM. Comparative effects of oral esterified estrogens with and without methyltestosterone on endocrine profiles and dimensions of sexual function in postmenopausal women with hypoactive sexual desire. Fertil Steril 2003; 79: 1341–52.

83. Bachmann G, Bancroft J, Braunstein JD et al. Female androgen insufficiency: the Princeton concensus statement on definition, classification and assessment. Fertil Steril 2002; 77: 660–5.

84. Simon JA, Nachtigall LE, Davis SR, Utian WH et al. Transdermal testosterone patch improves sexual activity and desire in surgically menopausal women. Obstet Gynecol 2004; 1003: 645–5.

85. Addis IB, Ireland CC Vittinghoff E, Lin F, Stuenkel CA, Hulley S. Sexual activity and function in postmenopausal women with heart disease. Obstet Gynecol 2005; 106: 121–7.

86. Davis SR, Davison SL, Donath S, Bell RJ. Circulating androgen levels and self-reported sexual function in women. JAMA 2005; 294: 91–6.

87. Harvey PJ, Picton PE, Su WS, Morris BL, Notarius CF, Floras JS. Exercise as an alternative to oral estrogen for amelioration of endothelial dysfunction in postmenopausal women. Am Heart J 2005; 149: 291–7.

88. Kuh D, Langenberg C, Hardy R et al. Cardiovascular risk at age 53 years in relation to the menopause transition and use of hormone replacement therapy: a prospective British birth cohort study. Br J Obstet Gynaecol 2005; 112: 476–85.

89. Ness J, Aronow WS, Newkirk E, McDanel D. Use of hormone replacement therapy by postmenopausal women after publication of the Women's Health Initiative Trial. J Gerontol A Biol Sci Med Sci 2005; 60: 460–2.

# Chapter 22

# Complementary and alternative therapies

Edzard Ernst

## INTRODUCTION

The definition adopted by the Cochrane Collaboration describes complementary/alternative medicine (CAM) as 'diagnosis, treatment and/or prevention which complements mainstream medicine by contributing to a common whole, by satisfying a demand not met by orthodoxy or by diversifying the conceptual frameworks of medicine'.[1] CAM entails a bewildering array of therapeutic and diagnostic modalities (Table 22.1). Some common features of CAM include:

- the emphasis is on holism
- treatments are alleged to be natural
- treatments are often assumed to be harmless
- treatments often need to be individualized
- the emphasis is on the body's power to heal itself
- a long tradition of usage exists
- by and large, CAM is private healthcare.

CAM has become increasingly important for most healthcare professionals simply because patients are voting with their feet in favour of it. Many doctors remain sceptical about its value, and few have in-depth knowledge about it. But, because of its popularity, it seems desirable that conventional healthcare providers know the basics of CAM.

## PREVALENCE

In each year, about 65% of all US citizens seem to try at least one form of CAM.[2] These figures can be even higher in patient populations, especially those suffering from chronic conditions. Virtually all surveys agree that women use CAM signifi-

cantly more often than men. Menopausal women frequently try CAM, and dietary supplements, spiritual approaches, exercise, herbal medicines, and homoeopathy are particularly popular options.[3]

## REASONS FOR POPULARITY

Many conventional healthcare providers are puzzled by the popularity and commercial success of CAM. Arguably, conventional drugs are more effective than ever before. So why do people turn towards 'alternatives'?

The first important point to make here is that CAM is not normally employed as an alternative. Usually it is used as an 'add on' to conventional healthcare. In the majority of instances the term 'alternative medicine' is therefore wrong.

The second important point is that no single reason or set of reasons for the popularity of CAM exists. It all depends on what CAM is being used for. Imagine a woman suffering from a potentially life-threatening condition, e.g. breast cancer, and someone with menopausal symptoms. Their reasons for trying CAM will evidently be dramatically different.

Notwithstanding these caveats, research has identified numerous reasons for trying such products. We tend to divide them into positive (pull) and negative (push) factors (Tables 22.1 and 22.2).[4] Depending on the precise circumstances, the relative importance of these factors will vary considerably.

Much of the current high popularity of complementary medicine amounts to a criticism of conventional healthcare. This can be seen as a

**Table 22.1**   The most important modalities in complementary and alternative medicine

| Name | Description |
| --- | --- |
| Acupuncture | Insertion of a needle into the skin and underlying tissues in special sites, known as points, for therapeutic or preventive purposes |
| Aromatherapy | The controlled use of plant essences for therapeutic purposes |
| Bach flower remedies | A therapeutic system that uses specially prepared plant infusions to balance physical and emotional disturbances |
| Biofeedback | The use of apparatus to monitor, amplify and feed back information on physiological responses so that a patient can learn to regulate these responses. It is a form of psychophysiological self-regulation |
| Chelation therapy | A method for removing toxins, minerals, and metabolic wastes from the bloodstream and vessel walls using intravenous EDTA (ethylene diamine tetra-acetic acid) infusions |
| Chiropractic | A system of health care which is based on the belief that the nervous system is the most important determinant of health, and that most diseases are caused by spinal subluxations which respond to spinal manipulation |
| Craniosacral therapy | A proprietary form of therapeutic manipulation which is tissue-, fluid-, membrane-, and energy-orientated, and more subtle than any other type of cranial work |
| Herbalism | The medical use of preparations that contain exclusively plant material |
| Homoeopathy | A therapeutic method using preparations of substances whose effects when administered to healthy subjects correspond to the manifestations of the disorder (symptoms, clinical signs, and pathological states) in the unwell patient |
| Hypnotherapy | The induction of a trance-like state to facilitate the relaxation of the conscious mind and make use of enhanced suggestibility to treat psychological and medical conditions, and effect behavioural changes |
| Massage | A method of manipulating the soft tissue of whole body areas using pressure and traction |
| Naturopathy | An eclectic system of health care, which integrates elements of complementary and conventional medicine to support and enhance self-healing processes |
| Osteopathy | A form of manual therapy involving massage, mobilization and spinal manipulation |
| Reflexology | A therapeutic method that uses manual pressure applied to specific areas, or zones, of the feet (and sometimes the hands or ears) that are believed to correspond to areas of the body, in order to relieve stress and prevent and treat physical disorders |
| Relaxation therapy | Techniques for eliciting the 'relaxation response' of the autonomic nervous system |
| Spiritual healing | The direct interaction between one individual (the healer) and a second (sick) individual, with the intention of bringing about an improvement or cure of the illness |
| Yoga | A practice of gentle stretching, exercises for breath control and meditation as a mind–body intervention |

backlash from the spirit of the mid-20th century when we expected science to achieve everything. Reality turned out to be different. Consumers now feel disappointed that so many medical conditions cannot be cured or adequately alleviated (i.e. without side-effects). Complementary medicines, on the other hand, are 'free' of safety problems – at least this is what proponents incessantly claim, and many consumers believe.

The delivery process of conventional healthcare is also often perceived as wanting. This includes the (allegation of) poor therapeutic relationships

**Table 22.2** Positive and negative motivations for trying complementary and alternative medicine

*Positive motivations*

- Hope for increased wellbeing and other positive outcomes
- Philosophical congruence:
  - spiritual dimension
  - emphasis on holism
  - active role of patient
  - explanation intuitively acceptable
  - natural treatments
- Personal control over treatment
- Good relationship with therapist:
  - on equal terms
  - time for discussion
  - allows for emotional factors
- Accessibility

*Negative motivations*

- Dissatisfaction with certain aspects of conventional medicine:
  - ineffective
  - adverse effects
  - poor communication with health care practitioner
  - insufficient time with health care practitioner
- Total rejection of conventional medicine:
  - anti-science or anti-establishment attitude
- Desperation

with conventional healthcare providers. Arthritis sufferers, who use both complementary and general practitioners for their condition, experience the therapeutic relationship much more satisfactorily with the former compared to the latter group of professionals.[5] Inadequate delivery of

healthcare also covers issues such as long waiting lists or too short consultation times.

Desperation can be another powerful push factor. Imagine a patient who has been given a diagnosis of cancer. Is it not understandable that she looks everywhere for help? And there are plenty of promises of a cure in complementary medicine![6] The fact that these are often false promises is usually not known by those who are led by desperation.

Users of CAM usually learn from friends or the media about the latest 'alternative'. The UK media seem to have jumped on the bandwagon of uncritical and often misleading promotion of unproven treatments. Who can blame the consumer (or politician) for being influenced by this incessant flow of misinformation? A recent UK government-sponsored patient guide, for instance, perpetuates the self-interested myths promoted by the 'alternative' industry, and is irresponsibly devoid of information on risk and benefit.[7] Consumers are seduced by promises of better health, fewer side-effects, and enhanced wellness.

Philosophical congruence with many aspects of CAM is another important 'pull factor'. Philosophical congruence essentially means that many messages of CAM ring intuitively true. We all want to be treated as whole human beings, take active roles in our healthcare, or feel that natural means benign. Again, these messages may not be totally correct (e.g. natural is not the same as harmless; think of hemlock!). And again, there is much criticism here of conventional healthcare delivery. For instance, all good medicine has always been (and should always be) 'holistic'.[8] Complementary medicine therefore has by no means a monopoly on holism. But consumers may well have a point when they experience their own healthcare as suboptimal and reductionist. People

**Table 22.3** Randomized controlled trials of herbal medicines lacking replication

| Herbal medicine | Sample size | Control intervention | Result | Reference |
|---|---|---|---|---|
| Dong quai (*Angelica sinensis*) | 71 | Placebo | No superiority over placebo | 27 |
| Evening primrose (*Oenothera biennis*) | 56 | Placebo | No superiority over placebo | 28 |
| Ginkgo biloba | 31 | Placebo | Modest effect on cognitive function | 29 |
| Ginseng (*Panax ginseng*) | 384 | Placebo | No superiority over placebo | 30 |
| Pueraria lobata | 129 | HRT | No significant improvements | 31 |
| Wild yam (*Dioscorea villosa*) | 23 | Placebo | No superiority over placebo | 32 |

are often attracted to complementary therapists by their human approach to healthcare delivery. Through them, patients experience all the sympathy, understanding, empathy, etc they crave.[5] However, I argue that we should not have to consult complementary practitioners to benefit from this; conventional healthcare should provide it as well.

## THE EVIDENCE FOR OR AGAINST CAM

Even though often denied by proponents of CAM, most therapies can be tested for effectiveness in randomized clinical trials (RCTs). Occasionally, the standard RCT design requires adaptation to fit the demands of CAM,[9] but there are no compelling reasons in principle why CAM should defy scientific testing. This discussion regarding the effectiveness of CAM will therefore be based on evidence from clinical trials and (where available) systematic reviews of such studies.

### Acupuncture

Acupuncture is often recommended for the management of menopausal symptoms such as hot flushes. RCTs have arrived at conflicting results; some concluding that acupuncture is useful,[10–12] others that it is not.[13] The totality of this evidence is therefore not convincing.[14]

Even though not devoid of serious adverse effects, acupuncture is by and large safe. The largest prospective study of almost 100 000 cases demonstrated that serious events (e.g. pneumothorax) are extreme rarities and mild, transient events (e.g. pain and bleeding) occur in about 7% of all patients.[15]

### Herbal medicine

Many herbal medicines contain phytoestrogens which theoretically could be useful in the treatment of menopausal complaints. Certainly they have become highly popular, particularly since the views of many women on hormone replacement therapy (HRT) have changed considerably.

Black cohosh (*Actaea racemosa*) is a herbal medicine that has long been associated with estrogenic effects, even though the evidence favors the hypothesis that it works via its activity on the central nervous system.[16] A systematic review included four RCTs of black cohosh, with a total of 226 patients. The methodologically best study was negative, while the less rigorous trials suggested beneficial effects on menopausal symptoms. The conclusions of this systematic review were therefore not strongly in favour of black cohosh's effectiveness.[17] Since the publication of this article, two further RCTs have emerged. Both are of adequate scientific rigor, and both suggest that black cohosh is effective in managing vasomotor symptoms of menopause.[18,19] Thus the totality of the evidence on this herbal remedy is encouraging but not compelling. The adverse effects of black cohosh are rare and usually mild: gastrointestinal complaints, hypotension, headache, dizziness, nausea, and allergic reactions.[4]

Kava (*Piper methysticum*) is a herbal medicine with well-established anxiolytic efficacy.[20] Three double-blind, placebo-controlled RCTs with menopausal women suggest that it improves mood and other symptoms in such patients.[21–23] Unfortunately kava has been associated with hepatotoxicity. About 80 cases, some of them severe, have been reported worldwide. For that reason, it has been withdrawn from the market in several countries.[24]

Red clover (*Trifolium pratense*) has estrogenic properties. Seventeen RCTs with a total of 1160 patients are available. A systematic review and meta-analysis of these studies showed a significant but modest effect on the frequency of hot flushes. On average a reduction of 1.5 hot flushes per day was noted.[25] Adverse effects of red clover are rare, transient and mild: breast tenderness, menstruation changes, and weight gain are the most frequently recorded adverse effects.[4]

Other isoflavones or phytoestrogens have also been tested for controlling menopausal symptoms. A systematic review of 25 RCTs with a total of 2348 patients found no overall effect on hot flushes or other menopausal symptoms.[26] It is as yet unclear whether or not phytoestrogens are burdened with adverse effects similar to those of synthetic estrogens.

Numerous other herbal treatments are often recommended. Table 22.3 summarizes the data from RCTs of further herbal medicines as treatments for menopause.[27–32] For all of them independent replications have yet to be published.

### Relaxation

Three RCTs have suggested that relaxation therapies, e.g. progressive muscle relaxation, convey beneficial effects on menopausal women.[33–35]

Specifically, hot flushes seem to be reduced by this approach.

## Supplements

A systematic review of soy supplements included 13 RCTs, some of which were rigorous.[36] The majority, but not all of these studies, showed significantly positive effects on hot flushes. The conclusion was therefore cautiously positive. Epidemiological data seem to imply that soy is not associated with major risks. An RCT of vitamin E did not suggest that this treatment was superior to placebo.[37]

## Other treatments

Preliminary data suggest that regular Tai Chi reduces postmenopausal bone loss.[38] It is, however, unclear whether this type of exercise is more effective than conventional types. An RCT of reflexology demonstrated that this treatment was not superior to sham-therapy for controlling menopausal symptoms.[39]

## CONCLUSION

CAM is used by many postmenopausal women. Numerous RCTs have tested the effectiveness of a range of CAM therapies. Encouraging, albeit not fully convincing, results have emerged for black cohosh, red clover, relaxation techniques, and soy. The effect sizes of all of these options are modest, and probably less than those of HRT. None of these treatments have been associated with serious adverse effects when used adequately. Therefore these treatments might be worth considering in some patients, particularly those who reject HRT.

## REFERENCES

1. Ernst E, Resch KL, Mills S et al. Complementary medicine – a definition. Br J Gen Pract 1995; 45: 506.
2. Barnes PM, Powell-Griner E, McFann K, Nahin RL. Complementary and alternative medicine use among adults: United States, 2002. Advance Data from Vital and Health Statistics. Hyattsville, Maryland: National Center for Health Statistics, 2004; 343: 1.
3. Kass-Annese B. Alternative therapies for menopause. Clin Obstet Gynecol 2000; 43: 163–83.
4. Ernst E, Pittler MH, Stevinson C, White AR. The desktop guide to complementary and alternative medicine. Edinburgh: Mosby, 2001.
5. Resch K, Hill S, Ernst E. Use of complementary therapies by individuals with 'arthritis'. Clin Rheumatol 1997; 16: 391–5.
6. Schmidt K, Ernst E. Assessing websites on complementary and alternative medicine for cancer. Ann Oncol 2004; 15: 733–42.
7. The Prince of Wales's Foundation for Integrated Health. The Prince of Wales's Foundation for Integrated Health: Complementary Healthcare: a Guide for Patients. www.fihealth.org.
8. Calman K. The profession of medicine. BMJ 1994; 309: 1140–3.
9. Ernst E. Randomised clinical trials: unusual designs. Perfusion 2004; 17: 416–21.
10. Wyon Y, Lindgren R, Hammar M, Lundeberg T. Acupuncture against climacteric disorders? Lower number of symptoms after menopause. Crit Care Clin 1994; 91: 2318–22.
11. Kraft K, Coulon S. Effect of a standardised acupuncture treatment on complaints, blood pressure and serum lipids of hypertensive postmenopausal women. A randomized controlled clinical study. Forsch Komplementärmed 1999; 6: 74–9.
12. Cohen SM, Rousseau ME, Carey BL. Can acupuncture ease the symptoms of menopause? Holist Nurs Pract 2003; 17: 295–9.
13. Sandberg M, Wijma K, Wyon Y, Nedstrand E, Hammar M. Effects of electro-acupuncture on psychological distress in postmenopausal women. Complement Ther Med 2002; 10: 161–9.
14. White AR. A review of controlled trials of acupuncture for women's reproductive healthcare. J Fam Plann Reprod Health Care 2003; 29: 233–6.
15. Melchart D, Weidenhammer W, Streng A et al. Prospective investigation of adverse effects of acupuncture in 97 733 patients. Arch Intern Med 2004; 164: 104–5.
16. Borrelli F, Izzo AA, Ernst E. Pharmacological effects of Cimicifuga racemosa. Life Sci 2003; 73: 1215–29.
17. Borrelli F, Ernst E. Cimifuga racemosa: a systematic review of its clinical efficacy. Eur J Clin 2002; 58: 235–41.
18. Wuttke W, Seidlová-Wuttke D, Gorkow C. The Cimicifuga preparation BNO 1055 vs. conjugated estrogens in a double-blind placebo-controlled study: effects on menopause symptoms and bone markers. Maturitas 2003; 44: S67–S77.
19. Liske E, Hanggi W, Henneicke-von Zepelin HH, Boblitz N, Wustenberg P, Rahlfs VW. Physiological investigation of a unique extract of black cohosh (Cimicifugae racemosae rhizoma): a 6-month clinical study demonstrates no systematic estrogenic effect. J Womens Health Gend Based Med 2002; 11: 163–74.
20. Pittler MH, Ernst E. Kava Extract for Treating Anxiety (Cochrane review). In: The Cochrane Library, Issue 1. Oxford: Update Software, 2002.
21. Warnecke G. Wirksamkeit von Kawa-Kawa-Extrakt beim klimakterischen Syndrom. Zeitschrift für Phytotherapie 1990; 11: 81–6.
22. Warnecke G. Psychosomatische Dysfunktionen im weiblichen Klimakterium: Klinische Wirksamkeit und Verträglichkeit von Kava-Extrakt WS 1490. Fortschr Med 1991; 109: 119–22.
23. De Leo V, La Marca A, Lanzetta D et al. Valutazione dell'associazione di estratto di kava-kava e terapia ormonale sostitutiva nel trattamento d'ansia in postmenopausa. Minerva Ginecol 2000; 52: 263–7.

24. Ernst E. Kava – update: a European perspective. N Z Med J 2004; 117: U1143.

25. Thompson Coon J, Pittler MH, Ernst E. The role of red clover isoflavones in women's reproductive health: a systematic review and meta-analysis of randomised clinical trials. Phytomedicine 2006 (submitted for publication).

26. Krebs EE, Ensrud KE, MacDonald R, Wilt TJ. Phytoestrogens for treatment of menopausal symptoms: a systematic review. Obstet Gynecol 2004; 104: 824–36.

27. Hirata JD, Swiersz LM, Zell B, Small R, Ettinger B. Does dong quai have estrogenic effects in postmenopausal women? A double-blind, placebo-controlled trial. Fertil Steril 1997; 68: 981–6.

28. Chenoy S. Effect of oral gamolenic acid from evening primrose oil on menopausal flushing. BMJ 1994; 308: 501–3.

29. Hartley DE, Heinze L, Elsabagh S, File SE. Effects on cognition and mood in postmenopausal women of 1-week treatment with Ginkgo biloba. Pharmacol Biochem Behav 2003; 75: 711–20.

30. Wiklund IK, Mattsson LA, Lindgren R, Limoni C. Effects of a standardized ginseng extract on quality of life and physiological parameters in symptomatic post-menopausal women: a double-bline, placebo-controlled trial. Swedish Alternative Medicine Group. Int J Clin Pharmacol Res 1999; 19: 89–99.

31. Woo J, Lau E, Ho SC et al. Comparison of *Pueraria lobata* with hormone replacement therapy in treating the adverse health consequences of menopause. Menopause 2003; 10: 352–61.

32. Komesaroff PA, Black CV, Cable V, Sudhir K. Effects of wild yam extract on menopausal symptoms, lipids and sex hormones in healthy menopausal women. Climacteric 2001; 4: 144–50.

33. Germaine LM, Freedman RR. Behavioral treatment of menopausal hot flashes: evaluation by objective methods. J Consult Clin Psychol 1984; 52: 1072–9.

34. Freedman RR, Woodward S. Behavioral treatment of menopausal hot flushes: evaluation by objective methods. Am J Obstet Gynecol 1992; 167: 436–9.

35. Irvin JH, Domar AD, Clark C, Zuttermeister PC, Friedman R. The effects of relaxation response training on menopausal symptoms. J Psychosom Obstet Gynaecol 1996; 17: 202–7.

36. Huntley AH, Ernst E. Soy for the treatment of peri-menopausal symptoms – a systematic review. Maturitas 2004; 47: 1–9.

37. Blatt MHG, Weisbader H, Kupperman HS. Vitamin E and climacteric syndrome. Arch Intern Med 1953; 91: 792–9.

38. Chan K, Qin L, Lau M et al. A randomized, prospective study of the effects of Tai Chi Chun exercise on bone mineral density in postmenopausal women. Arch Phys Med Rehabil 2004; 85: 717–22.

39. Williamson J, White A, Hart A, Ernst E. Randomised controlled trial of reflexology for menopausal symptoms. Br J Obstet Gynaecol 2002; 109: 1050–5.

# Chapter 23

# Nutritional aspects of the menopause

Mona R Sutnick and Donna H Mueller

## INTRODUCTION

Nutrition plays a vital role in the health of women of all ages. An extensive body of literature documents the role of diet and nutrients during growth and development, and during pregnancy and lactation. There is less information about the nutritional needs of women beyond the childbearing years. This situation is improving as a result of two trends: the aging of the American population has stimulated interest in changes in nutritional needs in adulthood, while concern about osteoporosis is focusing particular attention on certain of the nutritional needs of women during the peri- and postmenopausal periods.

## NUTRITIONAL REQUIREMENTS AND RECOMMENDATIONS

The commonly used nutrition intake standards for the US are developed by the Food and Nutrition Board, a division of the Institute of Medicine of the National Academy of Sciences. Since 1943 the recommendations have been revised periodically to reflect the latest nutrition research. The current standards are known as the Dietary Reference Intakes (DRIs). Detailed information may be accessed electronically.[1,2] With few exceptions, the recommendations are not averages, but are set high enough to fulfil the nutritional needs of two standard deviations above the mean of the healthy population. The DRIs are not intended to cover the requirements of ill people whose conditions may necessitate more or less of a nutrient. Also, since individual needs vary, the DRIs cannot be viewed as the exact requirements for any one person. Hence, there is a fine distinction between nutritional requirements (specific intakes of nutri-

ents for an individual at a given point in life) versus nutritional recommendations (suggested intakes of nutrients for a healthy individual or groups of healthy individuals over time).

The DRI categories are divided by sex and life stages. Perimenopausal women fall into the 31–50 years and the 51–70 years categories. Besides energy (kilocalories), recommendations are presented for the macronutrients (protein, carbohydrate, fat, water) and the micronutrients (vitamins and minerals).

There is a variety of nutrient levels. Those nutrients for which there is greatest knowledge have recommended dietary allowances (RDAs) established. The nutrients for which RDAs are available are most of the vitamins and minerals. These nutrient intakes are set to meet the needs of 97–98% of individuals in a healthy population. The term adequate intake (AI) is used for those nutrient levels believed to cover the needs of all individuals in the sex–age group, but for which there is lack of data or uncertainty in the data to prevent the recommended numbers from being more specific. Tolerable upper intake levels (UL) is the term applied to the maximum daily level of a nutrient that is likely to pose no risk of adverse effects. Unless specified, the UL represents total intake from food, water, and supplements.

Protein, fat, and carbohydrate intake values are set as acceptable macronutrient distribution ranges (AMDR). Ranges are used since healthy people can remain healthy at different levels. The important point to remember is that the energy-containing nutrients are carbohydrate, fats, protein, and ethanol. The total intake of kilocalories remains at 100% of those four energy-containing nutrients. Thus, at the end of the day, if the intake of one of those nutrients is more or less, then the intakes of the remainder make up a greater or smaller proportion of the woman's daily total caloric intake.

The term used for energy intake is estimated energy requirements (EER). The values are derived from regression equations. Metabolic rate and physical activity are included. Thermic effects of food and adaptive thermogenesis, although usually minor influences, are not included.

It is important to recognize that nutritional health is based on a lifetime of dietary intake, not just on the intake on a single day or week. Because of the day-to-day variability of any individual woman's nutrient intake, it is essential that the DRIs be applied to average intakes over a period of time. Also important is the recognition that there are multiple other chemical components in foods that may enhance, or impede, a particular nutrient's metabolism. Such components in plants are known as phytochemicals, and those in animal foods are known as zoochemicals. Finally, dietary supplements do not supply the full range of all nutrients and other beneficial substances, known and possibly unrecognized, which are obtained from a varied wholesome diet.

## NUTRITION CONCERNS

### Weight control

Weight control is a preoccupation of a majority of American women. In a culture which equates slenderness with attractiveness, over half of adult women report being 'on a diet' when surveyed.[3] They spend billions of dollars in pursuit of slimness each year. Despite their efforts at weight loss, women are obese more often than men, and the prevalence of obesity is rising. Between 1988 and 94, 60% of women aged 45 to 55 years were overweight, and 32% were obese. In the period 1999 to 2002, the proportions for the same groups had increased to 65% and 37%.[4]

Body mass index (BMI), a measure of relative weight calculated as weight (kilograms) divided by height squared (m²) is a useful replacement for height–weight tables, since it converts height and weight to a single number, enabling standards to be defined independently of height. BMI can also be calculated from pounds and inches using the formula BMI = (weight (pounds)/height (inches)² × 703). An expert panel of the National Heart, Lung and Blood Institute has set the following

standards for BMI: underweight, <18.5; normal weight, 18.5 to 24.9; overweight, 25.0 to 29.9, and obese, >30.0.[5]

Weight or BMI is only one consideration in assessing the importance of a woman's weight status. Waist circumference and overall risk status should also be assessed. Excessive abdominal fat is an independent predictor of risk factors and morbidity. A cutoff of >88 cm (>35 inches) has been recommended to identify increased relative risk of disorders associated with obesity in adult women. The presence of other risk factors, including smoking, hypertension, low high-density lipoprotein (HDL) cholesterol, elevated fasting glucose, and family history of premature coronary heart disease, should be considered in making decisions about weight control interventions.[5]

Middle-aged women often find, to their dismay, that they tend to gain weight more rapidly and have to work harder to lose it than had been the case in earlier years. While there is a common tendency to look at eating habits to explain weight gain, the difficulty experienced by these women may be more closely related to changes in energy expenditure than in energy intake. Resting energy needs decrease by about 2% per decade throughout adulthood. If not compensated for, this fairly small decline can lead to a gain of two to three pounds per year, or 20 to 30 pounds per decade. Furthermore, the decline in metabolic rate is often accompanied by a decrease in physical activity, the most important and controllable variable in determining energy need. While individuals will, of course, differ in their energy need, the average energy intake recommended for women over 50 years (1900 kcal) is about 14% lower than the calories suggested for women from 25 to 50 years (2200 kcal).[6] An excess intake of 300 kcal per day, if maintained over a year, can result in a weight gain of over 30 lb.

The two ways to counter the tendency to gain weight are to reduce caloric intake, and to maintain or increase physical activity.

Dietary control is a necessary part of weight control. The approximate rate of weight loss can be predicted based on the value of 3500 kcal per pound of adipose tissue. A deficit of 500 kcal/day will produce a loss of one pound per week. Using the RDA figure of 1900 kcal/day, a 51-year-old woman who made no changes in her physical activity would have to reduce her daily intake to about 1400 kcal to lose 1 lb/week. Since there is no evidence that requirements for protein and most vitamins and minerals decrease with age, there is less room in the diet for high-calorie, low-nutrient foods, and women should be instructed about food choices.

Decreasing energy density by increasing water-rich fruits and vegetables, cooked grains and soups while decreasing high fat foods can produce weight loss and good nutrition.[7]

For some women, the support of a weight loss group or consultation with a registered dietitian can be very helpful in making dietary changes.

Behavior therapy, employing strategies such as self-monitoring, stimulus control, stress management, and social support can also increase women's abilities to manage their eating.[8]

Another and different approach is the intuitive eating or 'health at every size' approach.[9] As described by Bacon, this 'model teaches people to support homeostatic regulation and eating intuitively (i.e. in response to internal cues of hunger, satiety and appetite) instead of cognitively controlling food intake through dieting'. The emphasis is on self-acceptance, improvement in health and fitness, and reduction in markers of health risk, rather than weight loss, In a well-controlled study, participants in a 'health at every size' program showed more sustained improvement in health risk and psychological measures at the end of two years than a comparable group offered a conventional, behavioral based weight loss program.

With our national penchant for dieting, it is equally important to emphasize the role of exercise in maintaining weight and health.[10,11] In an hour of brisk walking, a 60 kg woman will use up 200 kcal, in addition to the benefits of exercise for cardiopulmonary conditioning and maintenance of bone mass. And, if more persuasion is needed, we should note that when intakes are held too low – below 1000–1200 kcal – it is difficult to obtain adequate amounts of essential nutrients.

Drug therapy may be a useful adjunct, which can increase weight loss when combined with an appropriate diet and exercise program. Moyers has recently reviewed both approved and off-label agents in use for weight control.[12]

Panelists at a National Institutes of Health Technology Assessment Conference on Methods for Voluntary Weight Loss and Control concluded that, '. . . most people who achieve weight loss . . . regain weight. For many overweight persons, achieving and maintaining a healthy weight is a lifelong challenge', and emphasized the need for more research into the biological and social influences on weight and weight control.[13]

Whatever combination of physical activity, modification of food consumption, and drugs is used for weight loss, the approach should stress the need for permanent adjustment of eating and exercise habits to maintain desirable weight over the long term.

## Osteoporosis

The etiology, prevention, diagnosis, and treatment of osteoporosis are reviewed elsewhere in this book (Chapter 14). Thus, the emphasis here is on nutritional factors and dietary strategies that have either positive or negative effects on bone formation, mineralization, or demineralization.[14] Nutrients considered essential for promoting bone health include adequate amounts of the minerals calcium, magnesium, and fluoride; the vitamins D, C, and K; and the macronutrient protein. Detrimental effects have been observed with excessive amounts of phosphorus, sodium, protein, alcohol, and caffeine. The strongest evidence continues to be for women to have lifelong optimal intakes of calcium and vitamin D, with food being the best, or safest, source of nutrients. However, to determine an individual woman's course of nutritional medical care, the clinician must interpret a wide variety of confounding variables, such as the woman's weight, exercise habits, tobacco use, serum levels of calcium and 25-hydroxyvitamin D, the presence of chronic diseases, and medication prescription.

Although the precise mechanism by which calcium intake influences the genesis and progression of osteoporosis remains to be clarified, there is ample evidence to support recommendations for optimal dietary calcium, and/or the use of calcium supplements. The National Osteoporosis Foundation concurs with the National Academy of Sciences' recommendation of calcium intakes for 31–50-year-old women as 1000 mg/day, and for 51–70-year-old women as 1200 mg/day.[15] It is important to note that these recommendations are for healthy women rather than for women at risk, or under treatment, for osteoporosis.

Dietary surveys of American women indicate usual intakes of 450–550 mg, barely or less than half the amount needed to maintain bone mass, and that milk and dairy products supply 50% of the calcium in US diets.[16,17] To double her calcium intake, then, a woman must increase her use of dairy products, preferably vitamin D-fortified non-fat or low-fat milk, yogurt, and cheeses. Women who are lactase deficient may substitute lactose-modified products. There may be an advantage in using milk as the main source of calcium since it has been shown to lead to less suppression of remodeling than does calcium carbonate.[18]

Other foods also supply calcium, as shown in Table 23.1. Based on reports of typical diets, an American woman consumes about 200–300 mg calcium from foods other than dairy products. Careful selection of such foods can slightly raise that intake. Importantly, reliance on food sources of nutrients promotes a sound diet while striving against potential nutritional imbalances.[19]

Realistically, however, not all women can be expected to achieve the optimal amount of calcium from dietary sources alone. Moreover, for women who have multiple risk factors for osteoporosis, inclusion of calcium supplements in addition to optimal dietary calcium intake may be necessary. Numerous calcium-fortified food products and calcium supplements are on the market. (The percentage of calcium in several common supplements is listed in Table 23.2). When advising patients about supplementary calcium, it is helpful to clarify the difference between the total weight in milligrams of the calcium compound used in the product, versus the actual weight in milligrams of elemental calcium the product contains. For calcium tablets, this knowledge assists the woman in taking the proper number of tablets each day. Hence, if one pill contains 500 mg calcium carbonate, it only provides 200 mg elemental calcium. Also notable is the appearance of the acronym 'USP' on the supplement label. This indicates that the calcium tablet meets the United States Pharmacopeia's standards for label integrity, ingredient purity, ingredient dissolution and release in the body, and product safe manufacturing practices.[20] For calcium-fortified foods such as orange juice, the package nutrition facts panel states the amount of calcium in a serving as a percentage of the daily value standard. The daily value for calcium is set at 1000 mg, so the commonly seen '35% of daily value' equals 350 mg of calcium.

Another precaution concerns such 'natural' calcium supplement products as dolomite and bone meal. Samples of both products have been shown to be contaminated with lead and other heavy metals, and cases of toxicity have been reported.[21] Patients need to be apprised of this risk in any discussion about the choice of calcium supplements.

Adequate amounts of preformed vitamin D (calcitriol or 1,25-$(OH)_2D_3$) are needed for calcium absorption. The dietary requirement for vitamin D is variable, as the vitamin can be synthesized in the skin from 7-dehydrocholesterol with exposure to ultraviolet light. The DRI for vitamin D assumes women have an absence of adequate exposure to sunlight. The food source of vitamin D is cholecalciferol. Its DRI (adequate intake) for 31–50-year-old women is established at 5 µg (equivalent to 200 IU) per day, and for 51–70-year-old women at 10 µg (equivalent to 400 IU) per day.

Naturally occurring food sources of vitamin D are limited to fatty fish and their oils, and egg yolks, but nearly all milk and butter or margarine sold in the US is fortified with vitamin D at a level of 400 IU per quart, or equivalent. However, other dairy foods, such as yogurts or cheeses, may not be fortified. Soy products may or may not be fortified. Nevertheless, many food products, especially breakfast cereals and breakfast/sports/energy bars, may be fortified with vitamin D. The vitamin also is added to many calcium supplements, and is found in multivitamin preparations. Women who take supplements should be instructed about the potential for toxicity of vitamin D. Prolonged ingestion of excess vitamin D can cause hypercalcemia and hypercalciuria.[22] While the amount of vitamin D from any one of the usual sources usually is no more than the DRI, a combination of milk, a highly fortified cereal, a multivitamin, and a combined calcium and vitamin D supplement is quite possible, and would add up to excessive levels of this vitamin. A reasonable recommendation to patients is that they take no more than one supplementary source of vitamin D.

Physicians often care for women years prior to their entering menopause, and also are involved in the medical care of such women's daughters. Anticipatory nutritional guidance offered to all adolescent, young and middle-aged women may help them in the early adoption of optimal dietary practices and nutritional intakes aimed at promoting maximal bone accrual. Thus, bone health may be preserved for as long as possible.

## DIET AND DISEASE PREVENTION

Nutritional factors have been identified as either protective or risk factors for other diseases, including coronary heart disease, hypertension, and cancer at several sites.

| Table 23.1   Calcium value of selected foods | Amount | Calcium (mg) |
|---|---|---|
| **Dairy products** | | |
| Milk, whole, low-fat or skimmed | I cup | 300 |
| Yogurt, with added milk solids | I cup | 400 |
| Cheese | | |
|   hard | I oz | 200 |
|   cottage | I oz | 25 |
|   cream | I oz | 20 |
| Ice cream | ½ cup | 75 |
| **Vegetables** | | |
| High; broccoli, kale, mustard, collard, turnip, dandelion greens (note: beet greens and spinach contain calcium but it is not absorbed) | ½ cup | 175 |
| All others | ½ cup | 20 |
| **Fruits** | | |
| Juices | ½ cup | 10–30 |
| Fruits | I piece or ½ cup | 10–30 |
| **Meats and fish** | | |
| Canned salmon and sardines (with bones) | 3 oz | 200 |
| Bacon | 2 slices | 5 |
| All other meat and fish | 3 oz | 5–20 |
| **Legumes** | | |
| All | I cup | 100 |
| **Nuts** | | |
| Almonds, Brazil nuts | ¼ cup | 80 |
| All others | ¼ cup | 25 |
| Peanut butter | I tablespoon | 10 |
| **Starches** | | |
| Bread | I slice | 20 |
| Rice, pasta | ½ cup | 10 |
| Cereals | ½ cup | 10 |
| Miscellaneous | | |
| Eggs | I | 25 |
| Cake | I slice | 85 |
| Candy, chocolate | I oz | 60 |
| Molasses | I tablespoon | 60 |
| Pie | | |
|   fruit | I slice | 10 |
|   custard | I slice | 160 |
| Soup | | |
|   bean | I cup | 215 |
|   made with milk | I cup | 215 |
|   other | I cup | 15–50 |

**Table 23.2**  Calcium content of common supplements

| Calcium salt | Elemental calcium (%) |
| --- | --- |
| Calcium carbonate | 40 |
| Calcium gluconate | 9 |
| Calcium lactate | 13 |
| Calcium phosphate, dibasic | 23.3 |

## Coronary heart disease

Women lag about 10 years behind men in the incidence of coronary heart disease. After the menopause, the incidence increases so that women as well as men should benefit from nutritional guidance. Ample consumption of fruits, vegetables, beans, legumes (including intact soybeans), whole grains, non-fat/low-fat dairy foods, fish and lean meats are associated with cardiac benefits. All these kinds of foods provide a wide assortment of vitamins, minerals, fiber, and phytochemicals, or zoochemicals. Conversely, obesity, abdominal adiposity, and high intakes of saturated and trans fatty acids have been associated with elevated serum cholesterol levels, and increased risk of coronary heart disease.[23,24] Again, dietary sources of nutrients appear to be more beneficial than any nutrient ingested as an individual supplement. While there is no unequivocal proof of the effectiveness of dietary change in preventing atherosclerosis, there is a body of data that supports controlling calorie, fat (especially saturated and *trans* fatty acids as well as cholesterol), and disaccharides, as a means of reducing serum cholesterol levels and cardiovascular risk. The National Cholesterol Education Program, and the American Heart Association, have published similar nutritional recommendations.[25–28]

## Hypertension

The incidence of hypertension in women may increase after menopause. From a nutritional standpoint, when indicated, the usual recommendations include weight loss, decreased sodium intake, increased potassium and fiber intakes, possible increased calcium and magnesium intakes, along with limited ethanol consumption.[29] Dietary teaching is focused on decreasing calories, salt (NaCl) and salty foods, and alcohol, while increasing fruits, vegetables, and non-fat/low-fat dairy foods. This dietary pattern is based on the Dietary Approaches to Stop Hypertension (DASH) multicenter, randomized dietary study.[30] The study's purpose was to test the effects of combined dietary adjustments versus the simple alteration of individual nutrients in relationship to hypertension. The patient educational acronym is often known as the 'DASH diet', and materials useful to help with patient implementation of the diet are available.[31]

## Cancer

Research on the role of diet in cancer is more recent, and much more investigation is needed to define the mechanisms and importance of the associations which have been observed. Aromatic hydrocarbons and nitroso compounds in smoked and cured foods have been associated with cancer of the esophagus and stomach.[32,33] Investigations of meat and animal fat in relation to colon cancer have had inconsistent results.[34,35] Fruits, vegetables, and dietary fiber consistently appear to be protective.[36] Obesity and high dietary fat consumption, which often go together, appear to increase the risk of breast cancer in postmenopausal women.[37] Alcohol may also increase this risk.[38] Dietary fiber has been associated with a lower risk of breast cancer.[39]

Although current knowledge is inadequate to resolve debates over nutrient supplementation or fortification programs, diets containing liberal amounts of fruits and vegetables are clearly protective and should be encouraged. The Five a Day program, a collaborative public information and education effort of the National Cancer Institute and the Produce for Better Health Foundation has the goal of persuading all Americans to consume more fruits and vegetables.[40]

Similar recommendations are found in the guidelines recommended by the American Cancer Society,[41] shown in Table 23.3.

## HOT FLUSHES

Hot flushes are one of the most common annoyances associated with the perimenopause. They are not a nutritional problem but these authors have encountered many women who report that their hot flushes are relieved by eliminating caffeine, sugar and alcohol from their diets. The evidence, such as it is, is purely anecdotal, but the measure is simple and safe and can be offered to patients for a trial.

**Table 23.3**   American Cancer Society Guidelines

- Eat a variety of healthful foods, with an emphasis on plant sources.
- Eat five or more servings of a variety of vegetables and fruits each day:
  - include vegetables and fruits at every meal and for snacks
  - eat a variety of vegetables and fruits
  - limit French fries, snack chips, and other fried vegetable products
  - choose 100% juice if you drink fruit or vegetable juices.
- Choose whole grains in preference to processed (refined) grains and sugars:
  - choose whole grain rice, bread, pasta, and cereals
  - limit consumption of refined carbohydrates, including pastries, sweetened cereals, soft drinks, and sugars.
- Limit consumption of red meats, especially those that are processed and high in fat:
  - choose fish, poultry, or beans as an alternative to beef, pork, and lamb
  - when you eat meat, select lean cuts and smaller portions
  - prepare meat by baking, broiling, or poaching, rather than by frying or charbroiling.
- Choose foods that help maintain a healthful weight:
  - when you eat away from home, choose food low in fat, calories, and sugar, and avoid large portions
  - eat smaller portions of high-calorie foods. Be aware that 'low fat' or 'fat free' does not mean 'low calorie', and that low-fat cakes, cookies, and similar foods are often high in calories
  - substitute vegetables, fruits, and other low-calorie foods for calorie-dense foods such as French fries, cheeseburgers, pizza, ice cream, doughnuts, and other sweets.

Vitamins E and B$_6$ also appear in the folklore concerning menopausal symptoms. Again, the evidence is mostly anecdotal. One study of vitamin E in breast cancer survivors showed a statistically significant but clinically marginal benefit from the vitamin.[42] Dosing with vitamins, however, is not innocuous, so one should be cautious in advising it. Being fat soluble, vitamin E is stored in the body and, theoretically, could reach toxic levels. In fact, vitamin E is readily available and is often promoted in popular literature with few, if any, reports of toxicity.

Vitamin B$_6$, on the other hand, is water soluble so would be expected to be easily excreted. But in 1983, Schaumberg et al reported peripheral neuropathies in women who had been taking doses of 2–6 g daily for months.[43] Subsequent reports have attributed peripheral neuropathies to doses of 500 mg and doses closer to 100 mg.[44] Clearly, women should be warned about self-medicating with megadoses of vitamin B$_6$.

Soy foods and their isoflavone components are being evaluated as possible alternatives to hormone replacement therapy (HRT) since it was observed that Japanese women appear to have fewer hot flushes than American women. Recent reviewers have reached contradictory conclusions about their usefulness. [45–47]

In addition, the North American Menopause Society has issued a cautionary Consensus Statement which is quoted in the next section. (p. 316).

## COMPLEMENTARY AND ALTERNATIVE MEDICINE (See also Chapter 22)

The use of herbal and other alternative therapies is becoming increasingly common in North America. The National Center for Complementary and Alternative Medicine reports that 62% of American consumers tried some type of alternative therapy in 2002. In 1997 they spent an estimated amount between 36 and 47 billion dollars on these therapies.[48]

Seidl and Stewart conducted intensive interviews with 13 perimenopausal women who acknowledged using alternative therapies, mainly herbal preparations.[49] They found that women perceived the alternatives as 'natural' and, therefore, safe. They liked the sense of personal control that they felt in using alternatives, contrasted with what they felt was 'pressure' from their physicians to use HRT.

Alternative modalities which have been recommended for perimenopausal women include nutrient supplements, herbs, acupuncture, relaxation techniques, massage and chiropractic. It is difficult to find reliable evidence on acupuncture, massage, and chiropractic. Practitioners speak of energy and balance and offer anecdotal evidence, but controlled trials still need to be conducted.[50]

There are more data on phytoestrogens and herbal products. Phytoestrogens, lignans and isoflavones, are converted in the intestine to heterocyclic phenols with structures similar to estrogens, but their estrogenic activity is far lower than that of synthetic estrogens. Lignans are widely distributed in grains, fruits, and vegetables, with flaxseed having a particularly high concentration. Isoflavones are found in all legumes, with the highest concentrations in soy.[51] The observation that women in Asian countries, who consume larger amounts of soy foods than do Americans, report fewer hot flushes led to trials of isolated soy protein in postmenopausal women.[52] Murkies and colleagues supplemented subjects' diets with either soy or wheat flour and found decreases in hot flushes in both groups, with the soy groups having a more rapid response.[53] Albertazzi and coworkers compared isolated soy protein with placebo;[54] both groups reported a decrease in hot flushes, with the soy group having a significantly greater improvement. Several studies also suggest that soy protein may also improve cardiovascular risk profiles by decreasing the ratio of total to HDL cholesterol, and maintaining arterial elasticity.[55,56] There are some indications that soy protein may also be effective in decreasing bone loss; more, and longer, trials are needed to clarify this possibility.[51] It has also been suggested that soy consumption may play an important role in the well-known lower rate of breast cancer among Japanese women, compared to Americans.[51]

The North American Menopause Society, in its consensus statement on phytoestrogens, concluded that:

> Although the observed health effects in humans cannot be clearly attributed to isoflavones alone, it is clear that foods or supplements that contain isoflavones have some physiologic affects. Clinicians may wish to recommend that menopausal women consume whole foods that contain isoflavones, especially for the cardiovascular benefits of these foods; however, a level of caution needs to be observed in making these recommendations. Additional clinical trials are needed before specific recommendations can be made regarding increased consumption of foods or supplements that contain high amounts of isoflavones.[57]

A variety of herbal therapies has been recommended for alleviation of menopausal symptoms: black cohosh, vitex agnus castelli, rehmannia, siberian ginseng, dong quoi, fo ti, wild yam and St John's wort.[58,59] American law considers herbs to be food supplements, not drugs, and as such they are not subjected to review for safety and efficacy by the Food and Drug Administration. There is relatively little good scientific literature on the use of herbal remedies available in English. Two reliable references are Tyler's Honest Herbal: A Sensible Guide to the Use of Herbs and Related Remedies,[60] and Herbs of Choice: The Therapeutic Use of Phytomedicinals,[61] both by Varro E Tyler, PhD, and coauthors. Kronenberg and Fugh-Berman have recently reviewed randomized controlled trials of complementary and alternative medicine (CAM) for menopausal symptoms.[62]

The following are among the most popular CAM therapies for menopausal symptoms:

- black cohosh (*Cimicifuga racemosa*), sold as Remifemin, has been shown to suppress hot flushes. It is usually administered in an alcoholic extract equivalent to 40 mg daily. Because of the lack of long-term toxicity studies, Tyler recommends that it be used for no longer than six months.[60,61]
- dong quai (*Angelica polymorpha*) contains several coumarin derivatives and lacks evidence supporting its effectiveness
- evening primrose oil (*Oenothera biennis*) lacks evidence supporting its use, but has not produced untoward effects
- fo ti (*Polygonum multiforum*) is effective only as a laxative, with undetermined side-effects.

## PRACTICAL APPLICATIONS: DIETARY GUIDANCE

To be effective, dietary guidance should build, as indicated above, on each woman's current status and projected future needs. The bases for recommendations to ensure nutritional adequacy and reduce the risk of disease have been presented. The body of evidence relating diet to health promotion and disease risk reduction has been reviewed by expert panels from voluntary and government agencies.[1,2,15,17,25,26,28,31,57] While their recommendations vary in some particulars, creating a stir in the media and confusion for the public, there is a consensus around a dietary pattern that includes more whole grains, fruits, and vegetables, and fewer calories, lipids, and disaccharides. Ideally, energy intake is balanced with energy expenditure to achieve and maintain healthy weight throughout women's lives, including before, during, and after the menopause.

Two US government reports have recently been released that are pubic health outreach measures to educate and guide people to choose healthy foods and beverages. One is the Dietary Guidelines for Americans, published jointly by the United States Department of Health and Human Services and the United States Department of Agriculture.[63] The recommendations are summarized in Table 23.4. The other is the food pyramid (Figure 23.1), published by the Department of Agriculture.[64]

Both documents advise choosing a variety of foods each day, emphasizing whole grains and fruits and vegetables. Fats, sugars, salt and alcohol are limited. While these recommendations have been offered by the government for many years, the newest editions stress the need for physical activity to balance caloric intake and maintain a healthy weight.

These authors would add one more guideline: eat foods that you like, and enjoy them. The medical and nutrition communities have done such an energetic job of proclaiming the health values of food that eating in America has, too often, become 'medicalized'. Women need to understand how to balance appropriate amounts of all foods to make meals a source of pleasure as well as health.

Taken together, the dietary guidelines, food guide pyramid, and the accompanying websites can help women to eat well and be physically active during their perimenopausal years. Doing so will enable them to retain, or achieve, nutritional health and wellbeing.

## SUMMARY

Good nutrition is important in maintaining the health of menopausal women. Dietary advice should include the liberal use of low-fat dairy products, fresh fruits and vegetables, and whole grains and moderate amounts of lean meat, poultry, and fish. Unless the diet includes two to three cups of milk or its equivalent per day, calcium supplementation should be considered.

---

**Table 23.4**   2005 Dietary Guidelines for Americans (key recommendations for the general population)

**Adequate nutrients within calorie needs**
- Consume a variety of nutrient-dense foods and beverages within and among the basic food groups while choosing foods that limit the intake of saturated and trans fats, cholesterol, added sugars, salt, and alcohol.
- Meet recommended intakes within energy needs by adopting a balanced eating pattern, such as the US Department of Agriculture (USDA) Food Guide or the Dietary Approaches to Stop Hypertension (DASH) eating plan.

**Weight management**
- To maintain body weight in a healthy range, balance calories from foods and beverages with calories expended.
- To prevent gradual weight gain over time, make small decreases in food and beverage calories, and increase physical activity.

**Physical activity**
- Engage in regular physical activity and reduce sedentary activities to promote health, psychological wellbeing, and a healthy body weight:
  - to reduce the risk of chronic disease in adulthood, engage in at least 30 min moderate-intensity physical activity, above usual activity, at work or home on most days of the week
  - for most people, greater health benefits can be obtained by engaging in physical activity of more vigorous intensity or longer duration
  - to help manage body weight and prevent gradual, unhealthy body weight gain in adulthood, engage in approximately 60 min moderate- to vigorous-intensity activity on most days of the week, while not exceeding caloric intake requirements
  - to sustain weight loss in adulthood, Participate in at least 60 to 90 min daily moderate-intensity physical activity while not exceeding caloric intake requirements. Some people may need to consult with a healthcare provider before participating in this level of activity.
- Achieve physical fitness by including cardiovascular conditioning, stretching exercises for flexibility, and resistance exercises or calisthenics for muscle strength and endurance.

**Table 23.4**   2005 Dietary Guidelines for Americans (key recommendations for the general population) (*continued*)

**Food groups to encourage**
- Consume a sufficient amount of fruits and vegetables while staying within energy needs. Two cups of fruit and 2½ cups of vegetables per day are recommended for a reference 2 000 calorie intake, with higher or lower amounts depending on the calorie level.
- Choose a variety of fruits and vegetables each day. In particular, select from all five vegetable subgroups (dark green, orange, legumes, starchy vegetables, and other vegetables) several times a week.
- Consume three or more ounce-equivalents of whole-grain products per day, with the rest of the recommended grains coming from enriched or whole-grain products. In general, at least half the grains should come from whole grains.
- Consume 3 cups per day of fat-free or low-fat milk, or equivalent milk products.

**Fats**
- Consume less than 10% of calories from saturated fatty acids and less than 300 mg/day cholesterol, and keep trans fatty acid consumption as low as possible.
- Keep total fat intake between 20% and 35% of calories, with most fats coming from sources of polyunsaturated and monounsaturated fatty acids, such as fish, nuts, and vegetable oils.
- When selecting and preparing meat, poultry, dry beans, and milk or milk products, make choices that are lean, low-fat, or fat-free.
- Limit intake of fats and oils high in saturated and/or trans fatty acids, and choose products low in such fats and oils.

**Carbohydrates**
- Choose fiber-rich fruits, vegetables, and whole grains often.
- Choose and prepare foods and beverages with little added sugars or caloric sweeteners, such as the amounts suggested by the USDA Food Guide and the DASH eating plan.
- Reduce the incidence of dental caries by practicing good oral hygiene and consuming sugar- and starch-containing foods and beverages less frequently.

**Sodium and potassium**
- Consume less than 2300 mg (approximately 1 teaspoon of salt) of sodium per day.
- Choose and prepare foods with little salt. At the same time, consume potassium-rich foods, such as fruits and vegetables.

**Alcoholic beverages**
- Those who choose to drink alcoholic beverages should do so sensibly and in moderation – defined as the consumption of up to one drink per day for women and up to two drinks per day for men.
- Alcoholic beverages should not be consumed by some individuals, including those who cannot restrict their alcohol intake, women of childbearing age who may become pregnant, pregnant and lactating women, children and adolescents, individuals taking medications that can interact with alcohol, and those with specific medical conditions.
- Alcoholic beverages should be avoided by individuals engaging in activities that require attention, skill, or co-ordination, such as driving or operating machinery.

**Food safety**
- To avoid microbial food-borne illness:
  - clean hands, food contact surfaces, and fruits and vegetables. Meat and poultry should not be washed or rinsed
  - separate raw, cooked, and ready-to-eat foods while shopping, preparing, or storing foods
  - cook foods to a safe temperature to kill microorganisms
  - chill (refrigerate) perishable food promptly, and defrost foods properly
  - avoid raw (unpasteurized) milk or any products made from unpasteurized milk, raw or partially cooked eggs, or foods containing raw eggs, raw or undercooked meat, and poultry, unpasteurized juices, and raw sprouts.

**Note:**   The Dietary Guidelines for Americans 2005 contains additional recommendations for specific populations. The full document is available at www.healthierus.gov/dietaryguidelines.

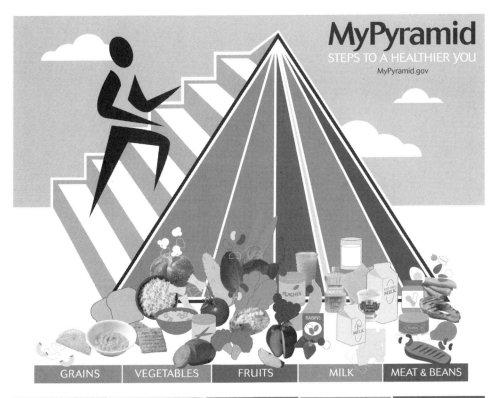

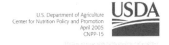

**Figure 23.1** MyPyramid: steps to a healthier you. (Reproduced courtesy of US Department of Agriculture Center for Nutritional Policy and Promotions.[64])

# REFERENCES

1. National Academies Press: Dietary Reference Intakes. Available at http://www/nap.edu. Accessed June 29 2005.
2. Institute of Medicine: Dietary Reference Intakes. Available at http://www.iom.edu. Accessed June 29 2005
3. Neumark Stainer D, Rock CL, Thornquist MD et al. Weight control behaviors among adults and adolescents: associations with dietary intake. Prev Med 2000; 30: 381–91.
4. National Center for Health Statistics: Health United States, 2004 With Chartbook on Trends in the Health of Americans. Hyattsville, MD, 2004.
5. The National Heart, Lung and Blood Institute Expert Panel on the Identification, Evaluation, and Treatment of Overweight and Obesity in Adults: Executive summary of the clinical guidelines on the identification, evaluation, and treatment of overweight and obesity in adults. J Am Dietet Assoc 1998; 98: 1178–91.
6. Durnin JUCA, Passmore R. Energy, Work and Leisure. London: Heinemann Educational Books, 1967.
7. Rolls BJ, Drewnowski A, Kadikwe JH. Changing the energy density of the diet as a strategy for weight management. J Am Diet Assoc 2005; 105: 98–105.
8. Wadden TA, Stunkard AJ. Handbook of Obesity Treatment. New York: Guildford Press, 2002.
9. Bacon L, Stern J, Van Loan M, Keim N. Size acceptance and intuitive eating improve health for obese, female chronic dieters. J Am Diet Assoc 2005; 105: 929–36.
10. Pi-Sunyer FX. Exercise in the treatment of obesity. In: Frankle R and Yang M-U, (eds). Obesity and Weight Control. Rockville, MD: Aspen Publishers, Inc., 1988.
11. Schoeller D. But how much physical activity? Am J Clin Nutr 2003; 78: 669–70.
12. Moyers SB. Medications as adjunct therapy for weight loss: approved and off-label agents in use. J Am Diet Assoc 2005; 105: 948–59.
13. National Institutes of Health Technology Assessment Conference Statement: Methods for Voluntary Weight Loss, 1992, Office of Medical Applications of Research, National Institutes of Health, Bethesda, MD.
14. US Department of Health and Human Services: Bone Health and Osteoporosis: a report of the surgeon general, 2004. Available at http://www.surgeongeneral.gov/library. Accessed June 29 2005.
15. National Osteoporosis foundation: Prevention, calcium and vitamin D. Available at http://nof.org/prevention/calcium.htm. Accessed June 29 2005.
16. Tranquilli AL, Lucino E, Garzettti GG, Romani C. Calcium, phosphorus and magnesium intakes correlate with bone mineral content in postmenopausal women. Gynecol endocrinol 1994; 8: 55–8.
17. Committee on Diet and Health, Food and Nutrition Boards, National Research Council: Diet and Health: implications for reducing chronic disease risk. Washington, DC: National Academy Press, 1989, p. 69.
18. Recker RR, Heaney RP. The effect of milk supplements on calcium metabolism, bone metabolism and calcium balance. Am J Clin Nutr 1985; 41: 254–63.
19. Heaney RR. The role of nutrition in prevention and management of osteoporosis. Clin Obstet Gynecol 1987; 50: 833–46.
20. United States Pharmacopeia. Available at www.osp.org/USPverified/dietaryStandards. Accessed June 29 2005.
21. Food and Drug Administration: Advice on limiting intake of bone meal, FDA Drug Bulletin 1982; 12: 5–6.
22. Food and Nutrition Board: Hazards of overuse of vitamin D. Nutr Revs 1975; 33: 61–3.
23. Manson JE, Colditz GA, Stampfer MJ. A prospective study of obesity and risk of coronary heart disease in women. N Engl J Med 1990; 322: 882–6.
24. Rexrode KM, Carey VJ, Hennekens CH et al. Abdominal adiposity and coronary heart disease in women. JAMA 1998; 280: 1843–8.
25. Expert Panel on Detection, Evaluation and Treatment of High Blood Cholesterol in Adults. Executive summary of the third report of the national cholesterol education program (NCEP) expert panel on detection, evaluation and treatment of high blood cholesterol inadults (adult treatment panel III). JAMA 2001; 285: 2486–97.
26. Consensus Panel Guide to Comprehensive Risk Reduction for Adult Patients Without Coronary or Other Atherosclerotic Vascular Diseases. AHA Guidelines for primary prevention of cardiovascular disease and stroke: 2002 update. Circulation 2002; 106: 388–91.
27. Kris-Etherton P, Lichenstein A, Howard BV et al. Antioxidant vitamin supplements and cardiovascular disease. Circulation 2004; 110: 637–41.
28. American Heart Association website. Available at http://americanheart.org. Accessed June 29 2005.
29. Chobanian AV, Bakris GL, Black HR et al. The seventh report of the joint national committee on prevention, detection evaluation and treatment of high blood pressure. JAMA 2003; 289: 2560–72.
30. Appel LJ, Moore TJ, Obarzanek E et al. A clinical trial of the effects of dietary patterns on blood pressure. NEJM 1997; 336: 1117–24.
31. National Institutes of Health, National Heart, Lung and Blood Institute: The DASH eating plan. Available at http://www.nhlbi.nih.gov/health/public/heart/hbp/dash/. Accessed June 29 2005.
32. Doll R, Peto R. The causes of cancer, quantitative estimates of available risks of cancer in the United States today. J Natl Cancer Inst 1981; 66: 1191–308.
33. Committee on Diet, Nutrition and Cancer, Assembly of Life Sciences, National Research Council: Diet, Nutrition, and Cancer. Washington, DC: National Academy Press, 1982.
34. Goldbohm RA, van den Brandt PA, van't Veer P et al. A prospective cohort study on the relation between meat consumption and the risk of colon cancer. Cancer Res 1994; 54: 718–23.
35. Willett WC, Stampfer MJ, Colditz GA et al. Relation of meat, fat and fiber intake to the risk of colon cancer in a prospective study among women. N Engl J Med 1990; 323: 1664–72.
36. Steinmetz KA, Kushi LH, Bostick RM et al. Vegetables, fruit and colon cancer in the Iowa Women's Health Study. Am J Epidemiol 1994; 139: 1–15.
37. Barrett-Connor E, Friedlander NJ. Dietary fat, calories, and the risk of breast cancer in postmenopausal women: a prospective population-based study. J Am Coll Nutr 1993; 12: 390–9.
38. Gapstur SM, Potter JD, Sellers TA et al. Increased risk of breast cancer with alcohol consumption in post-menopausal women. Am J Epidemiol 1992; 136: 541–2.
39. Rohan TE, Howe GR, Friedenreich CM. Dietary fiber, vitamins A, C, and E and risk of breast cancer. Cancer Causes Control 1993; 4: 29–37.

40. Produce for Better Health Foundation: Five a Day for Better Health, Newark, DE, 1991.

41. American Cancer Society. The Complete Guide – Nutrition and Physical Activity. Available at http://www.cancer.org. Accessed June 15 2005.

42. Barton DL, Loprinzi CL, Quella SK et al. Prospective evaluation of vitamin E for hot flashes in breast cancer survivors. J Clin Oncol 1998; 16: 495–500.

43. Schaumberg H, Kaplan J, Windebank N et al. Sensory neuropathy from pyridoxine abuse. N Engl J Med 1983; 309: 445–8.

44. Dalton K, Dalton MJT. Characteristics of pyridoxine overdose neuropathy syndrome. Acta Neurol Scand 1987; 76: 8–11.

45. Messina M, Hughes C. Efficacy of soy foods and soybean isoflavone supplements for alleviating menopausal symptoms in positively related to initial hot flush frequency. J Med Food 2003; 6: 1–11.

46. Krebs EE, Ensrud KE, MacDonald R, Wilt TJ. Phytoestrogens for treatment of menopausal symptoms: a systematic review. Obstet Gynecol 2004; 104: 824–36.

47. Vincent A, Fitzpatrick LA. Soy isoflavones: are they useful in menopause? Mayo Clin Proc 2000; 75: 1174–84.

48. National Center for Complementary and Alternative Medicine: The Use of Complementary and Alternative Medicine in the United States. Available at http://www.nnccam.nih.gov. Accessed June 15 2005.

49. Seidl, MM, Stewart, DE: Alternative treatments for menopausal symptoms. Can Fam Physician 1998; 44: 1271–6.

50. Seidl MM, Stewart DE. Alternative treatments for menopausal symptoms: Systematic review of scientific and lay literature. Can Fam Physician 1998; 44: 1299–308.

51. Murkies AL, Wilcox G, Davis S. Clinical review 92: Phytoestrogens. J Clin Endocrin Metab 1998; 83: 297–303.

52. Knight PC, Edden JA. Phytoestrogens – a short review. Maturitas 1995; 22: 167–75.

53. Murkies AL. Lonbard C, Strauss BJ et al. Dietary flour supplementation decreases post-menopausal hot flushes: effect of soy and wheat. Maturitas 1995; 21: 189–95.

54. Albertazzi P, Pansini F, Bonaccorsi G et al. The effect of dietary soy supplementation on hot flushes. Obstet Gynecol 1998; 91: 6–11.

55. Baum JA, Teng H, Erdman JW et al. Long-term intake of soy protein improves blood lipid profiles and increases mononuclear cell low-density lipoprotein receptor messenger RNA in hypercholesterolemic, post-menopausal women. Am J Clin Nutr 1998; 68: 545–51.

56. Nestel PJ, Yamashita T, Sasahara T et al. Soy isoflavones improve systemic arterial compliance but not plasma lipids in menopausal and perimenopausal women. Atheroscler Thromb Vasc Biol 1997; 17: 3392–8.

57. North American Menopause Society Consensus Statement. Menopause 2000; 7: 215–29.

58. Mayo JL. A natural approach to menopause. Clin Nutr Insights 1997; 5: 1–8.

59. Northrup C. Menopause. Prim Care 1997; 24: 921–48.

60 Foster S, Tyler V. Tyler's Honest Herbal: A Sensible Guide to the Use of Herbs and Related Remedies. New York: Haworth Press, 1999.

61. Robbers JE, Tyler, VE. Herbs of Choice: the Therapeutic Use of Phytomedicinals. New York: Haworth Press, 1999.

62. Kronenberg F, Fugh-Berman A. Complementary and alternative medicine for menopausal symptoms: a review of randomized, controlled trials. Ann Int Med 2002; 137: 805–14.

63. Dietary Guidelines for Americans 2005. Available at http://healthierus.gov/dietaryguidelines. Accessed June 29 2005.

64. My Pyramid 2005. Available at http://www.MyPyramid.gov. Accessed June 29 2005.

# Chapter 24

# Exercise in the menopause

Laura E Post Kornegay

In 1978, the American College of Sports Medicine (ACSM) published its original position statement on exercise. In the nearly three decades since then, the medical community has become increasingly aware of the multiple benefits of regular exercise through numerous studies that document the beneficial effects of activity on overall health. Indeed, this chapter should complement the preceding text by highlighting the effects of exercise on many of the conditions that have already been explored, including osteoporosis, cardiovascular disease, diabetes, neoplastic processes, and depression. While the thinking in regard to these processes shifts with advances in evidence-based medicine, participation in a regular exercise program remains a cost-effective intervention for reducing or preventing many of the functional declines associated with aging in women.

## SEDENTARY LIFESTYLE: A PUBLIC HEALTH THREAT

Unfortunately, despite growing awareness by both the lay community and medical professionals of the positive effects of exercise in maintaining health, a significant proportion of our population remains physically inactive. Studies have shown that 30–50% of the US population lead sedentary lifestyles, defined as no leisure-time physical activity in the past month.[1,2] It has been estimated that as many as 250 000 deaths per year in the US, approximately 12% of the total, are attributable to lack of regular exercise.[3] Because of this significant public health problem, a number of governing bodies, including the Centers for Disease Control and Prevention (CDC), the ACSM and the National Institutes of Health (NIH) have adopted

guidelines for the promotion of regular physical activity in the population.

## EXERCISE GOALS AND GUIDELINES

The ACSM, the CDC and the NIH recommend that every US adult should accumulate 30 min or more of moderate-intensity exercise on most, if not all, days of the week. Moderate-intensity exercise is that performed at an intensity of 3–6 metabolic equivalents of task or METs (work metabolic rate/resting metabolic rate). This would be the equivalent of brisk walking at 3–4 miles per hour for most healthy adults. Among women aged 50–64 years, a recent survey revealed that less than half of the women interviewed engaged in any regular recreational exercise, and that less than 25% followed the current guidelines.[4] Overall, women over 65 years have one of the lowest levels of physical activity of any demographic group.[5,6]

Previous exercise guidelines had advocated 20–60 min of moderate- to high-intensity exercise performed three or more times per week. The new recommendations not only emphasize the benefits of moderate-intensity exercise but also encourage the accumulation of activity in short bouts (minimum of 10 min sessions accumulated throughout the day). Evidence suggests that cumulative exercise sessions are as beneficial as longer, sustained periods of training, and they may have the additional benefit of improved patient compliance.

Table 24.1 gives intensity levels for some common activities. Walking, swimming, and aerobics are usually done as dedicated exercise, but daily activities, such as stair climbing, house cleaning and so on can also be used to achieve 30 min of physical activity. The 1990 National Health

Interview Study found that the most commonly reported recreational activities for adults age 65 years and older were walking and gardening; other less frequently reported activities included golf, biking, and bowling.[5]

In summary, there are many recreational and daily activities that can be used to fulfil the recommended exercise requirements. The ACSM position papers on exercise make no specific activity recommendations, but do advise aerobic activities in general for the maintenance of health in both young and older adults.[7,8] Clearly, the most effective program is one that a patient will maintain over time, and this is more easily accomplished by emphasizing activities that an individual enjoys doing, and that are compatible with their lifestyle. In approaching the menopausal female, suggesting activities that may have been part of her earlier adult life, such as dancing, walking or swimming, would be reasonable. A beginning exercise prescription for an office worker might include stair climbing; on the other hand, a nature enthusiast may enjoy exploring walking, and hiking trails. Whatever the activity, it is important that it will be a program that the patient will incorporate into their daily routine and continue on a regular basis.

## Components of an exercise program

The three components of an exercise program are aerobic activities, strength training, and flexibility training. Including all of these elements is particularly vital in designing a program for the menopausal female, as maximum cardiovascular function, muscle strength and flexibility all decline with age. Yet, despite these declines, the cardiovascular and strengthening responses to exercise by older adults are similar to those of younger adults. Maximal oxygen consumption ($\dot{v}O_2$) can be expected to increase by 10–30% with endurance exercise training in both younger

and older adults.[9,10] Likewise, two- to three-fold increases in muscle strength can be accomplished in response to resistance training in the older adult – a result similar to findings in a younger cohort.[11] Most studies of regular exercise in the older age group have shown that exercise in general increases the range of motion in multiple joints, even without a planned flexibility training program.[12,13] Thus, the benefits of exercise are achievable by all age groups, and exercise counseling should be an important element in the care of the menopausal woman.

## Contraindications to exercise or exercise testing

In a healthy postmenopausal female with no cardiovascular risk factors, there is no indication for exercise stress testing prior to embarking on a graded exercise program. The ACSM lists the following conditions as absolute contraindications to exercise testing or exercise training: new electrocardiogram (ECG) changes or recent myocardial infarction, unstable angina, uncontrolled arrhythmias, third-degree heart block, and acute congestive heart failure.[14] Major relative contraindications include uncontrolled hypertension, cardiomyopathies, valvular heart disease, complex ventricular arrhythmia, and uncontrolled diabetes, thyroid, or other metabolic diseases. The approach to each patient in regard to exercise and exercise testing should be individualized, and in approaching the menopausal female, atypical presentations of cardiac disease should also be kept in mind. The ACSM guidelines for exercise testing can be used as a general schema for evaluating the need for pre-exercise cardiac evaluation and for planning an exercise program.[14]

## Writing an exercise prescription

In developing a graded exercise program for a patient, it is important to set reasonable goals based on the baseline level of fitness of each patient. In general, the conditioning intensity of an exercise session is most easily expressed as a percentage of the individual's maximal functional capacity, and the most direct way to do this is through heart rate achieved (the maximum heart rate is approximately 220 minus the patient's age).

As discussed above, physical activities that use large muscle groups in a continuous, rhythmic manner should be encouraged. Activities such as walking, hiking, swimming, bicycling, rowing,

| Table 24.1 Exercise intensity | | |
|---|---|---|
| **~3 MET** | **3–6 MET** | **6+ MET** |
| Stroll (1–2 mph) | Brisk walk (3–4 mph) | Uphill walk |
| Slow swim | Moderate swim | Fast swim |
| Stretches | Aerobics | Stair climbing |

MET: metabolic equivalent of task.

skating, jump roping, skiing, and dancing are ideal. Each session should last between 15 and 60 min, with an aerobic component of at least 10 min per session. Ideally, an exercise session should include a 5–10 min warm-up, 10–60 min of aerobic exercise at an appropriate training level (3–6 METs or 60–90% of maximal heart rate), and a cooldown of 5–10 min. The function of the warm-up is to gradually increase the metabolic rate from the resting level to the MET level required for conditioning. Likewise, the cool-down phase should include exercise of diminishing intensity to return the body gradually to the resting state.

Static stretching exercises of the large muscle groups involved in the particular exercise can be used during the warm-up period, and would incorporate one of the three elements of an exercise program: flexibility training. The aerobic training portion can be graded over weeks to months, gradually increasing the session length (with a goal of 20 min to no more than 60 min) and, eventually, the intensity as well. Muscle strengthening exercises can be incorporated to complete the triad of strengthening, flexibility, and aerobic conditioning.

## Exercise counseling

Exercise guidelines urge physicians and other health professionals to counsel patients to adopt and maintain regular physical activity. As with counseling on tobacco cessation and other preventive and safety measures, a few studies have shown that counseling on physical inactivity as a modifiable risk factor does seem to be beneficial.[15] The 1990 National Health Interview Study looked at the prevalence of leisure-time physical activity among men and women advised to exercise by their physician as a means of lowering high blood pressure. The patients who received exercise advice from their physicians were 50–60% more likely to exercise than those who had not been counseled in the importance of exercise.[16]

As with most behavioral counseling, there are some barriers and misconceptions towards adopting exercise as a lifestyle change, and these need to be taken into account to obtain most effectively the objective of incorporating physical activity into our patients' daily routine. First, it should be recognized that many patients view exercise as an all-or-nothing venture. Many feel that the inability initially to sustain moderate-intensity exercise for a reasonable length of time makes any attempt at exercise almost futile. Hopefully, emphasizing the recommendations for the accumulation of activity over the course of the day will decrease this threshold mentality. Second, many patients consider only those activities typically done as dedicated exercise (swimming, jogging, aerobics, and so on) to be beneficial to their health. As previously discussed, it is important to also encourage the use of daily activities, such as stair climbing, house cleaning, and walking to achieve the 30 min of physical activity recommended in the new guidelines. By doing this, the impact on time management is lessened, as some of the activities are incorporated into the patient's usual routine. Emphasizing the benefits of even modest increases in physical activity, and providing positive reinforcement, is an important element in approaching exercise counseling. Another caveat to share with patients is that the health benefits gained from increased physical activity depend on the patient's initial activity level, with sedentary individuals expected to benefit most from increasing their activity to the recommended level. This steep initial response curve should certainly be a positive message for the more sedentary patient.

In directing exercise counseling efforts towards the groups most at risk, there are several factors that have been shown to correlate with sedentary lifestyles. The 1990 Behavioral Risk Factor Surveillance System reported that older age, African-American race, low education, smoking, alcohol use, and obesity were all positively correlated with physical inactivity.[17] Conversely, younger age, higher income, lower body mass index (BMI), and higher education levels have been shown to be associated with more physically active lifestyles.[18] Maximal efforts at achieving behavioral changes should probably be focused on African-American women, who meet some of the higher risk criteria for inactive lifestyles.

## SEDENTARY LIFE-STYLE: A PROTEAN RISK FACTOR

The remainder of this chapter is primarily devoted to discussing the role of exercise in reducing the risk of multiple, specific disease processes. The aim is to discuss general trends, highlighted by the results of selected studies. For a more comprehensive review of available literature, the reader is directed to other sources, an excellent example of which is the Surgeon General's 'Report of Physical Activity and Health'.[19]

Beginning with general effects on health, a large landmark study showed that exercise reduced overall mortality – a very positive message to relay to patients. This study looked at a group of over 10 000 men and 3000 women at the Cooper Clinic, Dallas, Texas, and followed them for over 8 years. Physical fitness was measured by a maximal exercise treadmill test, and patients were assigned to fitness categories based on their age, sex, and maximal time on the treadmill. Treadmill time 'quintiles' were determined, and subjects with a treadmill time in the first quintile were assigned to the low-fitness group. Those with scores in the second to the fifth quintiles were assigned to groups two to five, group five being the most fit group.

Overall, this study found a strong, inverse association between fitness and all-cause mortality.[20] Importantly, comparing overall mortality between fitness group one (least fit) and fitness group five (most fit), the major reduction in all-cause death rates was between the first and second fitness levels. This change in fitness would be attainable with only moderate exercise, again emphasizing the fact that even a small change in the level of fitness can lead to large health gains.

Obviously, there are multiple variables other than physical activity in a study looking at all-cause mortality. However, the general trends seemed to remain valid after adjustment for age, smoking, cholesterol levels, fasting glucose levels, and family history of heart disease. Low physical fitness was an important risk factor for both men and women, and higher levels of physical fitness appeared to delay all-cause mortality.

A recently published analysis of the effect of physical activity on mortality using data collected from the Nurse's Health Study was published by Hu et al.[21] This study examined the association of BMI and physical activity with death among over 10 000 women with no known cardiovascular disease or cancer. They found that both obesity and sedentary lifestyles were strong and independent predictors of mortality. Thus, over more than a decade of research, these same correlations hold true: physical inactivity remains an important risk factor for morbidity and mortality in women.

## CORONARY ARTERY DISEASE AND WOMEN'S HEALTH

Coronary artery disease (CAD) is the leading cause of death in women in the US. In 1991, the age-adjusted death rates per 100 000 from CAD were 197.4 for white women, and 129.1 for African-American women; this compares to breast cancer rates of 35.5 for white women and 29.3 for African-American women.[22] The incidence of myocardial infarction or death from CAD in premenopausal women is below 1/10 000 per year; one-third of all deaths occur from age 65 to age 74 years in women, and a majority of cardiovascular deaths occur after age 75.[23] As noted in the previously cited studies, the largest reduction in deaths due to higher levels of physical fitness resulted from a decrease in coronary events. Sedentary lifestyle is a well-defined cardiovascular risk factor, and it has been estimated that as many of 35% of excess deaths due to CAD could be eliminated by increasing physical activity.[24]

There are probably multiple mechanisms by which exercise may contribute to the primary or secondary prevention of CAD. These include delay of progression of coronary atherosclerosis by improving the lipoprotein profile (increasing high-density lipoprotein (HDL)/low-density lipoprotein (LDL) ratio), improving carbohydrate metabolism (increasing insulin sensitivity), and possibly decreasing platelet aggregation. In addition, enhanced physical fitness decreases myocardial work and oxygen demand, and has modest effects on reducing blood pressure.

Exercise may also affect CAD by producing a more favorable overall cardiac risk factor profile. One study examined the effects of fitness levels, again determined by maximal treadmill tests, on multiple cardiac risk factors in healthy women. They found that enhanced physical fitness was associated with lower body weight, a lower incidence of cigarette smoking, lower systolic and diastolic blood pressures, and a lower total cholesterol with an improved HDL/LDL ratio.[25] Not surprisingly, the more fit women also had a lower incidence of cardiovascular disease. A recent study looking at women who underwent coronary angiography for suspected ischemia showed that a higher level of self-reported fitness, but not a lower BMI, was associated with a lower incidence of coronary disease on angiography, fewer cardiac risk factors, and a lower incidence of cardiovascular events.[26]

## OBESITY

Along with being a comorbid factor for cardiovascular disease, obesity is at nearly epidemic proportions in the US. Approximately 33% of US adults are overweight,[27] and a tremendous number of healthcare dollars are spent on diseases associated with obesity. With estimated healthcare expenditures of over $US68 billion per year,[28] this problem clearly has economic as well as medical implications. Although an issue in all age groups, progressive weight gain is often a problem in the third to sixth decades of life, and is a common presenting problem in the perimenopausal and postmenopausal female. One contributor to this problem may be an age-related decline in energy expenditure,[29] but many other factors probably also contribute, including metabolic and hormonal changes associated with aging.

Obesity is most easily defined in terms of the BMI, calculated by dividing the patient's weight (kilograms) by her height (meters) squared. An acceptable BMI for women would be approximately 19–24 or 25. A BMI greater than 27 is associated with a three to four times greater risk of CAD, and is also linked to hypertension, type II diabetes and some types of cancer.[30] Data analyzed from the Nurse's Health Study found obesity to be a strong independent predictor of death. Even in physically active women, modest weight gain during adulthood was found to be associated with higher risks of death.[21]

Exercise probably has multiple benefits in weight control, including decreasing appetite and preserving lean body mass. Exercise is also useful in enhancing mood and improving self-image, and these can be useful motivators in maintaining diet programs.

Multiple trials have looked at the relationship of exercise to weight loss. The Minnesota Heart Health Program examined several interventions aimed at increasing physical activity for the purpose of weight loss. These included educational programs and even small financial incentives. Some were effective, and others showed no significant change in one year of follow-up.[31]

Adherence to exercise regimens is an obvious problem; one study that looked at the addition of a walking program for weight loss in obese women reported a 68% dropout rate.[32] However, those who did continue with the exercise regimen lost significant amounts of fat. Exercise also seems to be an important factor in the maintenance of weight loss over time.[33] Interestingly, adherence to exercise and weight loss and maintenance may be better in programs with low rather than high caloric expenditure.[34] This makes sense in that it is more likely that patients will be able to maintain a low- or moderate-intensity regimen over time, but may become discouraged or burned out with a more strenuous program.

Finally, preventing weight gain would eliminate the difficulties involved in treating obesity, and the perimenopausal period appears to be a time frame in which weight control interventions are particularly successful.[35] Many women seek advice from their physicians in realtion to weight control, and this affords an important opportunity for counseling on the importance of exercise in both improving and maintaining health.

## TYPE II DIABETES: A PREVENTABLE DISEASE

Recent projections predict that the number of individuals with type II diabetes will increase nearly 16-fold in the coming years. This trend is closely linked to the fact that nearly one-third of the American population is overweight. Weight is a major concern in both the development of and treatment strategies for type II diabetes. Exercise is an important, yet often neglected modality in the treatment of diabetes, and has been shown to decrease insulin requirements and improve glucose tolerance.[36,37] Along with diet and medical interventions, exercise needs to be a cornerstone in the treatment and, more importantly, the prevention of diabetes.

A 1991 study used data from the University of Pennsylvania Alumni Health Study to determine the effect of exercise on the subsequent development of type II diabetes.[38] The authors found that leisure-time physical activity was inversely related to the later development of diabetes. Moreover, the protective effect of exercise was strongest in the highest-risk patients: obese patients, hypertensive patients, and those with a family history of type II diabetes. Overall, the occurrence of type II diabetes was found to be reduced by 6% for every 500 kcal per week increase in physical activity. Sports activities such as jogging, bicycling, and swimming at moderate intensity were effective. This retrospective study of nearly 6000 male patients supports the hypothesis that regular physical activity lowers the risk of developing non-insulin-dependent diabetes. More recent studies exploring the effect of physical activity on the subsequent development of type II diabetes have also shown an inverse relationship between exercise and the risk of diabetes in women.[39] Therefore, it would seem reasonable that providing guidance and counseling on exercise would be a positive step in curbing the growing epidemic of type II diabetes.

As with CAD, obesity and overall mortality, no controlled clinical trials have been conducted on type II diabetes and physical activity. Large epidemiological studies, such as the University of Pennsylvania study, do support the role of exercise in the prevention of diabetes, and the Surgeon General has advocated this as a useful preventive strategy.[19] As with CAD, one of the benefits of exercise in diabetes is probably in producing an improved overall risk factor profile, that is, improving blood pressure, body fat composition, and lipoprotein profiles.

## OSTEOPOROSIS

A mounting concern in women's health over the past few years has been postmenopausal bone loss. This is probably attributable to several factors. First, there are higher percentages of women living to ages where the complications of osteoporosis become apparent. Second, the widespread availability of dual-energy X-ray absorbiometry (DEXA) scanners allows for the accurate quantitation of bone loss. Third, the advent of non-hormonal treatments and preventive strategies for osteoporosis has produced new medical interventions for this disease process. Finally, the social and economic impact of complications of osteoporosis, particularly hip fractures, is enormous. In the early 1980s alone, nearly US$4 billion per year were spent on the treatment of osteoporotic fractures. Additionally, hip fractures have a 15–20% 1-year mortality rate,[40] making the prevention of such events an important consideration in the care of the postmenopausal woman.

Bone mineral density is dependent on several factors, including hormonal milieu, calcium metabolism, and physical activity, among other things. The attention in this discussion is focused on the role that physical activity plays in bone remodeling. Unfortunately, there really are no simple answers regarding what types of exercise may be most beneficial in either maintaining or increasing bone mineral density. The multitude of published studies have differed greatly in the mode, intensity, and duration of exercise used, making it difficult to provide specific guidelines in prescribing exercise regimens. However, a few generalizations can be made.

Clearly, physical inactivity is a strong risk factor for bone loss. This has been demonstrated in subjects during extended periods of bed rest.[41] In addition, studies comparing the bone density of athletes to that of sedentary subjects support the concept of a higher bone density in the active versus the inactive population.[42,43] The type of exercise that may be most beneficial is unclear, but both resistance and endurance activities (weight lifting and aerobics, for example) seem to have positive effects on bone density.[44] In general, however, weight-bearing exercise is probably more beneficial than non-weight-bearing exercise. A study of female athletes ages 42–50 years found that bone mineral density in long-term swimmers did not differ significantly from that of sedentary subjects.[42]

Although the optimal exercise regimen for preserving and improving bone density is not known, a moderate intensity weight-bearing exercise program should be considered in most peri- and postmenopausal women. The role of bisphosphonates and selective estrogen receptor modulators in conjunction with physical activity has been less well explored at this point. The role of these agents combined with specific exercise regimens, along with further studies of the longitudinal effects of physical activity and the optimal types of activity to maintain bone mass may by avenues for future research.

### Fall prevention

A vital component in the treatment plan for a woman with osteoporosis is the prevention of falls that could lead to osteoporotic fractures. Exercise is not only an important modality in improving bone density, but exercise interventions in the elderly may also decrease fall frequency and thereby decrease the risk of hip fractures. Several studies have shown that physical activity may be useful in preventing falls; other studies have failed to show a significant effect. A meta-analysis of a series of large trials, the FICIT trials (Frailty and Injuries: Cooperative Studies of Intervention Techniques), found that assignment to an exercise group was associated with a decrease in the risk of falling.[45] The interventions used in these trials, however, were quite varied, and included non-exercise components, so the effect of exercise as a sole modality remains unclear but it may well be of benefit. Resistance training to improve overall strength has also been shown to be effective in decreasing fall risk, even in the frail elderly.[46]

Exercise probably affects muscle strength and balance, and in that way improves gait stability. The risk of falls in the elderly, however, is a multifactorial problem, and includes factors such as visual acuity, medications, environmental hazards (throw rugs, appliance cords, etc) and so on. Overall, the ACSM concurs that there is sufficient evidence that strength training and other forms of exercise may reduce fall risk, and recommends 'a broad based exercise program that includes balance training, resistive exercise, walking and weight transfer ... as part of a multifaceted intervention to reduce the risk of falling'.[9]

## CANCER PREVENTION

One of the less obvious benefits of exercise, and certainly a concern for most patients, is the correlation between exercise and several types of cancer. The most studied associations have been in the area of colon and breast cancer, but a small number of studies have also looked at the relationship between exercise and endometrial and ovarian cancer. In general, the mechanisms for the positive effects of exercise on neoplastic processes are unclear. However, sharing with patients some of the positive correlations may help to motivate a healthy move towards a more physically active lifestyle. Along with the standard American Cancer Society guidelines for screening for cancer, consideration should be given to emphasizing exercise as part of a healthy lifestyle, and possibly as a component in decreasing the risk of certain types of cancer.

### Colon cancer and exercise

The positive benefit of exercise for prevention of colon cancer in men has been well reported in the past. Previous studies looking at the correlation in women had not shown a significant association between colon cancer and exercise. However, recent large studies indicate that exercise may play a protective role in preventing development of colon cancer in women.

A look at the correlation between colon cancer and exercise using data from the Nurses' Health Study was published in the July 1997 issue of *Journal of the National Cancer Institute*. This study found a significant inverse association between leisure-time physical activity and the incidence of colon cancer in this large cohort of women. It found that moderate-intensity exercise for 1 h per day

decreased the risk of colon cancer by 46%. Significantly, this effect was independent and separate even from an elevated BMI, a previously known risk factor for colon cancer.[47] The mechanism for the positive effect of exercise in colon cancer is unclear. Some proposed theories include decreased gastrointestinal transit time, increased immune function and altered prostaglandin levels.

Likewise, the Cancer Prevention Study II Nutrition Cohort found that increasing amounts of recreational activity among both men and women were associated with a lower risk of colon cancer, even when the activity began later in life, a promising finding for menopausal women.[48] This study also reported an inverse relationship between rectal cancer and activity, an association that had not been found in previous studies.

### Breast cancer

The evidence for the role of exercise in decreasing breast cancer risk is inconsistent. Some studies have shown a protective effect, and others have shown no significant association. Specific findings are well outlined and reviewed in other sources.[19,49] While the data regarding an association between breast cancer and exercise are inconsistent, the yearly screening visit for this disease does afford the opportunity for counseling on other issues, such as the general health benefits of exercise.

## EXERCISE AND MOOD

Depression is one of the most common presenting problems in the outpatient primary care setting, and women tend to report a higher prevalence of depression and other affective disorders than do men. Exercise may have multiple psychological benefits, including improving self-esteem and body image, providing a sense of wellbeing, and improving mood, as well as decreasing mild stress and anxiety. Multiple studies suggest a positive correlation between physical activity and mood. A 1990 nationwide Canadian survey showed an inverse relationship between symptoms of depression and physical activity in adults over 25 years of age.[50] Another study compared 12 weeks of aerobic exercise to traditional psychotherapy in the treatment of mild to moderate depression, and found that exercise reduced depression symptoms to a greater degree than did therapy.[51] Several other large studies have revealed an inverse relationship between exercise and depression.[52,53] The Iowa 65+ Rural Health Study reported a decrease in depression symptoms in men and women aged 65 years and older, who walked on a daily basis.[54]

Mood swings and mild to moderate depression and anxiety may accompany the menopause. A recent study looked at the effects of exercise on both mood and reporting of menopausal vasomotor symptoms. The researchers found that exercise had a positive effect on mood, and that immediately after exercise women had a significant decrease in reported vasomotor symptoms.[55] In light of significant recent concerns regarding the safety of hormonal therapy, exercise may be an important adjunct in treating symptoms of menopause.

## ADVERSE EFFECTS OF EXERCISE

As discussed to this point, exercise may have multiple health benefits, but there are potential adverse effects of exercise. The most common are orthopedic injuries, and these tend to be sports-specific. Runners are subject to overuse injuries of the lower extremities. Conversely, swimmers more often suffer shoulder injuries. Compared with males, female athletes demonstrated similar sports-related injury rates overall.[56] Strains and sprains of the ankle and knee are the most commonly reported musculoskeletal injuries.[57] The majority of orthopedic injuries are self-limited and often related to overuse. Most are probably preventable with the use of a moderate-intensity, graded exercise program.

Adverse cardiac events, such as angina, acute myocardial infarction, arrhythmias and sudden death can be a concern with either starting a new exercise regimen, or increasing the intensity of an established program. However, as discussed above, the benefits of physical activity in reducing CAD and coronary risk factors probably far outweigh the potential for adverse cardiac events. As recommended by the ACSM, women over the age of 50 years who wish to embark on a new exercise regimen or women with risk factors for heart disease or other chronic medical problems should consult a physician prior to starting training.[7,8]

## CONCLUSION

A majority of patients lead a sedentary lifestyle, which has profound implications on the development of multiple disease processes. Exercise counseling should be an integral consideration in preventive health strategies. Women, particularly those over age 65, are at particular risk for an inactive lifestyle, and many of the physiological changes associated with aging and the menopause can be positively impacted upon by exercise. A recent (2004) collaboration between the American Cancer Society, the American Diabetes Association and the American Heart Association to help prevent cancer, cardiovascular disease and diabetes highlights the positive effects of weight loss and exercise on these disease processes and represents a growing awareness of the need to focus on exercise as an important component of health and disease prevention.

## REFERENCES

1. Centers for Disease Control. Sex-, age- and region-specific prevalence for sedentary lifestyle in selected states in 1985. The Behavioral Risk Factor Surveillance System. Morbid Mortal Weekly Rep 1987; 36: 195.
2. Centers for Disease Control. CDC Surveillance Summaries. Morbid Mortal Weekly Rep 1990; 39: 8.
3. Hahn RA, Teutsch SM, Rothenberg RB, Marks GS. Excess deaths from nine chronic diseases in the United States. JAMA 1986; 264: 2654–9.
4. McTeirnan A, Stanford JL, Daling J, Voigt LF. Prevalence and correlates of recreational physical activity in women aged 50–64 years. Menopause 1997; 5: 95–101.
5. Caspersen CJ, Christenson GM, Pollard RA. Status of the 1990 physical fitness and exercise objectives: evidence from the NHIS 1985. Public Health Rep: 1986; 101: 587–93.
6. Lee C. Factors related to adoption of exercise among older women. J Behav Med 1993; 16: 323–34.
7. American College of Sports Medicine. Position stand: the recommended quantity and quality of exercise for developing and maintaining cardio- respiratory and muscular fitness and flexibility in healthy adults. Med Sci Sports Exercise 1998; 30: 975–89.
8. American College of Sports Medicine. Position stand: exercise and physical activity for older adults. Med Sci Sports Exercise 1998; 30: 992–1008.
9. Kohrt W, Malley M, Coggan AR et al. Effects of gender, age and fitness level on response of $\dot{v}O_2$ max to training in 60–71 year olds. J Appl Physiol 1991; 71: 2004–11.
10. Seals D, Hagberg J, Jurley B, Ehsani A, Hollozy J. Endurance training in older men and women: I Cardiovascular responses to exercise. J Appl Physiol 1984; 57: 1 024–9.
11. Frontera WR, Meredith CN, O'Reilly KP, Knuttzen HG, Evans WJ. Strength conditioning in older men: skeletal muscle hypertrophy and improved function. J Appl Physiol 1988; 64: 1038–44.

12. Hubley-Kozcy CL, Wall JC, Hogan DB. Effects of a general exercise program on passive hip, knee and ankle range of motion of older women. Top Geriatr Rehabil 1995; 10: 33–44.

13. Leslie DK, Frekany GA. Effects of an exercise program on selected flexibility measures of senior citizens. Gerontologist 1975; 4: 182–3.

14. American College of Sports Medicine. ACSM's Guidelines for Exercise Testing and Prescription, 5th edn. Baltimore: Williams and Wilkins, 1995.

15. Lewis BS, Lynch WD. The effect of physician advice on exercise behaviour. Prev Med 1993; 22: 110–21.

16. Yusuf HR, Croft JB, Giles WH et al. Leisure-time physical activity among older adults United States, 1990. Arch Intern Med 1996; 156: 1321–6.

17. Simoes EJ, Byers T, Coates RJ et al. The association between leisure-time physical activity and dietary fat in American adults. Am J Public Health 1995; 85: 240–4.

18. Patterson RE, Haines PS, Popkin BM. Health life-style patterns of US adults. Prev Med 1194; 23: 453–60.

19. US Department of Health and Human Services. Physical Activity and Health: A Report of the Surgeon General. Atlanta, GA: US Department of Health and Human Services, Centers for Disease Control and Prevention, National Center for Chronic Disease Prevention and Health Promotion, International Medical Publishing, 1996.

20. Blair SN, Kohl HW, Paffenbarger RS, Clark DG, Cooper KH, Gibbons LW. Physical fitness and all cause mortality: a prospective study of healthy men and women. JAMA 1989; 262: 2395–401.

21. Hu FB, Willett WC, Li T, Stampfer MJ, Colditz GA, Manson JE. Adiposity as compared with physical activity in predicting mortality among women. N Engl J Med 2004; 351: 2694–703.

22. Vital Statistics of the United States, 199. Vol. II, Mortality Part A. DHHS Publication No. (PHS) 96–101. Hyattsville, MD: USDH&HS, PHS, CDC, NCHS, 1996.

23. Siegel AJ. Medical conditions arising during sports. In: Shangold M, Miran G, eds. Women and Exercise: Physiology and Sports Medicine, 2nd edn. Philadelphia, PA: FA Davis, 1994: 261–78.

24. Powell KE, Blair SN. The public health burdens of sedentary living habits: theoretical but realistic estimates. Med Sci Sports Exercise 1994; 26: 851–6.

25. Gibbons LW, Blair SN, Cooper KH et al. Association between coronary heart disease risk factors and physical fitness in healthy adult women. Circulation 1983; 67: 977–83.

26. Wessel TR, Arant CB, Olson MB et al. Relationship of physical fitness vs. body mass index with coronary artery disease in women. JAMA 2004; 292: 1179–87.

27. National Task Force on the prevention and treatment of obesity. Long term pharmacotherapy in the management of obesity. JAMA 1996; 276: 1907–15.

28. Kuczmarski RJ, Flegal KM, Campbell SM, Johnson CL. Increasing prevalence of overweight among US, adults. JAMA 1994; 272: 205–11.

29. Bray GA. The energetics of obesity. Med Sci Sports Exercise 1983; 15: 32–40.

30. Van Itallie T. Health implications of overweight and obesity in the United States. Ann Intern Med 1985; 103: 983–8.

31. Jeffery RW. Community programs for obesity prevention: the Minnesota Heart Health Program. Obesity Res 1995; Suppl 3: 283–8s.

32. Gwinup G. Effect of exercise alone on the weight of obese women. Arch Intern Med 1975; 135: 676.

33. Brownell KD. Behavioral, psychological and environmental predictors of obesity and success in weight reduction. Int J Obesity 1984; 8: 543.

34. Pavlou KN, Krey S, Stefee WP. Exercise as an adjunct to weight loss and maintenance in moderately obese subjects. Am J Clin Nutr 1989; 49: 1115.

35. Wing RR. Changing diet and exercise behaviors in individuals at risk for weight gain. Obesity Res 1995; Suppl 3: 277–82.

36. Soman VR, Koivisto VA, Deibert D, Felig P, DeFronzo RA. Increased insulin sensitivity and insulin binding to monocytes after physical training. N Engl J Med 1979; 301: 1200–4.

37. Rauramaa R. Relationship of physical activity, glucose tolerance and weight management. Prev Med 1984; 13: 37–46.

38. Helmrich SP, Ragland DR, Leung RW, Paffenbarger RS. Physical activity and reduced occurrence of non-insulin dependent diabetes mellitus. N Engl J Med 1991; 325: 147–51.

39. Hu FB, Sigal RJ, Rich-Edwards JW et al. Walking compared with vigorous physical activity and risk of type 2 diabetes in women: a prospective study. JAMA 1999; 282: 1433–9.

40. National Institutes of Health. Consensus Development Conference on Osteoporosis, Vol. 5, No.3. Washington, DC: Government Printing Office, 1984.

41. Donaldson CL, Hulley SB, Vogel JM, Hattner KS, Bayers JH, McMillan DE. Effect of prolonged bed rest on bone mineral. Metab Clin Exp 1970; 19: 1071–84.

42. Kirchner EM, Lewis RD, O'Connor PT. Effect of past gymnastics participation on adult bone mass. J Appl Physiol 1996; 80: 225–32.

43. Dook JE, James C, Henderson NK, Price RI. Exercise and bone mineral density in mature female athletes. Med Sci Sports Exercise 1997; 29: 291–6.

44. Nilsson BE, Westlin NE. Bone density in athletes. Clin Orthop 1971; 77: 179–82.

45. Province MA, Hadley EC, Hombrook MC et al. The effects of exercise on falls in elderly patients: a preplanned meta-analysis of the FICSIT trials – Frailty and Injuries: Cooperative Studies of Intervention Techniques. JAMA 1995; 273: 1341–7.

46. Fiatarone MA, O'Neill EF, Ryan ND et al. Exercise training and nutritional supplementation for physical frailty in very elderly people. N Engl J Med 1994; 330: 1769–75.

47. Martinez ME, Giovannucci E, Spiegelman D, Hunter DJ, Willet WC, Colditz GA. Leisure time physical activity. Body size and colon cancer in women. J Natl Cancer Inst 1997; 89: 948–54.

48. Chao A, Connell CJ, Jacobs EJ et al. Amount, type, and timing of recreational physical activity in relation to colon and rectal cancer in older adults: the Cancer Prevention Study II Nutrition Cohort. Cancer Epidemiol Biomarkers Prev 2004; Vol 13: 2187–95.

49. Gammon MD, Schoenberg JB, Britton JA et al. Recreational physical activity and breast cancer risk among women under 45 years. Am J Epidemiol 1998; 147: 273–80.

50. Stephens J, Craig CL. The Well Being of Canadians: Highlights of the 1988 Campbell's Survey. Ottawa: Canadian Fitness and Lifestyle Research Institute, 1990.

51. Griest JH, Klein MH, Eicchens RR et al. Running as a treatment for depression. Comp Psychiatry 1979; 20: 41.

52. Camacho JC, Roberts RE, Lazarus NB, Kaplan GA, Cahen RD. Physical activity and depression: evidence from the Alameda County study. Am J Epidemiol 1991; 134: 220–31.

53. Paffenbarger RS, Lee IM, Leung R. Physical activity and personal characteristics associated with depression and suicide in American college men. Acta Psychiatr Scand 1994; Suppl 377: 16–22.

54. Mobily KE, Rubenstein JH, Lemke JH, O'Hara MW, Wallace RB. Walking and depression in a cohort of older adults: the Iowa 65+ Rural Health Study. J Aging Physiol Activ 1996; 4: 119–35.

55. Slaven L, Lee C. Mood and symptom reporting among middle-aged women: the relationship between menopausal status, hormone replacement therapy and exercise participation. Health Psychol 1997; 16: 203–8.

56. Whiteside P. Men's and women's injuries in comparable sports. Physician Sports Med 1980; 8: 130.

57. Rettawen K. Athletic injuries: comparison by age, sport and gender. Am J Sports Med 1986; 14: 218.

# Chapter 25

# Vision in the menopausal woman

Parveen K Nagra

## INTRODUCTION

Cataracts, age-related macular degeneration, diabetic retinopathy and glaucoma are leading causes of visual impairment and blindness in the aging population throughout the world.[1] In addition, the incidence of dry eye syndrome, or keratoconjunctivitis sicca, is increased in postmenopausal women.[2-4] Associations, albeit controversial, between these conditions and sex hormones, including hormone replacement therapy (HRT), have been demonstrated. As postmenopausal women are enjoying increasing life expectancy, they have a high probability of developing some of these age-related ocular conditions.

## DRY EYES

Dry eye syndrome is one of the most common ocular conditions affecting the general population. Its refers to a heterogenous group of diseases that lead to decreased tear production, increased evaporative loss of tears, or instability of the tear film. Dry eye syndrome may be associated with debilitating symptoms such as ocular irritation, pain, redness, foreign body sensation, and blurry vision, and may lead to a diminished quality of life and high economic burden.[5-7] Signs and symptoms of dry eyes have been shown to occur more frequently in women and in older populations.[2-4] Sjögren's syndrome, an inflammatory condition marked by severe dry eyes, occurs almost exclusively in women. In addition, postmenopausal women and patients with premature ovarian failure have also been found to have a higher prevalence of dry eyes when compared to premenopausal controls.[8,9]

The tear film is primary composed of three layers. An inner mucin layer, formed by conjunctival goblet cells, a middle aqueous layer, formed by lacrimal glands, and an outer oily layer, formed by meibomian glands make up the tear film (Figure 25.1). Alterations in any of these layers can lead to dry eyes. All of these components of the tear film have been shown to be hormonally regulated. Cyclical changes in the maturity index of the conjunctival epithelium have been associated with hormonal changes during the menstrual cycles, suggesting the conjunctiva is an estrogen-sensitive tissue.[10] Androgen and prolactin receptors, but not estrogen receptors, have been found in lacrimal glands.[11-13] However, estrogen may play an indirect role on lacrimal gland function, suggested by sex- and age-related differences in the level of lacrimal gland peroxidase, an antioxidant and antimicrobial involved in protecting the ocular surface.[14]

Meibomian glands, which are specialized sebaceous glands, have been demonstrated to be androgen target organs.[15-16] Androgens have been shown

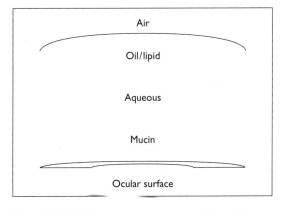

**Figure 25.1** Schematic representation of tear film.

to be involved in the development, differentiation, and lipid production of sebaceous glands throughout the body.[17–19] Androgen insensitivity and the use of anti-androgen medications have been associated with meibomian gland dysfunction and dry eyes.[20–23]

The different structures involved in tear production and their hormonal influences create a complex relationship between menopause and dry eyes. As menopause leads to alterations in hormonal levels, these changes may lead to alterations in tear production, stability and evaporation. Several studies have assessed the effect of HRT on the ocular surface with conflicting results. Some have found no significant correlation with HRT and self-reported dry eye symptoms,[3,4] while others have found a significant association between dry eye syndrome and hormone replacement therapy.[24] The largest study, the Women's Health Study, involving over 25 000 postmenopausal women, found those who used HRT, especially estrogen alone (odds ratio 1.69), were at higher risk of dry eye syndrome. Further, this study showed that the risk of dry eyes increased with the duration of HRT.[25]

However, other smaller studies have suggested that HRT may be beneficial for patients with dry eyes.[9,26–28] Given the possible benefit of hormone replacement in some studies, topical estrogen therapy has been proposed as a treatment for postmenopausal dry eyes.[29] Further clinical trials are needed to assess the role of topical estrogens and androgens in the treatment of dry eyes.

The treatment of dry eyes typically begins with topical artificial tears, used frequently throughout the day. Often, treatment of meibomitis, with warm compresses followed by lid scrubs with a mild soap or shampoo, is also recommended to improve production of the oily layer of tears and the quality of the tear film. For patients who require additional therapy, topical cyclosporin A has been shown to increase tear production by its anti-inflammatory properties. Another alternative is punctual occlusion, whereby punctual plugs are inserted into the lacrimal puncta to prevent drainage of tears. Punctal plugs can be inserted into the lower lid's punctum alone for mild to moderate cases of dry eye, or both the upper and lower lid puncta in moderate to severe cases, to achieve total occlusion of the puncta and prevention of tear drainage. Advanced dry eyes, in addition to all of the treatments mentioned, may require much less common approaches including autologous serum eyedrops and lateral tarsorrhaphy, to minimize the exposed surface area of the ocular surface.

## CATARACT

Cataracts remain the leading cause of blindness worldwide.[1] Cataracts, which most commonly affect people beginning in their fifth decade of life, are a result of natural clouding and opacification of the lens. This typically results in gradual, painless loss of vision. There are several subtypes of cataracts, including nuclear sclerosis, cortical, and posterior subcapsular, all of which may lead to decreased or blurred vision.

Estrogen-receptor RNA has been found in the natural lens, suggesting that this tissue may be hormonally influenced.[30,31] Several clinical studies have also exposed the possible hormonal influences in the lens. Older age at menarche has been associated with increased severity of nuclear sclerosis, while older age at menopause was associated with a decrease in cortical cataracts, and postmenopausal use of HRT was associated with less severe nuclear sclerosis.[32,33] A large epidemiological study, the Beaver Dam Eye Study, found a trend towards a protective effect of increasing number of live births with posterior subcapsular cataract, although another similar study, the Blue Mountain Eye Study did not confirm this association.[34–35] In addition, postmenopausal women, compared to men, have been shown to have a higher incidence of cataract formation, particularly cortical cataracts.[32,36,37]

The incidence of cataract among HRT users is controversial, with some studies demonstrating a decrease in the incidence of nuclear opacities and posterior subcapular opacities with the use of HRT,[38–39] while another suggests an increased incidence of posterior subcapsular opacities with HRT use,[34] and still others find little evidence of an association between HRT use and incidence of cataracts.[35,40] Clearly more research is indicated into the role of hormones in cataract formation, as well as the possible protective effect of HRT.

Cataracts usually progress slowly, and in their early stages are usually followed conservatively. When patients begin to notice visual compromise leading to difficulty with daily activities, intervention may be warranted. Cataract extraction is typically performed with the use of ultrasound, or phacoemulsification, and is followed by the placement of an intraocular lens. Modern-day cataract extraction is very successful in achieving reversal of visual loss. Newer intraocular lenses promise correction of both distance and near vision without the use of glasses.

## AGE-RELATED MACULAR DEGENERATION

Age-related macular degeneration (ARMD) is one of the leading causes of irreversible visual loss in industrialized nations among patients 65 years and older.[41–43] As the name implies, this condition predominantly affects older patients, leading to painless, loss of central vision. It may be more common in women.[44] There are two main subtypes, non-exudative ('dry') and exudative ('wet'). Non-exudative ARMD, the most common form, is characterized by intraretinal deposits called drusen, while exudative ARMD may lead to intraretinal bleeding and scarring, with significant visual consequences.

Similar to other ocular structures, estrogen receptors have also been found in the retina and retinal pigment epithelium, suggesting these structures may also be hormonally influenced.[45,46] In spite of this possible influence, however, there is conflicting data regarding the role of hormones in ARMD. A few studies have shown a decreased risk of ARMD associated with increasing years from menarche to menopause,[44] and among post-menopausal estrogen users and nulliparous women;[47,48] other studies have failed to confirm an association.[49–51] Given this conflicting picture, more studies are warranted to further investigate the influence of hormones and hormone replacement on this condition.

There is no treatment for non-exudative ARMD. Patients are typically observed closely, and instructed to perform frequent monocular testing of their central vision to assess for progression. Exudative changes can be treated with laser photocoagulation, photodynamic therapy, or intra-ocular injection of an anti-VEGF (vascular endothelial growth factor) molecule. A large, National Eye Institute-sponsored, multicenter study has demonstrated that a combination of vitamins and minerals (vitamin C, vitamin E, beta-carotene, zinc, and copper) may slow the progression of intermediate to advanced macular degeneration and its associated visual loss.[52] It should be stressed to the patient that ARMD cannot be cured, visual loss cannot be reversed, and treatments are aimed at slowing or stopping the progression of the disease and loss of vision.

## DIABETIC RETINOPATHY

Diabetic retinopathy, a microvasculopathy often associated with poor glucose control, can be divided into non-proliferative and proliferative changes. Non-proliferative diabetic retinopathy is characterized by microaneurysm, retinal hemorrhages and cotton-wool spots (small retinal infarcts), while the more advanced proliferative diabetic retinopathy is associated with optic nerve and retinal neovascularization, which leads to vitreous hemorrhages, retinal detachments and potentially significant visual loss. Diabetics are also at risk for macular edema, which may lead to loss of central vision, and can occur in either non-proliferative or proliferative retinopathy.

Sex hormones appear to have an influence on diabetes mellitus, which itself is a condition that is hormonally responsive to insulin. Glucose control has been show to vary during the menstrual cycle.[53] Type 1 diabetes may also be a risk factor for menstrual disturbances,[54] and long or highly irregular menstrual cycles have been suggested as a risk factor for the development of type 2 diabetes.[55] In addition, pregnancy has been shown to lead to increased insulin resistance and worsening of diabetic retinopathy. Similar to ARMD, as the retina and retinal pigment epithelium has estrogen receptors, diabetic retinopathy may be influenced by this hormone. Diabetic men under age 45 years have been shown to have a higher rate of diabetic retinopathy, which equalizes among the two sexes after age 45, suggesting sex hormones may have a protective effect.[56] Although few studies have looked directly at hormone replacement and diabetic retinopathy, several have suggested HRT may decrease the incidence of diabetes and improve glycemic control, which would indirectly positively influence the development and progression of diabetic retinopathy.[57,58]

It has been well-established that improved blood sugar control may decrease the onset and progression of diabetic retinopathy. In the management of these patients, counseling regarding improved diabetic control is imperative. There is no current treatment for non-proliferative diabetic retinopathy, and these patients are observed closely for signs of proliferative changes. Proliferative retinopathy is often treated with laser photocoagulation, and may require vitreoretinal surgery. Macular edema may benefit from laser photocoagulation treatment, intravitreal steroids or anti-VEGF therapy.

## GLAUCOMA

Glaucoma is a leading cause of irreversible blindness worldwide. This insidious optic neuropathy is often associated with elevated intraocular pressure, and may lead to loss of visual field. Glaucoma is often divided into open-angle and angle-closure, based on the anatomy of the anterior chamber and trabecular meshwork. Primary open-angle glaucoma is the most common type of glaucoma, and therefore an important subject of research.

The prevalence of glaucoma increases with age. Some studies have suggested a higher prevalence of primary open-angle glaucoma in men,[59–61] while other have reported no significant difference in the prevalences between men and women.[62,63] Intraocular pressure, a risk factor for glaucoma, has been found to fluctuate with the menstrual cycle in women, both with and without glaucoma.[64,65] In addition, primary open-age glaucoma has been associated with late menarche and increased parity as well as early menopause.[66,67] HRT has been shown to significantly decrease intraocular pressure in postmenopausal women in some studies,[68,69] with other suggesting no significant association.[70] While more evidence is necessary before a conclusion can be reached, the current data suggest a hormonal influence in intraocular pressure and glaucoma.

Glaucoma is evaluated and followed with frequent intraocular pressure evaluations, and regular dilated examinations of the optic discs with careful documentation of its appearance. Additional testing includes visual field testing, usually performed with automated perimetry, and optic disc documentation with traditional photographs or newer instruments that allow more detailed optic nerve analysis. Treatment of glaucoma is aimed at slowing or halting the progression of disease, and consists of topical medications, laser procedures or surgery.

## CONCLUSION

As the population continues to age, ocular conditions such as dry eyes, cataract, age-related macular degeneration, diabetic retinopathy, and glaucoma are becoming more prevalent. The onset of menopause also seems to influence the onset of these conditions independent of aging, as many ocular tissues have been found to be hormonally sensitive. While some preliminary evidence is available, there are many conflicting reports regarding the role of hormones and the benefits of HRT. Thus, more research is warranted to further detail the influence of hormones on these common ocular conditions, as well as the benefits and/or risks of HRT and the eye. Fortunately, successful treatment is available for many of these ocular conditions, with a growing ability to improve or preserve vision in menopausal women.

## REFERENCES

1. Resnikoff S, Pascolini D, Etya'ale D et al. Global data on visual impairment in the year 2002. Bull World Health Organ 2004; 82: 844–51.
2. Metka M, Enzelsberger H, Knogler W et al. Ophthalmic complaints as a climacteric symptom. Maturitas 1991; 14: 3–8.
3. McCarty CA, Bansal AK, Livingston PM et al. The epidemiology of dry eye in Melbourne, Australia. Ophthalmology 1998; 105: 1114–19.
4. Moss SE, Klein R, Klein BE. Prevalence of and risk factors for dry eye syndrome. Arch Ophthalmol 2000; 118: 1264–8.
5. Mertzanis P, Abetz L, Rajagopalan K et al. The relative burden of dry eye in patients' lives: comparisons to a U.S. normative sample. Invest Ophthalmol Vis Sci 2005; 46: 46–50.
6. Reddy P, Grad O, Rajagopalan K. The economic burden of dry eye: a conceptual framework and preliminary assessment. Cornea. 2004; 23: 751–61.
7. Nelson JD, Helms H, Fiscella R et al. A new look at dry eye disease and its treatment. Adv Ther 2000; 17: 84–93.
8. Smith JA, Vitale S, Reed GF et al. Dry eye signs and symptoms in women with premature ovarian failure. Arch Ophthalmol 2004; 122: 151–6.
9. Altintas O, Caglar Y, Yuksel N et al. The effects of menopause and hormone replacement therapy on quality and quantity of tear, intraocular pressure and ocular blood flow. Ophthalmologica 2004; 218: 120–9.
10. Kramer P, Lubkin V, Potter W, Jakobs M, Labay G, Silverman P. Cyclic changes in conjunctival smears from menstruating females. Ophthalmology 1990; 97: 303–7.
11. Rocha FJ, Wickham LA, Pena JD et al. Influence of gender and endocrine environment on the distribution of androgen receptors in the lacrimal gland. J Steroid Biochem Mol Biol 1993; 46: 737–49.
12. Warren DW. Hormonal influences on the lacrimal gland. Int Ophthalmol Clin 1994; 34: 19–25.
13. Wood RL, Zhang J, Huang ZM et al. Prolactin and prolactin receptors in the lacrimal gland. Exp Eye Res 1999; 69: 213–26.
14. Marcozzi G, Liberati V, Madia F et al. Age- and gender-related differences in human lacrimal fluid peroxidase activity. Ophthalmologica 2003; 217: 294–7.
15. Cermak JM, Krenzer KL, Sullivan RM, Dana MR, Sullivan DA. Is complete androgen insensitivity syndrome associated with alterations in the meibomian gland and ocular surface? Cornea 2003; 22: 516–21.
16. Sullivan DA, Hann LE, Yee L et al. Age- and gender-related influence on the lacrimal gland and tears. Acta Ophthalmol 1990; 68: 188–94.

17. Thody AJ, Shuster S. Control and function of sebaceous glands. Physiol Rev 1989; 69: 383–416.
18. Akamatsu H, Zouboulis CC, Orfanos CE. Control of human sebocyte proliferation in vitro by testosterone and 5-alpha-dihydrotestosterone is dependant on the localization of the sebaceous glands. J Invest Dermatol 1992; 99: 509–11.
19. Deplewski D, Rosenfled RL. Role of hormones in pilosebaceous unit development. Endocr Rev 2000; 21: 363–92.
20. Krenzer KL, Dana MR, Ullman MD et al. Effect of androgen deficiency on the human meibomian gland and ocular surface. J Clin Endocrinol Metab 2000; 85: 4874–82.
21. Sullivan BD, Evans JE, Krenzer KL, Reza Dana M, Sullivan DA. Impact of antiandrogen treatment on the fatty acid profile of neutral lipids in human meibomian gland secretions. J Clin Endocrinol Metab 2000; 85: 4866–73.
22. Sullivan DA, Sullivan BD, Evans JE et al. Androgen deficiency, meibomian gland dysfunction, and evaporative dry eye. Ann N Y Acad Sci 2002; 966: 211–22.
23. Cermak JM, Krenzer KL, Sullivan RM, Dana MR, Sullivan DA. Is complete androgen insensitivity syndrome associated with alterations in the meibomian gland and ocular surface? Cornea 2003; 22: 516–21.
24. Chia EM, Mitchell P, Rochtchina E et al. Prevalence and associations of dry eye syndrome in an older population: the Blue Mountains Eye Study. Clin Experiment Ophthalmol 2003; 31: 229–32.
25. Schaumberg DA, Buring JE, Sullivan DA et al. Hormone replacement therapy and dry eye syndrome. JAMA 2001; 286: 2114–19.
26. Jensen AA, Higginbotham EJ, Guzinski GM et al. A survey of ocular complaints in postmenopausal women. J Assoc Acad Minor Phys 2000; 11: 44–9.
27. Taner P, Akarsu C, Atasoy P et al. The effects of hormone replacement therapy on ocular surface and tear function tests in postmenopausal women. Ophthalmologica 2004; 218: 257–9.
28. Scott G, Yiu SC, Wasilewski D et al. Combined esterified estrogen and methyltestosterone treatment for dry eye syndrome in postmenopausal women. Am J Ophthalmol 2005; 139: 1109–10.
29. Sator MO, Joura EA, Golaszewski T et al. Treatment of menopausal keratoconjunctivitis sicca with topical oestradiol. Br J Obstet Gynaecol 1998; 105: 100–2.
30. Wickham LA, Gao J, Toda I et al. Identification of androgen, estrogen and progesterone receptor mRNA in the eye. Acta Ophthalmol Scand 2000; 78: 146–53.
31. Ogueta SB, Schwartz SD, Yamashita CK et al. Estrogen receptor in the human eye: influence of gender and age on gene expression. Invest Ophthalmol Vis Sci 1999: 40: 1906–11.
32. Klein BE, Klein R, Linton KL. Prevalence of age-related lens opacities in a population. The Beaver Dam Eye Study. Ophthalmology 1992; 99: 546–52.
33. Klein BEK, Klein R, Ritter LL. Is there evidence of an estrogen effect of age-related lens opacities? The Beaver Dam Eye Study. Arch Ophthalmol 1994; 112: 85–91.
34. Cumming RG, Mitchell P. Hormone replacement therapy, reproductive factors, and cataract. The Blue Mountains Eye Study. Am J Epidemiol 1997; 145: 242–9.
35. Klein BEK, Klein R, Lee KE. Reproductive exposures, incident age-related cataracts, and age-related maculopathy in women: The beaver dam eye study. Am J Ophthalmol 2000; 130: 322–6.
36. Maraini G, Pasquini P, Sperduto RD et al. Distribution of lens opacities in the Italian-American Case-Control Study of Age-Related Cataract. The Italian-American Study Group. Ophthalmology 1990; 97: 752–6.
37. Mitchell P, Cumming RG, Attebo K et al. Prevalence of cataract in Australia: the Blue Mountains eye study. Ophthalmology 1997; 104: 581–8.
38. Freeman EE, Munoz B, Schein OD et al. Hormone replacement therapy and lens opacities. The Salisbury Eye Evaluation Project. Arch Ophthalmol 2001; 119: 1687–92.
39. Aina FO, Smeeth L, Hubbard R et al. Hormone replacement therapy and cataract: a population-based case-control study. Eye 2005; April, e-publication ahead of print.
40. Weintraub JM, Taylor A, Jacques P et al. Postmenopausal hormone use and lens opacities. Ophthalmic Epidemiol 2002; 9: 179–90.
41. VanNewkirk MR, Nanjan MB, Wang JJ et al. The prevalence of age-related maculopathy: the visual impairment project. Ophthalmology 2000: 107: 1593–600.
42. Buch H, Vinding T, Nielsen NV. Prevalence and causes of visual impairment according to World Health Organization and United States criteria in an aged, urban Scandinavian population: The Copenhagen City Eye Study. Ophthalmology 2001; 108: 2347–57.
43. Klein R, Klein BEK, Linton KLP. Prevalence of age-related maculopathy. The Beaver Dam Eye Study. Ophthalmology 1992; 99: 933–43.
44. Smith W, Mitchell P, Wang JJ. Gender, oesterogen, hormone replacement and age-related macular degeneration: results from the Blue Mountain Eye Study. Aust N Z J Ophthalmol 1997; 25: S13–S15.
45. Munaut C, Lambert V, Noel A et al. Presence of oestrogen receptor type beta in human retina. Br J Ophthalmol 2001; 85: 877–82.
46. Kobayashi K, Kobayashi H, Ueda M et al. Estrogen receptor expression in bovine and rat retinas. Invest Ophthalmol Vis Sci 1998; 39: 2105–10.
47. Eye Disease Case control Study Group. Risk factors for neovascular age-related macular degeneration. Arch Ophthalmol 1992; 110: 1701–8.
48. Snow KK, Cote J, Yang W et al. Association between reproductive and hormonal factors and age-related maculopathy in postmenopausal women. Am J Ophthalmol 2002; 134: 842–8.
49. Defay R, Pinchinat S, Lumbroso S et al. Sex steroids and age-related macular degeneration in older French women: the POLA study. Ann Epidemiol 2004; 14: 202–8.
50. Abramov Y, Borik S, Yahalom C et al. The effect of hormone therapy on the risk for age-related maculopathy in postmenopausal women. Menopause 2004; 11: 62–8.
51. Freeman EE, Munoz B, Bressler SB et al. Hormone replacement therapy, reproductive factors, and age-related macular degeneration: the Salisbury Eye Evaluation Project. Ophthalmic Epidemiol 2005; 12: 37–45.
52. Age-Related Eye Disease Study Research Group. A randomized, placebo-controlled, clinical trial of high-dose supplementation with vitamins C and E, beta carotene, and zinc for age-related macular degeneration and vision loss: AREDS report no. 8. Arch Ophthalmol 2001; 119. 1417 36.
53. Goldner WS, Kraus VL, Sivitz WI et al. Cyclic changes in glycemia assessed by continuous glucose monitoring

system during multiple complete menstrual cycles in women with type 1 diabetes. Diabetes Technol Ther 2004; 6: 473–80.

54. Strotmeyer ES, Steenkiste AR, Foley TP Jr et al. Menstrual cycle differences between women with type 1 diabetes and women without diabetes. Diabetes Care 2003; 26: 1016–21.

55. Solomon CG, Hu FB, Dunaif A et al. Long or highly irregular menstrual cycles as a marker for risk of type 2 diabetes mellitus. JAMA 2001; 286: 2421–26.

56. Yuen KK, Kahn HA. The association of femal hormones with blindness from diabetic retinopathy. Am J Ophthalmol 1976; 81: 820–22.

57. Kanaya AM, Herrington D, Vittinghoff E et al. Glycemic effects of postmenopausal hormone therapy: the Heart and Estrogen/progestin Replacement Study. A randomized, double-blind, placebo-controlled trial. Ann Intern Med 2003; 138: 1–9.

58. Crespo CJ, Smit E, Snelling A et al. Hormone replacement therapy and its relationship to lipid and glucose metabolism in diabetic and nondiabetic postmenopausal women: results from the Third National Health and Nutrition Examination Survey (NHANES III). Diabetes Care 2002; 25: 1675–80.

59. Leske MC, Connell AM, Schachat AP et al. The Barbados Eye Study. Prevalence of open angle glaucoma. Arch Ophthalmol 1994; 112: 821–9.

60. Kini MM, Leibowitz HM, Colton T et al. Prevalence of senile cataract, diabetic retinopathy, senile macular degeneration, and open-angle glaucoma in the Framingham Eye Study. Am J Ophthalmol 1978; 85: 28–34.

61. Wolfs RC, Borger PH, Ramrattan RS et al. Changing views on open-angle glaucoma: definitions and prevalences – The Rotterdam Study. Invest Ophthalmol Vis Sci 2000; 41: 3309–21.

62. Klein BEK, Klein R, Sponsel WE et al. Prevalence of glaucoma. The Beaver Dam Eye Study. Ophthalmology 1992; 99: 1499–504.

63. Mitchell P, Smith W, Attebo K et al. Prevalence of open-angle glaucoma in Australia. The Blue Mountain Eye Study. Ophthalmology 1996; 103: 1661–9.

64. Salvati AL. Influence de la menstruation sur la tension oculaire. Ann Ocul 1923; 160: 568–9.

65. Dalton K. Influence of menstruation on glaucoma. Br J Ophthalmol 1967; 51: 692–5.

66. Lee AJ, Mitchell P, Rochtchina E et al. Blue Mountains Eye Study. Female reproductive factors and open angle glaucoma: the Blue Mountains Eye Study. Br J Ophthalmol 2003; 87: 1324–8.

67. Hulsman CA, Westendorp IC, Ramrattan RS et al. Is open-angle glaucoma associated with early menopause? The Rotterdam Study. Am J Epidemiol 2001; 154: 138–44.

68. Sator MO, Joura EA, Frigo P et al. Hormone replacement therapy and intraocular pressure. Maturitas 1997; 28: 55–8.

69. Affinito P, Di Spiezio Sardo A, Di Carlo C et al. Effects of hormone replacement therapy on ocular function in postmenopause. Menopause 2003; 10: 482–7.

70. Abramov Y, Borik S, Yahalom C et al. Does postmenopausal hormone replacement therapy affect intraocular pressure? J Glaucoma 2005; 14: 271–5.

# Chapter 26

# Hearing impairment in the menopause and beyond

Frank I Marlowe, Edward W Keels and Lenora R Johnson

In large series, approximately 30% of adults between the ages of 65 and 74 years have hearing loss, and this percentage rizes to 50% by age 75 years. In any consideration of menopause, it must be first recognized that women are part of the larger contingent of the human race, and are women firstly before they become menopausal.

In normal hearing, sound waves, which are alternating compressions and rarefactions of air, are conducted through the external ear canal to impinge on the eardrum or tympanic membrane. This causes a vibration motion in the drumhead which is then transmitted via a series of very small bones contained in the middle ear space, and ultimately these vibrations are conducted into the fluid-filled sac-like structure that constitutes the inner ear or cochlea. These vibrations cause undulating motions in the membrane contained within this cochlea, and these vibrations create an electrical stimulus in specialized cells, the most important of which are the outer hair cells, and, finally, these electrical impulses are conducted via the acoustic nerves to the appropriate auditory centers in the midbrain and the temporal lobe. Defective function at any site along this pathway results in hearing impairment.

Broadly, these types of impairment are divided into conductive, in which the sound signal is not transmitted appropriately to the inner ear, and sensorineural (SNHL), in which the sound signal is appropriately delivered to the inner ear, but there is a defect in processing at that point or in transmission along the nerve pathways to the brain. Combinations of these defects are also encountered, and are referred to as mixed hearing loss. In conductive hearing loss, the simplest example is an accumulation of wax impacted in the external ear canal. This is adequately handled by removal using water irrigation or debridement with instruments, frequently under the magnification and illumination provided by a microscope. A further example of a pure conductive loss would be extensive calcification in the tympanic membrane, referred to as tympanosclerosis, or a perforation in the eardrum that interferes with its vibratory characteristics. This type of loss would also be noted in necrosis or erosion of one of the bones in the middle ear, which is referred to as ossicular discontinuity, and in which the vibrations fail to cross the intervening middle ear space adequately. A further example would consist of an ankylosis of the bones of the middle ear, or a condition known as otosclerosis in which a calcium-like deposit is present in the area of the third bone in the ossicular chain, namely the stapes, and prevents adequate vibration of this bone. An infectious or inflammatory condition such as a cholesteatoma, which is a sac-like mass containing keratin or squamous debris, which by mass effect inhibits proper function of the middle ear, would also cause a conductive loss. Finally, a relatively rare middle ear vascular tumor such as a glomus tympanicum, or glomus jugulare, or a vascular anomaly such as a high-riding internal jugular vein or exposed internal carotid artery can by mass effect or erosion produce this type of loss. All of these conditions are amenable to medical or surgical intervention for correction.

Sensorineural hearing loss can occur as a genetic disorder or syndrome, but in most patients defects in this portion of the hearing mechanism are secondary to acquired causes such as aging, infection or metabolic diseases, or exposure to ototoxic drugs, most commonly antibiotics, or to excessive and/or prolonged high levels of noise. Common symptoms of this type of loss other than the obvious hearing impairment consist of difficulty in understanding spoken speech, even though the patient may well feel that he hears the sounds, and a condition of noise that appears to arise in the ears and can vary from a high-pitched squealing sound to a low-pitched somewhat hollow sound that simulates the sound noted when a seashell is placed to the ear. This noise is generally termed tinnitus and may have an origin within the inner ear or even at centers central to this. The problem with discriminating words is exemplified by the fact that many words within the English language sound similar. For example, cat, fat, mat, rat, sat, all have the same carrier sound, but if you miss the initial sound you lose the meaning of the word. Additionally, there is a not uncommon disease syndrome termed Menière's syndrome in which fluctuating hearing loss of the sensorineural type, and tinnitus along with vertigo are the three hallmark symptoms for the diagnosis. This syndrome is generally acknowledged to be a result of altered fluid mechanics within the inner ear in which the end result is endolymphatic hydrops, and even occurs in a rare form termed cochlear Menière's in which the vertiginous aspect is absent. This condition is usually managed medically, and, in severe cases unresponsive to medical management, occasionally by surgical intervention aimed at endolymphatic decompression.

Sophisticated hearing tests, referred to as audiometry, or audiological evaluation, can provide detailed information as to the type of hearing loss, and within the types possibly the area or site of the defect. Standard audiological testing consists of pure tones delivered via the air route, usually an earphone, and via the bone route, usually with a vibrator placed over the mastoid process. In addition, speech audiometry, which consists of word lists presented to the patient replicating the occurrence of the word sounds in the English language (referred to as spondee word lists), is carried out. The final portion of the standard audiological test is basically a pressure test to measure the function of the middle ear components, and this is referred to as tympanometry.

The most frequent hearing loss in the aging population, both male and female, is by far the sensorineural type, and is termed presbycusis. Noise-related hearing loss was initially almost exclusively limited to the male population and became a significant factor with the turn of the 20th century and the industrial revolution. Boilermakers' deafness from exposure to the noises of steel fabrication, and deafness in construction workers from exposure to pneumatic drills and large compressors were almost universal prior to our realization that these exposures to high noise levels for extended periods was the underlying cause. This was also noted during the World Wars, when ongoing exposure to machinery noises in the propulsion systems of ships, aircraft engines on airfields and the decks of aircraft carriers, and exposure to repeated small arms fire and artillery sounds resulted in massive disability. The cost of rehabilitation, hearing aids, and disability payments for hearing loss in all of the military far exceeds the cost of treatment for all other injuries, including amputations and paraplegia. Noise-induced or environmental hearing loss has now been noted in increasing frequency in the female population, as women began working in the textile industries as aptly demonstrated in the popular Academy Award-winning film *Norma Rae*. In addition, women working in the garment industries with constant unremitting exposure to sewing machine noises which began in the early years of this past century was a significant contributing factor. Even more recently during the World War II with women replacing men in historically male roles, such as riveting in the construction of ships and aircraft, we began to see the same noise-induced losses. For the sake of completeness, a relatively rare cause of unilateral sensorineural hearing loss or certainly asymmetrical hearing loss which is otherwise unexplained, is a small benign tumor of the acoustic nerve termed an acoustic neurinoma, and the most common form of treatment for this lesion is surgical excision, although recently specialized forms of X-ray therapy using the gamma knife have been employed.

With people living longer, and the increased incidence of chronic cardiovascular, pulmonary, and renal disease in both men and women, we have seen increases in age-related hearing loss which might be more properly subclassed as disease-related. It has been postulated that cardiovascular disease and/or associated peripheral vascular disease is associated with changes in the vascular supply to the tissues of the inner ear, and results in diminished oxygenation, which contributes to progressive hearing impairment. Pulmonary disease would have similar effects on oxygenation of the susceptible inner ear tissues as would diabetes through its multiple degenerative metabolic effects, such as vascular changes and even neuropathy. Bone loss or osteoporosis has been noted within the cochlear capsule, and it has been proposed that this change in and of itself can contribute to hearing impairment. Many of the medications that are used to treat disease processes are notorious for their ototoxic effects. Principal among these would be the aminoglycoside antibiotics which are employed for serious life-threatening conditions (streptomycin, tobramycin, vancomycin, and gentamicin). The physicians that usually deal with serious infectious problems in the population, and more particularly in the aging population, are well aware of these effects, and the best treatment is preventative. This is usually supervised by infectious disease personnel who will carefully monitor blood levels of the drugs which are delivered intravenously, usually in a hospital setting, and also by serial determinations of hearing to detect any early changes. This is also a problem with the use of certain anticancer drugs such as carboplatin and cisplatin, which are commonly employed in the chemotherapy of ovarian cancer. In addition, the so-called loop diuretics such as furosemide and ethacrynic acid which are used in many of the cardiovascular conditions, such as congestive heart failure, and in the more severe forms of hypertension and renal disease, have ototoxic properties.

Sex differences have been observed in longitudinal studies of age-associated hearing loss.[1] In these studies, hearing sensitivity declined more than twice as fast in men as in women at most ages and frequencies, which represents good news for women. Declines in hearing sensitivity are detectable at all frequencies among men by age 30 years, but the age of onset of decline is later in women at most frequencies, and in general women have more sensitive hearing than men at frequencies above 1000 Hz, which is the approximate middle of the speech frequency range. Although hearing ability declines with aging in everyone, the variation in degree is quite large. Some of this can be explained by medical conditions and different exposure to environmental factors, but virtually nothing is known about the genetic contribution. Hereditability accounts for approximately half of the variation in age-related hearing loss, but it is a very complex trait influenced by an interplay between genetics and environment.[2] This is what accounts for the fact that two women working side by side in a noisy factory setting would have one sustain a severe hearing impairment while the other sustains virtually none with the same length of exposure. Several genes for hearing impairment have indeed been identified both in mice and in man, but no susceptibility genes have been identified.

A hormonal mechanism for hearing loss in women has been suggested by the temporal relationship between the onset of the loss and the decline in reproductive hormone production. The problem is, however, that this association does not exist as an isolated finding but is confounded by the effect of aging itself, and the presence of other diseases and their associated medication regimens.[3,4] Hormone replacement therapy (HRT), designed to relieve the symptoms of hot flashes and unstable sleep patterns, has been linked at least in one study to high-frequency hearing loss and tinnitus. It has been suggested that high doses of estrogen may damage certain receptors in the ear.[5] Those using HRT had greater difficulty understanding speech in the presence of competing or background noise, and it has been recommended by some that baseline audiological evaluations be carried out prior to administration of HRT.

The treatment of sensorineural hearing loss secondary to disease processes and/or the medications used to treat disease is primarily preventative, and consists of early treatment and careful attention to the pharmacological effects of the medications. The treatment of noise-induced or environmental hearing loss is also largely preventative, and consists of monitoring of the noise levels, adequate use of ear protection in the form of noise abatement earplugs, ear-cups, and sophisticated noise cancellation ear-cups. In addition, every effort should be made to modify the factors producing the noise, to limit the overall levels, and this might consist of redesign of certain machinery, modification of certain industrial production processes, and even the extended use of robotics.

The treatment alternative for age-related hearing loss, the most common type encountered in menopausal and post menopausal women, referred to as presbycusis, is termed hearing rehabilitation. This consists of the use of hearing aids, of which there are many different types depending on the need for certain levels of amplification.

Digital amplification is a dynamic new technology which addresses many of the frustrations experienced by hearing aid users in the past. The sound is 'natural' because of digital processing. The hearing system has several programs which reduce ambient noise, and enable to the user to utilize directional or omnidirectional hearing. The hearing aids can be reprogrammed any number of times, in the office, to accommodate changes in hearing loss. In addition, these systems have feedback suppression circuits to eliminate whistling.

Hearing aids range in size from an instrument which fits totally within the ear canal CIC (completely in the canal), to instruments which fit within the cavity of the auricle – these are somewhat more powerful. These are referred to as ITCs (in the canal) or ITEs (in the ear). The most powerful, which provide the highest decibel output, are behind the ear hearing aids (BTE). Behind the ear hearing aids are commonly used in patients with 'chronic ears', where drainage could be a problem. Skeletal molds are made to aerate the external ear canal. There is one further type of aid, referred to as a body aid, which is very rarely used in current practice and would be used only in those instances where extreme levels of amplification are required. Within each of these categories there are different types of microprocessors that can be customized to provide the optimal amount of amplification at certain ranges of the speech frequencies, without causing over-boosting of the areas of the range that are relatively normal. In addition, some of the more sophisticated aids include computer-like circuitry which can help to differentiate background or unwanted sounds from the true speech sounds. In the majority of instances where the hearing loss is bilateral and symmetrical, the fitting with bilateral aids provides binaural hearing and markedly improves the ability to discriminate speech sounds. In patients unable to wear a hearing aid for various reasons such as chronic otitis media with drainage and moisture in the ear, or mastoid, implantable hearing aids of various types are available. In these, a magnetic device is implanted, which directly conducts sound impulses transcranially into the cochlea.

Another aspect of rehabilitation consists of assistive listening devices. A common example is infrared devices that consist of earphones connected to an amplifier with a detachable microphone placed near the sound source. These are useful in automobiles, restaurants, and at home for watching TV, and are widely available from hearing healthcare professionals as well as electronic stores. These devices are becoming more commonly available in concert halls, movies, churches, and theaters, whereby the building incorporates a telemagnetic loop system or FM system transmitting the sound to a receiver that the hearing impaired person wears. In addition, there are simple devices to amplify telephone receivers, and some of these are available directly incorporated in the telephone by various manufacturers. For persons with more severe degrees of hearing loss, light systems that flash when activated by a telephone, doorbell, or smoke detector are available, and finally, there are, for the profoundly impaired, telecommunication devices for the deaf (TDD) which allow communication via small typewriters to type messages that are then transmitted via the telephone.

A final augmenting technique for hearing impairment is speech reading, commonly called lipreading. This allows visual cues associated with speech gestures involving the facial structures, such as the lips, tongue, and teeth, to be interpreted, and clarify the spoken message. This technique requires training, dedication, and effort on the part of the hearing impaired party.

More recently, for profoundly hearing impaired persons, especially those with bilateral loss that has occurred after acquisition of normal speech, there is cochlear implantation. The technology for cochlear implants has improved immensely over the past several years. This technique involves an external speech processor and an array of implantable electrodes, which are surgically implanted directly into the cochlea. Extensive preoperative evaluation and postoperative training are required to obtain optimal benefits from this technology, but in appropriately selected patients, it is extremely effective. The implant enhances speech reading and identification of environmental sounds, with some possibility of significant improvement in the discrimination of words.

## REFERENCES

1. Pearson JD, Morrell CH, Gordon-Salant S et al. Gender differences in a longitudinal study of age-associated hearing loss. J Acoust Soc Am 1995; 97: 1196–205.
2. Fransen E, Lemkens N, Van Laer L, Van Camp G. Age-related hearing impairment (ARHI) environmental risk factors and genetic prospects. Exp Gerontol 2003; 38: 353–9.
3. Lim DP, Stephens SD. Clinical investigation of hearing loss in the elderly. Clin Otolaryngol 1991; 16: 288–93.
4. Kim SH, Kang BM, Chae HD et al. The association between serum estradiol level and hearing sensitivity in postmenopausal woman. Obstet Gynecol 2002; 99: 726–30.
5. Kilicday EB, Yavuz H, Bagis T et al. Effects of estrogen therapy on hearing in postmenopausal women. Am J Obstet Gynecol 2004; 190: 77–82.

# Chapter 27

# Epilogue

Bernard A Eskin

Since the previous edition of *The Menopause*, there has been an entirely new medical approach to the care of the maturing woman. Nothing has changed the characterization of the universal symptoms of the menopause, which interfere with her quality of life. However, new advances in endocrine, nutritional, physical and clinical attention have added years and improved enjoyment. Particularly impressive are the increases in longevity that have been predicted to result in an average life expectancy of 82 years by 2010. Thus, more of these specific treatments should be available for the pressing problems observed during this extension.

Some recent major modifications in medical advice lie in resolving which treatment improves the menopausal conditions resulting from the effects of estrogen loss. Correlation with changes from clinical aging requires further consideration and is more complex. Aging affects atrophy and metabolism universally in the cells and tissues. Anticipated cellular repair and function becomes much less efficient during the fifth and sixth decades. The endocrine glands are an important factor in causing the onset of enhanced deficiencies in the premenopausal, menopausal and geripausal phases of a woman's life.

This millennium began with promising results from clinical trials, which showed that hormonal replacement or therapies could restore function satisfactorily throughout most of the body. While tissue restoration was not totally effective, cosmetic and hormonal replacement improvement was offered by estrogen treatment (alone or accompanied by progesterone). The aging process in the premenopause was thought to slow down as well; however, aging continued relentlessly. Stemming the tide of serious degenerative

changes was not universally manageable with estrogen alone. Clinical studies showed that complete reversal of menopause was presently unlikely. While the use of estrogen had some successes, it was apparent that other medical treatment or replacements for related problems was necessary. The mechanism of estrogen treatments and particularly the dosage levels needed revision, and basically the design required some reconsideration. Particularly there is much debate about many conclusions of the Women's Health Initiative and the other related studies and trials. Serious complications were considered significant and the full trials cancelled before completion. Hopefully, new basic and clinical programs will be devised, carefully controlled and without untoward exposure which can provide an acceptable therapeutic regimen.

We recognize that during the menopausal transitions, both aging and specific hormonal loss problems must be re-evaluated in women. It becomes apparent after the vast research described, that women are confronted with an early loss of reproduction as well as the other systemic aging dysfunctions that are seen in men. Thus, she has the ongoing aging spiral with acute reproductive physiologic losses with which to contend as described throughout this textbook. However, all the separate cellular and functional losses are not completely known and need further study. Genetic factors, as an example, are mixed thoroughly into intracellular molecular metabolism and appear to follow a remarkably complex regulation. The dynamics for these activities have only recently begun to be understood.

The present supports and interventions for reconstitution remain ubiquitous for aging. Medical therapies for symptoms and maintenance treatments are described throughout the text. No overall recommendation fulfills all the needs, but a healthy life style and timely medical check-ups remain most advantageous.

While the process of aging remains unknown and persistent, menopause therapy continues to be partially remedial. Geriatric specialists and demographologists are describing these changes and provide new programs to assist in women's care. Once again, I look forward to the next edition where we may expect new exciting interventions and health methods for women to enjoy their increasing longevity. Women entering menopause will wisely continue to take an interest in her daily activities, and thus, pursue greater happiness and improved quality of life.

# Index